Polyomaviruses and Human Diseases

ADVANCES IN EXPERIMENTAL MEDICINE AND BIOLOGY

Recent Volumes in this Series

Polyomaviruses and Human Diseases

Edited by

Nasimul Ahsan, M.D., FACP

Mayo Clinic - College of Medicine, Mayo Clinic Transplant Center, Jacksonville, Florida, U.S.A.

Springer Science+Business Media
Landes Bioscience / Eurekah.com

Springer Science+Business Media
Eurekah.com / Landes Bioscience

Printed in the U.S.A.

Springer Science+Business Media, 233 Spring Street, New York, New York 10013, U.S.A.

Please address all inquiries to the Publishers:
Eurekah.com / Landes Bioscience, 810 South Church Street, Georgetown, Texas, U.S.A. 78626
Phone: 512/ 863 7762; FAX: 512/ 863 0081
http://www.eurekah.com
http://www.landesbioscience.com

Polyomaviruses and Human Diseases, edited by Nasimul Ahsan, Landes Bioscience / Eurekah.com /
Springer Science+Business Media dual imprint / Springer series: Advances in Experimental Medicine
and Biology

ISBN: 0-387-29233-0

While the authors, editors and publisher believe that drug selection and dosage and the specifications
and usage of equipment and devices, as set forth in this book, are in accord with current recommendations and practice at the time of publication, they make no warranty, expressed or implied, with
respect to material described in this book. In view of the ongoing research, equipment development,
changes in governmental regulations and the rapid accumulation of information relating to the biomedical
sciences, the reader is urged to carefully review and evaluate the information provided herein.

Library of Congress Cataloging-in-Publication Data

Polyomaviruses and human diseases / edited by Nasimul Ahsan.
     p. ; cm. -- (Advances in experimental medicine and biology ; v. 577)
     Includes bibliographical references and index.
     ISBN 0-387-29233-0
     1. Polyomavirus infections. 2. Polyomaviruses.   I. Ahsan, Nasimul.
     II. Series.
     [DNLM: 1. Polyomavirus Infections. 2. BK Virus. 3. JC Virus.
     QW 165.5P2 P783 2006]
     QR201.P732P65 2006
     616.9'1--dc22
                                        2005025594

DEDICATION

To the memories of Late Dr. Humayun Kabir who inspired me to study medicine and of Late Dr. Gerald Stoner, whose pioneering works inspired many scientists to study Polyomavirus.

To my parents for their everlasting support. To my family: Arzumand (wife), Shaon (daughter), and Naveed (son) for their love and sacrifice.

FOREWORD

Science never solves a pr oblem without creating ten more
Geor ge Bernard Shaw

How prophetic the above words prove to be when applied to the advances of 20th century medicine. Prior to Banting and Best, clinicians were unaware of the ravages of diabetes, patients simply wasted away and died. Following the purification of insulin, clinicians now had to deal with diabetic retinopathy, diabetic nephropathy and all the other complications of long-term diabetes. A little over 50 years ago, the first successful human kidney transplant was performed in Boston. The first 30 years of the experience had successes when compared to the alternative but were a constant struggle to get even 50% of the grafts from deceased donors to survive more than a year. However, the science continued to advance knowledge of the immune response. With this came more and increasingly powerful tools for the clinician. Suddenly, success rates of 80-90% at one year were attainable. With this success came new problems, new complications and clinicians now had to worry about the long-term consequences of their therapy as patients were surviving with functional grafts for extended periods. A particular infectious complication evolved with the application of ever more powerful immunosuppressant drugs.

Astute clinicians noted that occasionally cellular rejections seemed to get worse with steroids. Despite their best efforts and the use of powerful drugs, patients lost their grafts to overwhelming interstitial infiltrates not seen before. In the mid-1990s, investigators reported series of patients with BK nephropathy due to emergence of polyomavirus reactivation in the kidney. Polyomaviruses had been previously described and had been known to cause disease in immunocompromised hosts. These had included CNS disease due to the JC virus, association of cancer with members of the Polyoma family particularly JC and SV40, and hemorrhagic cystitis. However, the newly recognized entity of BK nephropathy began to reach epidemic proportions with some centers reporting infections in the 15-20% range. This was clearly a complication of powerful immunosuppressive drugs and sparked a renewed interest in the study of all members of this virus family.

This book is a compilation of that research explosion. The contributors have done a great service by compiling in one place the most complete collection of knowledge regarding the polyomaviruses. The clinical aspects of the disease affecting kidney transplant recipients including detection, diagnosis, monitoring and treatment are laid out for the reader in a rational and readable manner. Polyoma virus interaction with the central nervous system as well as their association with malignancy is covered as well. A compilation of the basic science aspects of this family of viruses is gathered in one place for the first time. This work should serve those interested in these viruses and the diseases caused by them. Understanding all aspects of a disease is the first step in conquering it. Many in the field of transplantation and virology should find this book useful in future endeavors and as with any good text, it should serve as a guide and as an inspiration to those who follow.

Thomas A. Gonwa, M.D., FACP

PREFACE

"Life is short; art is long; opportunity fugitive; experience delusive; judgment difficult. It is the duty of the physician not only to do that which immediately belongs to him, but likewise to secure the cooperation of the sick, of those who are in attendance, and of all the external agents."
Oenopieles Hippocrates

What prompted this book was a seeming imbalance, between advancements made in science and what appears to be known generally. We admit that only modest progress has been made in understanding many infectious diseases such as those caused by polyomavirus. In studying infectious diseases around the world, one ends by regarding them as biological individuals, which have survived centuries, spanning human generations. Polyomavirus lends itself to such treatment because of its life cycles in the animal (human) worlds, the salient facts of which have all been elucidated within the last 30 years. However, the means of diagnosis and treatment of this virus have become, if not perfect, at least somewhat effective, and they deserve as full an explication as possible.

Many valuable monographs we possess, and even volumes of admirable papers have been published on this virus, but the former are so scattered as to be out of reach for a great number of interested readers, and the latter so academically detailed as to be unsuitable except for basic scientists. Why, then, not write a succinct manual of practice, limited to the main theme of clinical care? Ah, but an explosion of information in this field mandates both a far-reaching scope of coverage and in-depth analysis to present the complete and current picture. To meet these objectives, this book has been arranged to contain an ample outline of the history, pathology, symptoms, and treatment of diseases induced by human polyomavirus, without any detail of controversies or conflicting opinions. The use of multiple authors was essential to ensure the all-inclusive nature of this text. Many of these authors are pioneers in the field, and all have extensive experience studying or treating this virus. Because it is comprehensive, this book has broad applications for a variety of readers, including medical students, virologists, pathologists, and transplant specialists, as well as patients.

The book is divided into four sections covering the entirety of polyomaviruses from basic science considerations to clinical implications. The first section begins with a general discussion of the virus including immunology, epidemiology, and molecular and experimental virology. Due to increasing interests in the diseases caused by Polyoma-BK virus in transplant recipients, an entire second section explores transplant-related pathobiology, histopathology, diagnosis, management, and pharmacotherapy. The third section discusses the afflictions and diseases caused by Polyoma-JC virus, particularly that of the central nervous system. The fourth section deals with neoplastic associations of polyomaviruses.

From the sketch just given, it is evident that the book has no higher goal than that of a compilation, with the addition of whatever information the distinguished authors may have from some of their own work. A few who read our book may be attracted to study the diseases that are caused by the polyomaviruses. Altogether it is earnestly hoped that the information contained in this book may be found useful, facilitating future research in this field.

We wish, as well, to recognize and honor the careers of several friends and colleagues who contributed unstintingly to research in the field of polyomavirus. To that end, the authors and editors have done what they can do, and tried to present the views and experiments of everyone, as best as they could. If any mistakes have occurred, and in a work like the present it is very possible, I shall thankfully receive notification of such errors, and shall take the earliest opportunity to correct them. If any apology be necessary for the publication of the following work, the editor accepts responsibility. Our book will be an agent of change and betterment. Even the best books have only a small effect on what people do. If our work benefits patients and draws investigators into our field, we are satisfied. That will be enough.

Nasimul Ahsan, M.D., FACP

PARTICIPANTS

Irfan Agha, M.D.
St. Louis University School
  of Medicine
St. Louis VA Medical Center
St. Louis, Missouri
USA

Nasimul Ahsan, M.D., FACP
Mayo Clinic - College of Medicine
Mayo Clinic Transplant Center
Jacksonville, Florida
USA

Aarthi Ashok, Ph.D.
Brown University
Providence, Rhode Island
USA

Walter J. Atwood Ph.D.
Brown University
Providence, Rhode Island
USA

Giuseppe Barbanti-Brodano, M.D.
University of Ferrara
Ferrara
Italy

Signy Bendiksen, Ph.D.
University of Trosm¿
Trosm¿
Norway

Daniel C. Brennan, M.D.
University St. Louis Medical School
St. Louis, Missouri
USA

Lukas Bubendorf, M.D.
Institute of Pathology
University Hospital of Basel
Basel
Switzerland

Ryan G. Christensen
Brigham Young University
Provo, Utah
USA

Barbara Clayman
Johns Hopkins University School
  of Medicine
Baltimore, Maryland
USA

Alfredo Corallini, Ph.D.
University of Ferrara
Ferrara
Italy

Keith A. Crandall, Ph.D.
Brigham Young University
Provo, Utah
USA

Christopher L. Cubitt, Ph.D.
Translational Research Laboratory
H. Lee Moffitt Cancer and Research
  Institute
Tampa, Florida
USA

Joakim Dillner, M.D.
Lund University
Malm University Hospital
Malm
Sweden

Kristina Doerries, Ph.D.
Institute for Virology
  and Immunobiology
University of Wuerzburg
Wuerzburg
Germany

Cinthia B. Drachenberg
University of Maryland School
  of Medicine
Baltimore, Maryland
USA

Richard J. Frisque, Ph.D.
Pennsylvania State University
University Park, Pennsylvania
USA

Thomas A. Gonwa, M.D.
Mayo Clinic - College of Medicine
Mayo Clinic Transplant Center
Jacksonville, Florida
USA

Jennifer Gordon, Ph.D.
Center for Neurovirology and Cancer
  Biology
Temple University
Philadelphia, Pennsylvania
USA

Abdolreza Haririan, M.D.
Wayne State University
Detroit, Michigan
USA

Hans H. Hirsch, M.D., M.S.
University of Basel
Basel
Switzerland

Catherine Hofstetter, Ph.D.
Pennsylvania State University
University Park, Pennsylvania
USA

Jean Hou
National Institute of Neurological
  Disorders and Stroke
Bethesda, Maryland
USA

Basit Javaid, M.D.
University of Chicago
Pritzker School of Medicine
Chicago, Illinois
USA

Michelle A. Josephson, M.D.
University of Chicago
Pritzker School of Medicine
Chicago, Illinois
USA

Pradeep V. Kadambi, M.D.
University of Chicago
Pritzker School of Medicine
Chicago, Illinois
USA

Kamel Khalili, Ph.D.
Center for Neurovirology and Cancer
   Biology
Temple University
Philadelphia, Pennsylvania
USA

David K. Klassen, M.D.
University of Maryland School
   of Medicine
Baltimore, Maryland
USA

Wendy A. Knowles, Ph.D.
Health Protection Agency
London
UK

Erik Langhoff, M.D., Ph.D.
Mount Sinai Medical School
New York, New York
USA

Winston Lee, M.D.
Mount Sinai Medical School
New York, New York
USA

Annika Lundstig, Ph.D.
Lund University
Malm University Hospital
Malm
Sweden

Eugene O. Major, Ph.D.
National Institute of Neurological
   Disorders and Stroke
National Institute of Health
Bethesda, Maryland
USA

Fernanda Martini, Ph.D.
University of Ferrara
Ferrara
Italy

David A. McClellan, Ph.D.
Integrative Biology
Brigham Young University
Provo, Utah
USA

Shane M. Meehan, M.B., B.Ch.
University of Chicago
Pritzker School of Medicine
Chicago, Illinois
USA

Michael J. Mihatsch, M.D.
University Hospital of Basel
Basel
Switzerland

Ugo Moens, Ph.D.
University of Trosm¿
Trosm¿
Norway

Massimo Negrini, Ph.D.
University of Ferrara
Ferrara
Italy

Volker Nickeleit, M.D.
University of North Carolina
   at Chapel Hill
Chapel Hill, North Carolina
USA

Martha Pavlakis, M.D.
Beth Israel Deaconess Hospital
Boston, Massachusetts
USA

Marcos P rez-Losada, Ph.D.
Brigham Young University
Provo, Utah
USA

Emilio Ramos
University of Maryland School
    of Medicine
Baltimore, Maryland
USA

Parmjeet Randhawa, M.D.
University of Pittsburgh Medical
    Center
Pittsburgh, Pennsylvania
USA

Ole Petter Rekvig, Ph.D.
University of Trosm¿
Trosm¿
Norway

Dana E.M. Rollison, Sc.M., Ph.D.
H. Lee Moffitt Cancer Center
    and Research Institute
Tampa, Florida
USA

Julie Roskopf, Pharm D.
Wake Forest University Baptist
    Medical Center
Winston-Salem, North Carolina
USA

Silvia Sabbioni, Ph.D.
University of Ferrara
Ferrara
Italy

Pankaj Seth, Ph.D.
National Brain Research Center
Manesar, Haryana
India

Keerti V. Shah, M.D., Dr.P.H.
Johns Hopkins Bloomberg School
    of Public Heath
Baltimore, Maryland
USA

Ron Shapiro, M.D.
University of Pittsburgh Medical
    Center
Pittsburgh, Pennsylvania
USA

Harsharan K. Singh, M.D.
University North Carolina
    at Chapel Hill
Chapel Hill, North Carolina
USA

Juerg Steiger, M.D.
University of Basel
Basel
Switzerland

Robert J. Stratta, M.D.
Wake Forest University Baptist
    Medical Center
Winston-Salem, North Carolina
USA

Mauro Tognon, Ph.D.
University of Ferrara
Ferrara
Italy

Jennifer Trofe, Pharm D., BCPS
Hospital of the University
    of Pennsylvania
Philadelphia, Pennsylvania
USA

Shiva K. Tyagarajan
Pennsylvania State University
University Park, Pennsylvania
USA

Abhay Vats, M.D.
Children s Hospital of Pittsburgh
University of Pittsburgh
Pittsburgh, Pennsylvania
USA

Raphael P. Viscidi, M.D.
Johns Hopkins University School
   of Medicine
Baltimore, Maryland
USA

Martyn K. White, Ph.D.
Center for Neurovirology and Cancer
   Biology, Temple University
Philadelphia, Pennsylvania
USA

James W. Williams, M.D.
University of Chicago
Pritzker School of Medicine
Chicago, Illinois
USA

CONTENTS

9. IMMUNITY AND AUTOIMMUNITY INDUCED BY POLYOMAVIRUSES: CLINICAL, EXPERIMENTAL AND THEORETICAL ASPECTS 117

Ole Petter Rekvig, Signy Bendiksen and Ugo Moens

10. THE PATHOBIOLOGY OF POLYOMAVIRUS INFECTION IN MAN 148

Parmjeet Randhawa, Abhay Vats and Ron Shapiro

11. POLYOMAVIRUS-ASSOCIATED NEPHROPATHY IN RENAL TRANSPLANTATION: CRITICAL ISSUES OF SCREENING AND MANAGEMENT 160

Hans H. Hirsch, Cinthia B. Drachenberg, Juerg Steiger and Emilio Ramos

23. BK VIRUS, JC VIRUS AND SIMIAN VIRUS 40 INFECTION IN HUMANS, AND ASSOCIATION WITH HUMAN TUMORS 319

Giuseppe Barbanti-Brodano, Silvia Sabbioni, Fernanda Martini,
  Massimo Negrini, Alfredo Corallini and Mauro Tognon

24. EPIDEMIOLOGIC STUDIES OF POLYOMAVIRUSES AND CANCER: PREVIOUS FINDINGS, METHODOLOGIC CHALLENGES AND FUTURE DIRECTIONS 342

Dana E.M. Rollison

ACKNOWLEDGMENTS

The editor is deeply indebted to each contributor to this first edition of "Polyomaviruses and Human Diseases". The painstaking revision and responses to suggestions for appropriate additions have also been important features of this edition. The willingness of the participants to adhere to a standard format in order to achieve a uniform style is gratefully acknowledged.

High Tribute is due to those members of the Landes Bioscience staff responsible for publication. Mr. Ronald G. Landes provided strong support and advice in the preparation of all aspects of this work, and his kind invitation, encouragement and enthusiasm have been very functional in making it a reality. The contribution of Ms. Cynthia Conomos, who has been involved in all aspects of this work with an impressive commitment to detail, is gratefully acknowledged. Appreciation is also expressed to Ms. Celeste Carlton and the rest of the dedicated staff of Landes Bioscience, who skillfully processed the illustrations and prepared the thorough index.

Special recognition must be given to Professor Keerti V. Shah, who contributed the leading chapter and very importantly, gave his unconditional guidance in every aspects including selection of the contributors and the chapters. To late Dr. Gerald Stoner, Professor Giuseppe Barbanti-Brodano and my many international colleagues, my gratitude cannot be overstated.

Finally, a thoroughly dedicated colleague and my loving wife Arzumand Ara has brought her many talents in editorial preparation to the compilation of this book. Her critical and assiduous review of every chapter has been extraordinary, and her commitment and excitement in developing this book has been prime stimulus deserving of the highest praise.

Nasimul Ashsan, M.D., FACP

CHAPTER 1

Polyomaviruses and Human Diseases

Nasimul Ahsan and Keerti V. Shah

Abstract

Polyomaviruses are small, nonenveloped DNA viruses, which are widespread in nature. In immunocompetent hosts, the viruses remain latent after primary infection. With few exceptions, illnesses associated with these viruses occur in times of immune compromise, especially in conditions that bring about T cell deficiency. The human polyomaviruses BKV and JCV are known to cause, respectively, hemorrhagic cystitis in recipients of bone marrow transplantation and progressive multifocal leukoencephalopathy in immunocompromised patients, for example, by HIV infection. Recently, transplant nephropathy due to BKV infection has been increasingly recognized as the cause for renal allograft failure. Quantitation of polyomavirus DNA in the blood, cerebrospinal fluid, and urine, identification of virus laden "decoy cells" in urine, and histopathologic demonstration of viral inclusions in the brain parenchyma and renal tubules are the applicable diagnostic methods. Genomic sequences of polyomaviruses have been reported to be associated with various neoplastic disorders and autoimmune conditions. While various antiviral agents have been tried to treat polyomavirus-related illnesses, current management aims at the modification and/or improvement in the hosts' immune status. In this chapter, we provide an overview of polyomaviruses and briefly introduce its association with human diseases, which will be covered extensively in other chapters by experts in the field.

History

The polyomaviruses and papillomaviruses were previously considered subfamilies of the family *Papovaviridae*, which derived its name from three of its members: rabbit papilloma virus, mouse polyomavirus, and simian vacuolating agent or simian virus 40 (SV 40). Recently, the International Committee on Taxonomy of Viruses has recognized polyomaviruses and papillomaviruses as independent virus families. Immunologically and genetically, viruses of these two families are unrelated and also have different biological characteristics. Thirteen members of the family *Polyomaviridae* have been identified, which includes two human pathogens, JC virus (JCV) and BK virus (BKV), both of which were first isolated in 1971 from immunocompromised patients. Padgett et al[1] isolated and partially characterized JCV from the brain of a patient (with the initials J.C.) with Hodgkin's lymphoma who died of progressive multifocal leukoencephalopathy (PML), a demyelinating disorder of the central nervous system (CNS). Prior to this discovery, a virus was suspected in the etiology of PML as early as 1958; in 1969 electron microscopy of PML tissue showed viral particles in the nucleus of the infected oligodendrocytes, which were structurally identical to polyoma virion. Gardner et al[2] isolated BKV from the urine of a Sudanese renal transplant patient (with the initials B.K.) who developed ureteral stenosis and was shedding inclusion-bearing epithelial cells in his urine. Initial electron microscopy demonstrated viral particles in the urine. Inoculation of the urine into rhesus monkey kidney cells and human embryonic kidney cells produced viral cytopathic

Polyomaviruses and Human Diseases, edited by Nasimul Ahsan. ©2006 Eurekah.com and Springer Science+Business Media.

Table 1. *Polyomaviruses and their natural hosts* [a]

Host	Virus	Characteristics
Human	BK virus (BKV)	Early childhood infection; persists in renal epithelium and lymphocytes; causes nephropathy and ureteritis in immunocompromised hosts
	JC virus (JCV)	Late childhood infection; persists in renal epithelium, lymphocytes, and brain; causes PML in immunocompromised hosts
Monkey	Simian virus 40(SV40)	Infects Asian macaques; persists in kidney; causes PML-like disease in immunocompromised animals
	Simian agent 12 (SA-12)	Infects African baboons
	Lymphotropic papovavirus (LPV)	Multiplies in B lymphoblasts of African green monkeys
	Cynomolgus polyoma virus (CPV)	Infects Cynomolgus monkeys; persists in renal epithelium and lymphocytes; causes nephropathy and ureteritis in immunocompromised hosts, similar to BKV nephropathy in humans
Cattle[b]	Bovine polyoma Virus (BpyV)	Infects cattle; persists in kidney
Rabbit	Rabbit kidney vacu-olating Virus (RKV)	Infects cottontail rabbits
Hamster	Hamster papovavirus (HaPV)	Produces cutaneous tumors in hamsters
Mouse	Mouse polyoma virus	Natural infection of wild mice and may infect laboratory mouse colonies; persists in kidneys
	K virus	Infects pulmonary epithelium of mice
Athymic rat	Rat polyomavirus	Affects parotid gland
Parakeet	Budgerigar fledging disease virus (BFDV)	Produces acute fatal illness in fledgling budgerigars

[a] Modified from reference 5. [b] A virus initially described as originating from stump-tailed macaques was subsequently identified as bovine polyomavirus

effects. The initial BKV isolate is known as the Gardner strain. In 1960, Sweet and Hilleman identified simian virus 40 (SV 40) which has rhesus macaques as the natural host.[3] Due to its ability to grow and induce characteristic cytopathic effect of cell vacuolization in African monkey kidney cells, SV 40 was initially designated as "vacuolating agent". In the late 1950s and early 1960s, millions of people were inadvertently exposed to SV 40 due to administration of SV 40-contaminated Salk polio vaccines, but this appeared to have insignificant clinical consequences.[4] Shortly, after its discovery, SV 40 was found to induce tumors in animals and to transform a variety of cell types from different species and has been periodically described to be associated with several human tumors.

Polyomavirus

Distributed widely in nature, polyomaviruses have been isolated from many species including humans (Table 1).[5] They are exquisitely adapted to grow in the species they infect and have

Table 2. Polyomavirus proteins [a]

Protein/ Region	Molecular Weight	No of Amino Acids JCV/BKV	Sequence Homology Shared with JCV [b]		Function
			BKV	SV40	
Early coding					
Large T	79,305	688/695	83	72	Initiates viral repli cation; stimulates host DNA synthesis; modulates early and late transcription; establishes and maintains host transformation
Small T	20,236	172/172	78	67	Facilitates viral DNA replication
Late coding					
VP1	39,606	354/362	78	75	Major capsid protein; forms viral ichosahedron, enables entry, mediates hemagglutination
VP2	37,366	344/351	79	72	Minor capsid protein
VP3	25,743	225/232	75	66	Minor capsid protein; subset of VP2
Agnoprotein	8,081	71/66	59	46	Facilitates capsid assembly

[a] Modified from reference 5. [b] Percent amino acids. Molecular weight and number of amino acids of JCV proteins deduced from nucleotide data. In addition to large T and small T, a middle T antigen is coded for by mouse polyomavirus and hamster papovavirus.

probably coevolved with their hosts. Each polyomavirus infects only one or a group of closely related species.

Viral Structure and Genome

Polyomaviruses have the following properties: small size of the virion (diameter 40-45 nm), naked icosahedral capsid, superhelical double-strand circular DNA genome of molecular weight 3.2×10^6, shared nucleotide sequences with other polyomaviruses, and nuclear site of multiplication. The nonenveloped virion has icosahedral symmetry and 72 pentameric capsomers. The virion is made up of protein (88%) and a single copy of a circular double-stranded DNA molecule (12%), which has about 5,300 base pairs. BKV, JCV, and SV40 display a high degree of nucleotide sequence homology. Overall, the JCV genome shares 75% of the sequences with the BKV genome and 69% of the sequences with the SV40 genome.[5,6]

The virus-coded proteins of polyomaviruses are listed in Table 2. BKV and JCV have both species-specific and cross-reactive antigenic determinants. The viral genome is functionally divided into (i) a noncoding control region (NCCR) (0.4 kb), (ii) an early coding region (2.4 kb), which codes for tumors antigens: large T (T-ag), middle T (in mouse and hamster viruses), and small T (t-ag), and (iii) a late coding region (2.3 kb), which codes for viral capsid proteins VP1, VP2, and VP3 and agnoprotein. The NCCR is located between the early and late regions and contains the T-ag binding sites. It contains (i) the origin of DNA replication (*ori*) and (ii) the regulatory regions for early and late transcription. The sequence blocks in NCCR are arbitrarily referred to by the alphabetical designations P, Q, R, and S. These blocks serve as regulatory regions, or enhancer elements, and contain several transcription factor binding sites, which putatively modulate viral transcription.[7-12] Naturally occurring SV40, BKV and JCV strains in the kidney and urine usually have an archetypal regulatory region. By contrast, JCV found in the brain tissue of PML usually shows a variety of point mutations, deletions, and duplications on the late side of *ori*.[13-15]

The early and late coding regions are transcribed from different strands of the DNA molecule and the direction of early and late transcription is divergent, with opposite strands participating in these processes, starting from the origin of replication.[16] T-ag is a multifunctional protein with helicase activity and distinct ability to bind host cell regulatory proteins. T-ag controls both viral DNA replication, and early and late gene transcription, and interferes with host cell transcription factors.[17] During replication, viral DNA associates with host cell histones H2A, H2B, H3, and H4 to form mini viral chromosomes, which are structurally indistinguishable from host cell chromatin.[18-21] Each pentamer of the viral icosahedron consists of five VP1 molecules and one molecule of VP2 or VP3. VP1 (molecular mass 39,600) is the major capsid protein and accounts for more than 70% of the virion protein mass. It mediates viral attachment to the receptors on susceptible cells and contains epitopes for neutralization, hemagglutination inhibition, and other virus-specific and shared immunologic determinants. VP2 (37,300) and VP3 (25,700) are minor capsid proteins.[22,23] JCV agnoprotein consists of 71 amino acid residues, with molecular weight of approximately 8 kDa. Agnoprotein differs from all other early and late proteins in that it localizes primarily in the cytoplasmic and perinuclear regions of the infected cell. Unlike viral capsid proteins, it is not detectable in the virion and its intracellular distribution has led to the suggestion that agnoprotein may promote release of virion from the cell. Agnoprotein also plays a role in the stability of microtubules and preservation of the infected cell via interaction with tubulin. BKV and JCV share a large umber of amino acids, ranging from 59% (agnoprotein) to 83% (T-ag). A greater homology exists between JCV and BKV than between JCV and SV 40.[24,25]

Isolation and Propagation

BKV can be propagated in human epithelial cells and fibroblasts. For isolation of BKV, human embryonic kidney (HEK) cells, diploid lung fibroblasts, and urothelial cells are suitable.[26] During the course of infection cytopathic effects typical of polyomavirus infections (rounding of cells containing cytoplasmic vacuoles) and formation of BKV plaques on HEK monolayers may take several weeks, whereas BKV-T antigen may be detected in infected cultures in 1 or 2 days.[27] In the case of JCV, primary human fetal glial (PHFG) cells are the most sensitive tissue culture system for isolation and propagation.[28] Human fetal Schwann cells[29] and astrocytes[30] also support JCV multiplication. Other cell types, which allow isolation of JCV, are urothelial cells, human amnion, adult brain, and HEK cells. Both BKV and JCV have been shown to produce plaques in HEK cells and can also be assayed by scoring for cytopathic effect in end-point titrations in tissue culture tubes. Because both BKV and JCV agglutinate human red blood cells of O blood type, hemagglutination can be used as a laboratory assay for quantifying virus. Both polyclonal and monoclonal antibodies to the viral T or capsid proteins are used in immunocytochemistry assays to follow the stages of BKV and JCV infection.[31-34]

Life Cycle

Depending on the host cell, polyomaviruses cause either permissive (host of origin, when all viral genes are expressed) or nonpermissive (host unrelated to species of origin) infections. All polyomaviruses multiply in the nucleus and during permissive infection the viruses cause characteristic, often pathognomonic, nuclear changes and result in cell death. Urothelial cells infected with BKV or JCV, oligodendrocytes infected with JCV, and mouse pulmonary endothelial cells infected with the mouse K virus display similar nuclear abnormalities and may result, in renal tubulo-interstitial changes, ureteral obstruction and tubular injury, PML, and pneumonia, respectively. BKV and JCV also undergo nonpermissive infection when only the viral T-ag and t-ag are made, resulting in cell transformation in tissue culture of rodent cells. In case of BKV, transformed cells exhibit BKV-T antigen and contain multiple copies of BKV-DNA. BKV-DNA is integrated into the host cell genome in rodent cells, but in human cells, it may remain as free unintegrated copies.[35-37] The transformed cells can induce tumors in the appropriate animal hosts. Both BKV and JCV can also induce clastogenic events in infected cells, resulting in chromosomal damage, translocations, and unstable multicentric chromosomes leading to further DNA damage and ultimately cell transformation and cell death.[38]

Pathogenesis and Pathology

BKV and JCV do not naturally infect any species other than humans. The host range and tissue specificity of polyomaviruses are determined by an interaction of cellular and viral factors. There are also significant differences between BKV and JCV with respect to their biological behavior and disease potential. When inoculated into a wide variety of laboratory animals, BKV and JCV produce serologic response and sometimes tumors, but do not result in infections similar to that seen in humans. Although BKV and JCV are latent in the kidney and are reactivated in immunosuppressed states, only JCV infects the CNS and produces PML. In renal transplant recipients and in pregnant women, both BKV and JCV are reactivated frequently and are excreted in the urine; however, in bone marrow transplant recipients, BKV reactivation is far more frequent than JCV reactivation.[39,40]

The pathogenesis of a polyomavirus infection involves the following sequence of events: (1) entry of virus into the body, (2) multiplication at the entry site, (3) viremia with transport of virus to the target organs, and (4) multiplication in the target organs. VP1 interacts with specific receptors present on susceptible cells, mediates virion entry into the cell by endocytosis; virus is then transported to the nucleus, where it is uncoated.[41] BKV enters into the host cell via α (2-3)-linked sialic acids receptor. In case of JCV, an N-linked glycoprotein containing α (2-6) linked sialic acids receptor has been described on the surface of B cells and glial cells. JCV appears to enter cells by clathrin-dependent endocytosis.[42] A caveolae-dependent endocytosis allows SV40 viral entry, which requires SV40 specific receptor comprising of MHC class I and O-linked proteins.[43,44] After multiplication in the nucleus, virus reaches the target organs by the hematogenous route. The viral determinants that affect host range and tissue specificity of BKV and JCV are located in the enhancer/promoter elements in the regulatory regions[45] and the early regions of these viruses.[46,47] With respect to BKV and JCV, the route of infection is not known. Recently, JCV DNA has been isolated from tonsillar stroma and in B-lymphocyte population within the tonsils.[48] Using PCR technique, JCV DNA is routinely identified in the peripheral blood of 5-40% of normal volunteers and in brains of nearly all patients with PML.[49] While BKV is seldom recovered from the respiratory tract, the rapid acquisition of antibodies in the first few years of life is consistent with virus transmission by the respiratory route.[50] Although BKV-IgM in cord blood and BKV-DNA in fetal and placental tissues have been reported, there is controversy about the role of transplacental transmission of BKV.[51-53] Other potential sources of BKV infection are blood products, and renal allografts.[54,55] Both JCV and BKV have also been identified in other organs including heart, spleen, lung, colon, and liver. Primary infection may be accompanied by transient viruria and in the immunocompetent host, BKV and JCV persist indefinitely as latent infections.[56] BKV and JCV also persist in the kidney and B-lymphocytes for an indefinite period of time.[57,58] Reactivation of BKV and JCV in the urinary tract occurs under a wide variety of conditions, including (i) kidney and bone marrow transplantation, (ii) primary immunodeficiency diseases, (iii) immunotherapy for malignancy and other disorders, (iv) pregnancy, (v) chronic diseases e.g., diabetes, (vi) infection with human immunodeficiency virus, and (vii) old age.

SV40-associated PML in a macaque colony and SV40-associated interstitial pneumonia and renal tubular necrosis in a rhesus macaque have been reported.[59,60] In the animal with renal disease, abundant numbers of SV40 particles and large intranuclear inclusions were seen in the renal tubular epithelial cells. The disease was similar to BKV-induced tubulointerstitial nephritis, described in a child with an inherited immunodeficiency disease.[61] SV40-associated PML occurred in immunosuppressed simian immunodeficiency virus (SIV)-infected rhesus macaques.

In a kidney transplant model, Gorder et al[62] described a new polyomavirus (cynomolgus polyoma virus—CPV) from renal tubules of cynomolgus monkeys (*Macaca fascicularis*) treated with cyclosporine and azathioprine. This virus has 84% DNA sequence homology to SV40. Most of the animals infected with polyomavirus developed lethargy, anorexia and had rising serum creatinine due to polyomavirus interstitial nephritis in the native kidney and/or the renal graft. In addition, several grafts had extensive rupture and destruction of collecting ducts and demonstrated endarteritis and focal hemorrhage indicative of active cellular rejection. None of the animals with detectable virus in the allograft had infections of the native kidney. In the renal graft, the peak frequency of infection was from day 21-48 after transplant and during this study, no particular association of polyomavirus with any of the immunosuppressive agents was evident.

Clinical Features

Primary Infection

In healthy children, primary infection with BKV and JCV is rarely associated with clinical disease. In a prospective study, 11 out of 66 children with respiratory illness demonstrated BKV seroconversion; seven of these children had mild respiratory disease and four were asymptomatic. BKV was isolated from the urine of one of the children showing seroconversion. Unintegrated BKV DNA was identified in the tonsillar tissue of five of 12 children with recurrent respiratory disease.[63] In immunocompromised children, primary BKV infection may cause cystitis or nephritis and primary JCV infection may lead to PML. Primary BKV infection may also present with encephalitis. Following primary infection viruses persist indefinitely as "latent" infections of the kidney.

Silent Viruria

BKV can be reactivated after many years, usually by states of acquired (cell-mediated) immunosuppression: pregnancy, HIV, neoplasm, systemic lupus erythematosus, nephrotic syndrome, bone marrow, and organ transplantation. Twenty per cent of immunocompetent patients are found to have JC viruria; in this situation whether viral shedding represents reactivation or new infection remains unclear.[64]

Pregnancy

Approximately 3.2% of pregnant women during second (late) and third trimesters show cytologic evidence of BKV and JCV excretion in urine.[65] In tests of paired sera spanning pregnancy, a rise in antibody titers to BKV or JCV was found in 14% of the women.[66] The viral reactivation may be induced by hormonal changes and shedding continues intermittently through the pregnancy until the postpartum period. While controversy exists about trans-placental transmission to fetus, viral excretion does not appear to be associated with any ill effect to the mother.[67]

Systemic Lupus Erythematosus (SLE)

The prevalence of BKV genome is significantly higher than JCV in the serum of patients with SLE.[68] Christie et al[69] observed that rabbits inoculated with BKV particles produced antibodies directed to both viral structural protein and host histones. It has been suggested that BKV infection may contribute to the development of SLE as supported by the findings that patients with BKV infection with expression of large T-ag develop anti-DNA antibodies and anti-BKV antibodies have some cross reactivity with DNA.[70] Indeed, using PCR, Sundsfjord et al[71] have identified BKV genomic sequences in 16% of 44 patients with SLE. In another study, 80% (16/20) of SLE patients showed at least one or several episodes of BKV (12 patients) or JCV (4 patients) reactivation, while control group did not have any viral replication.[72] Similarly, several other investigators reported that reactivation of polyomavirus in patients with auto-immune diseases including SLE.[73,74] In these reports, observed viruria was found to be independent of immunosuppressive therapy suggesting that an unknown inherent immunologic defect in SLE patients might be the contributing factor. In this book, Rekvig and colleagues have discussed the association between polyomavirus and auto-immunity in great detail in a subsequent chapter.

HIV Disease and Polyomavirus

The major polyomavirus associated disease in HIV infected patients is JCV mediated PML (*vide infra*) which occurs in about 1.6% of the cases. The role of polyomavirus infection in kidneys was examined in a retrospective study using immunohistochemistry for T-ag and PCR.[75] Multifocal polyomavirus replication was diagnosed in 6.3% (7/111) of the patients. Cytopathic changes of limited necrosis, interstitial infiltrates, and intratubular casts were noted. Surprisingly, JCV genomes were identified in five of these seven patients. Several studies have demonstrated that 20-30% of patients with HIV disease also excrete BKV in the urine without any symptom.[76-78] The frequency of BK viruria increases with decreasing CD4 count when the prevalence of BKV shedding increases from 4-8% to 27-51% when CD4 counts fall below 200/μL.[76,78,79] Despite frequent reactivation in AIDS, clinical manifestations BKV are rare. In patients with AIDS, BKV has been reported to cause fatal tubulointerstitial nephropathy, disseminated pulmonary infection, retinitis, and meningoencephalitis.[78,80-82] Others have reported hemorrhagic cystitis similar to that observed in bone marrow transplant recipients.[83,84]

Renal Transplant Recipients—Polyomavirus-Associated Nephropathy

Infections in renal transplant recipients have been studied by several investigators[85-91] and have been frequently reviewed.[92-103] In a multicenter serologic study of nearly 500 renal allograft recipients in the United States, BKV and JCV infections occurred, in 22% and 11% of the patients, respectively.[88] Coexistence of SV40 infection has also been described.[104] Virus shedding in urine of renal transplant recipients has been monitored by a variety of techniques, including urinary cytology, immunoassay, electron microscopy, virus isolation, ELISA assays, nucleic acid hybridization, and PCR.[105-119] In prospective studies, 25-44% of renal transplant patients excrete virus in their urine in the posttransplant period. The duration of excretion ranges widely, from transient viruria to excretion over several weeks or several months. The kidney of a seropositive donor may initiate infections in the recipient.[120] Infections may be either reactivations or primary infections affecting up to 5% of renal allograft recipients in about 40 weeks (range 6-150) post-transplantation. More than 50% of the patients show serologic evidence of infection with the virus. Persistent BKV infections have been associated with irreversible graft loss in more than 50% of the cases over 12-240 weeks of follow-up.[97,117] The infections appear to be responsible for some of the cases of ureteral obstruction.[121,122] Risk factors include treatment of rejection episodes and increasing viral replication under potent immunosuppressive drugs such as tacrolimus, sirolimus, or mycophenolate mofetil.[92,94-98,101,123] The histological presentation of BKV nephropathy has been described recently[88,94,95] (Fig. 1). Cytopathic changes in renal tubules reflecting viral multiplication consist of enlarged nuclei with smudgy chromatin, intranuclear inclusions, rounding and detachment. These have been classified into: (a) stage A: focal medullary involvement of tubular cells, (b) stage B: extensive renal involvement with multifocal or diffuse cytopathic alterations, necrosis, profound inflammatory response, and early fibrosis, and (c) stage C: characterized by interstitial fibrosis, scarring, and calcification.[98] BKV related vasculopathy, a new tropism, has been described recently, in which a fatal case of disseminated BKV infection in a renal transplant recipient was associated with BKV multiplication in endothelial cells.[124] In subsequent chapters, several authors have also discussed polyomavirus related infections particularly in the setting of organ transplantations.

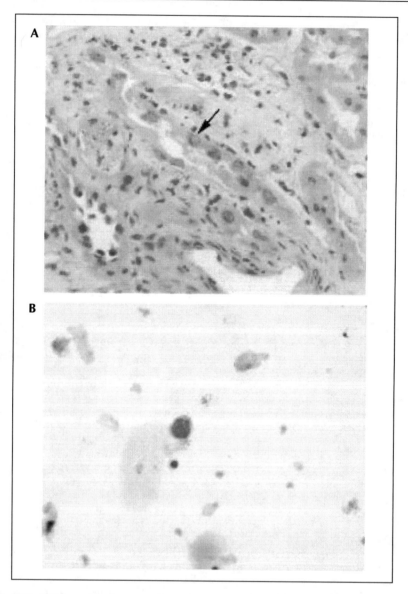

Figure 1. BKV nephropathy: A) Light microscopy of transplant kidney tissue: BKV laden renal tubular epithelial cells with intranuclear inclusion (hematoxylin-eosin stain, x 200). B) Urinary cytology showing BKV infected urothelial cell, so called "decoy cell". Note rounded nucleus with smudgy, glassy intra nuclear inclusion and margination of nuclear chromatin (Papanicolaou stain, x 400).

Bone Marrow Transplantation and Hemorrhagic Cystitis

Hemorrhagic cystitis (HC) is not an uncommon complication affecting more than 10% of the recipients of bone marrow transplantation (BMT).[125-128] Transient HC occurring in the first few days after transplantation usually represents drug toxicity. About one-half of the BMT patients shed BKV without any symptoms of HC in the posttransplant period, which is higher in recipients of allogeneic marrow. Late onset HC (2-12 weeks post-transplant) that lasts more than 7 days is associated with BK viruria.[129,130] In one study, HC occurred four times more frequently in BKV excreters than in nonBKV excreters, and in these patients, BK viruria was associated with 16 out of 18 cases of HC.[129] The onset and termination of BK viruria often coincided with the onset and termination of HC. BKV was recovered far more frequently in urine collected during the episodes of hemorrhagic cystitis (55%) than in urine collected in cystitis-free periods (8-11%). In another study, BK viruria in BMT recipients was associated with gross or microscopic hematuria but without evidence of clinical cystitis.[131]

JCV Related Disease—Progressive Multifocal Leukoencephalopathy

Progressive multifocal leukoencephalopathy (PML) is a rare, subacute, demyelinating disease of the central nervous system (CNS) primarily affecting individuals who have impaired immunity.[132-134] PML, previously a disease of the fifth and sixth decades of life, is now recognized in younger patients. PML is recognized in as many as 3.8% of patients with AIDS who have neurologic abnormalities.[135,136] The disease was reported more frequently in those who were exposed to HIV by blood transfusion than in those in all other exposure categories. In addition to AIDS, PML also occurs in patients with (i) lymphoproliferative disorders, (ii) sarcoidosis and tuberculosis, (iii) inherited primary immunodeficiency diseases, and (iv) in those under prolonged immunosuppression and chemotherapies.

In PML, JCV causes a cytocidal infection of oligodendrocytes leading to demyelination. Neurons are unaffected and morphologic changes in JCV-T antigen containing astrocytes probably represent nonpermissive infection.[132] The widespread and multifocal distribution of demyelination in PML suggests a hematogenous spread. JCV genome has also been isolated in B-lymphocytes of individuals previously infected with JCV.[137] It has been proposed that during multiplication of JCV, infected B-lymphocytes transport the virus to the CNS and initiate PML.[138] Alternatively, reactivation of JCV seeded in the brain during primary infection may also lead to PML as seen in older patients.[139]

The onset of the disease is insidious and may occur at any time during the course of the underlying condition. Early signs and symptoms point to multifocal, asymmetric lesions in the brain when patients present with impaired speech, vision, and mentation. As the disease progresses rapidly, paralysis, blindness, and sensory abnormalities develop. Death occurs within 3-6 months after onset of symptoms. Lesions are usually localized in the cerebral hemispheres, cerebellum and brain stem and can be diagnosed by neuro-imaging studies (MRI or CT) of the brain.[140]

Macroscopically, the PML brain shows widespread foci of demyelination of varying sizes (2-3 cm in diameter) distributed mainly in the subcortical white matter. In advanced cases, the lesions show central necrosis and cavitary changes. Histopathology demonstrates loss of myelin and presence of macrophages, reactive astrocytes, and enlarged oligodendrocytes containing basophilic or eosinophilic inclusion bodies. Greatly enlarged, bizarre, giant astrocytes with pleomorphic, hyperchromatic nuclei resembling the malignant astrocytes are additional findings.[141]

Abundant amounts of JCV particles are often found in dense crystalline arrays in the altered oligodendrocyte nuclei. JCV in PML brains has been routinely identified by a variety of techniques, including (i) immune electron microscopy, (ii) immunofluorescence or immunoperoxidase tests, (iii) cultivation of virus, and (iv) Southern blot, in situ hybridization, or PCR. In PML brains, viral DNA is distributed more extensively than viral antigen and may be found in cytologically unaffected oligodendrocytes. In cases of PML, JCV is also found in the cerebrospinal fluid[139-141] and extraneural sites e.g., kidney, liver, lung, lymph node, and spleen.[142] The amount of DNA in these tissues is significantly less than that in the brain.

SV40 Related Disease

Naturally occurring SV40, a polyomavirus of rhesus macaques was inadvertently entered into the human population through contaminated polio vaccines.[4] Whether SV40 circulates in humans currently is controversial. A large scale population based study in England reported that there was no serological evidence suggesting that SV40 entered the human population during the past 40 years.[143] In studies of urines from HIV seropositive and HIV seronegative individuals, almost 50% of specimens had BKV or JCV or both, but none had SV40.[144] On the other hand, David et al[145] found that 16% of peripheral blood lymphocytes from noncancer patients were positive for SV40 genome and SV40 DNA sequences were identified in PBMC and sperm of 25% and 40% of healthy volunteers, respectively.[146] Li et al[147] have detected SV40 genome from PBMC and urinary cells and renal tissues from kidney diseases e.g., focal segmental glomerulosclerosis. These investigators have observed a considerable diversity in the regulatory region of human SV40 showing both archetypal and nonarchetypal regulatory regions. Recently, Butel and colleagues[148] found SV40 seropositivity in children in association with renal transplantation, and amplified SV40 genome from renal allograft.

Polyomaviruses and Human Malignancies

Polyomaviruses are oncogenic for laboratory animals and are capable of transforming human cells.[149,150] Tumors or tumor-derived cells have been examined for viral particles, viral T antigen, and viral genomes; moreover, sera from cancer patients have been screened for the presence of antibodies to capsid and T antigens. Genomic sequences of BKV, JCV and SV 40 have been variably reported from a wide variety of human cancers including mesothelioma, pediatric and adult brain tumors, osteosarcoma, and nonHodgkin lymphomas.[151-162] The significance of these observations is unclear. The possibilities being examined include (i) they are laboratory artifacts, (ii) they represent passenger viruses, and (iii) the infections contribute to the development of these cancers. A discussion of the association between polyomavirus and human malignancies can be found in several chapters in this book.

Prevention and Control

BKV and JCV infections are extremely common and are essentially harmless except when the host is immunologically impaired. Infection with BKV occurs at an earlier age than that with JCV. In the United States, antibodies to BKV are acquired by 50% of the children by the age of 3-4 years, whereas antibodies to JCV are acquired by 50% of the children by the age of 10-14 years. The antibody prevalence to BKV reaches nearly 100% by the age of 10-11 years and then declines to around 70-80% in the older age groups.[163] The antibody prevalence to JCV reaches a peak of about 75% by adult age.

Primary infections with BKV and JCV in healthy children are rarely associated with illness. BKV seroconversion is associated with mild respiratory illness. Reactivations are brought about not only by significant immunosuppression, as in renal transplant recipients and HIV-infected individuals,[164] but also by more subtle factors, such as pregnancy, diabetes, and old age. There have been no attempts to devise strategies for the prevention and control of these infections.

Serial monitoring of the BKV load in plasma and performing urinary cytology for BK viruria are helpful in early diagnosis of BKV nephropathy. At this time, due to continued shortage of organs, discarding organs from BKV-seropositive donors is an unacceptable proposal.

Diagnosis and Treatment

BKV

Cytomorphology of urinary epithelial cells is helpful as an indication of polyomavirus excretion in urine.[88,94-97,113,165,166] Virus-infected epithelial cells are enlarged "decoy cells", and their nuclei contain a single, homogeneous, large, pale basophilic inclusion that may occupy the entire nuclear area. Polyomavirus-infected urinary cells should not be mistaken for cells infected with CMV, which are generally smaller, basophilic or eosinophilic, and surrounded by a halo and contains intracytoplasmic inclusions. The rough-textured nuclear chromatin of a malignant cell differs greatly from the structureless inclusion in a polyomavirus-infected cell. The cytologic findings by themselves are not definitive because they cannot distinguish between BKV and JCV infections, and virus excretion in urine may occur without marked cytologic abnormalities. The presence of virus in the blood and urine has been demonstrated by a variety of techniques, including (i) tissue culture, (ii) electron-microscopic, (iii) ELISA assays, (iv) Southern hybridization, and (v) polymerase chain reaction (PCR).[105-112,114-120] Currently, PCR methodology is universally used for polyomavirus diagnosis.

Although experience is limited, current management strategies aim at the judicious lowering, switching and discontinuation of the dosage of the immunosuppressive therapy to allow clearance of BKV. Individual case reports and reports from single centers support the view that early stages of BKV nephropathy might be more readily reversible.[85,86,89,94,95,97,100,103,167,168] Ramos et al[168] reported their experience in 67 kidney transplant patients with BKV nephropathy. 52 patients underwent decrease in immunosuppression and in 15 patients no intervention was made. There were 14 cases of nephropathy, in 15% of the reduction group and in 20% of the "no intervention" group. This difference was (not) statistically significant. In another report, renal graft loss was 10% (1/10) when this strategy of lowering immunosuppression was applied.[169] In case of coexisting acute rejection, a two-step procedure of immediate antirejection treatment followed by reducing the maintenance immunosuppression might be indicated.[170] In some situations, allograft and native nephrectomies were carried out in order to remove the source of infection and then successful retransplantation was performed.[171] More, recently, antiviral treatment has been employed with variable results.[172] Retinoic acid, DNA gyrase inhibitors, Cidofovir and 5'-brome2'-deoxyuridine inhibit polyoma virus replication in vitro. In clinical trials, Cidofovir was effective when administered at 20% of the dosage recommended for treatment of CMV.[173-176] In clinical trial 5'-brome2'-deoxyuridine has been ineffective but vidarabine has reportedly produced dramatic remission in a patients with post-BMT HC.[177] There are several recent reports of successful reversal of renal allograft function in patients with BKV nephropathy, the largest of which was published by University of Pittsburgh Transplant Program.[173,175] Cidofovir was administered at doses 0.2-1 mg/kg every 1-4 weeks intervals, renal function improved in 31% (5/16) and stabilized in another 31% (5/16) patients. Intravenous immunoglobulin (IVIG) has been shown to contain antibodies against BKV and clinical reduction in BK viremia had been demonstrated when IVIG was administered at a dose of 500 mg/kg/day for seven days.[178] Interferon has some activity against BKV in vitro but has no effect on BK viruria in renal transplant patients.[179] Early results with two malonoitrilamide compounds, FK-778 and FK-779 showed that these agents demonstrated anti-polyomavirus (simian and murine) activity and were able to decrease free virus production.[180] Recently several centers have reported that treatment with leflunomide, the parent compound of malonoitrilamide resulted in improved graft function in patients with biopsy proven BK nephropathy.[181,182]

JCV

Signs and symptoms of asymmetric multifocal brain disease without signs of increased intracranial pressure in an immunocompromised person would suggest the diagnosis of PML. Computed tomographic scan or magnetic resonance imaging of the brain is effective in establishing the diagnosis, however, stereotactic biopsies may be needed to distinguish PML from other conditions.[183] Serologic studies are not helpful as JCV antibodies levels tend not to increase in the course of the disease. Viral antibodies are not detected in the cerebrospinal fluid. The unique histopathologic features of PML can be identified by light microscopy and can be confirmed by demonstration of JCV particles, antigen, or DNA in the brain. JCV DNA can be amplified from the cerebrospinal fluid of PML patients.

Attempts to treat PML have not been generally successful, although some remissions have been reported.[132] The general strategy has been to discontinue, if possible, immunosuppressive drugs and treatments and to attempt to inhibit viral multiplication by chemotherapy. The drugs most frequently tried are nucleic acid base analogues, adenine arabinoside, cytosine arabinoside, and alpha-interferon. Patients most likely to benefit by therapy are those whose basic defense mechanisms are relatively intact (e.g., renal allograft recipients) and in whom it would be possible to eliminate or reduce iatrogenic immunosuppression. Patients with inflammatory response in the PML lesions,[184] and patients who have JCV-specific CD8+ cytotoxic T lymphocytes[185] appear to survive longer than patients without such response. Unfortunately, early detection of PML and aggressive symptomatic treatment do not seem to extend the survival time of PML patients.

Summary

Infections with human polyomaviruses are ubiquitous. Illnesses with these infections occur almost exclusively in immunosuppressed individuals. BKV infection is associated with hemorrhagic cystitis in bone marrow transplant recipients and nephropathy in renal transplant recipients. JCV infection is responsible for progressive multifocal leukoencephalopathy, which is a complication of diseases, which lead to immunologic impairment. Whether the human polyomaviruses BKV and JCV and the simian virus 40 of rhesus macaques have any role in human cancer is at present unclear.

References

1. Padgett BL, Walker DL, Zu Rhein GM et al. Cultivation of papova-like virus from human brain with progressive multifocal leucoencephalopathy. Lancet 1971; i:1257-1260.
2. Gardner SD, Field AM, Coleman DV et al. New human papovavirus (B.K.) isolated from urine after renal transplantation. Lancet 1971; i:1253-1257.
3. Sweet BH, Hillemean MR. The vacuolating virus, SV 40. Proc Soc Exp Biol Med 1960; 105:420-427.
4. Mortimer EA, Lepow ML, Gold E et al. Long-term follow-up of persons inadvertently inoculated with SV40 as neonates. N Engl J Med 1981; 305:1517-1518.
5. Ahsan N, Shah KV. Polyomaviruses: An overview. Graft 2002; 5:S9-18.
6. Walker DL, Frisque RJ. The biology and molecular biology of JC virus. In: Salzman NP, ed. The papovaviridae, the polyomaviruses. New York: Plenum Press, 1986:1:327-377.
7. Moens U, Johansen T, Johansen JI et al. Noncoding control region of naturally occurring BK virus variants: Sequence comparison and functional analysis. Virus Genes 1995; 10:261-75.
8. Kristoffersen AK, Johnsen JI, Seternes OM et al. The human polyomavirus BK T antigen induces genes expression in human cytomegalovirus. Virus Res 1997; 52:61-71.
9. Cubitt c, Stoner G. Molecular genetics of the BK virus. Graft 2002; 5:S20-28.
10. Imagawa M, Chiu R, Karin M. Transcription factor AP-2 mediates induction by two different signal-transduction pathways: Protein kinase C and cAMP. Cell 1987; 51:251-260.
11. Moens U, Sundsfjord A, Flaegstad T et al. BK virus early RNA transcripts in stably transformed cells: Enhanced levels induced by dibutyryl cyclic AMP, forskolin and 12-O-tetradecanoylphorbol-13-acetate treatment. J Gen Virol 1990; 71:1461-1471.
12. Knepper JE, DiMayorca G. Cloning and characterization of BK virus-related DNA sequences from normal and neoplastic human tissues. J Med Virol 1987; 21:289-299.
13. Newman JT, Frisque RJ. Detection of archetype and rearranged variants of JC virus in multiple tissues from a pediatric PML patient. J Med Virol 1997; 52:243-52.
14. Loeber G, Dorries K. DNA rearrangements in organ-specific variants of polyomavirus JC strain GS. J Virol 1988; 62:1730-5.
15. Ault GS, Stoner GL. Brain and kidney of progressive multifocal leukoencephalopathy patients contain identical rearrangements of the JC virus promoter/enhancer. J Med Virol 1994; 44:298-304.
16. Moens U, Rekvig OP. Molecular biology of BK virus and clinical and basic aspects of BK virus renal infection. In: Khalili K, Stoner GL, ed. Human polyomaviruses. Molecular and clinical perspectives. New York: Willey-Liss Inc., 2001:359-408.
17. Moens U, Seternes OM, Johansen B et al. Mechanism of transcriptional regulation of cellular genes SV40 larger T- and small t-antigens. Virus Genes 1997; 15:135-154.
18. Kornberg RD. Structure of chromatin. Annu Rev Biochem 1977; 46:931-954.
19. McGhee JD, Felsenfeld G. Nucleosome structure. Annu Rev Biochem 1980; 49:1115-1156.
20. Kornberg RD, Lorch Y. Twenty-five years of nucleosome, fundamental particle of the eukaryotic chromosome. Cell 1999; 98:285-294.
21. Andreassen K, Bredholt G, Moens U et al. T cell lines specific for polyomavirus T-antigen recognize T-virus complexed with nucleosomes: A molecular basis for anti-DNA antibody production. Eur J Immunol 1999; 29:2715-2728.
22. Liddington RC, Yan Y, Moulat J et al. Structure of seminal virus 40 at 3.8—A resolution. Nature 1991; 554:278-294.

23. Rayment I, Baker TS, Casper DL et al. Polyoma virus capsis structure at 22.5 A resolution. Nature 1982; 295:13-31.
24. Resnick J, Shenk T. Simian virus 40 agnoprotein facilitates normal nuclear location of the major capsid polypeptide and cell-to-cell spread of virus. J Virol 1986; 60:1098-1106.
25. Endo S, Okada Y, Nishihara H et al. JC virus agnoprotein co localizes with tubulin. J Neuro Virol 2003; 9:10-14.
26. Beckmann A, Shah K. Propagation and primary isolation of JCV and BKV in urinary epithelial cell cultures. In: Sever JL, Madden DL, eds. Polyomaviruses and human neurological diseases. New York: Alan R Liss, 1983:3-14.
27. Marshall WF, Telenti A, Proper J et al. Rapid detection of polyomavirus BK by a shell vial cell culture assay. J Clin Microbiol 1990; 28:1613-1615.
28. Padgett B, Walker D. Natural history of human polyomavirus infections. In: Stevens JG, Todaro GJ, Fox CF, eds. Persistent viruses. New York: Academic Press, 1978:751-758.
29. Assouline JG, Major EO. Human fetal Schwann cells support JC virus multiplication. J Virol 1991; 65:1001-1006.
30. Major EO, Vacante D. Human fetal astrocytes in culture support the growth of the neurotropic human polyomavirus JCV. J Neuropathol Exp Neurol 1989; 48:425-436.
31. Aoki N, Mori M, Kato K et al. Antibody against synthetic multiple antigen peptides (MAP) of JC virus capsid protein (VP1) without cross reaction to BK virus: A diagnostic tool for progressive multifocal leukoencephalopathy. Neurosci Lett 1996; 205:111-114.
32. Knowles WA, Gibson PE, Gardner SD. Serological typing scheme for BK-like isolates of human polyomavirus. J Med Virol 1989; 28:118-123.
33. Knowles WA, Gibson PE, Hand JF et al. An M-antibody capture radioimmunoassay (MACRIA) for detection of JC virus-specific IGM. J Virol Mehtods 1992; 40:95-105.
34. Marshall J, Smith AE, Cheng SH. Monoclonal antibody specific for BK virus large T antigens. Oncogene 1991; 6:1673-1676.
35. Frisque RJ, Rifkin DB, Walker DL. Transformation of primary hamster brain cells with JC virus and its DNA. J Virol 1980; 35:265-269.
36. Pater MM, Pater A, di Mayorca G et al. BK virus-transformed inbred hamster brain cells: Status of viral DNA in subclones. Mol Cell Biol 1982; 2:837-844.
37. Takemoto KK, Linke H, Miyanura T et al. Persistent BK papovavirus infection of transformed human fetal brain cells. J Virol 1979; 29:1177-1185.
38. Thiele M, Grabowski G. Mutagenic activity of BKV and JCV in human and other mammalian cells. Arch Virol 1990; 113:221-233.
39. Apperly JF, Rice SJ, Bishop JA et al. Late-onset hemorrhagic cystitis associated with urinary excretion of polyomaviruses after bone marrow transplantation. Transplantation 1987; 43:108-112.
40. Arthur RR, Shah KV, Charache P et al. BK and JC virus infections in recipients of bone marrow transplants. J Infect Dis 1988; 158:563-569.
41. Atwood WJ. Cellular receptors for the polyomaviruses. In: Khallili K, Stoner GL, eds. Human polyomaviruses: Molecular and clinical perspectives. New York: Wiley-Liss, 2001:179-96.
42. Liu CK, Wei G, Atwood WJ. Infection of glial cells by the human polyomavirus JC is mediated by an N-linked glycoprotein containing terminal alpha (2-6) linked sialic acids. J Virol 1998; 72:4643-9.
43. Breau WC, Atwood WJ, Norkin LC. Class I major histocompatibility proteins are an essential component of the simian virus 40 receptor. J Virol 1992; 66:2037-2045.
44. Atwood WJ, Norkin LC. Class I major histocompatibility proteins as cell surface receptors for simian virus 40. J Virol 1989; 63:4474-7.
45. Kenney S, Natarajan V, Strike D et al. JC virus enhancer-promoter active in human brain cells. Science 1984; 226:1337-1339.
46. Corallini A, Pagnani M, Caputo A et al. Cooperation in oncogenesis between BK virus early region gene and the activated human c-Harvey ras oncogene. J Gen Virol 1988; 69:2671-2679.
47. Knepper JE, di Mayorca G. Cloning and characterization of BK virus-related DNA sequences from normal and neoplastic human tissues. J Med Virol 1987; 21:289-299.
48. Monaco MC, Jensen PN, Hou J et al. Detection of JC virus DNA in human tonsil tissue: Evidence for site of initial viral infection. J Virol 1998; 72:9918-9923.
49. Weber T, Major EO. Progressive multifocal leukoencephalopathy: Molecular biology, pathogenesis, and clinical impact. Intervirology 1997; 40:98-111.
50. Sundsfjord A, Spein AR, Lucht E et al. Detection of human polyomavirus BK DNA in nasopharyngeal aspirates from children with respiratory infections but not in saliva from immunodeficient and immunocompetent patients. J Clin Microbiol 1994; 32:1390-1394.

51. Taguchi F, Nagaki D, Saito M et al. Transplacental transmission of BK virus in human. Jpn J Micrbiol 1975; 19:395-398.
52. Pietropaolo V, Di Taranto C, Degener AM et al. Transplacental transmission of human polyomavirus BK. J Med Virol 1998; 56:372-376.
53. Shah K, Daniel R, Madden D et al. Serological investigation of BK papovavirus infection pregnant women and their offspring. Infect Immun 1980; 30:29 (in recipients of renal allografts. J Infect Dis 1998; 158:176-181.
54. Arthur RR, DagostinS, Shah KV. Detection of BK virus and JC virus in urine and brain tissue by polymerase chain reaction. J Clin Microbiol 1989; 27:1174-1179.
55. Andrews CA, Shah KV, Daniel RW et al. A serological investigation of BK virus and JC virus infections in recipients of renal allografts. J Infect Dis 198; 158:176-181
56. Major EO, Amemiya K, Tornatore CS et al. Pathogenesis and molecular biology of progressive multifocal leukoencephalopathy, the JC virus-induced demyelinating disease of the human brain. Clin Microbiol Rev 1992; 5:49-73.
57. Dorries K, Vogel E, Gunther S et al. Infection of human polyomaviruses JC and BK in peripheral blood leukocytes from immunocompetent individuals. Virology 1994; 198:59-70.
58. Tornatore C, Berger JR, Houff SA et al. Detection of JC virus DNA in peripheral lymphocytes from patients with and without progressive multifocal leukoencephalopathy. Ann Neurol 1992; 31:454-462.
59. Holmberg C, Gribble D, Takernoto K et al. Isolation of simian virus 40 from rhesus monkeys (Macacca mulatta) with spontaneous progressive multifocal leukoencephalopathy. J Infect Dis 1977; 136:593-596.
60. Horvath CJ, Simon MA, Bergsagel DJ et al. Simian virus 40-induced disease in rhesus monkeys with simian acquired immunodeficiency syndrome. Am J Pathol 1992; 140:1431-1440.
61. Rosen S, Harmon W, Krensky A et al. Tubulo-interstitial nephritis associated with polyomavirus (BK type) infection. N Engl J Med 1983; 308:1192-1196.
62. Gorder MA, Pelle PD, Henson JW et al. A new member of the polyoma virus family causes interstitial nephritis, ureteritis, and enteritis in immunocompromised cynomolgus monkeys. Am J Pathol 1999; 154:1273-1284.
63. Goudsmit J, Wertheim-van Dillen P, van Strein A et al. The role of BK virus in acute respiratory tract disease and the presence of BKV DNA in tonsils. J Med Virol 1982; 10:91-99.
64. Mantyjarvi R, Meumian 0, Vihma L et al. Human papovavirus (B.K.), biological properties and seroepidemiology. Ann Dis Res 1973; 5:283-287.
65. Coleman D, Wolfendale M, Daniel R et al. A prospective study of human polyomavirus infection in pregnancy. J Infect Dis 1980; 142:1-8.
66. Arthur RR, Shah KV. The occurrence and significance of papovaviruses BK and JC in the urine. Prog Med Virol 1989; 36:42-61.
67. Chang D, Wang M, Ou WC et al. Genotypes of human polyomaviruses in urine samples of pregnant women in Taiwan. J Med Virol. 1996; 48:95-101.
68. Rekvig OP, Moens U. Polyoma BK and autoimmunity to nucleosomes. Graft 2002; 5:S36-S45.
69. Christie KE, Flaegstad T, Traavik T. Characterization of BK virus-specific antibodies in human sera by Western immunoblotting, native DNA are produced during BK virus infection, but not after immunization with noninfectious BK DNA. Scand J Immunol 1992; 36:487-95.
70. Rekvig OP, Moens U, Fredriksen K et al. Human polyomavirus BK and immunogenicity of mammalian DNA: A conceptual framework. Methods 1997; 11:44-54.
71. Sundsfjord A, Osei A, Rosenqvist H et al. BK and JC viruses in patients with systemic lupus erythematosus: Prevalent and persistent BK viruria, sequence stability of the viral regulatory regions, and nondetectable viremia. J Infect Dis 1999; 180:1-9.
72. Gheule MV, Moens U, Beniksen S et al. Autoimmunity to nucleosomes related to viral infection: A focus on hapten-carrier complex formation. J Autoimmunity 2003; 20:171-182.
73. Chang D, Tsai RT, Wang M et al. Different genotypes of human polyomaviruses found in patients with autoimmune diseases in Taiwan. J Med Virol 1996; 48(2):204-9.
74. Tsai RT, Wang M, Ou WC et al. Incidence of JC viruria is higher than that of BK viruria in Taiwan. J Med Virol 1997; 52(3):253-7.
75. Boldorini R, Omodeo-Zorini E, Nebuloni M et al. Lytic JC virus infection in the kidneys of AIDS subjects. Mod Pathol 2003; 16(1):35-42.
76. Markowitz RB, Thompson HC, Mueller JF et al. Incidence of BK virus and JC virus viruria in human immunodeficiency virus-infected and uninfected subjects. J Infect Dis 1993; 167:13-20.
77. Shah KV, Daniel RW, Stricker HD et al. Investigation of human urine for genome sequences of the primate polyomaviruses simian 40, BK virus, and JC virus. J Infect Dis 1997; 176:1618-21.

78. Sundsfjord A, Flaegstad T, Flo R et al. BK and JC viruses in human immunodeficiency virus 1 infected persons: Prevalence, excretion, viremia, and viral regulatory regions. J Infect Dis 1994; 169:485-90.
79. Knowles WA, Pillay D, Johnson MA et al. Prevalence of long term BK and JC excretion in HIV-infected adults and lack of correlation with serological markers. J Med Virol 1999; 59:474-79.
80. Bratt G, Hammarin AL, Grandien M et al. BK virus as the cause of meningoencephalitis, retinitis and nephritis in a patient with AIDS. AIDS 1999; 18:1071-5.
81. Cubukcu-Dimopulo O, Greco A, Kumar D et al. BK virus infection in AIDS. Am J Surg Pathol 2002; 24:145-9.
82. Vallbracht A, Lohler J, Gossmann J et al. Disseminated BK type polyomavirus infection in an AIDS patient associated with central nervous system disease. Am J Pathol 1993; 143:29-39.
83. Gluck TA, Knowles WA, Johnson MA et al. BK virus-associated haemorrhagic cystitis in an HIV-infected man. AIDS 1994; 8(3):391-2.
84. Barouch DH, Faquin WC, Chen Y et al. BK virus-associated hemorrhagic cystitis in a Human Immunodeficiency Virus-infected patient. Clin Infect Dis 2002; 35(3):326-9.
85. Hirsch HH, Knowles W, Dickenmann M et al. Prospective study of polyomavirus type BK replication and nephropathy in renal-transplant recipients. N Engl J Med 2002; 347(7):488-96.
86. Ramos E, Drachenberg CB, Portocarrero M et al. BK virus nephropathy diagnosis and treatment: Experience at the University of Maryland Renal Transplant Program. Clin Transpl 2002; 143-53.
87. Schmitz M, Brause M, Hetzel G et al. Infection with polyomavirus type BK after renal transplantation. Clin Nephrol 2003; 60(2):125-9.
88. Randhawa PS, Finkelstein S, Scantlebury V et al. Human polyoma virus-associated interstitial nephritis in the allograft kidney. Transplantation 1999; 67:103-9.
89. Ginevri F, De Santis R, Comoli P et al. Polyomavirus BK infection in pediatric kidney-allograft recipients: A single-center analysis of incidence, risk factors, and novel therapeutic approaches. Transplantation 2003; 75(8):1266-70.
90. Lin PL, Vats AN, Green M. BK virus infection in renal transplant recipients. Pediatr Transplant 2001; 5(6):398-405.
91. Lee JM, Park JH, Kim SK. BK polyomavirus interstitial nephritis in a renal allograft recipient. Ultrastruct Pathol 2003; 27(1):61-4.
92. Hirsch HH. Polyomavirus BK nephropathy: A (re)emerging complication in renal transplantation. Am J Transplant 2002; 2(1):25-30.
93. Randhawa P, Vats A, Shapiro R et al. BK virus: Discovery, epidemiology, and biology. Graft 2002; 5:S 19-S27.
94. Nickleit V, Steiger J, Mihatsch M. BK virus infection after kidney transplantation. Graft 2002; 5:S46-S57.
95. Randhawa PS, Demetris AJ. Nephropathy due to polyomavirus type BK. N Engl J Med 2000; 342(18):1361-3.
96. Nickeleit V, Singh HK, Mihatsch MJ. Polyomavirus nephropathy: Morphology, pathophysiology, and clinical management. Curr Opin Nephrol Hypertens 2003; 12(6):599-605.
97. Binet I, Nickeleit V, Hirsch HH. Polyomavirus infections in transplant recipients. Curr Opin Organ transplant 2000; 5:210-216.
98. Hirsch HH, Steiger J. Polyomavirus BK. Lancet Infect Dis 2003; 3(10):611-23.
99. Kazory A, Ducloux D. Renal transplantation and polyomavirus infection: Recent clinical facts and controversies. Transpl Infect Dis 2003; 5(2):65-71.
100. Mylonakis E, Goes N, Rubin RH et al. BK virus in solid organ transplant recipients: An emerging syndrome. Transplantation 2001; 72(10):1587-92.
101. Fishman JA. BK virus nephropathy-polyomavirus adding insult to injury. N Engl J Med 2002; 347(7):527-30.
102. Pahari A, Rees L. BK virus-associated renal problems-clinical implications. Pediatr Nephrol 2003; 18(8):743-8.
103. Reploeg MD, Storch GA, Clifford DB. BK virus: A clinical review. Clin Infect Dis 2001; 33(2):191-202.
104. Li RM, Mannon RB, Kleiner D et al. BK virus and SV40 coinfection in polyomavirus nephropathy. Transplantation 2002; 74(11):1497-504.
105. Ding R, Medeiros M, Dadhania D et al. Noninvasive diagnosis of BK virus nephritis by measurement of messenger RNA for BK virus VP1 in urine. Transplantation 2002; 74(7):987-94.
106. Randhawa P, Zygmunt D, Shapiro R et al. Viral regulatory region sequence variations in kidney tissue obtained from patients with BK virus nephropathy. Kidney Int 2003; 64(2):743-7.
107. Randhawa PS, Vats A, Zygmunt D et al. Quantitation of viral DNA in renal allograft tissue from patients with BK virus nephropathy. Transplantation 2002; 74(4):485-8.

108. Randhawa PS, Khaleel-Ur-Rehman K, Swalsky PA et al. DNA sequencing of viral capsid protein VP-1 region in patients with BK virus interstitial nephritis. Transplantation 2002; 73(7):1090-4.
109. Leung AY, Chan M, Tang SC et al. Real-time quantitative analysis of polyoma BK viremia and viruria in renal allograft recipients. J Virol Methods 2002; 103(1):51-6.
110. Bergallo M, Merlino C, Bollero C et al. Human polyoma virus BK DNA detection by nested PCR in renal transplant recipients. New Microbiol 2002; 25(3):331-4.
111. CF, Randhawa P. Molecular genotyping of BK and JC viruses in human polyomavirus-associated interstitial nephritis after renal transplantation. Am J Kidney Dis 2001; 38(2):354-65.
112. Boldorini R, Zorini EO, Fortunato M et al. Molecular characterization and sequence analysis of polyomavirus BKV-strain in a renal-allograft recipient. Hum Pathol 2001; 32(6):656-9.
113. Fogazzi GB, Cantu M, Saglimbeni L. 'Decoy cells' in the urine due to polyomavirus BK infection: Easily seen by phase-contrast microscopy. Nephrol Dial Transplant 2001; 16(7):1496-8.
114. Randhawa P, Baksh F, Aoki N et al. JC virus infection in allograft kidneys: Analysis by polymerase chain reaction and immunohistochemistry. Transplantation 2001; 71(9):1300-3.
115. Limaye AP, Jerome KR, Kuhr CS et al. Quantitation of BK virus load in serum for the diagnosis of BK virus-associated nephropathy in renal transplant recipients. J Infect Dis 2001; 183(11):1669-72.
116. Chen CH, Wen MC, Wang M et al. A regulatory region rearranged BK virus is associated with t tubulointerstitial nephritis in a rejected renal allograft. J Med Virol 2001; 64(1):82-8.
117. Nickeleit V, Hirsch HH, Zeiler M et al. BK-virus nephropathy in renal transplants-tubular necrosis, MHC-class II expression and rejection in a puzzling game. Nephrol Dial Transplant 2000; 15(3):324-32.
118. Nickleit V, Klimkait T, Binet IF et al. Testing for polyomavirus type BK DNA in plasma to identify renal-allograft recipients with viral nephropathy. N Engl J Med 2000; 342:1309-15.
119. Jin L. Molecular methods for identification and genotyping of BK virus. Methods Mol Biol 2001; 165:33-48.
120. Andrews CA, Shah KV, Daniel RW et al. A serologic investigation of BK virus and JC virus infections in recipients of renal allografts. J Infect Dis 1988; 158:176-181.
121. Coleman D, Mackenzie S, Gardner S et al. Human polyomavirus (BK) infection and ureteral stenosis in renal allograft recipients. J Clin Pathol 1978; 31:338-347.
122. Constantinescu A, Ahsan N, Lim JW. Polyomavirus allograft nephropathy – parenchymal and extra-parenchymal manifestations. GRAFT 2002; 5:S98-S103.
123. Agha IA, Brennan DC. BK virus and current immunosuppressive therapy. Graft 2002; 5:S65-S72.
124. Petrogiannis-Haliotis T, Sakoulas G, Kirby J et al. BK-related polyomavirus vasculopathy in a renal-transplant recipient. N Engl J Med 2001; 345:1250-5.
125. Bedi A, Miller CB, Hanson JL et al. Association of BK virus with failure of prophylaxis against hemorrhagic cystitis following bone marrow transplantation. J Clin Oncol 1995; 13(5):1103-9.
126. Nevo S, Swan V, Enger C et al. Acute bleeding after bone marrow transplantation (BMT) incidence and effect on survival. A quantitative analysis in 1,402 patients. Blood 1998; 91(4):1469-77.
127. Seber A, Shu XO, Defor T et al. Risk factors for severe hemorrhagic cystitis following BMT. Bone Marrow Transplant 1999; 23(1):35-40.
128. Kondo M, Kojima S, Kato K et al. Late-onset hemorrhagic cystitis after hematopoietic stem cell transplantation in children. Bone Marrow Transplant 1998; 22(10):995-8.
129. Arthur RR, Shah KV, Baust SJ et al. Association of BK viruria with hemorrhagic cystitis in recipients of bone marrow transplants. N Engl J Med 1986; 315:230-234.
130. Chapman C, Flower AJ, Dunant ST. The use of vidarabine in the treatment of human polyomavirus associated acute haemorrhagic cystitis. Bone Marrow Transplant 1991; 7:481-482.
131. Cottler-Fox M, Lynch M, Deeg JH et al. Human polyomavirus: Lack of relationship of viruria to prolonged or severe hemorrhagic cystitis after bone marrow transplant. Bone Marrow Transplant 1989; 4:279-282.
132. Johnson R. Progressive multifocal leukoencephalopathy. In: Johnson R, ed. Viral infections of the nervous system. New York: Raven Press, 1982:255-263.
133. Richardson EP. Progressive multifocal leukoencephalopathy 30 years later. N Engl J Med 1988; 318:315-316.
134. Walker DL. Progressive multifocal leukoencephalopathy. Demyelinating diseases. In: Vinken PJ, Bruyn GW, Klawans HL, Koetsier JC, eds. Handbook of Clinical Neurology. Amsterdam: Elsevier Biomedical Press, 1985:4(7):503-524.
135. Berger JR, Kaszovita B, Donovan Post J et al. Progressive multifocal leukoencephalopathy associated with human immunodeficiency virus infection. Ann Intern Med 1987; 107:78-87.
136. Berger JR, Levy RM. The neurologic complications of human immunodeficiency virus infections. Med Clin North Am 1993; 77:1-23.

137. Major EO, Amemiya K, Tornatore CS et al. Pathogenesis and molecular biology of progressive multifocal leukoencephalopathy, the JC virus-induced demyelinating disease of the human brain. Clin Microbiol Rev 1992; 5:49-73.
138. White IIIrd FA , Ishaq M, Stoner GL et al. JC virus DNA is pre sent in many human brain samples from patients without progressive multifocal leukoencephalopathy. J Virol 1992; 66:5726-5734.
139. von Giesen HJ, Neuen-Jacob E, Dorries K et al. Diagnostic criteria and clinical procedures in HIV-1 associated progressive multifocal leukoencephalopathy. J Neurol Sci 1997; 147(1):63-72.
140. Berger JR, Major EO. Progressive multifocal leukoencephalopathy. Semin Neurol 1999; 19(2):193-200.
141. Gibson PI, Knowles WA, Hand JF et al. Detection of JC virus DNA in the cerebrospinal fluid of patients with progressive multifocal leukoencephalopathy. J Med Virol 1993; 39:278-281.
142. Grinnell B, Padgett B, Walker D. Distribution of nonintegrated DNA from JC papovavirus in organs of patients with progressive multifocal leukoencephalopathy. J Infect Dis 1983; 147:669-675.
143. Knowles WA, Pipkin P, Andrews N et al. Population-based study of antibody to the human polyomaviruses BKV and JCV and the simian polyomavirus SV40. J Med Virol 2003; 71(1):115-23.
144. Shah KV, Daniel RW, Strickler HD et al. Investigation of human urine for genomic sequences of the primate polyomaviruses simian virus 40, BK virus, and JC virus. J Infect Dis 1997; 176:1618-1621.
145. David H, Mendoza S, konishi T et al. Simian virus 40 is present in human lymphomas and normal blood. Cancer let 2001; 162:57-64.
146. Martini F, Iaccheri L, Lazzarin L et al. SV40 early region and large T antigen in human brain tumors, peripheral blood cells, and sperm fluids from healthy individuals. Cancer Res 1996; 56(20):4820-5.
147. Li RM, Branton MH, Tanawattanacharoen S et al. Molecular identification of SV40 infection in human subjects and possible association with kidney disease. J Am Soc Nephrol 2002; 13(9):2320-30.
148. Butel JS, Jafar S, Wong C et al. Evidence of SV40 infections in hospitalized children. Hum Pathol 1999; 30(12):1496-502.
149. Shah K, Nathanson N. Human exposure to SV40: Review and comment. Am J Epidemiol 1976; 103:1-12.
150. Lee W, Langhoff E. polyomavirus and human cancer. Graft 2002; 5:S73-S81.
151. Mayall F, Barratt K, Shanks J. The detection of Simian virus 40 in mesotheliomas from New Zealand and England using real time FRET probe PCR protocols. J Clin Pathol 2003; 56(10):728-30.
152. Reiss K, Khalili K. Viruses and cancer: Lessons from the human polyomavirus, JCV. Oncogene 2003; 22(42):6517-23.
153. Tognon M, Corallini A, Martini F et al. Oncogenic transformation by BK virus and association with human tumors. Oncogene 2003; 22(33):5192-200.
154. Khalili K, Del Valle L, Otte J et al. Human neurotropic polyomavirus, JCV, and its role in carcinogenesis. Oncogene 2003; 22(33):5181-91.
155. Carbone M, Pass HI, Miele L et al. New developments about the association of SV40 with human mesothelioma. Oncogene 2003; 22(33):5173-80.
156. Vilchez RA, Butel JS. SV40 in human brain cancers and nonHodgkin's lymphoma. Oncogene 2003; 22(33):5164-72.
157. MacKenzie J, Wilson KS, Perry J et al. Association between simian virus 40 DNA and lymphoma in the United kingdom. J Natl Cancer Inst 2003; 95(13):1001-3.
158. Vilchez RA, Kozinetz CA, Arrington AS et al. Simian virus 40 in human cancers. Am J Med 2003; 114(8):675-84.
159. Carbone M, Bocchetta M, Cristaudo A et al. SV40 and human brain tumors. Int J Cancer 2003; 106(1):140-2, author reply 143-5.
160. Rinaldo CH, Myhre MR, Alstad H et al. Human polyomavirus BK (BKV) transiently transforms and persistently infects cultured osteosarcoma cells. Virus Res 2003; 93(2):181-7.
161. Rinaldo CH, Myhre MR, Alstad H et al. Human polyomavirus BK (BKV) transiently transforms and persistently infects cultured osteosarcoma cells. Virus Res 2003; 93(2):181-7.
162. Vilchez RA, Kozinetz CA, Butel JS. Conventional epidemiology and the link between SV40 and human cancers. Lancet Oncol 2003; 4(3):188-91.
163. Gardner SD. Prevalence in England of antibody to human polyomavirus BK. Br Med J 1973; 1:77-78.
164. Shah K, Daniel R, Warszawski R. High prevalence of antibodies to BK virus, an SV40-related papovavirus, in residents of Maryland. J Infect Dis 1973; 128:784-787.

165. Drachenberg CB, Beskow CO, Cangro CB et al. Human polyoma virus in renal allograft biopsies: Morphological findings and correlation with urine cytology. Hum Pathol 1999; 30:970-977.
166. Purighalla R, Shapiro R, McCauley J et al. BK virus infection in a kidney allograft diagnosed by needle biopsy. Am J Kidney Dis 1995; 26:671-73.
167. Ginevri F, Pastorino N, De Santis R et al. Retransplantation after kidney graft loss due to polyoma BK virus nephropathy: Successful outcome without original allograft nephrectomy. Am J Kidney Dis 2003; 42(4):821-5.
168. Ramos E, Drachenberg CB, Papadimitriou JC et al. Clinical course of polyoma virus nephropathy in 67 renal transplant patients. J Am Soc Nephrol 2002; 13(8):2145-51.
169. Trofe J, Cavallo T, First MR et al. Polyomavirus in kidney and kidney-pancreas transplantation: A defined protocol for immunosuppression reduction and histologic monitoring. Transplant Proc 2002; 34(5):1788-9.
170. Hirsch HH, Mohaupt M, Klimkait T. Prospective monitoring of BK virus load after discontinuing sirolimus treatment in a renal transplant patient with BK virus nephropathy. J Infect Dis 2001; 184:1494-6.
171. Poduval RD, Meehan SM, Woodle ES et al. Successful retransplantation after renal allograft loss to polyoma virus interstitial nephritis. Transplantation 2002; 73:1166-69.
172. Fishman JA. BK nephropathy: What is the role of antiviral therapy? Am J Transplant 2003; 3(2):99-100.
173. Scantlebury V, Shapiro R, Randhawa P et al. Cidofovir: A method of treatment for BK virus-associated transplant nephropathy. Graft 2002; 5:S82-S87.
174. Kadambi PV, Josephson MA, Williams J et al. Treatment of refractory BK virus-associated nephropathy with cidofovir. Am J Transplant 2003; 3(2):186-91.
175. Vats A, Shapiro R, Singh Randhawa P et al. Quantitative viral load monitoring and cidofovir therapy for the management of BK virus-associated nephropathy in children and adults. Transplantation 2003; 75(1):105-12.
176. Bjorang O, Tveitan H, Midtvedt K et al. Treatment of polyomavirus infection with cidofovir in a renal-transplant recipient. Nephrol Dial Transplant 2002; 17(11):2023-5.
177. Held TK, Biel SS, Nitsche A et al. Treatment of BK virus-associated hemorrhagic cystitis and simultaneous CMV reactivation with cidofovir. Bone Marrow Transplant 2000; 26:347-50.
178. Cibrik DM, O'Toole JF, Norman SP et al. IVIG for the treatment of BK nephropathy. Am J Transplantation 2003; 3:370,(abstract).
179. Cheesman SH, Black PH, Rubin RH et al. Interferon and BK Papovavirus—clinical and laboratory studies. J Infect Dis 1980; 141:157-61.
180. Snoeck R, Andrei G, Lilja HS et al. Activity of malonoitrilamide compounds against murine and simian polyomavirus. Switzerland: 5th International conference on New Trends in Clinical and experimental immunosuppression, 2002, (Abstract).
181. Poduval RD, Kadambi PV, Javaid B et al. Leflunomide – a potential new therapeutic agent for BK nephropathy. Am J Transplantation 2003; 3:189,(abstract).
182. Foster PF, Wright F, McLean D et al. Leflunomide administration as an adjunct in treatment of BK-polyoma viral disease in kidney allografts. Am J Transplantation 2003; 3:421,(abstract).
183. Feiden W, Bise K, Steude U et al. The stereotactic biopsy diagnosis of focal intracerebral lesions in AIDS patients. Acta Neurol Scand 1993; 87:228-233.
184. Hair LS, Nuovo G, Powers JM et al. Progressive multifocal leukoencephalopathy in patients with human immunodeficiency virus. Hum Pathol 1992; 23:663-667.
185. Koralnik IJ, Du Pasquier RA, Kuroda MJ et al. Association of prolonged survival in HLA-A2+ progressive multifocal leukoencephalopathy patients with a CTL response specific for a commonly recognized JC virus epitope. J Immunol 2002; 168:499-504.

Discovery and Epidemiology of the Human Polyomaviruses BK Virus (BKV) and JC Virus (JCV)

Wendy A. Knowles

Abstract

Although discovered over thirty years ago, many aspects of the epidemiology of BKV and JCV in the general population, such as the source of infectious virus and the mode of transmission, are still unknown. Primary infection with both BKV and JCV is usually asymptomatic, and so age seroprevalence studies have been used to indicate infection. BKV commonly infects young children in all parts of the world, with the exception of a few very isolated communities, adult seroprevalence rates of 65-90% being reached by the age of ten years. In contrast, the pattern of JCV infection appears to vary between populations; in some anti-JCV antibody is acquired early as for BKV, but in others anti-JCV antibody prevalence continues to rise throughout life. This indicates that the two viruses are probably transmitted independently and by different routes. Whilst BKV DNA is found infrequently in the urine of healthy adults, JCV viruria occurs universally, increasing with age, with adult prevalence rates often between 20% and 60%. Four antigenic subtypes have been described for BKV and eight genotypes are currently recognized for JCV. The latter have been used to trace population movements and to reconstruct the population history in various communities.

Discovery of BKV and JCV

In the late 1960s only four polyomaviruses were known, polyoma and K virus of mice, simian virus 40 (SV40) of rhesus macaques, and rabbit kidney vacuolating virus (RKV). However, within 5 years the two human members of the polyomavirus genus, BKV and JCV, had been described. BKV was first isolated in London, England and JCV in Madison, Wisconsin, each group of workers being unknown to the other and each sending their findings to The Lancet, where they were published as consecutive papers in 1971.[1,2]

Histology or cytology followed by electron microscopy provided the first indications of the existence of each virus. The demyelinating disease progressive multifocal leukoencephalopathy (PML) was first described in 1958 as a distinct entity occurring in patients with leukaemia or lymphoma.[3] Intranuclear inclusions seen in enlarged oligodendrocytes, and the abnormal astrocytes, led investigators to propose a viral etiology for the disease.[4,5] Seven years later icosahedral-shaped virus particles, suggestive of a papovavirus, were reported within oligodendrocytes in thin sections of brain material from patients with PML.[6,7] Efforts were subsequently made by a number of laboratories to obtain material from this rare disease in order to culture the virus. All isolation attempts proved unsuccessful until Billie Padgett in Wisconsin succeeded in producing good cultures of human fetal spongioblasts (thought to

Polyomaviruses and Human Diseases, edited by Nasimul Ahsan. ©2006 Eurekah.com and Springer Science+Business Media.

be the precursors of oligodendrocytes) and astrocytes, and demonstrated virus replication in these cells.[2] The virus was named JC after the initials of the patient.

Unlike JCV, the discovery of BKV was an unexpected finding during a study on another virus, cytomegalovirus, in renal transplant recipients. Although BKV was associated with ureteric stenosis in the original patient (initials B.K), it was many years before further specific disease associations were found. Large numbers of papovavirus particles were seen in a high-speed pellet of a urine sample which had been taken three and a half months post-transplant and was known to contain many inclusion-bearing cells.[1] The presence of papovavirus particles was confirmed by thin sectioning of enlarged cell nuclei in a second urine sample taken from the same patient several days later. Inoculation of the original urine into cultures of secondary rhesus monkey kidney cells produced a cytopathic effect on day 19, with confirmation of virus particles in the culture fluid, but the virus died out on passage. However, subsequent inoculation of Vero cell cultures led to isolation of the virus and cultivation through many passages, although several weeks incubation was necessary for each subculture.

The same problems faced both groups of workers. Each laboratory raised animal antisera to their respective isolate and carried out initial characterization of the biological properties. The only human papovavirus known at the time was human wart virus, but on size it seemed that the new viruses were polyomaviruses and not papillomaviruses. Mouse polyoma, SV40, and human wart virus were also excluded by cross testing with specific antisera using indirect immunofluorescence (IFA), immune electron microscopy (IEM) and hemagglutination inhibition (HI), by growth characteristics in cell culture, and by hemagglutinating properties.[1,2] Later work confirmed the oncogenic nature of BKV and JCV in experimental animals, which was consistent with their classification as polyomaviruses. The isolates were subsequently exchanged and it was confirmed that they were, indeed, two different and new polyomaviruses. Detailed first-hand accounts of the discovery of JCV and BKV have previously been published.[8-11]

Epidemiology

More than thirty years after their discovery in immunocompromised patients, many aspects of the epidemiology of both BKV and JCV in the general population are unknown, e.g., the source of infectious virus, the route of natural transmission, and the site of initial virus replication within the body, although the presence of BKV and JCV DNA in tonsillar tissue may indicate this as a site of initial replication or later persistence.[12,13] Both viruses are endemic in almost all populations, and infection is not thought to be seasonal, although in one study it was reported that JCV was shed more frequently in the autumn and winter.[14] Man is the sole host for both BKV and JCV. Antibody to BKV is undetectable in chimpanzees, rhesus monkeys and owl monkeys,[15,16] and the anti-BKV HI antibody reported in rabbits and swine[17] was probably due to nonspecific activity.[18] Similarly, sera from a range of primates and domestic animals were negative for antibody to JCV.[19]

BKV and JCV circulate independently at both the individual and population level.[15] Individuals with antibody to BKV are often seronegative to JCV and vice versa,[20-22] and a negative association was noted between both the presence and titre of antibody to BKV and JCV.[23,24]

Neither BKV nor JCV produces a distinct, recognisable disease on primary infection and, indeed, most infection with these viruses in immunocompetent individuals is subclinical or may be associated with mild, nonspecific symptoms. A rise in BKV antibody or detection of the virus has temporally been associated with fever, and respiratory, neurological or urinary tract symptoms, mainly in children but also in adults.[12,25-33] There is one report of meningoencephalitis in a 13 year-old immunocompetent girl associated with serological evidence of current JCV infection.[34]

Primary infection with BKV and JCV must be followed by a period of viremia as both viruses persist for life in the kidney.[35-37] Peripheral blood leukocytes may be a site of latency or persistence in immunocompetent adults. However, even allowing for variation in the sensitivity of the techniques used, studies from various laboratories have reported widely differing frequencies of BKV and JCV DNA in peripheral blood leukocytes from immunocompetent individuals (Table 1).

An indication of a population's exposure to BKV and JCV may be more reliably made by assaying for antiviral antibodies.

Seroepidemiology

The virus neutralization test (VN) is recognised as the 'gold standard' for detecting past infection with many viruses, but with both BKV and JCV this is too laborious and impractical to be used as a large-scale assay. Several early BKV seroprevalence studies were done using complement fixation (CF),[47-49] indirect immunofluorescence (IFA),[50] or immunoelectroosmophoresis (IEOP).[51] However, the hemagglutination-inhibition assay (HI), which measures both IgG and IgM antibody to BKV capsid antigen,[49,52-54] has been used for most seroprevalence studies with the human polyomaviruses. HI shows a linear relationship with VN,[55] although VN may be more sensitive.[56] HI titres varying from 1:10 to 1:128 have been taken as the cut-off for positivity, due to the presence of nonspecific glycoprotein inhibitors of hemagglutination in human sera which may not be completely removed by the treatment methods used.[57,58] Later, enzyme-linked immunosorbent assays (ELISAs) were developed for BKV[23,59-64] and JCV[23,63,65] antibody detection, and recently recombinant antigens have been used in these tests.[66-71] ELISAs are applicable to large scale testing, and the results correlate with antibody titres measured by HI or VN, although ELISA may be more sensitive than HI.[23,43,60,61,63,67,72] The recent availability of virus-like particles (VLPs) of both BKV and JCV has overcome the problems of producing antigen in cell culture (particularly for JCV), and means that more information on the seroepidemiology of JCV in various populations can now be obtained.

BKV Seroprevalence

BKV is a common infection in all parts of the world, in both developed and developing countries. In most studies covering all age groups of healthy individuals or unselected patient groups the overall seroprevalence to BKV is between 55% and 85% (Table 2). There were differences in sensitivity between the assays used in each study, and some figures may represent an underestimate of the percentage of the population infected with BKV. However, in isolated populations BKV seroprevalence was found to vary from 0% to 100% (Table 3), indicating that BKV is absent from or infrequent in a few small, extremely remote Indian or aboriginal tribes in Brazil, Paraguay and Malaysia,[15,77] and may only recently have been introduced to others.[87] Generally no difference was found in seroprevalence between males and females, except for two studies in which a slightly higher seroprevalence was reported in adult males.[50,70]

The seroprevalence to BKV in different population groups within a country has only rarely been investigated. Whereas in Athens, where only small numbers of samples were tested, anti-BKV seroprevalence and titres were reported to be higher than in rural Greece,[88] no significant difference was found between urban and rural residents in Portugal.[64]

BKV Age Seroprevalence

The first age seroprevalence study of BKV in England showed that anti-BKV antibody was acquired in early childhood.[47] Maternal antibody, present at birth, was lost during the first few months of life, so that between 4 and 11 months of age only 5% of infants had anti-BKV antibody. Thereafter seroprevalence rose rapidly from the second year of life to reach 83% by late childhood. Subsequent studies from many other countries confirmed BKV as a common infection of early childhood (Fig. 1), which was also true in isolated communities,[15] near adult levels of seroprevalence of 65-90% being reached between 5 and 10 years of age, with a further slight increase during adolescence. In some studies a gradual decline in antibody prevalence was then seen throughout adulthood, probably due to waning titres that become undetectable using the HI test[24,25,50,73,83] or ELISA.[64,70] This may indicate a lack of BKV antigenic stimulation in most older immunocompetent individuals. The geometric mean titre (GMT) of anti-BKV antibody was highest during the first five years of life, confirming that this is the age at which most BKV infection is acquired, and declined with age.[24,64,85]

Table 1. Detection of BKV and JCV DNA by PCR in peripheral blood leukocytes of immunocompetent subjects

Subjects	Age (Years)	Genome Region Amplified	Sensitivity of Detection	Number Tested	Number Positive (%)		Reference
					BKV	JCV	
Patients with Parkinson's disease, U.S.A.	N.S.	NCCR (HN), T, VP1	10fg viral DNA = 1000 genome copies	30		0	38
Umbilical cord blood, Germany	Newborn	NCCR, T		10	0	0	39
Healthy adults, Germany	23-60	NCCR, T		18	17 (94)	15 (83)	39
Patients with Huntington's disease, Germany	27-69	NCCR, T		11	9 (82)	9 (82)	39
HIV-negative patients (38) and healthy volunteers (30), Houston	N.S.	NCCR, VP1	100-1000 genome copies	68		0	40
Adults, Houston (serial samples), 1998-1999	> 18		10 genome copies/ 500-ng test DNA	30	0	0	14
Healthy blood donors and operators, Sassari and Rome	18-63	NCCR (N)	10 ag viral DNA	231	50 (22)	2 (0.9)	41
		VP1 (N)	10 ag viral DNA	231	17 (7)	2 (0.9)	
Blood donors, Florence	N.S.	NCCR (N)	0.01 fg viral DNA	36	19 (53)	14 (39)	42
Students and employees, Pennsylvania	19-60	NCCR (N)	1-10 genome copies	40	22 (55)		43
Healthy blood donors, Bordeaux, 1995	22-51	T, VP1 (N)	7.8 genome copies	50		4 (8)	44
Blood donors, Bordeaux, 1996	18-50	T (N)		50		2 (4)	45
Cord blood, China	Newborn	T (HN)	3-5 genome copies	25	0	0	46
Blood donors (40), hospital employees (36), China	20-65	T (HN)	3-5 genome copies	76	32 (42)	6 (8)	46

N.S. = not stated; NCCR = non-coding control region; T = T antigen; VP1 = virion polypeptide 1; N = nested; HN = hemi-nested

Table 2. BKV seroprevalence in various populations

Country	Study Subjects	Age Range (Years)	Assay Used (Serum Dilution)	Number of Sera Tested	Number Positive (%)	Reference
U.S.A.	Healthy subjects in rubella vaccine study	1 to > 36	HI (1/20)	334	248 (74)	73
	Unselected donors	1 to > 80	HI (1/32)	993	902 (91)	74
	Patients for Wasserman testing	Young adults	HI (1/10)	400	375 (94)	75
	Patients for Wasserman testing	Young adults	HI (1/20)	400	325 (81)	75
	Donors for renal transplant	N.S.	VN (1/5)	496	392 (79)	63
	Healthy donors, Maryland; 1974 and 1989	13-87	ELISA (1/400)	130	117 (85)	68
	Controls for anogenital cancer patients, 1987-1999	19-78	ELISA (1/100)	415	262 (63)	70
	Controls for prostate cancer patients	40-64	ELISA (1/100)	72	42 (58)	70
Mexico	Rural highland community, 1968	1 to 4		139	78 (56)	76
	Rural highland community, 1968	5 to 9		249	204 (82)	76
Brazil	Cosmopolitan group	N.S.	HI (1/40)	N.S	N.S (70)	77
England	Healthy children and adults, and patients tested for	0 to > 50	HI (1/40)	409	254 (62)	47
	CMV or ASO titres	0 to > 50	CF (1/2)	508	276 (54)	47
	Residual sera, 1995	9/12 to 96	HI (1/8)	282	219 (78)	78
	Residual sera, 1991	1-69	HI (1/10)	2435	1965 (81)	24
	Healthy employees, controls for patients with malignant disease	Adults	HI (1/40)	66	44 (67)	79
Finland	Trauma patients, controls for SSPE cases	8 to 20	HI (1/10)	30	21 (70)	80
	Routine hospital patients with nonviral etiology, mostly trauma	2 to > 60	HI (1/10)	203	117 (58)	25
	Controls for MS patients	Mean 38	HI (1/10)	50	23 (46)	80
	Pregnant women	14 to 31	ELISA (1/40)	150	128 (85)	71

continued on next page

Table 2. Continued

Country	Study Subjects	Age Range (Years)	Assay Used (Serum Dilution)	Number of Sera Tested	Number Positive (%)	Reference
Norway	Healthy adults and pediatric patients	0 to 82	IgG ELISA (1/160)	461	340 (74)	62
Sweden	Unselected patients	1 to 13	ELISA (1/40)	288	206 (71)	71
Italy	Consecutive patients with various diagnoses at a childrens' hospital	0 to > 12	IEOP (N)	984	486 (49)	51
	Healthy children, adolescents, and blood donors	0.5 to 65	HI (1/128)	453	305 (67)	50
	Healthy children, adolescents, and blood donors	0.5 to 65	IFA (1/2)	311	197 (63)	50
	Healthy subjects and pediatric trauma patients	1 to > 50	HI (1/10)	582	380 (65)	48
	Healthy blood donors, controls for tumor and transplant patients	Adult	HI (1/128)	501	201 (40)	81
Switzer-land	Healthy blood donors	Adult	HI (1/10)	158	134 (85)	82
Hungary	Selected surgical patients and healthy subjects	0 to > 60	HI (1/10)	949	604 (64)	83
France	Children and blood donors	0 to > 15	HI (1/40)	183	126 (69)	84
Portugal	Healthy subjects	1 to 82	IgG ELISA (1/160)	320	218 (68)	64
Japan	Serum banks, Tokyo; 1978-1979	1 to > 51	HI (1/8)	136	110 (81)	21
	Controls from plasma bank, 1967-1984	15 to 33	HI (1/20)	100	77 (77)	85
	Healthy pregnant and nonpregnant women	20 to 29	HI (1/40)	214	158 (74)	86
	Parents of children in genetic study 1967-1984	39 to 81	HI (1/20)	98	64 (65)	85

HI = hemagglutination inhibition; VN = virus neutralization; ELISA = enzyme-linked-immunosorbent assay; CF = complement fixation; IEOP = immunoelectroosmophoresis; IFA = indirect fluorescent antibody

Table 3. BKV and JCV seroprevalence in isolated populations

Location	Population	Number of Sera Tested	Percentage Positive for BKV	Percentage Positive for JCV
Brazil	Ewarhoyana Indians, 1970[15]	9	0	0
Brazil	Mekranoti Indians, 1969[15]	60	2	8
Brazil	Diauarum Indians[77]	39	2.5	0
Paraguay	Guayaki Indians, 1963[15]	58	5	0
Brazil	Alto Xingú Indians[77]	68	5.8	4.4
Brazil	Kuben Kran Kegn Indians, 1970[15]	47	6	
Brazil	Tiriyo Indians, 1966[15]	49	6	
Brazil	Kren-Akorore Indians[77]	66	6.1	0
Brazil	Xikrin Indians, 1970[15]	53	11	
Malaysia	Semnoi aborigines, 1958[15]	20	15	75
	Piaroa[87]	23		8.7
Brazil	Kaxuyana Indians, 1970[15]	18	28	
	Makiritare[87]	21	29	19
Iran	Persian Gulf villagers, 1960[15]	23	30	
Iceland	South Thingeyarsysla farmers, 1963[15]	101	30	
West New Guinea	Tjitak group in Abau village, 1969[15]	22	41	0
Papua New Guinea	Onabasulu group in Waragu village, 1969[15]	46	41	31
Papua New Guinea	Moni group in Bilogai village, 1969[15]	60	53	
Canada	Foxe Basin Eskimos, 1971[15]	15	53	
Australia	Cape York aborigines, 1956[15]	34	62	
West New Guinea	Casuarine Coast villagers, 1969[15]	47	62	
Colombia	Siguirisua and Putumayo Indians, 1970[15]	130	68	
Brazil	Southern Pano[87]	10	70	70
Alaska	St. George Eskimos (Pribilofs), 1965[15]	59	73	
Western Caroline Islands	Fais Island Micronesians, 1964[15]	84	73	
Papua New Guinea	South Fore group in Weya village, 1969[15]	54	74	
Western Caroline Islands	Ifaluk Atoll Micronesians, 1963-1966[15]	77	75	
Panama	Guaymi[87]	24	87.5	75
British Solomon Islands	Anuta Island Polynesians, 1972[15]	88	88	5
New Hebrides	Merig Island Melanesians, 1972[15]	20	85	50
Brazil	Kraho[87]	20	90	50
	Wapishana[87]	21	90.5	76
Central Amazonas	Ticuna[87]	18	94	94
Panama	Cuna[87]	21	100	81
Brazil	Baniwa[87]	16	100	87.5
	Macushi[87]	20	100	90
Brazil	Kanamari[87]	18	100	94
Brazil	Northern Pano[87]	12	100	100
Costa Rica	Boruca[87]	18	100	100

From Brown et al,[15] Candeias et al,[77] and Major and Neel.[87]

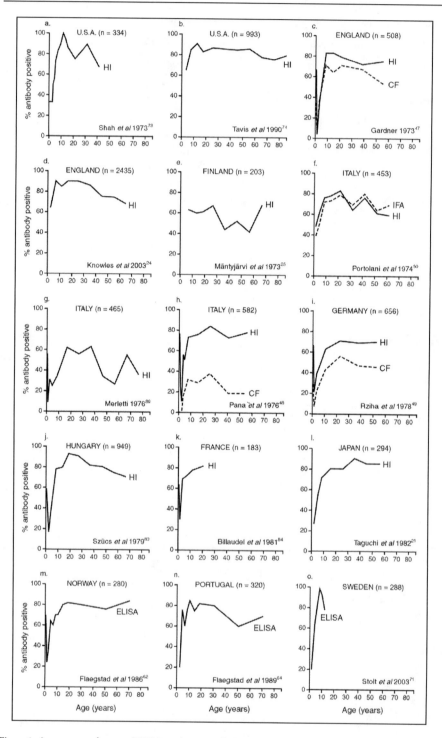

Figure 1. Age seroprevalence to BKV in various populations.

BKV-specific IgM antibody was not detected in infants during the first year of life whereas 3% of asymptomatic children between 5 and 15 years of age were positive.[62,90] When either healthy or unwell children under 5 years of age were included, between 11 and 21% had anti-BKV IgM consistent with BKV infection occurring in young children.[62,91] In some studies of healthy adults or blood donors anti-BKV IgM antibody was not detected,[54,86] whereas in others a rate of between 3.6 and 5.7 % was reported,[62,91] and even as high as 19.5% in a further study.[79] However, the methods used to detect IgM antibody varied in sensitivity and specificity, and it is not known whether these results represent primary BKV infection or reinfection in adulthood or are due to persistent IgM production in a few individuals.[79]

JCV Seroprevalence

Seroprevalence rates for JCV in various populations, and including various age ranges, are shown in Table 4. The percentage seropositivity in adults ranged from 44-77% in the U.S.A. and England and up to 85-92% in Brazil, Japan and Germany. When the overall seroprevalence rates covering all ages were recorded for a population, e.g., England, the figures were often lower and depended on the proportion of children included. As with BKV, isolated populations vary greatly in their seropositivity to JCV, with some apparently free of JCV and in others the JCV seroprevalence reaching 100% (Table 3).[15,77,87] However, there was often no correlation between a population's exposure to BKV and JCV. In some studies significantly more males than females had anti-JCV antibody[24,70] or the GMT was higher for males.[55]

JCV Age Seroprevalence

The results of seven JCV age seroprevalence studies from five countries are shown in Figure 2. More variation is apparent in the age at which JCV is acquired than with BKV. Whilst in some populations most JCV infection is acquired in early childhood as is BKV, in others the JCV seroprevalence rises more gradually even continuing into old age. These variations could indicate that the transmission of JCV is more dependent on differences between cultures or socio-economic conditions than is BKV, in which case it may be important to state the particular groups from which the sera were collected. Furthermore, a cohort effect may be seen over time if conditions change and studies done many years apart may not be comparable.[24]

In contrast to BKV, anti-JCV antibody titres do not decrease with age, indicating that there may be continuing JCV stimulation throughout life, either by virus reactivation or reinfection.[85]

Low-level anti-JCV IgM antibody was found in 15% of unselected blood donors in England,[97] which was calculated to represent up to 28% of seropositive individuals. IgM antibody may represent primary JCV infection in this population, sporadic virus reactivation in most or all seropositive adults, or a longer term inability to suppress JCV replication in a few individuals. It is not known whether or not the presence of IgM antibody indicates viral shedding in healthy adults or how the presence of JCV-specific IgM relates to age.

Virus Excretion and Source of Infectious Virus

The methods used to detect the presence of the polyomaviruses have evolved and with them has come a better understanding of the distribution of BKV and JCV in the general population. The original methods of cytology and electron microscopy (EM) were insensitive and usually did not differentiate between BKV and JCV,[90,94,98-101] although BKV- and JCV-induced inclusion-bearing cells may be distinguished cytologically[102] or by indirect immunofluorescence,[99,103] and virus particles identified by immune EM respectively.[1,104-106] Virus isolation, although specific, was always slow and laborious, antigen detection by ELISA[103,107,108] and DNA detection by hybridization[101,108-111] were more rapid, but many more sensitive methods now exist for the detection of subgenomic DNA fragments by polymerase chain reaction (PCR). With the newer techniques our views on BKV and JCV excretion have changed. The early insensitive methods were useful for diagnosis where high titres of virus are associated with disease, but more sensitive techniques are needed to detect low level viral loads in immunocompetent individuals.

Table 4. JCV seroprevalence in various populations

Country	Study Subjects	Age Range (Years)	Assay Used (Serum Dilution)	Number of Sera Tested	Number Positive (%)	Reference
U.S.A.	Routine serology, Wisconsin	0 to > 80	HI (1/32)	406	235 (58)	55
	Healthy donors, Maryland; 1974 and 1989	13 to 87	ELISA (1/400)	130	100 (77)	68
	Controls for anogenital cancer patients; 1987-1999	19 to 78	ELISA (1/100)	415	181 (44)	70
	Controls for prostate cancer patients; 1987-1999	40 to 64	ELISA (1/100)	72	46 (64)	70
	Southern California	Adults	HI (1/32)	180	135 (75)	16
	New York City	Adults	HI (1/32)	142	94 (66)	16
	Early pregnancy	N.S.	HI (1/20)	100	53 (53)	92
	Pre-renal transplant recipients and controls	Mostly adult	HI (1/32)	77	58 (55)	93
	Neurological patients; 1971-1973	N.S.	HI (1/40)	70	50 (72)	15
	Renal transplant donors	N.S.	VN (1/5)	496	372 (75)	63
Mexico	Rural highland community; 1968	1 to 4		139	44 (32)	76
		5 to 9		249	172 (69)	76
Brazil	Cosmopolitan group	Adults	HI (1/40)	N.S.	N.S.(85)	77
	Urban Brazil	N.S.	HI (1/32)	48	44 (92)	16
England	Unselected patients	0 to > 50	HI	409	105 (26)	32
	Residual sera; 1995	9/12 to 96	HI (1/8)	282	116 (41)	78
	Residual sera; 1991	1 to 69	HI (1/10)	2435	855 (35)	24
	Early pregnancy	15 to 46	HI (1/20)	429	208 (48)	94
	Pre-renal transplant	11 to 55	HI (1/20)	48	26 (54)	95
Finland	Pregnant women	14 to 31	ELISA (1/40)	150	99 (66)	71
Sweden	Unselected patients	1 to 13	ELISA (1/40)	288	91 (32)	71
Germany	Normal controls	N.S.	IgG ELISA	50	43 (86)	67
Japan	Serum banks, Tokyo; 1978-1979	1 to > 51	HI (1/8)	136	95 (70)	21
	Controls from plasma bank; 1967-1984	15 to 33	HI (1/20)	100	80 (80)	85
	Parents of children in genetic study; 1967-1984	39 to 81	HI (1/20)	99	85 (85)	85
Taiwan	Unselected patients	0 to 94	HI	1938	1228 (63)	96

HI = hemagglutination inhibition; ELISA = enzyme-linked-immunosorbent assay; VN = virus neutralization.

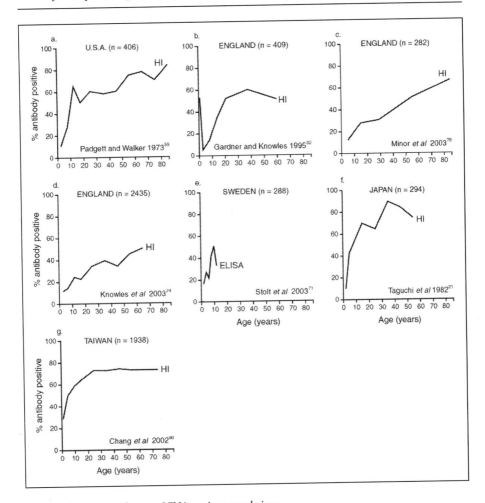

Figure 2. Age seroprevalence to JCV in various populations.

As both BKV and JCV are latent in the kidney and are excreted in the urine of many immunocompromised patients,[112] most studies on excretion have investigated the prevalence of BKV and JCV viruria. However, this may not be the only, or most appropriate, site relevant to virus transmission in healthy individuals.

BKV Excretion

Urinary excretion of BKV has been reported in immunocompetent subjects in association with urinary tract symptoms in children,[26,29-32] and adults.[101,110] However, BKV is generally not detected in the urine of immunocompetent healthy adults although a low percentage (<10%) of nonimmunosuppressed clinic patients or HIV-seronegative homosexual men may have BKV viruria (Table 5). A few laboratories have reported rates of BKV viruria greater than 16% in nonimmunosuppressed groups of adults but clinical details of the study subjects were generally not given and may have included those with subtle immunosuppression. Patients immunocompromised following renal (RT) or bone marrow (BMT) transplantation frequently excrete BKV,[93,95,108,111,112,138] as well as those with malignancy and other chronic or autoimmune diseases such as systemic lupus erythematosus (SLE).[90,98,128,133,139,140] There is an inverse relationship between the incidence of BKV viruria and CD4 cell count in HIV-infected

Table 5. BKV and JCV DNA in the urine of non-immunocompromised individuals

Subjects	Age (Years)	BKV DNA		JCV DNA		Reference
		Number Tested	Number Positive (%)	Number Tested	Number Positive (%)	
AMERICA						
Patients and healthy controls for BMT patients	0-39	125	0[a]			108
Healthy individuals (urine negative by ISH)	Adult	30	2 (6.7)			113
Normal subjects	N.S.	12	0	12	0	114
Male HIV negative patients at infectious diseases clinic	N.S.	34	6 (17.6)	34	9 (26.5)	115
General medical clinic patients (89) and healthy volunteers (16)	10 -20			6	0	116
"	21-30			14	3 (21.4)	"
"	31-40			21	8 (38.1)	"
"	41-50			25	14 (56.0)	"
"	51-60			21	7 (33.3)	"
"	61-70			9	6 (66.7)	"
"	71-94			9	5 (55.5)	"
General medical clinic patients (89), healthy volunteers (16)	N.S			105	43 (40.9)	117
General medical outpatients from New Mexico (Navaho)	12-83			68	45 (66.2)	118
General medical outpatients from Montana (Flathead)	19-88			25	14 (56.0)	118
HIV negative homosexual men, 1986-1988	28-69	78	4 (5.1)	78	29 (37.2)	119
HIV uninfected patients (38) and healthy volunteers (30), Houston	< 40			43	3 (7.0)	40
Adults, Houston (serial samples)	> 40			25	10 (40.0)	40
"	18-40	13	0	13	3 (23.1)	14
"	> 40	17	0	17	11 (64.7)	14

continued on next page

Table 5. *Continued*

Subjects	Age (Years)	BKV DNA		JCV DNA		Reference
		Number Tested	Number Positive (%)	Number Tested	Number Positive (%)	
EUROPE						
Genitourinary clinic patients (8 with hematuria), England	19-87	50	10 (20.0)[a]	50	6 (12.0)[a]	101
Outpatients, The Netherlands	N.S.			50	13 (26.0)[a]	120
Healthy volunteers, Germany	N.S.			50	8 (16.0)	"
Pediatric patients, England	5-9	100	5 (5.0)			121
Laboratory staff, England	Adult	29	0			"
Healthy laboratory staff, Sweden	Adult	14	0	14	7 (50.0)	122
Hospital patients, controls for HIV-positive group, Norway	16-64	56	0	56	12 (21.4)	123
Pediatric patients, England	<5	100	4 (4.4)	100	0	124
Pediatric patients, England	2-5	15	4 (26.7)			125
Healthy adults, England	N.S.	18	0			"
Blood donors, Florence	Adult	30	5 (16.7)	30	7 (23.3)	42
Healthy schoolchildren, Italy	3-5	134	7 (5.2)			126
Healthy schoolchildren, Italy	6-7	77	1 (1.3)			"
HIV negative children in ENT ward, Italy	6-12	56	0			"
HIV negative heterosexual patients at STD clinic, Italy	Mean 33.8	26	0			127
Healthy controls for SLE patients, Norway	23-75	88	0	88	18 (20.5)	128
Immunocompetent subjects, Italy	N.S.	62	25 (40.3)			129
Basque (San Sebastian)	31->70			25	13 (52.0)	130
Spanish controls (San Sebastian)	31->70			25	13 (52.0)	"
Gitano (Badalona)	<21-50			21	14 (67.0)	"
Spanish controls	<21-50			25	12 (48.0)	"

continued on next page

Table 5. Continued

Subjects	Age (Years)	BKV DNA		JCV DNA		Reference
		Number Tested	Number Positive (%)	Number Tested	Number Positive (%)	
Sinti GP patients (Freiburg)	<21-60			16	6 (37.5)	"
German eye patients and controls	<21- >70			103	32 (31.1)	"
Roma neurology patients (Budapest)	21- >70			19	16 (84.2)	"
Hungarian MS patients and controls	<21-70			60	25 (41.7)	"
Eye patients (Warsaw)	<21- >70			56	22 (39.3)	"
Healthy individuals, Italy	N.S.			211	97 (46.0)	140
ASIA						
Urology clinic outpatients, Tokyo	0-29	38	1 (2.6)[a]	38	5 (13.2)[a]	110
"	30-59	38	0[a]	38	10 (26.3)[a]	"
"	60-89	44	4 (9.1)[a]	44	20 (45.5)[a]	"
Patients without urological symptoms, Tokyo	60-90	23	2 (8.7)[a]	23	12 (52.2)[a]	"
Outpatients, Taipei	N.S.			50	9 (18.0)	120
Urology clinic patients and healthy volunteers, Tokyo	13-65	65	1 (1.5)[a]	65	15 (23.1)[a]	111
Urology outpatients (239) and healthy volunteers (76), Tokyo	0-9			35	3 (8.6)	132
"	10-19			35	6 (17.1)	"
"	20-29			35	16 (45.7)	"
"	30-39			35	20 (57.1)	"
"	40-49			35	19 (54.3)	"
"	50-59			35	21 (60.0)	"
"	60-69			35	22 (62.9)	"
"	70-79			35	22 (62.9)	"
"	80-89			35	23 (65.7)	"

continued on next page

Table 5. *Continued*

Subjects	Age (Years)	BKV DNA Number Tested	BKV DNA Number Positive (%)	JCV DNA Number Tested	JCV DNA Number Positive (%)	Reference
Neurology clinic patients from Guam (Chamorro), 1980	26-68			29	20 (69.0)	118
Healthy students, Taiwan	20-26	75	0	75	10 (13.3)	133
Bunun aborigines, Southern Lake village, Central Taiwan, 1997	0-19			9	3 (33.3)	134
	20-39			29	7 (24.1)	"
	40-59			22	16 (72.7)	"
	> 60			10	7(70.0)	"
Bunun aborigines, Double Dragon village, Central Taiwan, 1997	0-19			13	3 (23.1)	"
	20-39			14	5 (35.7)	"
	40-59			24	19 (79.2)	"
	> 60			13	8 (61.5)	"
Highlands of Papua New Guinea, 1998 (several ethnic groups)	Adults			32	20 (62.5)	135
Baining from New Britain	Adults			14	14 (100)	"
Tolai from New Britain	Adults			34	21 (62.5)	"
Native inhabitants of Hanoi, Vietnam	> 40			48	25 (52.1)	136
Native inhabitants of Danang, Vietnam	> 40			48	28 (58.3)	"
Native inhabitants of Peinnebeen, Myanmar	> 40			34	22 (64.7)	"

continued on next page

Table 5. *Continued*

Subjects	Age (Years)	BKV DNA		JCV DNA		Reference
		Number Tested	Number Positive (%)	Number Tested	Number Positive (%)	
Native inhabitants of Lhasa, China	> 40			31	16 (51.6)	"
Native inhabitants of Kathmandu, Nepal	> 40			65	32 (49.2)	"
Native inhabitants of Tashkent, Uzbekistan	> 40			50	27 (54.0)	"
Healthy individuals, Taiwan	3-7	135	0	135	3 (2.2)	96
	8-13	209	0	209	6 (2.9)	"
	14-19	237	0	237	16 (6.7)	"
	20-30	81	0	81	10 (12.3)	"
	31-40	58	0	58	16 (27.6)	"
	41-50	55	0	55	18 (32.7)	"
	51-60	62	0	62	26 (41.9)	"
	61-70	91	0	91	43 (47.3)	"
	71-84	84	0	84	55 (65.5)	"
AFRICA						
Healthy Biaka Pygmies from Central Africa	< 18			10	0	137
"	25-55			23	5 (21.7)	"
Healthy Bantu villagers from Central Africa	4-18			8	0	"
"	21-55			20	4 (20)	"

a = detected by DNA hybridization.

subjects,[115,119,125,141]and BKV viruria has also been reported in up to 47% of pregnant women, the percentage of excretors increasing as pregnancy progresses.[125,133,140,142,143]

It might be expected that children would frequently excrete BKV following primary infection, but the percentage with BKV viruria exceeded 5.2% in only one very small study group which included children as young as 2 years of age.[125] Maybe BKV viruria following childhood infection is short lived; inclusion-bearing cells containing papovavirus particles became undetectable in the urine of a 5 year-old boy with acute hemorrhagic cystitis when the symptoms subsided, and in a 3.5 year-old boy with transient nonhemorrhagic cystitis BKV was isolated from the urine on day 2, but not day 7, of the illness.[26,29,30] Urinary BKV excretion may occasionally increase in individuals over 60 years of age, possibly due to lowered immunity, and may persist for several months.[110] This may indicate that if BKV reactivation or reinfection occurs in later life it leads to prolonged shedding in contrast to primary infection in children.

BKV excretion.has rarely been investigated from sites other than the urinary tract. One report documented BKV DNA in a throat washing,[144] but the virus was not detected in saliva from 10 healthy adults or 60 HIV-infected patients, and BKV DNA was reported in only 2 nasopharyngeal aspirates from 201 hospitalised children, aged 7 and 8 months, with severe respiratory infection.[145] In neither of these children, however, could infectious virus be demonstrated. BKV was isolated from the urine, but not the throat, on day 3 of illness in a 2 year-old boy with a rise in antibody to BKV, dyspnea, high fever, cervical lymphadenopathy, conjunctival irritation, and tonsillitis.[28]

JCV Excretion

JCV viruria has been investigated in many different communities (due to the interest in molecular epidemiology, see later), including isolated populations, and data are shown in Table 5. In contrast to BKV, JCV viruria is almost universally present with an overall prevalence rate ranging from 12% to 100%. The differing excretion rates seen between various groups may be due to host factors, to the different JCV genotypes present, or both.[146] JCV viruria increases markedly with age,[14,40,96,110,116] and so the overall excretion rate reported from a community would also depend on the age range of the subjects. It was estimated that in the U.S.A about 40% of JCV seropositive individuals excrete the virus,[147] and in Taiwan the rate was found to increase from <5% in seropositive children to 80% in those over 70 years of age.[96] As for antibody, several studies have reported a higher excretion rate for JCV in males than in females.[14,116,117] Prolonged JCV excretion was documented in several studies with identical genotypes being shed for up to 7 years.[14,110,147,148]

JCV viruria has been documented in patients immunocompromised following renal and bone marrow transplantation,[93,95,111,112,138] and those with chronic or autoimmune diseases.[117,128,133,139,140,149] However, unlike BKV, the incidence of JCV urinary excretion does not vary with the CD4 cell count in HIV-infected patients,[115,119,123,141] and in studies where a control group was included the excretion rate in the patient group was not significantly higher than in the controls. The excretion rate therefore appears to represent the normal background for the population irrespective of the clinical state.

In a very large study of pregnant women 40 (3.2%) were found to excrete polyomavirus inclusion-bearing cells in the urine, excretion increasing as pregnancy progressed.[94] Subsequent testing of the urine by PCR in 38 of these cytologically positive women detected BKV DNA in 6 and JCV DNA in 36.[124] These results may indicate that JCV is preferentially detected by cytological screening. In further studies JCV DNA was reported in the urine of up to 34% of pregnant women, but again the figures may simply represent the background JCV excretion rate in each population.[133,140,142,143]

Transmission of BKV and JCV in the General Population

Seroprevalence studies in which the same sera were tested for antibody to both BKV and JCV indicate that in the U.S.A., England and Sweden the viruses are probably naturally transmitted by different routes (Fig. 3). In contrast in Japan and Mexico the acquisition of antibody

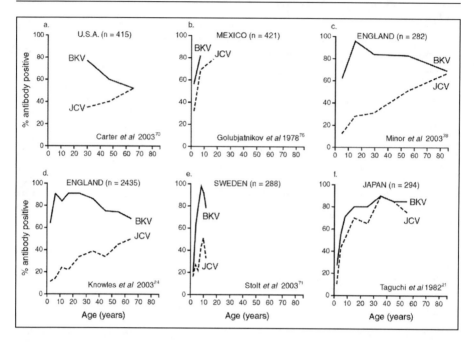

Figure 3. Comparative age seroprevalence to BKV and JCV in various populations.

to each virus follows a much more similar pattern. Whilst BKV infection occurs readily in all populations, JCV transmission appears to be relatively inefficient in some communities but much more efficient in others. This may imply that the route of transmission for JCV is one that depends much more on socio-economic or cultural differences between groups. It may also suggest that virus is transmitted from an environmental source as well as by direct contact. Frequent shedding of virus would be required if transmission is inefficient.[148]

The early detection of BKV viruria in immunocompromised patients led to the assumption that urine was the most likely vehicle for virus transmission,[15] although a respiratory route of spread was suggested by others.[12,25,27,28] However, failure to detect BKV in the respiratory tract later led to a suggestion that a fecal-oral route of transmission should be investigated.[145] Recently evidence has been presented that both BKV DNA and JCV DNA are frequently found in sewage in widely differing locations: Spain, France, Sweden, South Africa, Egypt, Greece, and U.S.A.[150,151] thus identifying an environmental source for both viruses. Most genomes were archetypal or archetype-like, supporting reports on urinary DNA from normal adults that this is probably the transmissible form of virus.[14,120,130,131,152-154] The DNA of both viruses was detectable for up to 3 months in sewage, although it is not known whether or not this represents infectious virus. JCV DNA, but not BKV DNA, was also detected in oysters and mussels from fecally polluted waters of the Ebro River delta.[151] The DNA of both BKV and JCV is resistant to low pH which would be compatible with oral transmission and passage through the digestive tract. Reports of both BKV and JCV DNA in peripheral blood leukocytes (Table 1) would suggest the possibility of transmission by blood transfusion, and a report on the presence of BKV and JCV DNA in sperm[155] would suggest also the possibility of sexual transmission of the polyomaviruses.

Transplacental transmission has also been considered for both BKV and JCV. However, this route of transmission may not be apparent except in very large studies if it is a rare event, or occurs only as a result of primary infection in the mother during pregnancy,[92] as is the case for mouse polyoma.[156,157]

BKV Transmission

The age of antibody acquisition would indicate that BKV is readily transmitted between young children or to young children, and that little if any BKV infection or reinfection occurs later in life. BKV infection probably occurs between as well as within families.[15] Specific studies on the effect of factors such as socio-economic status or breast feeding on the early acquisition of BKV infection have not been done. BKV seroprevalence in children from a rural highland community in central Mexico with low socio-economic status, large family size and a low level of sanitation was reported to be similar to children in countries with high standards of hygiene.[76] Although the acquisition of BKV by single children compared to those with siblings has not been investigated, there is some evidence that BKV is acquired earlier by children in a residential nursery than by those living at home.[25] Sexual transmission of BKV may be suggested by the rise in antibody or titre seen in some adolescents and young adults (Fig. 1).[83] It is unlikely that reinfection often occurs naturally with BKV, although there is a report of different BKV types, MM and JL, being present in sequential samples from 2 SLE patients.[140] Whilst it was suggested by one group that working at a blood transfusion centre may be a risk factor for BKV reinfection,[41] there was felt by others to be no occupational risk from working in a chronic hemodialysis center or a renal transplant unit.[59]

The possibility of congenital BKV infection was investigated by several groups. Anti-BKV IgM antibody was reported in cord blood samples in two studies,[49,86] but could subsequently not be confirmed in a large number of infants including some whose mothers had anti-BKV IgM antibody at term or excreted inclusion-bearing cells during pregnancy,[56,91,94,158,159] and the earlier positive findings were regarded as nonspecific.[56] However, the possibility remains that primary BKV infection during pregnancy may lead to infection of the fetus. BKV DNA was detected in the brain and kidney of aborted fetuses and in placental tissue from cases of abortion as well as pregnancies with a normal outcome.[160,161] Isolation of BKV was also reported from the urine of a 1 month-old boy with multiple dysplasias and hepatosplenomegaly.[90]

JCV Transmission

Molecular typing of urinary JCV strains showed that the virus is probably transmitted horizontally both within families and outside the family group.[132] Either the mother or father appeared to be the source of virus, or possibly a sibling.[162] Early transmission of JCV within the family or the immediate community is also supported by the presence of characteristic genotypes in certain population groups after many years of close contact or cohabitation with other groups,[163,164] and JCV appeared not to have spread between neighboring American and Japanese communities in Okinawa Island, Japan.[165] The excretion of a stable genome over time suggests persistence of virus rather than reinfection in most people,[14,148] although the simultaneous excretion of two different genotypes, even in immunocompetent individuals, is occasionally seen.[116,118,130,166] Type 4 appears to be a recombinant between Types 1 and 3 and so probably arose in an individual during dual infection at some time in the past.[116,163]

There is so far no evidence for JCV infection of the fetus.[161] JCV-specific IgM antibody was not detected in cord blood of over 300 infants, including 6 whose mothers had a rise in anti-JCV HI antibody during pregnancy,[92] although very low level anti-JCV IgM antibody was found in the cord blood of one infant whose mother was excreting inclusion-bearing cells during pregnancy.[159]

Molecular Epidemiology

Two types of molecular variation are seen in both BKV and JCV. Firstly, nucleotide deletions and duplications occur in the archetypal regulatory region of the genome; unique changes arise in the individual host and are probably not transmitted.[167] Secondly, nucleotide substitutions are seen in the coding regions of the genome, which may or may not lead to amino acid changes, and produce antigenic variation in BKV and multiple genotypes in JCV. These two types of changes occur independently from one another.[152,153,168,169]

BKV Subtypes

Four antigenic subtypes (BK, SB, AS, IV) were described for BKV,[170] and the molecular basis for this variation was shown to reside in the BC loop of the VP1 coding region of the genome.[171,172] Prototype BKV (genotype I) is by far the commonest type found by either serological or molecular typing in all categories of patients. Peripheral blood lymphocytes of blood donors and healthy adults contained only genotype I, whereas in urine or renal tissue from patients with malignant disease, HIV infection, and post renal or bone marrow transplantation, a few genotype II (SB) and genotype IV (IV) strains were also detected. Genotype III (AS) was found in pregnant women and HIV-infected patients. Healthy young children were found to excrete genotypes I, III and IV. Dual infection between genotype I and one other genotype was also documented in HIV-infected patients and pregnant women.[32,41,121,125-127,173-176] Although stable genotypes were reported to be excreted for up to 3 months in BMT patients, in some RT recipients sequential sequence modification in VP1 was seen and some strains were nontypable.[125,174,176]

JCV Genotypes

Only one serologically distinct JCV isolate (Mad-11) has been reported.[177] However, very few amino acid changes are seen between JCV strains in the VP1 region of the genome, especially in the BC loop, as most nucleotide changes in this region are silent, and so antigenic variants of JCV would not generally be expected to occur.[66,178,179]

However, nucleotide changes occur elsewhere in the JCV genome and sequencing, particularly in the intergenic region between VP1 and T and within VP1, have so far allowed the identification of 8 major genotypes of JCV, differing by 1-2.6%; types 1, 2, 3, 7 and 8 are further subdivided.[145] The association of JCV with humans may date back more than 50,000 years, coevolution occurring, and stable genotypes arising in geographically isolated populations. Broadly Types 1 and 4 are found in Europe and North America, Types 2,5 and 7 in Asia, Types 3 and 6 in Africa, and Type 8 in Papua New Guinea. The transmission of JCV from parent to offspring would allow the same genotype to persist for generations within a population,[162,164] and the frequent excretion of JCV by healthy adults has enabled many genotyping studies to be carried out in diverse population groups. JCV subtyping has been used to identify the racial composition of modern China,[180] in reconstructing the population history of Taiwanese aborigines[134] and ethnic groups in Puerto Rico[181] and Europe,[130] to elucidate the Asian origin of ethnic groups in North and South America[118,182] and the European origin of populations in Siberia and Canada,[183] the distribution of ethnic groups in Asia,[136] migration to the Pacific islands,[135,184] and aboriginal population group movements in Africa,[137] and also for tracing the origin of unidentified cadavers.[185]

References

1. Gardner SD, Field AM, Coleman DV et al. New human papovavirus (B.K.) isolated from urine after renal transplantation. Lancet 1971; I:1253-1257.
2. Padgett BL, Walker DL, Zu Rhein GM et al. Cultivation of papova-like virus from human brain with progressive multifocal leucoencephalopathy. Lancet 1971; i:1257-1260.
3. Åström KE, Mancall EL, Richardson EP. Progressive multifocal leukoencephalopathy. A hitherto unrecognised complication of chronic lymphatic leukaemia and Hodgkin's disease. Brain 1958; 81:93-111.
4. Cavanagh JB, Greenbaum D, Marshall AHE et al. Cerebral demyelination associated with disorders of the reticuloendothelial system. Lancet 1959; 2:524-529.
5. Richardson EP. Progressive multifocal leukoencephalopathy. New Engl J Med 1961; 265:815-823
6. ZuRhein GM, Chou SM. Particles resembling papova viruses in human cerebral demyelinating disease. Science 1965; 148:1477-1479.
7. Silverman L, Rubinstein LJ. Electron microscopic observations on a case of progressive multifocal leukoencephalopathy. Acta neuropathol (Berl) 1965; 5:215-224.
8. Åström KE. Progressive multifocal leukoencephalopathy: The discovery of a neurologic disease. In: Khalili K, Stoner GL, eds. Human Polyomaviruses: Molecular and Clinical Perspectives. New York: Wiley-Liss, 2001:1-10.

9. ZuRhein GM. Papova virions in progressive multifocal leukoencephalopathy: A discovery at the interface of neuropathology, virology, and oncology. In: Khalili K, Stoner GL, eds. Human Polyomaviruses: Molecular and Clinical Perspectives. New York: Wiley-Liss, 2001:11-23.

10. Walker DL. Progressive multifocal leukoencephalopathy: Cultivation and characterization of the etiologic agent. In: Khalili K, Stoner GL, eds. Human Polyomaviruses: Molecular and Clinical Perspectives. New York: Wiley-Liss, 2001:25-43.

11. Knowles WA. Serendipity – the fortuitous discovery of BK virus. In: Khalili K, Stoner GL, eds. Human Polyomaviruses: Molecular and Clinical Perspectives. New York: Wiley-Liss, 2001:45-51.

12. Goudsmit J, Wertheim-van Dillen P, van Strien A et al. The role of BK virus in acute respiratory tract disease and the presence of BKV DNA in tonsils. J Med Virol 1982; 10:91-99.

13. Monaco MCG, Jensen PN, Hou J et al. Detection of JC virus DNA in human tonsil tissue: Evidence for site of initial viral infection. J Virol 1998; 72:9918-9923.

14. Ling PD, Lednicky JA, Keitel WA et al. The dynamics of herpesvirus and polyomavirus reactivation and shedding in healthy adults: A 14-month longitudinal study. J Infect Dis 2003; 187:1571-1580.

15. Brown P, Tsai T, Gajdusek DC. Seroepidemiology of human papovaviruses. Amer J Epidem 1975; 102:331-340.

16. Padgett BL, Walker DL. New human papovaviruses. Prog Med Virol 1976; 22:1-35.

17. Iwasaki K, Yano K, Yanagisawa Y et al. Incidence of antibody against BK virus among Tokyoites and animals in Tokyo. Ann Rep Tokyo Metr Res Lab 1974; 25:69-72.

18. Seganti L, Mastromarino P, Superti F et al. Comparative study of nonantibody inhibitors present in plasma of different animal species and active towards BK virus, a human papovavirus. Microbiologica 1981; 4:395-402.

19. Padgett BL, Rogers CM, Walker DL. JC virus, a human polyomavirus associated with progressive multifocal leukoencephalopathy: Additional biological characteristics and antigenic relationships. Inf Immun 1977; 15:656-662.

20. Gardner SD. Implication of papovaviruses in human diseases. In: Kurstak E, Kurstak C, eds. Comparative Diagnosis of Viral Diseases. I. Human and Related Viruses. Part A. Chapter 3. New York: Academic Press, 1977:41-84.

21. Taguchi F, Kajioka J, Miyamura T. Prevalence rate and age of acquisition of antibodies against JC virus and BK virus in human sera. Microbiol Immunol 1982; 26:1057-1064.

22. Walker DL, Padgett BL. The epidemiology of human polyomaviruses. In: Sever JL, Madden DL, eds. Polyomaviruses and Human Neurological Disease. Prog Clin Biol Res 105. New York: A.R.Liss, 1983:99-106.

23. Hamilton RS, Gravell M, Major EO. Comparison of antibody titers determined by hemagglutination inhibition and enzyme immunoassay for JC virus and BK virus. J Clin Microbiol 2000; 38:105-109.

24. Knowles WA, Pipkin P, Andrews N et al. Population-based study of antibody to the human polyomaviruses BKV and JCV and the simian polyomavirus SV40. J Med Virol 2003; 71:115-123.

25. Mäntyjärvi RA, Meurman OH, Vihma L et al. A human papovavirus (B.K.), biological properties and seroepidemiology. Ann Clin Res 1973; 5:283-287.

26. Hashida Y, Gaffney PC, Yunis EJ. Acute hemorrhagic cystitis of childhood and papovavirus-like particles. J Pediat 1976; 89:85-87.

27. van der Noordaa J, Wertheim-van Dillen P. Rise in antibodies to human papova virus BK and clinical disease. BMJ 1977; 1:1471.

28. Goudsmit J, Baak ML, Slaterus KW et al. Human papovavirus isolated from urine of a child with acute tonsillitis. BMJ 1981; 283:1363-1364.

29. Mininberg DT, Watson C, Desquitado M. Viral cystitis with transient secondary vesicoureteral reflux. J Urol 1982; 127:983-985.

30. Padgett BL, Walker DL, Desquitado MM et al. BK virus and nonhaemorrhagic cystitis in a child. Lancet 1983; I:770.

31. Saitoh K, Sugae N, Koike N et al. Diagnosis of childhood BK virus cystitis by electron microscopy and PCR. J Clin Path 1993; 46:773-775.

32. Gardner SD, Knowles WA. Human polyomaviruses. In: Zuckerman AJ, Banatvala JE, Pattison JR, eds. Principles and Practice of Clinical Virology. 3rd ed. UK: John Wiley, 1995:635-651.

33. Voltz R, Jäger G, Seelos K et al. BK virus encephalitis in an immunocompetent patient. Arch Neurol 1996; 53:101-103.

34. Blake K, Pillay D, Knowles W et al. JC virus associated meningoencephalitis in an immunocompetent girl. Arch Dis Childhood 1992; 67:956-957.

35. Heritage J, Chesters PM, McCance DJ. The persistence of papovavirus BK DNA sequences in normal human renal tissue. J Med Virol 1981; 8:143-150.

36. Chesters PM, Heritage J, McCance DJ. Persistence of DNA sequences of BK virus and JC virus in normal human tissues and in diseased tissues. J Infect Dis 1983; 147:676-684.
37. Grinnell BW, Padgett BL, Walker DL. Distribution of nonintegrated DNA from JC papovavirus in organs of patients with progressive multifocal leukoencephalopathy. J Infect Dis 1983; 147:669-675.
38. Tornatore C, Berger JR, Houff SA et al. Detection of JC virus DNA in peripheral lymphocytes from patients with and without progressive multifocal leukoencephalopathy. Ann Neurol 1992; 31:454-462.
39. Doerries K, Vogel E, Günther S et al. Infection of human polyomaviruses JC and BK in peripheral blood leukocytes from immunocompetent individuals. Virology 1994; 198:59-70.
40. Lednicky JA, Vilchez RA, Keitel WA et al. Polyomavirus JCV excretion and genotype analysis in HIV-infected patients receiving highly active antiretroviral therapy. AIDS 2003; 17:801-807.
41. Dolei A, Pietropaolo V, Gomas E. et al. Polyomavirus persistence in lymphocytes from blood donors and healthy personnel of a blood transfusion centre. J Gen Virol 2000; 81:1967-1973.
42. Azzi A, De Santis R, Ciappi S et al. Human polyomaviruses DNA detection in peripheral blood leukocytes from immunocompetent and immunocompromised individuals. J Neurovirol 1996; 2:411-416.
43. Chatterjee M, Weyardt TB, Frisque RJ. Identification of archetype and rearranged forms of BK virus in leukocytes from healthy individuals. J Med Virol 2000; 60:353-362.
44. Dubois V, Dutronc H, Lafon M-E et al. Latency and reactivation of JC virus in peripheral blood of human immunodeficiency virus type 1-infected patients. J Clin Microbiol 1997; 35:2288-2292.
45. Lafon M-E, Dutronc H, Dubois V et al. JC virus remains latent in peripheral blood B lympho-cytes but replicated actively in urine from AIDS patients. J Infect Dis 1998; 177:1502-1505.
46. Gu Z-Y, Li Q, Si Y-L et al. Prevalence of BK virus and JC virus in peripheral blood leucocytes and normal arterial walls in healthy individuals in China. J Med Virol 2003; 70:600-605.
47. Gardner SD. Prevalence in England of antibody to human polyomavirus (B.K.). BMJ 1973; i:77-78.
48. Panà A, Di Arca SU, Castello C et al. Prevalence in the Rome healthy population of antibodies to a human polyoma-virus (BK-strain). Boll Ist Sieroter Milan 1976; 55:18-22.
49. Rziha H-J, Bornkamm GW, zur Hausen H. BK virus. I. Seroepidemiologic studies and serologic response to viral infection. Med Microbiol Immunol 1978; 165:73-81.
50. Portolani M, Marzocchi A, Barbanti-Brodano G et al. Prevalence in Italy of antibodies to a new human papovavirus (BK virus). J Med Microbiol 1974; 7:543-546.
51. Dei R, Marmo F, Corte D et al. Age-related changes in the prevalence of precipitating antibodies to BK virus in infants and children. J Med Microbiol 1982; 15:285-291.
52. Mäntyjärvi RA, Arstila PP, Meurman OH. Hemagglutination by BK virus, a tentative new mem-ber of the papovavirus group. Infect Immun 1972; 6:824-828.
53. Takemoto KK, Mullarkey MF. Human papovavirus, BK strain: Biological studies including anti-genic relationship to simian virus 40. J Virol 1973; 12:625-631.
54. Jung M, Krech U, Price PC et al. Evidence of chronic persistent infections with polyomaviruses (BK type) in renal transplant recipients. Arch Virol 1975; 47:39-46.
55. Padgett BL, Walker DL. Prevalence of antibodies in human sera against JC virus, an isolate from a case of progressive multifocal leukoencephalopathy. J Infect Dis 1973; 127:467-470.
56. Shah K, Daniel R, Madden D et al. Serological investigation of BK papovavirus infection in preg-nant women and their offspring. Infect Immun 1980; 30:29-35.
57. De Stasio A, Orsi N, Panà A et al. The importance of pretreatment of human sera for the titration of hemagglutination-inhibiting antibodies towards BK virus. Ann Sclavo 1979; 21:249-257.
58. De Stasio A, Mastromarino P, Panà A et al. Characterization of a glycoprotein inhibitor present in human serum and active towards BK virus hemagglutination. Microbiologica 1980; 3:293-305.
59. Burguière AM, Fortier B, Bricout F et al. Control of BK virus antibodies in contacts of patients under chronic hemodialysis or after renal transplantation (by an enzyme linked immunosorbent assay). Path Biol 1980; 28:541-544.
60. Iltis JP, Cleghorn CS, Madden DL et al. Detection of antibody to BK virus by enzyme-linked immunosorbent assay compared to hemagglutination inhibition and immunofluorescent antibody staining. In: Sever JL, Madden DL, eds. Polyomaviruses and Human Neurological Disease. Prog Clin Biol Res 105. New York: A.R.Liss, 1983:157-168.
61. Flaegstad T, Traavik T. Detection of BK virus antibodies measured by enzyme-linked immunosorbent assay (ELISA) and two haemagglutination inhibition methods: A comparative study. J Med Virol 1985; 16:351-356.
62. Flaegstad T, Traavik T, Kristiansen B-E. Age-dependent prevalence of BK virus IgG and IgM antibodies measured by enzyme-linked immunosorbent assays (ELISA). J Hyg Camb 1986; 96:523-528.

63. Andrews CA, Shah KV, Daniel RW et al. A serological investigation of BK virus and JC virus infections in recipients of renal allografts. J Infect Dis 1988; 158:176-181.
64. Flaegstad T, Rönne K, Filipe AR et al. Prevalence of anti BK virus antibody in Portugal and Norway. Scand J Infect Dis 1989; 21:145-147.
65. Frye S, Trebst C, Dittmer U et al. Efficient production of JC virus in SVG cells and the use of purified viral antigens for analysis of specific humoral and cellular immune response. J Virol Methods 1997; 63:81-92.
66. Chang D, Liou Z-M, Ou W-C et al. Production of the antigen and the antibody of the JC virus major capsid protein VP1. J Virol Methods 1996; 59:177-187.
67. Weber T, Trebst C, Frye S et al. Analysis of the systemic and intrathecal humoral immune response in progressive multifocal leukoencephalopathy. J Infect Dis 1997; 176:250-262.
68. Rollison DE, Helzlsouer KJ, Alberg AJ et al. Serum antibodies to JC virus, BK virus, simian virus 40, and the risk of incident adult astrocytic brain tumors. Cancer Epidemiol Biomarkers Prev 2003; 12:460-463.
69. Viscidi RP, Rollison DEM, Viscidi E et al. Serological cross-reactivities between antibodies to simian virus 40, BK virus, and JC virus assessed by virus-like-particle-based enzyme immunoassays. Clin Diag Lab Immunol 2003; 10:278-285.
70. Carter JJ, Madeleine MM, Wipf GC et al. Lack of serologic evidence for prevalent simian virus 40 infection in humans. J Natl Cancer Inst 2003; 95:1522-1530.
71. Stolt A, Sasnauskas K, Koskela P et al. Seroepidemiology of the human polyomaviruses. J Gen Virol 2003; 84:1499-1504.
72. Flaegstad T, Traavik T, Christie KE et al. Neutralization test for BK virus: Plaque reduction detected by immunoperoxidase staining. J Med Virol 1986; 19:287-296.
73. Shah KV, Daniel RW, Warszawski RM. High prevalence of antibodies to BK virus, an SV40-related papovavirus, in residents of Maryland. J Infect Dis 1973; 128:784-787.
74. Tavis JE, Frisque RJ, Walker DL et al. Antigenic and transforming properties of the DB strain of the human polyomavirus BK virus. Virology 1990; 178:568-572.
75. Dougherty RM, DiStefano HS. Isolation and characterization of a papovavirus from human urine. Proc Soc Exp Biol Med 1974; 146:481-487.
76. Golubjatnikov et al. cited in Padgett BL, Walker DL. Natural History of Human Polyomavirus Infections. In: Stevens JG, Todaro GJ, Fox CF, eds. Persistent Viruses. ICN-UCLA Symposia on Molecular and Cellular Biology XI. Chapter 54. New York: Academic Press, 1978:751-758.
77. Candeias JAN, Baruzzi RG, Pripas S et al. Prevalence of antibodies to the BK and JC papovaviruses in isolated populations. Rev Saúde públ, S Paulo 1977; 11:510-514.
78. Minor P, Pipkin P, Jarzebek Z et al. Studies of neutralising antibodies to SV40 in human sera. J Med Virol 2003; 70:490-495.
79. Flower AJE, Banatvala JE, Chrystie IL. BK antibody and virus-specific IgM responses in renal transplant recipients, patients with malignant disease, and healthy people. BMJ 1977; ii:220-223.
80. Meurman OH, Mäntyjärvi RA, Salmi AA et al. Prevalence of antibodies to a human papova virus (BK virus) in subacute sclerosing panencephalitis and multiple sclerosis patients. Z Neurol 1972; 203:191-194.
81. Corallini A, Barbanti-Brodano G, Portolani M et al. Antibodies to BK virus structural and tumor antigens in human sera from normal persons and from patients with various diseases, including neoplasia. Infect Immun 1976; 13:1684-1691.
82. Krech U, Jung M, Price PC et al. Virus infections in renal transplant recipients. Z Immun-Forsch 1975; 148:S341-355.
83. Szücs Gy, Kende M, Új M. Haemagglutination-inhibiting antibodies to B.K. virus in Hungary. Acta microbiol Acad Sci Hung 1979; 26:173-178.
84. Billaudel S, Le Bris JM, Soulillou JP et al. Anticorps inhibant l'hémagglutination du virus BK: brève surveillance de 52 transplantés rénaux et prévalence dans différents groupes d'âge de l'ouest de la France. Ann Virol (Inst. Pasteur) 1981; 132E:337-345.
85. Neel JV, Major EO, Awa AA et al. Hypothesis: "Rogue cell"-type chromosomal damage in lymphocytes is associated with infection with the JC human polyoma virus and has implication for oncogenesis. Proc Natl Acad Sci USA 1996; 93:2690-2695.
86. Taguchi F, Nagaki D, Saito M et al. Transplacental transmission of BK virus in human. Japan J Microbiol 1975; 19:395-398.
87. Major EO, Neel JV. The JC and BK human polyoma viruses appear to be recent introductions to some South American Indian tribes: There is no serological evidence of cross-reactivity with the simian polyoma virus SV40. Proc Natl Acad Sci 1998; 95:15525-15530.

88. Markoulatos P, Spirou N, Ghubril V et al. Données préliminaires sur la présence d'anticorps antivirus BK (groupe papova) dans deux populations différentes de la Grèce. Arch Inst Past Hellén 1981; 27:45-51.
89. Merletti L. Sieroepidemiologia umana del polyoma virus BK in Umbria. Boll Ist Sieroter Milan 1976; 55:573-576.
90. Rziha H-J, Belohradsky BH, Schneider U et al. BK virus: II. Serologic studies in children with congenital disease and patients with malignant tumors and immunodeficiencies. Med Microbiol Immunol 1978; 165:83-92.
91. Brown DWG, Gardner SD, Gibson PE et al. BK virus specific IgM responses in cord sera, young children and healthy adults detected by RIA. Arch Virol 1984; 82:149-160.
92. Daniel R, Shah K, Madden D et al. Serological investigation of the possibility of congenital transmission of papovavirus JC. Inf Immun 1981; 33:319-321.
93. Hogan TF, Borden EC, McBain JA et al. Human polyomavirus infections with JC virus and BK virus in renal transplant patients. Ann Intern Med 1980; 92:373-378.
94. Coleman DV, Wolfendale MR, Daniel RA et al. A prospective study of human polyomavirus infection in pregnancy. J Infect Dis 1980; 142:1-8.
95. Gardner SD, Mackenzie EFD, Smith C et al. Prospective study of the human polyomaviruses BK and JC and cytomegalovirus in renal transplant recipients. J Clin Pathol 1984; 37:578-586.
96. Chang H, Wang M, Tsai RT et al. High incidence of JC viruria in JC-seropositive older individuals. J Neurovirol 2002; 8:447-451.
97. Knowles WA, Gibson PE, Hand JF et al. An M-antibody capture radioimmunoassay (MACRIA) for detection of JC virus-specific IgM. J Virol Methods 1992; 40:95-106
98. Reese JM, Reissig M, Daniel RW et al. Occurrence of BK virus and BK virus-specific antibodies in the urine of patients receiving chemotherapy for malignancy. Infect Immun 1975; 11:1375-1381.
99. Hogan TF, Padgett BL, Walker DL et al. Rapid detection and identification of JC virus and BK virus in human urine by using immunofluorescence microscopy. J Clin Microbiol 1980; 11:178-183.
100. Kahan AV, Coleman DV, Koss LG. Activation of human polyomavirus infection- detection by cytologic technics. Amer J Clin Path 1980; 74:326-332.
101. Cobb JJ, Wickenden C, Snell ME et al. Use of hybridot assay to screen for BK and JC polyomaviruses in nonimmunosuppressed patients. J Clin Pathol 1987; 40:777-781.
102. Itoh S, Irie K, Nakamura Y et al. Cytologic and genetic study of polyomavirus-infected or polyomavirus-activated cells in human urine. Arch Path Lab Med 1998; 122:333-337.
103. Marrero M, Pascale F, Alvarez M et al. Dot ELISA for direct detection of BK virus in urine samples. Acta Virol 1990; 34:563-567.
104. Penney JB, Narayan O. Studies of the antigenic relationships of the new human papovaviruses by electron microscopy agglutination. Infect Immun 1973; 8:299-300.
105. Albert AE, ZuRhein GM. Application of immune electron microscopy to the study of the antigenic relationships between three new human papovaviruses. Int Arch Allergy 1974; 46:405-416.
106. Gardner SD. The new human papovaviruses: Their nature and significance. In: Waterson AP, ed. Recent Advances in Clinical Virology. No.I. Chapter 6. Edinburgh: Churchill Livingstone, 1977:93-115.
107. Arthur RR, Shah KV, Yolken RH et al. Detection of human papovaviruses BKV and JCV in urines by ELISA. In: Sever JL, Madden DL, eds. Polyomaviruses and Human Neurological Disease. Prog Clin Biol Res 105. New York: AR Liss, 1983:169-176.
108. Arthur RR, Beckmann AM, Li CC et al. Direct detection of the human papovavirus BK in urine of bone marrow transplant recipients: Comparison of DNA hybridization with ELISA. J Med Virol 1985; 16:29-36.
109. Gibson PE, Gardner SD, Porter AA. Detection of human polyomavirus DNA in urine specimens by hybridot assay. Arch Virol 1985; 84:233-240.
110. Kitamura T, Aso Y, Kuniyoshi N et al. High incidence of urinary JC virus excretion in nonimmunosuppressed older patients. J Infect Dis 1990; 161:1128-1133.
111. Kitamura T, Yogo Y, Kunitake T et al. Effect of immunosuppression on the urinary excretion of BK and JC polyomaviruses in renal allograft recipients. Int J Urol 1994; 1:28-32.
112. Arthur RR, Shah KV. Occurrence and significance of papovaviruses BK and JC in the urine. Prog Med Virol 1989; 36:42-61.
113. Arthur RR, Dagostin S, Shah KV. Detection of BK virus and JC virus in urine and brain tissue by the polymerase chain reaction. J Clin Microbiol.1989; 27:1174-1179.
114. Marshall WF, Telenti A, Proper J et al. Survey of urine from transplant recipients for polyomaviruses JC and BK using the polymerase chain reaction. Mol Cell Probes 1991; 5:125-128.
115. Markowitz R-B, Thompson HC, Mueller JF et al. Incidence of BK virus and JC virus viruria in human immunodeficiency virus-infected and –uninfected subjects. J Infect Dis 1993; 167:13-20.

116. Agostini HT, Ryschkewitsch CF, Stoner GL Genotype profile of human polyomavirus JC excreted in urine of immunocompetent individuals. J Clin Microbiol 1996; 34:159-164.
117. Stoner GL, Agostini HT, Ryschkewitsch CF et al. Characterization of JC virus DNA amplified from urine of chronic progressive multiple sclerosis patients. Mult Scler 1996; 1:193-199
118. Agostini HT, Yanagihara R, Davis V et al. Asian genotypes of JC virus in Native Americans and in a Pacific Island population: Markers of viral evolution and human migration. Proc Nat Acad Sci USA 1997; 94:14542-14546.
119. Shah KV, Daniel RW, Strickler HD et al. Investigation of human urine for genomic sequences of the primate polyomaviruses simian virus 40, BK virus, and JC virus. J Infect Dis 1997; 176:1618-1621.
120. Yogo Y, Iida T, Taguchi F et al. Typing of human polyomavirus JC virus on the basis of restriction fragment length polymorphisms. J Clin Microbiol 1991; 29:2130-2138.
121. Jin L, Gibson PE, Booth JC et al. Genomic typing of BK virus in clinical specimens by direct sequencing of polymerase chain reaction products. J Med Virol 1993; 41:11-17.
122. Bogdanovic G, Brytting M, Cinque P et al. Nested PCR for detection of BK virus and JC virus DNA. Clin Diagn Virol 1994; 2:127-136.
123. Sundsfjord A, Flaegstad T, Flø R et al. BK and JC viruses in human immunodeficiency virus type 1-infected persons: Prevalence, excretion, viremia, and viral regulatory regions. J Infect Dis 1994; 169:485-490.
124. Gibson PE. Detection of human polyomaviruses by PCR. In: Clewley JP, ed. The Polymerase Chain Reaction (PCR) for Human Viral Diagnosis. Chapter 14. Florida: CRC Press, 1995:14:197-203.
125. Jin L, Pietropaolo V, Booth JC et al. Prevalence and distribution of BK virus subtypes in healthy people and immuncompromised patients detected by PCR-restriction enzyme analysis. Clin Diag Virol 1995; 3:285-295.
126. Di Taranto C, Pietropaolo V, Orsi GB et al. Detection of BK polyomavirus genotypes in healthy and HIV-positive children. Europ J Epidem 1997; 13:653-657.
127. Degener AM, Pietropaolo V, Di Taranto C et al. Detection of JC and BK viral genome in specimens of HIV-1 infected subjects. Microbiologica 1997; 20:115-122.
128. Sundsfjord A, Osei A, Rosenqvist H et al. BK and JC viruses in patients with systemic lupus erythematosus: Prevalent and persistent BK viruria, sequence stability of the viral regulatory regions, and nondetectable viremia. J Infect Dis 1999; 180:1-9.
129. Azzi A, Cesaro S, Laszlo D et al. Human polyomavirus BK (BKV) load and haemorrhagic cystitis in bone marrow transplantation patients. J Clin Virol 1999; 14:79-86.
130. Agostini HT, Deckhut A, Jobes DV et al. Genotypes of JC virus in east, central and southeast Europe. J Gen Virol 2001; 82:1221-1231.
131. Pagani E, Delbue S, Mancuso R et al. Molecular analysis of JC virus genotypes circulating among the Italian healthy population. J Neurovirol 2003; 9:559-566.
132. Kitamura T, Kunitake T, Guo J et al. Transmission of the human polyomavirus JC virus occurs both within the family and outside the family. J Clin Microbiol 1994; 32:2359-2363
133. Tsai R-T, Wang M, Ou W-C et al. Incidence of JC viruria is higher than that of BK viruria in Taiwan. J Med Virol 1997; 52:253-257.
134. Chang D, Sugimoto C, Wang M et al. JC virus genotypes in a Taiwan aboriginal tribe (Bunun): Implication for its population history. Arch Virol 1999; 144:1081-1090.
135. Ryschkewitsch CF, Friedlaender JS, Mgone CS et al. Human polyomavirus JC variants in Papua New Guinea and Guam reflect ancient population settlement and viral evolution. Microbes and Infection 2000; 2:987-996.
136. Saruwatari L, Sugimoto C, Kitamura T et al. Asian domains of four major genotypes of JC virus, Af2, B1-b, CY and SC. Arch Virol 2002; 147:1-10.
137. Chima SC, Ryschkewitsch CF, Stoner GL. Molecular epidemiology of human polyomavirus JC in the Biaka Pygmies and Bantu of Central Africa. Mem Inst Oswaldo Cruz, Rio de Janeiro 1998; 93:615-623.
138. Arthur RR, Shah KV, Charache P et al. BK and JC virus infections in recipients of bone marrow transplants. J Infect Dis 1988; 158:563-569.
139. Chang D, Tsai R-T, Wang M et al. Different genotypes of human polyomaviruses found in patients with autoimmune diseases in Taiwan. J Med Virol 1996; 48:204-209.
140. Bendiksen S, Rekvig OP, Van Ghelue M et al. VP1 DNA sequences of JC and BK viruses detected in urine of systemic lupus erythematosus patients reveal no differences from strains expressed in normal individuals. J Gen Virol 2000; 81:2625-2633.
141. Knowles WA, Pillay D, Johnson MA et al. Prevalence of long-term BK and JC excretion in HIV-infected adults and lack of correlation with serological markers. J Med Virol 1999; 59:474-479.

142. Markowitz R-B, Eaton BA, Kubik MF et al. BK virus and JC virus shed during pregnancy have predominantly archetypal regulatory regions. J Virol 1991; 65:4515-4519.
143. Chang D, Wang M, Ou W-C et al. Genotypes of human polyomaviruses in urine samples of pregnant women in Taiwan. J Med Virol 1996; 48:95-101.
144. Jin L. Rapid genomic typing of BK virus directly from clinical specimens. Mol Cell Probes 1993; 7:331-334.
145. Sundsfjord A, Spein A-R, Lucht E et al. Detection of BK virus DNA in nasopharyngeal aspirates from children with respiratory infections but not in saliva from immunodeficient and immuno-competent adult patients. J Clin Microbiol 1994; 32:1390-1394.
146. Agostini HT, Jobes DV, Stoner GL. Molecular evolution and epidemiology of JC virus. In: Khalili K, Stoner GL, eds. Human Polyomaviruses: Molecular and Clinical Perspectives. New York: Wiley-Liss, 2001:491-526.
147. Arthur RR. Detection of JC and BK viruses in pathological specimens by polymerase chain reaction. In: Becker Y, Daria G, eds. Frontiers of Virology I Diagnosis of human viruses by polymerase chain reaction technology. Chapter 17. Springer-Verlag, 1992:219-227.
148. Kitamura T, Sugimoto C, Kato A et al. Persistent JC virus (JCV) infection is demonstrated by continuous shedding of the same JCV strains. J Clin Microbiol 1997; 35:1255-1257.
149. Agostini HT, Ryschkewitsch CF, Baumhefner RW et al. Influence of JC virus coding region genotype on risk of multiple sclerosis and progressive multifocal leukoencephalopathy. J Neurovirol 2000; 6:S101-108.
150. Bofill-Mas S, Pina S, Girones R. Documenting the epidemiologic patterns of polyomaviruses in human populations by studying their presence in urban sewage. Appl Environ Microbiol 2000; 66:238-245.
151. Bofill-Mas S, Formiga-Cruz M, Clemente-Casares P et al. Potential transmission of human polyomaviruses through the gastrointestinal tract after exposure to virions or viral DNA. J Virol 2001; 75:10290-10299.
152. Ault GS, Stoner GL. Human polyomavirus JC promoter/enhancer rearrangement patterns from progressive multifocal leukoencephalopathy brain are unique derivatives of a single archetypal structure. J Gen Virol 1993; 74:1499-1507.
153. Iida T, Kitamura T, Guo J et al. Origin of JC polyomavirus variants associated with progressive multifocal leukoencephalopathy. Proc Nat Acad Sci 1993; 90:5062-5065.
154. Agostini HT, Ryschkewitsch CF, Stoner GL. Rearrangements of archetypal regulatory regions in JC virus genomes from urine. Res Virol 1998; 149:163-170.
155. Monini P, Rotola A, de Lellis L et al. Latent BK virus infection and Kaposi's sarcoma pathogenesis. Int J Cancer 1996; 66:717-722.
156. McCance DJ, Mims CA. Transplacental transmission of polyoma virus in mice. Infect Immun 1977; 18:196-202.
157. McCance DJ, Mims CA. Reactivation of polyoma virus in kidneys of persistently infected mice during pregnancy. Infect Immun 1979; 25:998-1002.
158. Borgatti M, Costanzo F, Portolani M et al. Evidence for reactivation of persistent infection during pregnancy and lack of congenital transmission of BK virus, a human papovavirus. Microbiologica 1979; 2:173-178.
159. Gibson PE, Field AM, Gardner SD et al. Occurrence of IgM antibodies against BK and JC polyomaviruses during pregnancy. J Clin Path 1981; 34:674-679.
160. Pietropaolo V, Di Taranto C, Degener AM et al. Transplacental transmission of human polyomavirus BK. J Med Virol 1998; 56:372-376.
161. Penta M, Lukic A, Conte MP et al. Infectious agents in tissues from spontaneous abortions in the first trimester of pregnancy. Microbiologica 2003; 26:329-337.
162. Kunitake T, Kitamura T, Guo J et al. Parent-to-child transmission is relatively common in the spread of the human polyomavirus JC virus. J Clin Microbiol 1995; 33:1448-1451.
163. Agostini HT, Ryschkewitsch CF, Stoner GL. JC virus Type 1 has multiple subtypes: Three new complete genomes. J Gen Virol 1998; 79: 801-805.
164. Suzuki H, Zheng H-Y, Takasaka T.et al. Asian genotypes of JC virus in Japanese-Americans suggest familial transmission. J Virol 2002; 76:10074-10078.
165. Kato A, Kitamura T, Sugimoto C et al. Lack of evidence for the transmission of JC polyomavirus between human populations. Arch Virol 1997; 142:875-882.
166. Agostini HT, Ryschkewitsch CF, Singer EJ et al. Co-infection with two JC virus genotypes in brain, cerebrospinal fluid or urinary tract detected by direct cycle sequencing of PCR products. J Neurovirol 1996; 2:259-267.

167. Yogo Y, Sugimoto C. The archetype concept and regulatory region rearrangement. In: Khalili K, Stoner GL, eds. Human Polyomaviruses: Molecular and Clinical Perspectives. New York: Wiley-Liss, 2001:127-148.
168. Kato K, Guo J, Taguchi F et al. Phylogenetic comparison between archetypal and disease-associated JC virus isolates in Japan. Jpn J Med Sci Biol 1994; 47:167-178.
169. Agostini HT, Ryschkewitsch CF, Singer EJ et al. JC virus regulatory region rearrangements and genotypes in progressive multifocal leukoencephalopathy: Two independent aspects of virus variation. J Gen Virol 1997; 78:659-664.
170. Knowles WA, Gibson PE, Gardner SD. Serological typing scheme for BK-like isolates of human polyomavirus. J Med Virol 1989; 28:118-123.
171. Tavis JE, Walker DL, Gardner SD et al. Nucleotide sequence of the human polyomavirus AS virus, an antigenic variant of BK virus. J Virol 1989; 63:901-911.
172. Jin L, Gibson PE, Knowles WA et al. BK virus antigenic variants: Sequence analysis within the capsid VP1 epitope. J Med Virol 1993; 39:50-56.
173. Agostini HT, Brubaker GR, Shao J et al. BK virus and a new type of JC virus excreted by HIV-1 positive patients in rural Tanzania. Arch Virol 1995; 140:1919-1934.
174. Baksh FK, Finkelstein SD, Swalsky PA et al. Molecular genotyping of BK and JC viruses in human polyomavirus-associated interstitial nephritis after renal transplantation. Amer J Kid Dis 2001; 38:354-365.
175. Priftakis P, Bogdanovic G, Kalantari M et al. Overrepresentation of point mutations in the Sp1 site of the noncoding control region of BK virus in bone marrow transplanted patients with haemorrhagic cystitis. J Clin Virol 2001; 21:1-7.
176. Randhawa PS, Khaleel-Ur-Rehman K, Swalsky PA et al. DNA sequencing of viral capsid protein VP-1 region in patients with BK virus interstitial nephritis. Transplantation 2002; 73:1090-1094.
177. Padgett BL, Walker DL. Virologic and serologic studies of progressive multifocal leukoencephalopathy. In: Sever JL, Madden DL, eds. Polyomaviruses and Human Neurological Disease. Prog Clin Biol Res 105. New York: A R Liss, 1983:107-117.
178. Ault GS, Stoner GL. Two major types of JC virus defined in progressive multifocal leukoencephalopathy brain by early and late coding region DNA sequences. J Gen Virol 1992; 73:2669-2678.
179. Sala M, Vartanian J-P, Kousignian P et al. Progressive multifocal leukoencephalopathy in human immunodeficiency virus type 1-infected patients: Absence of correlation between JC virus neurovirulence and polymorphisms in the transcriptional control region and the major capsid protein loci. J Gen Virol 2001; 82:899-907.
180. Guo J, Sugimoto C, Kitamura T et al. Four geographically distinct genotypes of JC virus are prevalent in China and Mongolia: Implication for the racial composition of modern China. J Gen Virol 1998; 79:2499-2505.
181. Fernandez-Cobo M, Jobes DV, Yanagihara R et al. Reconstructing population history using JC virus: Amerinds, Spanish, and Africans in the ancestry of modern Puerto Ricans. Hum Biol 2001; 73:385-402.
182. Fernandez-Cobo M, Agostini HT, Britez G et al. Strains of JC virus in Amerind-speakers of North America (Salish) and South America (Guarani), Na-Dene-speakers of New Mexico (Navajo), and modern Japanese suggest links through an ancestral Asian population. Amer J Phys Anthropol 2002; 118:154-168.
183. Sugimoto C, Hasegawa M, Zheng HY et al. JC virus strains indigenous to northeastern Siberians and Canadian Inuits are unique but evolutionally related to those distributed throughout Europe and Mediterranean areas. J Mol Evol 2002; 55:322-335.
184. Yanagihara R, Nerurkar VR, Scheirich I et al. JC virus genotypes in the western Pacific suggest Asian mainland relationships and virus association with early population movements. Hum Biol 2002; 74:473-488.
185. Ikegaya H, Iwase H, Sugimoto C et al. JC virus genotyping offers a new means of tracing the origins of unidentified cadavers. Int J Legal Med 2002; 116:242-245.

CHAPTER 3

Phylogenomics and Molecular Evolution of Polyomaviruses

**Keith A. Crandall, Marcos Pérez-Losada, Ryan G. Christensen,
David A. McClellan and Raphael P. Viscidi**

Abstract

We provide in this chapter an overview of the basic steps to reconstruct evolutionary relationships through standard phylogeny estimation approaches as well as network approaches for sequences more closely related. We discuss the importance of sequence alignment, selecting models of evolution, and confidence assessment in phylogenetic inference. We also introduce the reader to a variety of software packages used for such studies. Finally, we demonstrate these approaches throughout using a data set of 33 whole genomes of polyomaviruses. A robust phylogeny of these genomes is estimated and phylogenetic relationships among the polyomaviruses determined using Bayesian and maximum likelihood approaches. Furthermore, population samples of SV40 are used to demonstrate the utility of network approaches for closely related sequences. The phylogenetic analysis suggested a close relationship among the BK viruses, JC viruses, and SV40 with a more distant association with mouse polyomavirus, monkey polymavirus (LPV) and then avian polyomavirus (BFDV).

Introduction

Polyomaviruses are small, nonenveloped, double-stranded DNA viruses that are widely distributed among vertebrates. Each polyomavirus is exquisitely adapted to a single species, or to a group of closely related species. The polyomaviruses are often described as having coevolved with their hosts. As a rule, primary infections occur early in life and are asymptomatic and harmless. The viruses remain latent in the kidney after primary infection, and are reactivated in conditions associated with T-cell deficiency. Almost all the diseases caused by these viruses occur in immunodeficient hosts. The viruses multiply in the nucleus and virus-induced pathology is characterized by nuclei that are enlarged and have basophilic inclusions.

The human polyomaviruses, BKV and JCV, and macaque polyomavirus, SV40, are very similar biologically, and each virus has over 70 % nucleotide sequence similarity with the other two. In its natural host, SV40 produces an illness similar to JCV-PML in humans, while the cynomolgus virus produces a nephropathy similar to BKV-nephropathy in humans. Other viruses that might be biologically similar, although little is actually known about them, are SA12 of the chacma baboon, the recently described cynomolgus macaque virus, the bovine and the rabbit polyomaviruses, and perhaps the mouse polyoma virus. The avian budgerigar virus, which produces liver and spleen necrosis, and a rat polyomavirus, which produces salivary gland pathology in athymic animals, both produce lesions that are characteristic of viruses of the polyomavirus family.

Polyomaviruses and Human Diseases, edited by Nasimul Ahsan. ©2006 Eurekah.com
and Springer Science+Business Media.

The simian lymphotropic polyomavirus of African green monkeys seems to have a different biology from these viruses. In the mouse, the mouse polyomavirus (referred to above) seems biologically very different from K virus, which grows in endothelial cells of the lung. The tropism of K virus-infected endothelial cells is unique among polyomaviruses. The oddest polyomavirus is the hamster polyomavirus, which produces skin tumors and was at one time thought to be a papillomavirus. Thus, lymphotropic virus of African green monkeys, K virus of mouse and the hamster polyomavirus seem not to fit the general pattern.

In order to explore the diversity of polyomaviruses, both genomic diversity at the molecular level and diversity in host specificity, a phylogenetic perspective is essential. A phylogeny represents the evolutionary history among organisms or their parts. In our case, we will attempt to reconstruct evolutionary histories using whole genome analyses. Our analysis will provide a robust estimate of phylogenetic relationships among the polyomaviruses. Additionally, we will examine the population dynamics of SV40 in particular using only partial sequence and a network genealogical approach. We discuss the basics of sequence alignment, model selection, and recombination detection and their importance in terms of phylogenetic estimation. We introduce the reader to a variety of useful software packages for performing these analyses. Throughout this chapter, we demonstrate these important components of evolutionary analyses using the polyomaviruses as our model system. Our study results in a robust estimate of the evolutionary relationships among the polyomaviruses based on both maximum likelihood and Bayesian analyses. Finally, we introduce the reader to network approaches to estimating gene genealogies using an SV40 data set and suggest approaches for testing hypotheses of this virus associated with cancer.

Sequence Alignment

Perhaps the most difficult and underappreciated aspects of phylogeny estimation is the sequence alignment phase. For population genetic studies using single gene regions, alignments are often trivial, especially for conserved gene regions. However, for whole genome analysis across the phylogenetic diversity shown in the polyomaviruses, alignment is far from trivial. A standard approach is to use the popular alignment tool Clustal X[1] with the default parameters and then start using the output alignment for phylogeny estimation. One of the difficulties with this approach is that Clustal X does not take into account an amino acid reading frame. Thus gaps can be inserted within a genetic codon triplet breaking up an otherwise reasonable reading frame. Therefore, for coding sequences, it is important to review an alignment using a sequence editor that allows one to toggle between amino acids and nucleotides, for example Se-Al[2] (Fig. 1). Needless to say, the hand proofing of sequence alignments for large data sets becomes quickly unwieldy. An alternative is to use an alignment software that takes into account coding frame for nucleotide data, aligns by the amino acid sequence, and then converts back to the nucleotides. To our knowledge, such software does not exist that can handle a reasonable number of whole genomes. However, our group is currently developing software called AlignmentHelper that can perform this task. Even with the aid correcting for codons, there can still be significant ambiguity in the resulting alignment. The alignment provides the basis of positional homology (the assumption that each nucleotide in the same column of data

Sequence 1	AACCCAGATGAGTACTAT	N	P	D	E	Y	Y
Sequence 2	AACCCAGATGAGTACTAT	N	P	D	E	Y	Y
Sequence 3	AATCCC---GAAGATTAT	N	P	-	E	D	Y
Sequence 4	AATCCAGAAGACTACTAT	N	P	E	D	Y	Y
Sequence 5	AATCCAGAAGACTACTAT	N	P	E	D	Y	Y

Figure 1. Sample alignment with conversion to amino acids demonstrating the importance of this conversion for accurate alignment and the importance of positional homology for phylogeny estimation.

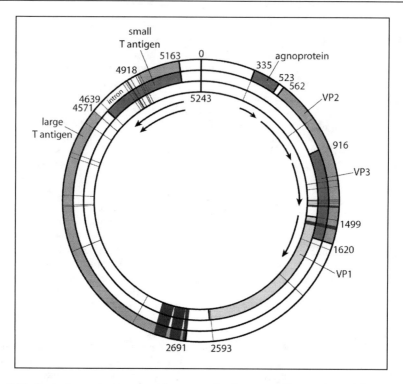

Figure 2. Idealized polyomavirus genome with genes, reading frames, and direction (arrows) shown. Vertical bars indicate regions from the coding sequence that were eliminated using GBlocks as questionably aligned areas. The remainder of the coding sequences were used in the subsequent phylogenetic analyses.

shares a common ancestor) for phylogeny estimation. If the alignment is questionable in any region, the inferred phylogeny may be in error as a result. For example, in Figure 1, we have some assurance of the positioning of the gaps as a triplet due to the translation to amino acids. However, it is impossible to reasonably choose where that gap should be in sequence 3. As shown, it tends to link sequence 3 with sequences 1 and 2 (this is indeed the Clustal X output). An alternative would be to slide the gap to the right (3') two or even three amino acids to link sequence 3 with sequences 4 and 5. This ambiguity (and often even greater ambiguity exists especially for nonprotein coding regions) can lead to spurious inferred relationships. Therefore it is important to have some assessment of positional homology before attempting phylogeny estimation. A quick assessment can be accomplished using the software Gblocks.[3] This software uses the number of contiguous conserved positions, lack of gaps, and high conservation of flanking positions to assess the "goodness" of different blocks of nucleotides within an alignment. Using this approach, one can quickly define regions of suspect positional homology and eliminate them from subsequent analyses.

For our analysis of polyomavirus phylogeny, we selected 33 sequences from GenBank (Table 1). These sequences were aligned (each gene being aligned independently) using T-Coffee,[4] which performs more accurate alignments than Clustal W although at a much slower speed for these large data sets. The resulting alignment was then adjusted using Se-Al and AlignmentHelper. Then GBlocks was used to identify regions of confident alignment throughout the genome of the polyomaviruses. Our final alignment included 8916 positions (larger than the average genome size!). After excluding blocks of ambiguous alignment as defined by GBlocks, our data set consisted of a total of 5298 nucleotides. Figure 2 shows the idealized polyomavirus genome with

Table 1. Summary of the polyomavirus sequence data used in this analysis

GenBank Accession #	Virus	Specific Host/Source Information from GenBank Record	First Reference in GenBank Accession
NC_004763	African green monkey polyomavirus		Pawlita M, Clad A, zur Hausen H. Complete DNA sequence of lymphotropic papovavirus: prototype of a new species of the polyomavirus genus. Virology 1985; 143(1):196-211.
AF118150	Budgerigar fledgling disease virus	Pteroglossus viridis	Lafferty SL, Fudge AM, Schmidt RE et al. Direct submission.
NC_004764	Budgerigar fledgling disease virus		Stoll R, Dong L, Kouwenhoven B et al. Molecular and biological characteristics of avian polyomaviruses: Isolares from different species of birds indicate that avian polyomaviruses form a distinct subgenus within the polyomavirus genus. J Gen Virol 1993; 74:229-237.
AF241168	Budgerigar fledgling disease virus - 1		Rott O, Kroger M, Muller H et al. The genome of budgerigar fledgling disease virus, an avian polyomavirus. Virology 1988; 165(1):74-86.
AF241169	Budgerigar fledgling disease virus - 4		Rott O, Kroger M, Muller H et al. The genome of budgerigar fledgling disease virus, an avian polyomavirus. Virology 1988; 165(1):74-86.
AF241170	Budgerigar fledgling disease virus - 5		Rott O, Kroger M, Muller H et al. The genome of budgerigar fledgling disease virus, an avian polyomavirus. Virology 1988; 165(1):74-86.
NC_001538	BK		Ryder K, DeLucia AL, Tegtmeyer P. Binding of SV40 a protein to the . K virus origin of DNA replication. Virology 1983; 129(1):239-245.
V01109	BK strain: MM		Yang RC, Wu R. BK virus DNA: complete nucleotide s. quence of a human tumor virus. Science 1979; 206(4417):456-462.
NC_001442	Bovine polyomavirus	From infected monkey kidney cell cultures	Schuurman R, Sol C, van der Noordaa J. The complete nucleotide sequence of bovine polyomavirus. J Gen Virol 1990; 71(Pt 8):1723-1735.
NC_004800	Goose hemorrhagic polyomavirus		Johne R, Muller H. The genome of goose hemorrhagic polyomavirus, a new member of the proposed subgenus Avipolyomavirus. Virology 2003; 308(2):291-302.
NC_001663	Hamster papovavirus		Delmas V, de La Roche Saint Andre C, Gardes M et al. Early gene expression in lymphoma-associated hamster polyomavirus viral genomes. Oncogene 1992; 7(2):295-302.

continued on next page

Table 1. Continued

GenBank Accession #	Virus	Specific Host/Source Information from GenBank Record	First Reference in GenBank Accession
NC_001699	JC		Miyamura T, Furuno A, Yoshiike K. DNA rearrangement in the control region for early transcription in a human polyomavirus JC host range mutant capable of growing in human embryonic kidney cells. J Virol 1985; 54(3):750-756.
AB038252	JC, isolate: GH-1	Cloned from urine of a healthy Ghanian	Kato A, Sugimoto C, Zheng HY et al. Lack of disease-specific amino acid changes in the viral proteins of JC virus isolates from the brain with progressive multifocal leukoencephalopathy. Arch Virol 2000; 145(10):2173-2182.
AB038254	JC, isolate: Tky-1	Cloned from brain of a Japanese PML (progressive multifocal leukoencephalopathy) patient.	Kato A, Sugimoto C, Zheng HY et al. Lack of disease-specific amino acid changes in the viral proteins of JC virus isolates from the brain with progressive multifocal leukoencephalopathy. Arch Virol 2000; 145(10):2173-2182.
AB038255	JC, isolate: Tky-2a	Cloned from brain of a Japanese PML (progressive multifocal leukoencephalopathy) patient.	Kato A, Sugimoto C, Zheng HY et al. Lack of disease-specific amino acid changes in the viral proteins of JC virus isolates from the brain with progressive multifocal leukoencephalopathy. Arch Virol 2000; 145(10):2173-2182.
AF295732	JC, strain: 310A	Homo sapiens; isolated from urine type: 3A.	Agostini HT, Ryschkewitsch CF, Brubaker GR et al. Five complete genomes of JC virus type 3 from Africans and African Americans. Arch Virol 1997; 142(4):637-655.
U61771	JC, strain: Taiwan-3		Ou WC, Tsai RT, Wang M et al. Genomic cloning and sequence analysis of Taiwan-3 human polyomavirus JC virus. J Formos Med Assoc 1997; 96(7):511-516.
M30540	Monkey B-lymphotropic papovavirus		Furuno A, Kanda T, Yoshiike K. Monkey B-lymphotropic papovavirus genome: the entire DNA sequence and variable regions. Jpn J Med Sci Biol 1986; 39(4):151-161.
K02737	Mouse polyomavirus, strain: Crawford small-plaque		Rothwell VM, Folk WR. Comparison of the DNA sequence of the Crawford small-plaque variant of polyomavirus with those of pol. omaviruses A2 and strain 3. J Virol 1983 48(2):472-480.
NC_001515	Murine polyomavirus, strain: A2		De Simone V, La Mantia G, Lania L et al. Polyomavirus mutation that confers a cell-specific cis advantage for viral DNA replication. Mol Cell Biol 1985; 5(8):2142-2146.
J02289	Murine polyomavirus, strain: A3		Friedmann T, Doolittle RF, Walter G. Amino acid sequence homology between polyoma and SV40 tumour antigens deduced from nucleotide sequences. Nature 1978; 274(5668):291-293.

continued on next page

Table 1. Continued

GenBank Accession #	Virus	Specific Host/Source Information from GenBank Record	First Reference in GenBank Accession
J02289	Murine polyomavirus, strain: A3		Friedmann T, Doolittle RF, Walter G. Amino acid sequence homology between polyoma and SV40 tumour antigens deduced from nucleotide sequences. Nature 1978; 274(5668):291-293.
AF442959	Murine polyomavirus, strain: BG	Mouse	Clark BE, Griffin BE. Direct submission.
NC_001505	Murine polyomavirus, strain: Kilham		Mayer M, Dorries K. Nucleotide sequence and genome organization of the murine polyomavirus, Kilham strain. Virology 1991; 181(2):469-480.
M23122	Polyoma virus AS		Tavis JE, Walker DL, Gardner SD et al. Nucleotide sequence of the human polyomavirus AS virus, an antigenic variant of BK virus. J Virol 1989; 63(2):901-911.
U27813	Polyomavirus sp., strain: LID		Bauer PH, Bronson RT, Fung SC et al. Genetic and structural analysis of a virulence determinant in polyomavirus VP1. J Virol 1995; 69(12):7925-7931.
U27812	Polyomavirus sp., strain: PTA		Bauer PH, Bronson RT, Fung SC et al. Genetic and structural analysis of a virulence determinant in polyomavirus VP1. J Virol 1995; 69(12):7925-7931.
Sa12	Sa12		Unpublished; Not yet submitted.
J02400	SV40		Dhar R, Zain S, Weissman SM et al. Nucleotide sequences of RNA transcribed in infected cells and by Escherichia coli RNA polymerase from a segment of simian virus 40 DNA. Proc Natl Acad Sci USA 1974; 71(2):371-375.
AF332562	SV40, strain: 777	Contains archetypal regulatory region variant 1.	Lednicky JA, Butel JS, Lewis AM. Direct submission.
AF345345	SV40, strain: GM00637H defective variant 12	Defective variant 12 predominant defective genome isolated from cell line GM00637H.	Lednicky JA, Butel JS, Lewis AM. Direct submission.
AF038616	SV40, strain: K661	SIV-infected monkey that had SV40 brain disease.	Lednicky JA, Arrington AS, Stewart AR et al. Natural isolates of simian virus 40 from immunocompromised monkeys display extensive genetic heterogeneity: new implications for polyomavirus disease. J Virol 1998; 72(5):3980-3990.
AF180737	SV40, strain: MC-028846B		Rizzo P, Di Resta I, Powers A et al. Unique strains of SV40 in commercial poliovaccines from 1955 not readily identifiable with current testing for SV40 infection. Cancer Res 1999; 59(24):6103-6108.
AF156107	SV40, strain: VA45-54-1		Lednicky JA, Butel JS. Tissue culture adaptation of natural isolates of simian virus 40: changes occur in viral regulatory region but not in carboxy-terminal domain of large T-antigen. J Gen Virol 1997; 78(Pt 7):1697-1705.

shading across the reading frames to indicate those sections eliminated by GBlocks analysis. The remainder of the coding sequence across the genome was then used for phylogenetic analysis. With a robust alignment, we moved to testing for recombination, since most phylogenetic approaches assume that recombination has not occurred throughout the history of the sequences under study. Thus, we must first statistically test for the possibility of recombination.

Recombination

Recombination in polyomaviruses, at least in JC viruses, has been controversial but seemingly does occur.[5,6] Recombination can have a large impact on our ability to accurately estimate evolutionary relationships[7] and population genetic parameters such as genetic diversity and substitution rates.[8] Furthermore, recombination can be an important evolutionary force that should be taken into account when considering drug and vaccine design.[9] Thus it is essential to test for recombination in a given data set. The question then becomes, what test should be used? There are a wide variety of methods for detecting recombination. Many of them are easily fooled by other phenomena such as population structure or rate heterogeneity. Posada and Crandall[10] evaluated a number of different methods that claim to detect recombination using a computer simulation approach. They found that phylogenetic methods (those most commonly used to test for recombination in viral sequences) typically performed poorer than methods that use substitution patterns or incompatibility among sites as a criterion for the inference of recombination. The "best" method for detecting recombination also greatly depended on the overall amount of genetic diversity in the sample. Posada[11] found similar results using empirical data sets. Therefore, there is still no easy guideline for choosing a method to apply to any particular data set to detect recombination. We therefore ran our 33-sequence data set through a variety of recombination detection algorithms and found no evidence for recombination (at least among the major clades). Given a lack of evidence for recombination coupled with a robust model of evolution, we can now proceed to estimation the evolutionary relationships among these viruses via phylogeny reconstruction.

Phylogeny Estimation

Our first decision in reconstructing evolutionary histories is what optimality criterion we should use. There are both algorithmic methods like neighbor-joining[12] and methods that optimize solutions based on some criterion like parsimony (minimizing the branch length) or likelihood (maximizing the likelihood). Optimality methods are generally better than algorithmic methods because they find not only the optimal solution but a variety of solutions close to the optimum whereas algorithmic methods provide simply a point estimate of the solution. There could possibly be a number of solutions that look quite different that are just as good as the point estimate provided by the algorithmic approach. Unfortunately, because the algorithmic approaches like neighbor-joining are computationally very fast, many researchers choose this approach despite its limitations. We highly recommend to the reader to use the more thorough optimality methods discussed below.

Optimality Criteria

There are two fundamentally different optimality criteria that are typically used in phylogeny estimation, minimize the branch lengths (parsimony) or maximize the likelihood scores. There are a variety of ways to implement these different criteria. Maximum parsimony can be performed with a "weighting matrix" that effectively incorporates a more realistic model of evolution within the parsimony framework. Such weighting matrices can be justified by using empirical estimates from the data for observed patterns of nucleotide substitutions. This approach has the advantage of being able to take into account gaps as characters in phylogeny estimation. However, the parsimony approach cannot accommodate rate heterogeneity (different substitution rates at different sites along the sequence) and it therefore performs poorly when there is great rate heterogeneity.[13] The alternative then becomes maximum likelihood.[14] This approach does incorporate a model of evolution (see below) allowing for rate heterogeneity, invariable sites, differences in base frequencies (none of which are accommodated in a parsimony frame-work), as well as differences in substitution rates. This approach does not, however, accommo-date gap characters. These are typically treated as missing data. The other weakness of the maxi-mum likelihood approach is in computational time. It is a very slow approach in general, especially with reasonably large data sets. However, alternative methods have been developed to speed the likelihood searches including genetic algorithms,[15,16] parallel algorithms,[17] and Bayesian ap-proaches to assess relative likelihoods.[18] We have used both standard maximum likelihood as implemented by PAUP*,[19] as well as a Bayesian approach implemented in Mr. Bayes.[20]

Bayesian analysis differs from maximum likelihood in that the standard likelihood is defined as the probability of the data given the tree and the model, or L = Prob(Data | Tree).[21] The Bayesian inference of phylogeny, on the other hand, is based on the posterior probability of a tree defined as. pr(Tree |Data) = Pr(Data |Tree)×Pr(Tree)/Pr(Data)Both methods incorporate mod-els of evolution as discussed above. One great advantage of the Bayesian approach is that the posterior probability is also used as a confidence assessment (see below), thus eliminating the need to repeat an analysis 100s-1000s of times to obtain a bootstrap value as an assessment of nodal confidence. Computationally, Bayesian approaches tend to be much faster and find very similar trees (both in terms of the topology as well as branch lengths). Bayesian approaches have also been implemented in a variety of other contexts including detecting selection, estimating divergence times, testing for a molecular clock, and evaluating models of evolution (see Huelsenbeck et al[18] for a review). Our preferred optimality criteria require some way of model-ing the evolutionary changes in the sequence data along a tree. We need to not only model the changes, but determine if our selected model is a reasonable estimate of the true underlying changes. The next section offers insights into models of evolution and model selection.

Models of Evolution

Models of evolution represent a probability statement for the change from one nucleotide to another (e.g., G $\Rightarrow$ A). The model is often represented as a relative rate of change from one nucleotide to another, leaving five free rates with one fixed at a relative rate of 1.0 in a symmetrical model (e.g., G $\Rightarrow$ A) (Fig. 3). The first model of evolution developed was that of Jukes and Cantor,[22] which accounted for multiple changes at a single site with equal rate parameters for all rates of change. Later, Kimura noticed that in many data sets transitions (change from purine to purine or pyrimidine to pyrimidine) occurred much more frequently than transversions (changes from purine to pyrimidine or vise versa). He then developed the Kimura 2-parameter model to

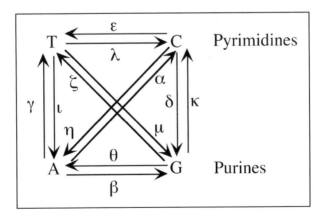

Figure 3. Models of evolution represent rate changes along the arrows changing a nucleotide from one to another. Often these rates are different and there is often a difference between transitions (changes within pyrimidines or purines) and transversions (changes among class).

allow for differences in the transition and transversion rates.[23] Subsequent models have been developed that incorporate differences for all relative rates (the general time reversible or GTR model)[24] as well as differences in nucleotide frequencies among base pairs,[14] rate heterogeneity among sites,[25] invariable sites,[26] and even codon position.[27,28] While the Kimura 2-parameter model is the default model for many studies for both historical reasons and simply because it is the default model in the population software package PHYLIP,[29] it has often been shown to be too simplistic to reasonably model the molecular evolution of viral systems.[30]

Given this plethora of models to choose from, one is left with a decision on how to make a reasonable choice of models. One could simply choose the most complex model of evolution available knowing that models by definition are simplifications of biological reality thereby hoping that the most complex model might come closest to a true underlying model. One problem with this approach is that highly complex models require many parameters. All these parameters need to be estimated from the data. One then needs to worry about having enough data to accurately estimate all these parameters. The errors in these estimates are typically not incorporated into a model of evolution that is subsequently used for phylogeny estimation. Therefore, an alternative is to fit the model to the data using some criterion like maximum likelihood through likelihood ratio testing,[31] an Akaike information criterion, or a Bayesian information criterion.[32] This approach allows one to determine statistically the relative gain in likelihood for adding more parameters to the model. There is now software available, for example ModelTest,[33] to assist in the evaluation of different models for a given data set.

One might ask if the model of evolution can really make much of a difference in the resulting estimated phylogeny and conclusions based on that tree. In a study on the origins of primate T-cell leukemia/lymphoma viruses (PTLVs), Kelsey et al[34] found that previous researchers had used the Kimura 2-parameter model without justification but that a model selected using ModelTest resulted in not only a different model of evolution, it changed the conclusion of the origin of PTLVs from Asia to Africa. Thus the main conclusions of studies can be severely affected by the wrong choice of model of evolution. It is therefore essential to justify one's choice in model and demonstrate that that model reasonably fits the data.

We used ModelTest to select a model of evolution for our 33-sequence data set of polyomaviruses. The resulting model was the general-time reversible model (GTR) with invariable sites and rate heterogeneity. The model parameters for this analysis were as follows: Base frequencies (A, C, G, T) = (0.3166 0.1973 0.2273), Nst = 6, Rmat = (1.8508 2.8908 1.5896 2.0755 3.9402), Rates = gamma, Shape = 1.5685, Pinvar = 0.1011. Now that we have a model of evolution in hand, it is time to estimate a phylogeny.

Here we used both maximum likelihood and Bayesian approaches to estimate phylogenetic relationships among the polyomaviruses. Both methods used the same model of evolution (see above) and both methods estimated the same tree (with an identical likelihood score) (Fig. 4). The comparative speeds, however, were quite different. The Bayesian analysis took 24.5 hours to run on a Lunix 3.0 GHz Xeon PC computer, whereas the maximum likelihood analysis took ~79.5 hours. The resulting tree shows a major grouping of each of the well-characterized polyomaviruses, e.g., JCVs form a clade sister to the BK viruses. The (BK, JCV) clade is sister to the SV40 clade. There is a robust clade of mouse polyomavirus related to the hamster papovavirus (HaPV). That clade is then sister to a clade of virus infecting monkeys. More distantly related are the goose hemorrhagic polyomavirus (GHPV) and the avian polyomaviruses (BFPV).

Confidence Assessment

Many studies mistakenly stop at this point (having a tree) and start telling stories about their tree and its wonderful significance, as we have just done. However, it is important to recognize that phylogeny estimation is a difficult problem and a single point estimate is not to be trusted, even when using a robust optimality criterion. Therefore, some measure of confidence is desired to judge the statistical validity of the inferred relationships. Confidence assessment is typically performed by using either posterior probabilities (for Bayesian approaches), or through a bootstrap[35] or jackknife procedure. Bootstrapping is the most common form of

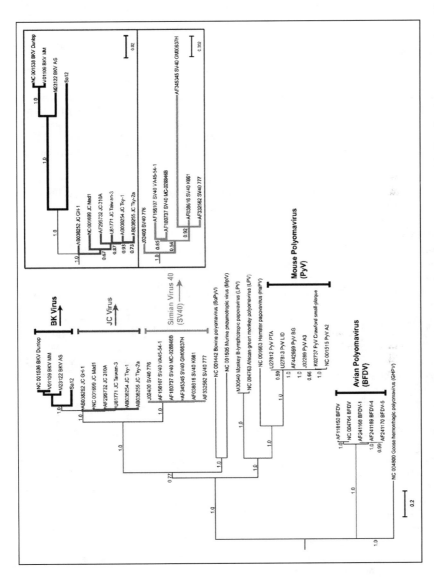

Figure 4. Estimated phylogeny of the polyomaviruses. The same topology was obtained from both a maximum likelihood and a Bayesian analysis. The numbers on the branches represent posterior probabilities in the Bayesian framework. The branch lengths are drawn proportional to the amount of change along that branch (scale shown).

confidence assessment and consists of resampling the data with replacement, reevaluating that new (resampled) data set using the same optimality criterion and same model of evolution and then repeating this many times. The resulting trees are then evaluated by a majority-rule consensus procedure with the bootstrap proportions being associated with the number of times that node is represented in the family of bootstrapped trees. Bootstrap values have been shown to be highly biased (seemingly in a conservative way).[36] The obvious difficulty with bootstrap values (as mentioned above) is that one needs to reestimate a phylogeny for each resampled data set. For reasonable bootstrap values, typically 100 – 1000 bootstrap replications are required. Thus if your original search takes any time at all (in our case 79.5 hours), your bootstrap evaluation of confidence will simply take too long (~9 years!).

The alternative approach then is to use a method like Bayesian analysis that performs an assessment of confidence at the same time as estimating the tree. In the Bayesian analysis, the search continues until the likelihood score plateaus, including the tree and substitution parameters. At this point there is typically a large set of trees with very similar likelihood scores. These trees are then used to create consensus trees with the percentage of times a particular node shows up in that group of trees related as the posterior probably. In our Figure 4, these posterior probabilities are shown on the major branches and range from 0.29 to 1.0. All of the major clades (those nodes leading to monophyletic groups of distinct viruses, e.g., BK) are supported by posterior probabilities of 1.0. There is a growing literature on the relationship between posterior probabilities and bootstrap values[37,38] and no consensus seems to have been reached at the moment.[39,40]

Population Variation of SV40

Notice that in Figure 4, there is very little resolution within the SV40 clade and parts of the JCV clade. Most of the nodes have no posterior probabilities associated with them (because we did not label nodes with less than 0.5 posterior probability). When one is working with closely related sequences with little divergence (and a greater potential for recombination), network approaches for visualizing genealogical relationships become preferred representations.[41] These network approaches allow for the simultaneous visualization of multiple solutions, the biological reality of nonbifurcating genetic exchange (e.g., through recombination, hybridization, etc.). They also allow for greater resolution when sequence divergences are low.[42,43]

We, therefore, used the statistical parsimony approach[44] as implemented in the software TCS[45] to estimate evolutionary relationships among the SV40 viruses. Using this approach, minimum connections are made using a 95% confidence assessment based on a statistical assessment of the conditional probability of the change of more than one nucleotide at a particular site. With a high probability (>95%) that a multiple change has not occurred, minimum connections are made to infer genealogical relationships. This approach has been tested using empirical data from a known bacteriophage phylogeny and shown to be robust and outperform other approaches such as parsimony,[42] likelihood and distance[46] approaches. Indeed, the resulting relationships (Fig. 5) show a great more resolution that the SV40 clade in Figure 4. One can also use the network structure to help interpret the data. For example, population genetic theory argues that sequences with high frequency in the sample and those in the interior of the network are older in evolutionary age.[47,48] Thus we can infer that isolates OPC/MEN, Rh911, and some of 777* are older in age (perhaps the oldest in the sample) relative to the other haplotypes that appear on the tips of the network. Using such reasoning it becomes possible to test hypotheses, for example, about the association with SV40 with cancer.[49] Clearly the methodology for testing such hypotheses is available. We only await an appropriate data set for such an analysis.

Summary

Phylogenetic methods are of great utility for a wide variety of hypotheses in infectious disease studies.[50] Here we have hopefully provided a useful introduction to a variety of phylogenetic methods and the complexity of phylogenetic analyses in general. We have done so using the polyomavirus

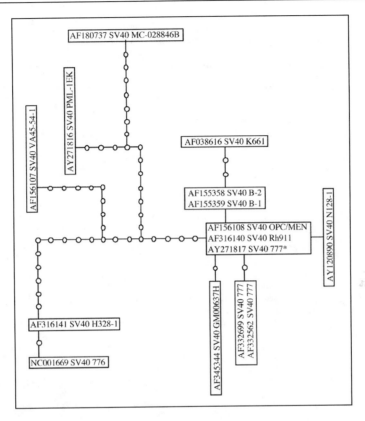

Figure 5. A network of genealogical relationships among the SV40 viruses where zeros are missing intermediates and each line represents a single mutational change.

as a model system and generated a novel phylogeny for the relationships among the viruses associated with this group. We hope that this work will stimulate further interest in phylogenetic inference with infectious diseases and in the proper use of phylogenetic methodology. We refer the reader to the new (and excellent) text by Felsenstein[21] for further details on phylogenetic inference.

Acknowledgements

We thank Nasimul Ahsan for the invitation to present this chapter and his patience in editing. We would also like to thank the NIH for supporting our work through grants R01 AI50217 (RPV, KAC) and GM66276 (KAC). This work was also supported by the Brigham Young University Cancer Research Center (RGC).

References

1. Thompson JD, Gibson TJ, Plewniak F et al. The clustalX windows interface: Flexible strategies for multiple sequence alignment aided by quality analysis tools. Nuc Acid Res 1997; 24:4876-4882.
2. Se-A. Sequence Alignment Editor [computer program]. Version 2.0. Oxford: http://evolve.zoo.ox.ac.uk. 2002.
3. Castresana J. Selection of conserved blocks from multiple alignments for their use in phylogenetic analysis. MBE 2000; 17(4):540-552.
4. Notredame C, Higgins D, Heringa J. T-Coffee: A novel method for multiple sequence alignments. J Mol Biol 2000; 302:205-217.
5. Hatwell JN, Sharp PM. Evolution of human polyomavirus JC. J Gen Virol 2000; 81:1191-1200.

6. Jobes DV, Chima SC, Ryschkewitsch CF et al. Phylogenetic analysis of 22 complete genomes of the human polyomavirus JC virus. J Gen Virol 1998; 79:2491-2498.
7. Posada D, Crandall KA. The effect of recombination on the accuracy of phylogeny estimation. JME 2002; 54:396-402.
8. Schierup MH, Hein J. Consequences of recombination on traditional phylogenetic analysis. Genetics 2000; 156:879-891.
9. Rambaut A, Posada D, Crandall KA et al. The causes and consequences of HIV evolution. Nat Rev Genet 2004; 5(1):52-61.
10. Posada D, Crandall KA. Evaluation of methods for detecting recombination from DNA sequences: Computer simulations. PNAS 2001; 98(24):13757-13762.
11. Posada D. On the performance of methods for detecting recombination from DNA sequences: Real data. MBE 2002; 19(5):708-717.
12. Saitou N, Nei M. The neighbor-joining method: A new method for reconstructing phylogenetic trees. MBE 1987; 4(4):406-425.
13. Huelsenbeck JP, Hillis DM. Success of phylogenetic methods in the four-taxon case. Syst Biol 1993; 42(3):247-264.
14. Felsenstein J. Evolutionary trees from DNA sequences: A maximum likelihood approach. JME 1981; 17:368-376.
15. Lewis PO. A genetic algorithm for maximum-likelihood phylogeny inference using nucleotide sequence data. MBE 1998; 15(3):277-283.
16. Lemmon AR, Milinkovitch MC. The metapopulation genetic algorithm: An efficient solution for the problem of large phylogeny estimation. PNAS 2002; 99(16):10516-10521.
17. Brauer MJ, Holder MT, Dries LA et al. Genetic algorithms and parallel processing in maximum-likelihood phylogeny inference. MBE 2002; 19(10):1717-1726.
18. Huelsenbeck JP, Ronquist F, Nielsen R et al. Bayesian inference of phylogeny and its impact on evolutionary biology. Science 2001; 294:2310-2314.
19. PAUP*. Phylogenetic analysis using parsimony (*and other methods) [computer program]. Version 4. Sunderland: Sinauer Associates, 2000.
20. Huelsenbeck JP, Ronquist F. MRBAYES: Bayesian inference of phylogenetic trees. Bioinformatics 2001; 17(8):754-755.
21. Felsenstein J. Inferring phylogenies. Sunderland: Sinauer Associates, 2003.
22. Jukes TH, Cantor CR. Evolution of protein molecules. In: Munro HM, ed. Mammalian Protein Metabolism. New York: Academic Press, 1969:21-132.
23. Kimura M. A simple method for estimating evolutionary rate of base substitutions through comparative studies of nucleotide sequences. JME 1980; 16:111-120.
24. Rodríguez F, Oliver JL, Marin A et al. The general stochastic model of nucleotide substitution. J Theor Biol 1990; 142:485-501.
25. Yang Z. Among-site rate variation and its impact on phylogenetic analyses. Trends Eco Evol 1996; 11(9):367-372.
26. Steel M, Huson D, Lockhart P. Invariable sites models and their use in phylogeny reconstruction. Syst Biol 2000; 49(2):225-232.
27. Muse SV, Gaut BS. A likelihood approach for comparing synonymous and nonsynonymous nucleotide substitution rates, with application to the chloroplast genome. MBE 1994; 11(5):715-724.
28. Yang Z, Goldman N, Friday A. Comparison of models for nucleotide substitution used in Maximum-likelihood phylogenetic estimation. MBE 1994; 11(2):316-324.
29. PHYLIP [computer program]. Version 3.6. Seattle: Department of Genome Sciences, University of Washington, 2002.
30. Posada D, Crandall KA. Selecting models of nucleotide substitution: An application to human immunodeficiency virus 1 (HIV-1). MBE 2001; 18(6):897-906.
31. Huelsenbeck JP, Crandall KA. Phylogeny estimation and hypothesis testing using maximum likelihood. Ann Rev Ecol Syst 1997; 28:437-466.
32. Posada D, Crandall KA. A comparison of different strategies for selecting models of DNA substitution. Syst Biol 2001; 50(4):580-601.
33. Posada D, Crandall KA. Modeltest: Testing the model of DNA substitution. Bioinformatics 1998; 14(9):817-818.
34. Kelsey CR, Crandall KA, Voevodin AF. Different models, different trees: The geographic origin of PTLV-I. Mol Phylogenet Evol 1999; 13(2):336-347.
35. Felsenstein J. Confidence limits on phylogenies: An approach using the bootstrap. Evolution 1985; 39:783-791.
36. Hillis DM, Bull JJ. An empirical test of bootstrapping as a method for assessing confidence in phylogenetic analysis. Syst Biol 1993; 42:182-192.

37. Erixon P, Svennnblad B, Britton T et al. Reliability of bayesian posterior probabilities and bootstrap frequencies in phylogenetics. Syst Biol 2003; 52(5):665-673.
38. Cummings M, Handley S, Myers D et al. Comparing bootstrap and posterior probability values in the four-taxon case. Syst Biol 2003; 52(4):477-487.
39. Alfardo M, Zoller S, Lutzoni F. Bayes or bootstrap? A simulation study comparing the performance of bayesian markov chain monte carlo sampling and boostrapping in assessing phylogenetic confidence. MBE 2003; 20(2):255-266.
40. Douady C, Delsue F, Boucher Y et al. Comparison of bayesian and maximum likelihood bootstrap measures of phylogenetic reliability. MBE 2003; 20(2):248-254.
41. Posada D, Crandall KA. Intraspecific gene genealogies: Trees grafting into networks. Trends Ecol Evol 2001; 16(1):37-45.
42. Crandall KA. Intraspecific cladogram estimation: Accuracy at higher levels of divergence. Syst Biol 1994; 43(2):222-235.
43. Crandall KA. Intraspecific phylogenetics: Support for dental transmission of human immunodeficiency virus. J Virol 1995; 69(4):2351-2356.
44. Templeton AR, Crandall KA, Sing CF. A cladistic analysis of phenotypic associations with haplotypes inferred from restriction endonuclease mapping and DNA sequence data. III. Cladogram estimation. Genetics 1992; 132:619-633.
45. Clement M, Posada D, Crandall KA. TCS: A computer program to estimate gene genealogies. Molecular Ecology 2000; 9:1657-1659.
46. Crandall KA. Multiple interspecies transmissions of human and simian T-cell leukemia/lymphoma virus type I sequences. MBE 1996; 13(1):115-131.
47. Crandall KA, Templeton AR. Empirical tests of some predictions from coalescent theory with applications to intraspecific phylogeny reconstruction. Genetics 1993; 134:959-969.
48. Castelloe J, Templeton AR. Root probabilities for intraspecific gene trees under neutral coalescent theory. Mol Phylogenet Evol 1994; 3(2):102-113.
49. Ferber D. Monkey virus link to cancer grows stronger. Science 2002; 296:1012-1015.
50. Crandall KA, Posada D. Phylogenetic approaches to molecular epidemiology. In: Leitner T, ed. The Molecular Epidemiology of Human Viruses: Kluwer Academic Publishers, 2002:25-39.

CHAPTER 4

Virus Receptors and Tropism

Aarthi Ashok and Walter J. Atwood

Abstract

Polyomaviruses are small, tumorigenic, nonenveloped viruses that infect several different species. Interaction of these viruses with cell surface receptors represents the initial step during infection of host cells. This interaction can be a major determinant of viral host and tissue tropism. This chapter reviews what is currently known about the cellular receptors for each of five polyomavirus family members: Mouse polyomavirus (PyV), JC virus (JCV), BK virus (BKV), Lymphotropic papovavirus (LPV) and Simian virus 40 (SV40). These polyomaviruses serve to illustrate the enormous diversity of virus-cell surface interactions and allow us to closely evaluate the role of receptors in their life cycles. The contribution of other factors such as transcriptional regulators and signaling pathways are also summarized.

Introduction

The polyomavirus family consists of small, tumorigenic, nonenveloped viruses that infect several different species, but are, in general, species-specific[1] (Table 1). They contain a double-stranded DNA genome of about 5200 base pairs complexed with cellular histones H2A, H2B, H3 and H4 within an icosahedral viral capsid.[2,3] The capsid is composed of 72 pentamers of the major capsid protein, VP1, each associated with one of the minor capsid proteins, VP2 or VP3[1] (Fig. 1). The viral genome is organized such that the bi-directional promoter and enhancer elements are contained within a regulatory region and the early genes (regulatory proteins) are transcribed off of one strand while the late genes (structural proteins) are transcribed off of the complementary strand in the opposite direction.[3] This capsid structure and genomic organization is conserved between all polyomaviruses.[4]

During viral infection, polyomaviruses interact with cell surface receptor molecules and gain entry into the host cell via endocytic mechanisms.[5-8] Upon entry, the virions exploit the cellular transport pathways to travel to the nuclear periphery, where they have been shown to interact with nuclear pores, to gain access to the nucleus.[9-15] Within the nucleus, the early viral genes are transcribed, followed by replication of the viral genome and expression of the late viral structural genes.[4] New capsids are assembled within the nucleus and are released upon lysis of the host cell. This lytic viral infection occurs in the permissive host cells, while nonpermissive or semi-permissive cells establish a block to viral replication, which may result in an abortive infection or tumorigenesis.[3]

Interaction of a virus with its cell surface receptor is the initial step during infection of a host cell. In the case of nonenveloped viruses such as polyomaviruses, the viral capsid proteins interact directly with the receptor molecules in order to gain entry into the cell. This interaction is often a major determinant of viral host and tissue tropism. However, there is emerging evidence that coreceptor or psuedoreceptor molecules as well as events downstream of cell surface interactions such as endocytosis, virus-induced signaling, intracellular trafficking as well as transcriptional regulators may also significantly contribute to viral tropism.

Polyomaviruses and Human Diseases, edited by Nasimul Ahsan. ©2006 Eurekah.com and Springer Science+Business Media.

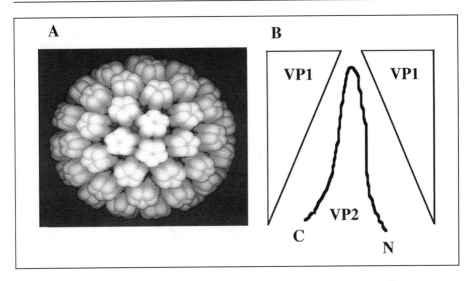

Figure 1. The polyomavirus capsid structure. A) Computer generated reconstruction of a polyomavirus capsid. B) Schematic of the association of VP1 pentamers with the minor capsid protein VP2. From: Khalili K, Stoner GL, eds. Human Polyomaviruses: Molecular and Clinical Perspectives. ©2001 John Wiley & Sons, Inc., with permission.

Table 1. Polyomaviruses and their host species

Polyomavirus Family Member	Host
JC virus (JCV)	Human
BK virus (BKV)	Human
Simian virus 40 (SV40)	Monkey
Lymphotropic papovavirus (LPV)	Monkey
Mouse polyomavirus (PyV)	Mouse
Bovine polyomavirus	Cattle
Hamster polyomavirus	Hamster
Budgerigar fledgling disease virus (BFDV)	Bird

This review will detail the identity, distribution, and contributions to tropism of specific receptor molecules or components of receptors, for each of these 5 polyomavirus family members: Mouse polyomavirus (PyV), JC virus (JCV), BK virus (BKV), Lymphotropic papovavirus (LPV) and Simian virus 40 (SV40). These polyomaviruses serve to illustrate the enormous diversity of virus-cell surface interactions and allow us to closely evaluate the role of receptors in their life cycles. The contribution of other factors such as transcriptional regulators and signaling pathways will also be summarized.

Mouse Polyomavirus (PyV)

Mouse polyomavirus has an unusually broad tropism in its natural host, *Mus musculus*, where it induces neoplasms in greater than 30 different cell types of mesenchymal and epithelial origin. For a detailed listing of these cell types, the reader is referred to Dawe et al.[16] Early experiments suggested a role for sialic acids during infection by mouse polyomavirus, as neuraminidase treated murine cells did not support infection by crude virus stocks.[17] The 2 major strains of mouse polyomavirus differ in their sialic acid binding specificities in addition to the extent of their virulence and spread in the host. The small plaque (SP), or less virulent strain, binds the unbranched terminal α 2,3 linkage: NeuAcα2,3Galβ1,3GalNAc as well as the branched disialyl structure:

Neu Acα2,3Galβ1,3

GalNAc.[18-20]

NeuAcα2,6

The large plaque (LP), or more virulent strain, also recognizes both structures of terminal sialic acid, but has a far lower affinity for the branched structure compared to the unbranched type.[18,19] Freund et al,[21] have mapped this difference in receptor specificity to a single amino acid change at position 92 of the outer capsid protein, VP1. The LP strain has a glutamic acid at this position, while the SP strain has a glycine and the crystal structure of mouse polyomavirus complexed with disialyl lactose has shown that while glycine at position 92 can accommodate the branched chain, glutamic acid would sterically hinder such a structure.[22-24] This led the authors to propose that the branched structure containing both α2-3 and α2-6 linked sialic acid acted as a pseudoreceptor for mouse polyomavirus, while the α 2-3 linked sialic acid alone acted as the productive entry receptor.[24] Studies with specific glycosylation inhibitors have shown that N-linked glycoproteins and not O-linked glycoproteins or glycolipids, can serve as receptors for mouse polyomavirus on mouse fibroblast cell lines.[25] However, the branched sialic acid structure recognized by the SP stain is normally only found in the context of O-glycoproteins, and it is hence thought that while the productive viral receptor is an N-linked glycoprotein, the psuedoreceptor is likely an O-linked glycoprotein or a glycolipid.

The identity of the proteinaceous component of the mouse polyomavirus receptor is unknown. Chemical crosslinking of the virus to mouse cells, followed by coimmunoprecipitation using anti-PyV antisera, resulted in the purification of a 120 KDa protein.[26,27] Antibodies against this protein, blocked infection by PyV in vitro, but the identity of this 120KDa protein remains to be described.[28] Attempts to clone the receptor through incubation of hamster anti-mouse cell hybridoma supernatants with mouse fibroblasts prior to assaying infection, have been unsuccessful in describing a single receptor molecule and it is therefore thought that several N-linked glycans may be capable of mediating entry and infection by PyV. This idea is consistent with the fact that polyoma infects a wide variety of cell types in its natural host.

The binding of mouse polyomavirus to host cells has been described in quantitative terms. There are an estimated 25, 000 receptor molecules per cell and the interaction with these receptors is of high affinity (K_d = 1.8 x 10^{-11} M), is fast (association and dissociation rate constants of 1.7 x 10^{7}M^{-1}s^{-1} and 3.1 x 10^{-4} s^{-1} respectively) and stable (t$_{1/2}$ = 38 minutes).[29] Previous crystal soaking experiments have suggested a K_d of between 5 x 10^{-3} and 10x 10^{-3}M for the binding of sialic acid -α2,3-galactose to PyV, which is far lower than the affinity calculated for the binding of PyV to its complete cellular receptor, suggesting a role for other components of the receptor in virus binding. This could be interpreted as the contribution of the proteinaceous component of the receptor complex or the contribution of several terminal sialic acid chains that are exposed by multiple members of the receptor complex.[29]

Integrin ligand binding sites, DLXXL, LDV and DGE, have been identified in the VP1 and VP2 proteins and a role for α4β1 integrin during infection by PyV was established by observing the inhibitory effect of preincubating host cells with natural integrin ligands, prior to infection by PyV. Caruso et al[30] have elegantly shown that while PyV does not bind to neuraminidase treated cells, it does bind to these cells if preincubated with soluble N-acetylneuraminic acid (NANA), suggesting that perhaps initial viral binding to sialylated receptor components, subsequently allowed binding to sialic acid-independent receptors. A two-step mechanism of viral is thought to occur though the initial interaction of PyV with sialic acid, followed by binding to α4β1 integrin, prior to gaining entry into the host cell. Interestingly, the authors have shown that transfection of a poorly susceptible murine cell line (BALB/c 3T3) with a cDNA encoding the α4 subunit, significantly enhances infection of this cell line.[30] This is the first direct demonstration that receptor usage is a critical determinant of PyV cellular tropism.

Recently, the addition of gangliosides GD1a and GT1b to phospholipid vesicles have been shown to allow specific binding of LP and SP strains of PyV to these vesicles during flotation in a discontinuous sucrose gradient.[31] Delivery of GD1a and GT1b in glycolipid micelles to a nonpermissive rat glioma cell line deficient in ganglioside synthesis, allows a dramatic enhancement of infection by PyV and allows normal transport to the endoplasmic reticulum (ER), suggesting that gangliosides are indeed involved in viral entry and may determine the cellular tropism of the virus.[31]

It now remains to be understood whether N-glycans, integrins and glycolipids can all function as receptors for PyV, or a certain combination of these form a PyV receptor complex, or whether the receptor choice depends on the cell type infected. The third possibility is also consistent with recent findings that PyV uses distinct endocytic pathways during infection of different cells types.[6,7,11] Comparative studies of the LP and SP strains of polyoma virus illustrate the idea that virus –receptor interactions may also be critical in virus dissemination throughout the host. For example, the recognition of vascular epithelial cell receptors by the virus, required for entry into and egress from the circulatory system, would be essential for the virus to then gain access to its permissive cell types.[32] The tropism of PyV has been attributed, at least in part, to post-entry events in the viral life cycle that include regulation by the enhancer/promoter elements and early regions of the viral genome. Mutant virus strains that are capable of replication in resistant cell types have been found to have rearrangements or point mutations within the enhancer region.[33-35] One such rearrangement has been characterized in detail to reveal the creation of a NF-1 transcription factor binding site as well as a binding site for a unique mouse transcription factor, named NF-D.[30] Another study has found that mutant virus strains that carry a deletion in one domain (Domain B) of the enhancer region are able to overcome the block to replication in certain neuroblastoma cell types.[36] This suggests that the creation or removal of binding sites in the viral enhancer for certain trans-acting factors can control cell type specific tropism of PyV.

Therefore, the presence of N-linked glycoprotein receptors, O-linked pseudoreceptors, gangliosides GT1b and GD1a, expression of integrins that could act as coreceptors and the presence of certain enhancer binding factors, could all contribute to the tropism of PyV (Table 2).

JC Virus (JCV)

There has been considerable interest in understanding the tissue tropism of JCV, due to the discovery that it is the etiological agent of the fatal disease, progressive multifocal leukoencephalopathy (PML), which is characterized by a lytic destruction of the myelin producing oligodendrocytes of the brain.[37] JCV infection is restricted to oligodendrocytes, astrocytes, tonsillar stromal cells, CD34+ hematopoietic progenitor cells, and a few established glial cell lines.[38,39] Some nonpermissive cell types, such as the HeLa cell, do not support infection by JC virions but can transcribe early viral genes when JCV DNA is transfected into them.[40] This suggested that there is a block very early during infection of a nonpermissive cell, perhaps at the level of viral receptors. Another clue that early events in the viral life cycle may contribute to tropism, came from the recent construction of a JCV-SV40 chimeric virus (JCSV) that contained the regulatory and early genes from SV40 and the late structural genes of JCV.[41] JCSV displayed biological and physical characteristics of both polyomaviruses, but maintained the host range of JCV, suggesting that the capsid-host cell interactions regulate viral tropism.[41]

Similar to most other polyomaviruses, JCV was found to hemagglutinate red blood cells in a sialic-acid dependent manner, which suggested that sialic acid may be important in virus-cell interactions.[42] Consistent with this notion, it has been shown that the closely related sialic-acid independent virus, SV40, did not share receptor specificity with JCV.[43] In these experiments, JC virions competed much more effectively with prebound labeled JCV on glial cells, than with SV40 virions. Additionally, incubation of anti-MHC class 1 antibody, did not inhibit

Table 2. Summary: polyomavirus receptors

Virus Name	Receptor	Number per Cell	Affinity of Binding (K_d)	Tropism	Remarks
PyV (small plaque)	N-linked glycoprotein with α2,3 linked sialic acids. Gangliosides GD1a and GT1b also act as receptors on certain rat glioma cells.	25,000	1.8×10^{-11} M	Broad	Pseudoreceptors are O-linked glycoproteins. α4β1 integrin may serve as co-receptor.
PyV (large plaque)	N-linked glycoprotein with α2,3 linked sialic acid and branched α2,6 linked sialic acid.	25,000	1.8×10^{-11} M	Broad	Pseudoreceptors are O-linked glycoproteins. α4β1 integrin may serve as co-receptor.
JCV	N-linked glycoprotein with α2,6 linked sialic acid. GT1b has been shown to play a role in one susceptible cell line.	50,000	Unknown	Restricted	Pseudoreceptors may be trypsin sensitive.
BKV	Gangliosides with a R_f lower than GM1. Phospholipids also shown to be required for entry.	Unknown	Unknown	Broad	The receptor complex is thought to be primarily composed of glycolipids and partially of phospholipids.
LPV	O-linked glycoprotein or glycolipid with α2,6 linked sialic acid.	600 - 1875	2.9×10^{-12} M	Very restricted	Trypsin sensitivity of LPV infection suggests that the receptor is likely a glycoprotein.
SV40	MHC class I molecules. GM1 has also been shown to regulate viral entry into glioma cells.	90,000	3.8×10^{-12} M	Broad	MHC class 1 is not the sole component of the receptor, as its distribution does not correlate with cellular susceptibility.

infection of these cells by JCV.[43] These experiments also showed that JC virus binding to glial cells was saturable, with an estimated 50,000 receptors per cell.[43]

Further studies have shown that infection by JCV was sensitive to treatment of glial cells with crude neuraminidase but not to α2,3 specific neuraminidase, and to treatment with the N-linked glycosylation inhibitor, tunicamycin.[44] JCV infection was resistant to treatment with chymotrypsin, the O-linked glycosylation inhibitor, BenzylGalNac, and phospholipases A2 and C.[44] Trypsin, treatment inhibits virus binding to glial cells, but enhances infection, leading to the hypothesis that trypsin may remove psuedoreceptors that would otherwise impede the efficient interaction of JCV with its receptor.[44] It is therefore thought that an N-linked glycoprotein with terminal α2,6 linked sialic acid is an important component of the JC virus receptor, but the nature of this glycoprotein remains to be established.[44] These studies have also hypothesized the existence of a trypsin-sensitive family of pseudoreceptors, but this remains to be proven. Eash et al[45] have recently shown that the expression of the α2,6 linkage of sialic acid on various human tissues can be completely correlated with the susceptibility of that tissue to infection by JCV, emphasizing the critical role of this linkage of sialic acid in virus-host cell interactions. Studies examining the binding of JC virus-like particles (VLPs) to various sialic acid linkages, have shown that in addition to sialic acid linkages on glycoproteins, gangliosides such as GT1b can also contribute to VLP binding.[46] Moreover, incubation of intact JC virions with GT1b led to inhibition of infection of the permissive cell line, IMR-32.[46] This suggests that oligosaccharides of both glycoproteins and glycolipids can act as JCV receptors on IMR-32 cells. The role of GT1b in mediating infection of glial cells by JCV has not yet been evaluated.

Despite this clear evidence for regulation of viral tropism at the level of cellular receptors, there is additional evidence for a role of cellular transcription factors in determining the host range of JCV. This idea was originally proposed by studies that reported a higher expression level of a reporter gene under the control of the JCV promoter in glial cells as opposed to nonglial cells.[47] More recently, one study has shown that JCV virus-like particles (VLPs) can be localized to the nucleus of nonpermissive cells within 10 minutes post infection and viral DNA from JCV virions could be detected equally well in the nuclei of all permissive and nonpermissive cell types examined.[48] The authors have also shown that despite the nuclear accumulation of virions, viral transcription and replication is limited to permissive cell types, thereby implicating host cell nuclear factors in the tropism of JCV.[48] A JCV-resistant glial cell line (SVGR2) derived from the permissive human glial cell line, SVG-A, after multiple rounds of infection, has been found to be blocked in early viral gene transcription, again suggesting that tropism is regulated at the level of viral gene expression.[49] Several efforts have identified a number of cis-regulatory regions in the JCV promoter, which are potential binding sites for NF-κB, NF-1, Sp-1, GBP-i, YB-1, Purα, Tst-1 and c-Jun.[50-56] Although there is no definitive evidence for regulation of JCV tropism by a single transcription factor, ectopic expression of NF-1X, one of the four members of the NF-1 family of transcription factors, appears to confer susceptibility to one resistant cell line.[57] Consistent with a role for DNA binding proteins in determining viral tropism, different JCV genotypes, that are classified by differences in the regulatory region, are consistently associated with different human tissues.[58] Differences in the regulatory region lead to changes in the types of binding sites available for various transcriptional regulators, which may then impact viral tropism.[59] Interestingly, one study has found that PML patients harboring a certain type of JCV viral variant with tandem repeats within the regulatory region, showed a consistently poor clinical outcome compared to patients infected with other JCV genotypes.[60]

In addition to the cell types previously mentioned in this section, JCV also infects B lymphocytes to a limited extent. Indirect infectivity assays and RT-PCR analysis have shown that the majority of JC virions remain cell-surface associated with B lymphocytes and only a minority of these virions can initiate an infection.[61] It is therefore thought the interaction of virus with these cells is inherently less efficient. It will be interesting to determine in future studies, if this inefficient viral entry can be attributed to the presence of a large number of psuedoreceptors that may sequester the virus at the cell surface. These studies would also add credence to the idea that JCV traffics to the CNS on the surface of activated B cells in the immunocompromised host.[61,62] Interestingly, lymphocytes express NF-1 proteins to similar levels as the glial cells, suggesting that regulation of viral tropism does not solely occur at the level of viral transcription.[63]

Therefore JCV tropism is likely governed by the presence of α2,6 sialic acid containing cellular receptors, the presence of trypsin-sensitive pseudoreceptors, the cell type specific expression of transcription factors as well as the genotype of the infecting JCV strain (Table 2).

BK Virus (BKV)

There is an emerging interest in understanding the biology of BK virus infection, due to its association with hemorrhagic cystitis in bone marrow recipients and ureteric stenosis as well as BKV nephropathy (BKN), which are the major cause of graft dysfunction and rejection in renal transplant recipients.[64-66] Human fibroblasts, epithelial cells, fetal brain cells (spongioblasts and astrocytes), human embryonic kidney cells (HEK), embryonic lung cells (HEL), and monkey kidney cells are highly susceptible to infection by BKV.[67,68] BKV virions have also been detected in association with lymphocytes, suggesting a hematogenous mechanism of viral spread.[69] Initial studies with this virus investigated the nature of the interaction between BKV and lymphocytes. Possatti et al[70] demonstrated the presence of cell surface receptors for BKV on B cells through a rosetting technique. Treatment of lymphocytes with various proteolytic enzymes, glycosidase and phospholipases revealed that the BK virus interaction was most sensitive to the removal of terminal sialic acid by neuraminidase and was only mildly affected by the action of both proteolytic enzymes and phosopholipases.[71] This implied that the BK virus receptor was a sialylated moiety on the surface of lymphocytes. It was later shown that polysialylated gangliosides on lymphocytes that have an R_f lower than that of GM1, are involved in BK virus binding, by examining the ability of crude ganglioside preparations as well as gangliosides inserted into liposomes, to inhibit hemagglutination by BK virus.[72] BK virus infection of Vero cells has also been shown to be affected by preincubation of the virus with preparations of free or liposome-incorporated gangliosides from Vero cells, prior to attachment to the host cells.[73] Incubation of BK virus with phospholipids extracted from Vero cells has been found to moderately inhibit adsorption of BK virus to Vero cells as well as its haemgglutination activity.[74] This inhibition was also seen upon treatment of Vero cells with phospholipases A2 and D, suggesting that phospholipids may act as a component of the BKV receptor.[74] These studies have therefore proposed that a receptor complex for BKV infection would be composed primarily of glycolipids and partially of phospholipids. Future studies designed to characterize the BKV receptor complex on Vero cells are required to confirm this hypothesis.

Given the hypothesis that the BK virus receptor complex may be comprised of ubiquitously and abundantly expressed cell surface molecules, it may be important to consider the contribution of transacting factors to the tropism of BKV. The noncoding control region (NCCR) contains the origin of replication and the enhancer/promoter elements of the BKV genome. This region is highly variable between different isolates of BKV and comparative studies have suggested that the sequence of the NCCR may regulate host cell tropism perhaps due to the rearrangement, duplication or deletion of transcription factor binding sites.[75,76] We could therefore extrapolate that the presence or absence of certain cellular trans factors may regulate the transcriptional activity of wild-type BKV. DNase I protection assays have identified 6 different regions within the BKV NCCR that are bound by HeLa cell nuclear factors. Two of the footprints were assigned to the binding of proteins from the nuclear factor 1 (NF-1) family, thereby implicating this protein family in the control of BK virus tropism.[77] This also draws an interesting parallel between the transcriptional regulation of both BK and JC virus genomes and the contribution of this regulation to viral tropism.[57,77]

In summary, the presence of gangliosides and phospholipids as well as the expression of transcriptional regulators such as NF-1, all contribute to the tropism of BKV (Table 2).

B-Lymphotropic Papovavirus (LPV)

African green monkey B-lymphotropic papovavirus (LPV), originally isolated from EBV-transformed African green monkey B-lymphoblasts, has a highly restricted tropism: it infects some Burkitt's lymphoma derived cell lines and a few EBV-immortalized human B-lymphoblastoid cells but is unable to infect any cultured malignant or normal human cells.[78,79] It has been shown that the noncoding control region of the BKV genome has tissue-specific enhancer elements that allows viral gene expression in all human hematopoietic cells.[80-82] Transfection of viral DNA into all types of hematopoietic cells, allows proper expression of viral genes and progression of the viral life cycle.[83] However, LPV particles display a very restricted tropism within the hematopoietic cell types, suggesting that early events in the viral life cycle, prior to expression of viral genes, are a major determinant of LPV tropism. Consistent with this notion, binding of LPV to several cell lines of hematopoeitic origin, correlated with permissivity, suggesting that tropism was likely determined at the level of the cellular receptor for LPV.[84] One study comparing an LPV-mutant capable of growing in T-lymphoblastoid cells to a wild type virus only capable of replication in B-lymphoblastoid cells, has shown that this change in host range can be attributed to mutations in the VP1 coding region, suggesting that virus-receptor interactions do indeed control the tropism of LPV.[85,86] Treatment of a permissive human B-lymphoma cell line, BJA-B, with trypsin and sialidases, indicated that LPV binding required the presence of α2,6-linked terminal sialic acid as well as a proteinaceous cell surface component.[84] Quantitative analysis of LPV binding to BJA-B cells indicated that there were between 600 and 1875 receptors for LPV per cell, the affinity of binding was high ($K_d = 2.9 \times 10^{-12}$M) and very stable (t $_{1/2}$ = 70minutes).[84,87] Treatment of susceptible cells with the N-glycosylation inhibitor, tunicamycin, led to an increase in the number of LPV infected cells and this has been attributed to the enhanced binding of LPV to these treated cells.[88] This effect suggests that the LPV receptor components are not likely to be N-linked glycoproteins, but are rather O-linked glycoproteins or glycolipids. The trypsin sensitivity of LPV infection, however, suggests that the former possibility is more likely, although this remains to be established.[84,88] It will be interesting to determine in the future whether the enhanced binding of LPV to susceptible cells treated with tunicamycin is due to an increase in the number or the affinity of cell surface receptors for the virus, or if indeed, N-linked glycoproteins can act as psuedoreceptors, thereby sequestering LPV at the cell surface. This would then draw an interesting parallel between LPV and PyV binding to their respective host cells.

Despite this clearly established role of the receptor in LPV tropism, there is additional evidence for cell type specific trans-acting factors that bind the Pu box motif within the enhancer of the LPV genome. Studies have shown that different nuclear factors footprint this site in different cell types and that this relates to the extent of viral transcriptional activation.[89,90]

Thus, the tropism of LPV appears to be controlled at two levels: viral interactions with either O-linked glycoprotein or glycolipid receptors as well as cell type specific trans factors that bind the Pu box motif of the viral enhancer (Table 2).

Simian Virus 40 (SV40)

Simian virus 40 was originally isolated from the rhesus kidney cells that were being used to cultivate the vaccine strains of poliovirus in the 1960s, which was inadvertently administered to innoculated individuals worldwide.[91] SV40 has since been implicated in the development of several human cancers including mesotheliomas and osteosarcomas and hence, the biology and seroepidemiology of this polyomavirus has been extensively studied.[92,93]

The natural hosts for SV40 are the Asian macaque monkeys, especially the rhesus and the African green monkey, in which it causes a widespread infection of the brain, lung, kidney, lymph node, and spleen.[94-96] Many human cell lines are susceptible to SV40 infection, including human fetal and newborn tissues and tumor cell lines but human fibroblasts are not susceptible to infection.[97-99] SV40, unlike the other polyomaviruses, does not bind sialic acid and treatment of monkey kidney cells with sialidases does not alter the infectivity of SV40.[100] Further characterization of the interaction of SV40 with monkey kidney cells showed that SV40 binding was of high affinity ($K_d = 3.76$ pM), with an estimated 9×10^4 receptors per cell.[100] SV40 infection was found to be resistant to treatment of the host cells with trypsin, chymotrypsin, phospholipases and glycopeptidases, but was sensitive to the removal of O-linked surface glycoproteins.[100] A study designed to determine the effect of SV40 infection on the expression levels of cell surface MHC-class 1 molecules, led to the identification of class I MHC protein as the primary receptor for SV40 on monkey kidney cells.[101] This discovery confirmed previous findings that the SV40 receptor is resistant to cleavage by trypsin and chymotrypsin as MHC-I is resistant to these proteases.[100,102] Further experiments showed that ectopic expression of class I MHC molecules in a null cell line, restored virus binding but not infectivity, suggesting that while MHC-I may be the major component of the receptor, additional factors also contributed to the cellular tropism of SV40.[103] Consistent with these results, the expression level and pattern of class I MHC molecules does not necessarily coincide with the pattern of SV40 binding to various cell types, again pointing to the involvement of other factors in determining susceptibility.[104] A recent study has shown that the delivery of ganglio-side GM1, to a glioma cell line, led to a significant increase in the number of SV40 infected cells, suggesting that gangliosides may also play a role in determining the tropism of SV40.[31] It is interesting to note that glycolipids also play a role during infection by PyV, BKV and JCV, in addition to SV40.[31,46,72,73] Moreover, GT1b has been implicated in both PyV and JCV entry but not in SV40 entry, correlating the presence of an additional sialic acid in the right branch residue of GT1b, with infection by sialic-acid dependent viruses.[31,46] It remains to be tested if GM1 also plays a role during infection of other permissive cell types by SV40.

Some early studies that examined the enhancer sequences of SV40 have shown that the 72-base pair tandem repeat sequences found in the enhancer of SV40 activate gene expression of a reporter construct much more efficiently in monkey kidney cells when compared to the moloney murine sarcoma virus enhancer, but expression of the same reporter gene from these promoters was reversed in mouse cells.[105] This led to the suggestion that host cell specific factors that bind the enhancer elements may control the host range of these viruses.[105] In addition, studies have shown that cells differ in factors that bind to the hormone response elements (HREs) found in the late promoter of SV40 that controls the expression of the late structural genes, and this variability contributes to defining the host range of SV40.[106]

Our current understanding of the tropism of SV40 appears to suggest the presence of a as yet unidentified coreceptor complex that in concert with the class I MHC molecules, mediates binding and entry into permissive cells. In addition, to these cell surface molecules, transcriptional regulators also contribute to the cell type specific tropism of this virus (Table 2).

Conclusions

Interaction of virions with receptors may have additional functions apart from mediating entry into the host cell, such as induction of signaling cascades and physiological changes in the cell that aid in the later stages of the viral life cycle. Purified VP1 from mouse polyomavirus has been shown to induce transient c-myc and c-fos expression upon binding to mouse fibroblasts in G_0, thereby rendering the cells competent for DNA replication.[107] Both SV40 and JCV have been shown to induce signals that can be inhibited by the tyrosine kinase inhibitor, genistein, suggesting a ligand-induced uptake mechanism utilized by both viruses.[108,109] In the case of SV40, virions could be seen stalled at the mouths of caveolae and labeled JC virions appeared sequestered at the cell surface upon genistein treatment of permissive cells.[109,110] In these studies, the MAP kinases ERK1 and ERK2 have been found to be downstream targets of the JCV induced signal and this activation is required for normal virus entry by clathrin dependent endocytosis.[109] In the case of SV40 internalization, genistein is thought to block phosphorylation of caveolin-1, which is critical for normal virus entry through caveolae.[111]

Upon entry of the virions into the host cells, there are additional factors that make the definition of viral tropism very complex. Some host range mutants of SV40 have suggested that nonpermissive cell types were deficient in proper virion assembly and release from the cell, suggesting that there may be other cytoplasmic factors that contribute to viral tropism.[112] Cross talk between different pathogens may further complicate the issue of viral tropism in vivo. For example, it has been shown that the human cytomegalovirus immediate-early transactivator 2 (IE2) is sufficient to activate JCV early gene expression in nonpermissive cell types, thereby overriding the restricted tropism of JCV.

Detailed biochemical characterization of the receptor or receptor complexes for the members of this virus family, will greatly improve our understanding of the tissue tropism of these polyomaviruses. These future studies will likely reveal a complex cellular pathway whereby the expression of cell surface viral receptors and the trans-acting factors required for normal viral gene expression are carefully coordinated in permissive cells, perhaps with the aid of the intricate cellular signaling pathways. Moreover, dissecting these pathways may lead to the development of effective anti-viral therapies which will aid in the prevention or cure of the human diseases associated with some of these polyomaviruses.

References

1. Eckhart W. Polyomavirinae and their replication. In: Fields BN, Knipe DM, eds. Virology Raven Press, 1994.
2. Keller W, Muller U, Eicken I et al. Biochemical and ultrastructural analysis of SV40 chromatin. Cold Spring Harb Symp Quant Biol 1978; 42(Pt 1):227-44.
3. Imperiale MJ. The human polyomaviruses, BKV and JCV: Molecular pathogensis of acute disease and potential role in cancer. Virology 2000; 267:1-7.
4. Frisque RJ, Bream GL, Cannella MT. Human polyomavirus JC virus genome. J Virol 1984; 51(2):458-69.
5. Pho MT, Ashok A, Atwood WJ. JC Virus enters human glial cells by clathrin dependent receptor mediated endocytosis. J Virol 2000; 74(5):2288-92.
6. Gilbert JM, Benjamin TL. Early steps of polyomavirus entry into cells. J Virol 2000; 74(18):8582-8.
7. Richterova Z, Liebl D, Horak M et al. Caveolae are involved in the trafficking of mouse polyomavirus virions and artificial VP1 pseudocapsids toward cell nuclei. J Virol 2001; 75(22):10880-91.
8. Anderson HA, Chen Y, Norkin LC. Bound simian virus 40 translocates to caveolin enriched membrane domains, and its entry is inhibited by drugs that selectively disrupt caveolae. Molecular Biology of the Cell 1996; 7:1825-34.
9. Ashok A, Atwood WJ. Contrasting roles of endosomal pH and the cytoskeleton in infection of human glial cells by JC virus and simian virus 40. J Virol 2003; 77(2):1347-56.
10. Pelkmans L, Kartenbeck J, Helenius A. Caveolar endocytosis of simian virus 40 reveals a new two-step vesicular-transport pathway to the ER. Nat Cell Biol 2001; 3(5):473-83.
11. Gilbert JM, Goldberg IG, Benjamin TL. Cell penetration and trafficking of polyomavirus. J Virol 2003; 77(4):2615-22.
12. Kasamatsu H, Lin W, Edens J et al. Visualization of antigens attached to cytoskeletal framework in animal cells: Colocalization of simian virus 40 Vp1 polypeptide and actin in TC7 cells. Proc Natl Acad Sci USA 1983; 80(14):4339-43.
13. Nakanishi A, Clever J, Yamada M et al. Association with capsid proteins promotes nuclear targeting of simian virus 40 DNA. Proc Natl Acad Sci USA 1996; 93(1):96-100.
14. Yamada M, Kasamatsu H. Role of nuclear pore complex in simian virus 40 nuclear targeting. J Virol 1993; 67(1):119-30.
15. Nakanishi A, Shum D, Morioka H et al. Interaction of the Vp3 nuclear localization signal with the importin alpha 2/beta heterodimer directs nuclear entry of infecting simian virus 40. J Virol 2002; 76(18):9368-77.
16. Dawe CJ, Freund R, Mandel G et al. Variations in polyoma virus genotype in relation to tumor induction in mice. Characterization of wild type strains with widely differing tumor profiles. Am J Pathol 1987; 127(2):243-61.
17. Fried H, Cahan LD, Paulson JC. Polyoma virus recognizes specific sialyligosaccharide receptors on host cells. Virology 1981; 109(1):188-92.
18. Cahan LD, Singh R, Paulson JC. Sialyloligosaccharide receptors of binding variants of polyomavirus. Virology 1983; 130:281-89.
19. Fried H, Cahan LD, Paulson JC. Polyomavirus recognizes specific sialyligosaccharide receptors. Virology 1981; 109:188-92.
20. Diamond L, Crawford LV. Some characteristics of large plaque and small plaque lines of polyomavirus. Virology 1964; 22:235-44.
21. Freund R, Calderone A, Dawe CJ et al. Polyomavirus tumor induction in mice, effects of polymorphisms of VP1 and large T antigen. J Virol 1991; 65:335-41.
22. Stehle T, Yan Y, Benjamin TL et al. Structure of murine polyomavirus complexed with an oligosaccharide receptor fragment. Nature 1994; 369(6476):160-3.
23. Stehle T, Harrison SC. High-resolution structure of a polyomavirus VP1-oligosaccharide complex: Implications for assembly and receptor binding. EMBO J 1997; 16(16):5139-48.
24. Bauer PH, Cui C, Stehle T et al. Discrimination between sialic acid containing receptors and pseudoreceptors regulates polyomavirus spread in the mouse. J Virol 1999; 73:5826-32.
25. Chen MH, Benjamin T. Roles of N-glycans with alpha 2,6 as well as alpha 2,3 linked sialic acid in infection by polyoma virus. Virology 1997; 233:440-42.
26. Griffith GR, Consigli RA. Cross-Linking of a polyoma attachment protein to its mouse kidney cell receptor. J Virol 1986; 58:773-81.
27. Marriott SJ, Griffith GR, Consigli RA. Octyl-B-D-glucopyranoside extracts polyomavirus receptor moieties from the surfaces of mouse kidney cells. J Virol 1987; 61:375-82.
28. Marriott SJ, Roeder DJ, Consigli RA. Anti-idiotypic antibodies to a polyomavirus monoclonal antibody recognize. J Virol 1987; 61:2747-53.

29. Herrmann M, von der Lieth CW, Stehling P et al. Consequences of a subtle sialic acid modification on the murine polyomavirus receptor. J Virol 1997; 71(8):5922-31.
30. Caruso M, Iacobini C, Passananti C et al. Protein recognition sites in polyomavirus enhancer: Formation of a novel site for NF-1 factor in an enhancer mutant and characterization of a site in the enhancer D domain. Embo J 1990; 9(3):947-55.
31. Tsai B, Gilbert JM, Stehle T et al. Gangliosides are receptors for murine polyoma virus and SV40. Embo J 2003; 22(17):4346-55.
32. Dubensky TW, Freund R, Dawe CJ et al. Polyomavirus replication in mice: Influences of VP1 type and route of innoculation. J Virol 1991; 65:342-49.
33. Amati P. Polyoma regulatory region: A potential probe for mouse cell differentiation. Cell 1985; 43(3 Pt 2):561-2.
34. Katinka M, Yaniv M, Vasseur M et al. Expression of polyoma early functions in mouse embryonal carcinoma cells depends on sequence rearrangements in the beginning of the late region. Cell 1980; 20(2):393-9.
35. De Simone V, La Mantia G, Lania L et al. Polyomavirus mutation that confers a cell-specific cis advantage for viral DNA replication. Mol Cell Biol 1985; 5(8):2142-6.
36. Maione R, Passananti C, De Simone V et al. Selection of mouse neuroblastoma cell-specific polyoma virus mutants with stage differentiative advantages of replication. Embo J 1985; 4(12):3215-21.
37. Padgett B, ZuRhein G, Walker D et al. Cultivation of papova-like virus from human brain with progressive multifocal leukoencephalopathy. Lancet 1971; I:1257-60.
38. Monaco MGC, Atwood WJ, Gravell M et al. JCV infection of hematopoetic progenitor cells, primary B lymphocytes, and tonsillar stromal cells: Implication for viral latency. J Virol 1996; 70:7004-12.
39. Houff SA, Major EO, Katz DA et al. Involvement of JC virus-infected mononuclear cells from the bone marrow and spleen in the pathogenesis of progressive multifocal leukoencephalopathy. N Engl J Med 1988; 318(5):301-5.
40. Schweighardt B, Atwood WJ. Glial cells as targets of viral infection in the human central nervous system. In: Nieto-Sampedro M, Castellano Lopez B, eds. Glial Cell Function in Health and Disease. Amsterdam: Elsevier Press, 2001:731-45.
41. Chen BJ, Atwood WJ. Construction of a novel JCV/SV40 hybrid virus (JCSV) reveals a role for the JCV capsid in viral tropism. Virology 2002; 300(2):282-90.
42. Padgett BL, Walker DL. Virologic and serologic studies of progressive multifocal leukoencephalopathy. Prog Clin Biol Res 1983; 105:107-17.
43. Liu CK, Hope AP, Atwood WJ. The human polyomavirus, JCV, does not share receptor specificity with SV40 on human glial cells. J Neurovirol 1998; 4:49-58.
44. Liu CK, Wei G, Atwood WJ. Infection of glial cells by the human polyomavirus JC is mediated by an N-linked glycoprotein containing terminal alpha 2-6 linked sialic acids. J Virol 1998; 72:4643-49.
45. Eash S, Tavares R, Stopa EG et al. Differential distribution of the JC virus receptor-type sialic acid in normal human tissues. American Journal of Pathology (In Press).
46. Komagome R, Sawa H, Suzuki T et al. Oligosaccharides as receptors for JC virus. J Virol 2002; 76(24):12992-3000.
47. Feigenbaum L, Khalili K, Major E et al. Regulation of the host range of human papovavirus JCV. Proc Natl Acad Sci USA 1987; 84(11):3695-8.
48. Suzuki S, Sawa H, Komagome R et al. Broad distribution of the JC virus receptor contrasts with a marked cellular restriction of virus replication. Virology 2001; 286(1):100-12.
49. Gee GV, Manley K, Atwood WJ. Derivation of a JC virus-resistant human glial cell line: Implications for the identification of host cell factors that determine viral tropism. Virology 2003; 314(1):101-9.
50. Amemiya K, Traub R, Durham L et al. Adjacent nuclear factor-1 and activator protein binding sites in the enhancer of the neurotropic JC virus. A common characteristic of many brain-specific genes. J Biol Chem 1992; 267:14204-11.
51. Chen N, Khalili K. Transcriptional regulation of human JC polyomavirus promoters by cellular proteins YB-1 and Pur alpha in glial cells. J Virol 1995; 69:5843-48.
52. Henson JW. Regulation of the glial-specific JC virus early promoter by the transcription factor Sp 1. J Biol Chem 1994; 269:1046-50.
53. Raj GV, Khalili K. Identification and characterization of a novel GGA/C-binding protein, GBP-i, that is rapidly inducible by cytokines. Mol Cell Biol 1994; 14(12):7770-81.
54. Kerr D, Chang C, Chen N et al. Transcription of a human neurotropic virus promoter in glial cells: Effect of YB-1 on expression of the JC virus late gene. J Virol 1994; 68:7637-43.
55. Ranganathan PN, Khalili K. The transcriptional enhancer element, kappa B, regulates promoter activity of the human neurotropic virus, JCV, in cells derived from the CNS. Nucleic Acids Res 1993; 21(8):1959-64.

56. Wegner M, Drolet DW, Rosenfeld MG. Regulation of JC virus by the POU-domain transcription factor Tst-1: Implications for progressive multifocal leukoencephalopathy. Proc Nat Acad Sci 1993; 90:4743-47.
57. Monaco MC, Sabath BF, Durham LC et al. JC virus multiplication in human hematopoietic progenitor cells requires the NF-1 class D transcription factor. J Virol 2001; 75(20):9687-95.
58. Elsner C, Dorries K. Human polyomavirus JC control region variants in persistently infected CNS and kidney tissue. J Gen Virol 1998; 79(Pt 4):789-99.
59. Shinohara T, Matsuda M, Yasui K et al. Host range bias of the JC virus mutant enhancer with DNA rearrangement. Virology 1989; 170(1):261-3.
60. Pfister LA, Letvin NL, Koralnik IJ. JC virus regulatory region tandem repeats in plasma and central nervous system isolates correlate with poor clinical outcome in patients with progressive multifocal leukoencephalopathy. J Virol 2001; 75(12):5672-6.
61. Wei G, Liu CK, Atwood WJ. JC Virus binds to primary human glial cells, tonsillar stromal cells, and B-lymphocytes, but not to T-lymphocytes. J Neurovirol 2000; 6(2):127-36.
62. Andreoletti L, Dubois V, Lescieux A et al. Human polyomavirus JC latency and reactivation status in blood of HIV-1-positive immunocompromised patients with and without progressive multifocal leukoencephalopathy. Aids 1999; 13(12):1469-75.
63. Atwood WJ, Amemiya K, Traub R et al. Interaction of the human polyomavirus, JCV, with human B-lymphocytes. Virology 1992; 190:716-23.
64. Hashida Y, Gaffney PC, Yunis EJ. Acute hemorrhagic cystitis of childhood and papovavirus-like particles. J Pediatr 1976; 89(1):85-7.
65. Binet I, Nickeleit V, Hirsch HH et al. Polyomavirus disease under new immunosuppressive drugs: A cause of renal graft dysfunction and graft loss. Transplantation 1999; 67(6):918-22.
66. Nickeleit V, Singh HK, Mihatsch MJ. Polyomavirus nephropathy: Morphology, pathophysiology, and clinical management. Curr Opin Nephrol Hypertens 2003; 12(6):599-605.
67. Takemoto KK, Mullarkey MF. Human papovavirus, BK strain: Biological studies including antigenic relationship to simian virus 40. J Virol 1973; 12(3):625-31.
68. Yoshiike K, Takemoto KK. Studies with BK virus and monkey lymphotropic papovavirus. In: Salzman NP, ed. The Papovaviridae. New York and London: Plenum Press, 1986:295-326.
69. Lecatsas G, Schoub BD, Rabson AR et al. Papovavirus in human lymphocyte cultures. Lancet 1976; 2(7991):907-8.
70. Possati L, Rubini C, Portolani M et al. Receptors for the human papovavirus BK on human lymphocytes. Arch Virol 1983; 75(1-2):131-6.
71. Seganti L, Mastromarino P, Superti F et al. Receptors for BK virus on human erythrocytes. Acta Virol 1981; 25(4):177-81.
72. Sinibaldi L, Viti D, Goldoni P et al. Inhibition of BK virus haemagglutination by gangliosides. J Gen Virol 1987; 68(Pt 3):879-83.
73. Sinibaldi L, Goldoni P, Pietropaolo V et al. Involvement of gangliosides in the interaction between BK virus and Vero cells. Arch Virol 1990; 113(3-4):291-6.
74. Sinibaldi L, Goldoni P, Pietropaolo V et al. Role of phospholipids in BK virus infection and haemagglutination. Microbiologica 1992; 15(4):337-44.
75. Johnsen JI, Seternes OM, Johansen T et al. Subpopulations of noncoding control region variants within a cell culturepassaged stock of BK virus: Sequence comparisons and biological characteristics. J Gen Virol 1995; 76(Pt 7):1571-81.
76. Moens U, Johansen T, Johnsen JI et al. Noncoding control region of naturally occurring BK virus variants: Sequence comparison and functional analysis. Virus Genes 1995; 10(3):261-75.
77. Chakraborty T, Das GC. Identification of HeLa cell nuclear factors that bind to and activate the early promoter of human polyomavirus BK in vitro. Mol Cell Biol 1989; 9(9):3821-8.
78. zur Hausen H, Gissmann L. Lymphotropic papovavirus isolated from African green monkey and human cells. Microbio Immunol 1979; 167:137-53.
79. Takemoto KK, Furuno A, Kato K et al. Biological and biochemical studies of African green monkey lymphotropic papovavirus. J Virol 1982; 42(2):502-9.
80. Mosthaf Luitgard, Pawlita Michael, Gruss Peter. A viral enhancer element specifically active in human haematopoietic cells. Science 1985; 315:587-600.
81. Pawlita M, Clad A, Hausen H. Complete DNA sequence of lymphotropic papovavirus: Prototype of a new. Virology 1985; 143:196-211.
82. Pawlita M, Mosthaf L, Clad A et al. Genome structure and host range restriction of the lymphotropic papovavirus (LPV): Identification of a viral lymphocyte specific enhancer element. Curr Top Microbiol Immunol 1984; 113:26-30.
83. Pawlita M, Lenoir G, zur Hausen H. Host range restriction of the lymphotropic papova virus (LPV) in cells of human hematopoietic origin. Haematologica 1987; 72(6 Suppl):71.

84. Haun G, Keppler OT, Bock CT et al. The cell surface receptor is a major determinant restricting the host range of the B-lymphotropic papovavirus. J Virol 1993; 67:7482-92.
85. Kanda T, Furuno A, Yoshiike K. Mutation in the VP-1 gene is responsible for the extended host range of a monkey B-lymphotropic papovavirus mutant capable of growing in T-lymphoblastoid cells. J Virol 1986; 59(2):531-4.
86. Kanda T, Takemoto KK. Monkey B-lymphotropic papovavirus mutant capable of replicating in T-lymphoblastoid cells. J Virol 1985; 55(1):96-100.
87. Herrmann M, Oppenlander M, Pawlita M. Fast and high affinity binding of B-lymphotropic papovavirus to human B-lymphoma cell lines. J Virol 1995; 69:6797-804.
88. Keppler OT, Herrmann M, Oppenlander M et al. Regulation of susceptibility and cell surface receptor for the B-lymphotropic papovavirus by N glycosylation. J Virol 1994; 68:6933-39.
89. Erselius JR, Jostes B, Hatzopoulos AK et al. Cell-type-specific control elements of the lymphotropic papovavirus enhancer. J Virol 1990; 64(4):1657-66.
90. Petterson M, Schaffner W. A purine-rich DNA sequence motif present in SV40 and lymphotropic papovavirus binds a lymphoid-specific factor and contributes to enhancer activity in lymphoid cells. Genes Dev 1987; 1(9):962-72.
91. Sweet B, Hilleman M. The vacuolating virus, SV40. Proc Soc Exp Biol Med 1960; 105:420.
92. Barbanti-Brodano G, Trabanelli C, Lazzarin L et al. [SV40 as a possible cofactor in the etiopathogenesis of mesothelioma and other human tumors]. G Ital Med Lav Ergon 1998; 20(4):218-24.
93. Carbone M, Rizzo P, Procopio A et al. SV40-like sequences in human bone tumors. Oncogene 1996; 13(3):527-35.
94. Ilyinskii PO, Daniel MD, Horvath CJ et al. Genetic analysis of simian virus 40 from brains and kidneys of macaque monkeys. J Virol 1992; 66(11):6353-60.
95. Horvath CJ, Simon MA, Bergsagel DJ et al. Simian virus 40-induced disease in rhesus monkeys with simian acquired immunodeficiency syndrome. Am J Pathol 1992; 140(6):1431-40.
96. Lednicky JA, Arrington AS, Stewart AR et al. Natural isolates of simian virus 40 from immunocompromised monkeys display extensive genetic heterogeneity: New implications for polyomavirus disease. J Virol 1998; 72(5):3980-90.
97. Shein HM, Enders JF. Multiplication and cytopathogenicity of Simian vacuolating virus 40 in cultures of human tissues. Proc Soc Exp Biol Med 1962; 109:495-500.
98. O'Neill FJ, Carroll D. Amplification of papovavirus defectives during serial low multiplicity infections. Virology 1981; 112(2):800-3.
99. O'Neill FJ, Xu XL, Miller TH. Host range determinant in the late region of SV40 and RF virus affecting growth in human cells. Intervirology 1990; 31(2-4):175-87.
100. Clayson ET, Compans RW. Characterization of simian virus 40 receptor moieties on the surfaces of Vero C1008 cells. J Virol 1989; 63:1095-100.
101. Atwood WJ, Norkin LC. Class I major histocompatibility proteins as cell surface receptors for simian virus 40. J Virol 1989; 63:4474-77.
102. Wong GH, Bartlett PF, Clark-Lewis I et al. Inducible expression of H-2 and Ia on brain cells. Nature 1984; 310:688-91.
103. Breau WC, Atwood WJ, Norkin LC. Class I major histocompatibility proteins are an essential component of the simian virus 40 receptor. J Virol 1992; 66:2037-45.
104. Basak S, Turner H, Compans RW. Expression of SV40 receptors on apical surfaces of polarized epithelial cells. Virology 1992; 190:393-402.
105. Laimins LA, Khoury G, Gorman C et al. Host-specific activation of transcription by tandem repeats from simian virus 40 and Moloney murine sarcoma virus. Proc Natl Acad Sci USA 1982; 79(21):6453-7.
106. Farrell ML, Mertz JE. Cell type-specific replication of simian virus 40 conferred by hormone response elements in the late promoter. J Virol 2002; 76(13):6762-70.
107. Zullo J, Stiles CD, Garcea RL. Regulation of c-myc and c-fos mRNA levels by polyomavirus: Distinct roles for the capsid protein VP1 and the viral early proteins. Proc Natl Acad Sci USA 1987; 84:1210-14.
108. Dangoria NS, Breau WC, Anderson HA et al. Extracellular simian virus 40 induces an ERK/MAP kinase-independent signalling pathway that activates primary response genes and promotes virus entry. J Gen Virol 1996; 77(Pt 9):2173-82.
109. Querbes W, Benmerah A, Tosoni D et al. A JC virus induced signal is required for infection of glial cells by a clathrin and eps15 dependent pathway. J Virol 2004; 78(1):250-256.
110. Chen Y, Norkin LC. Extracellular Simian Virus 40 transmits a signal that promotes virus enclosure within caveolae. Exp Cell Res 1999; 246(1):83-90.
111. Pelkmans L, Puntener D, Helenius A. Local actin polymerization and dynamin recruitment in SV40-induced internalization of caveolae. Science 2002; 296(5567):535-9.
112. Spence SL, Pipas JM. Simian virus 40 large T antigen host range domain functions in virion assembly. J Virol 1994; 68(7):4227-40.

CHAPTER 5

Serological Cross Reactivity between Polyomavirus Capsids

Raphael P. Viscidi and Barbara Clayman

Abstract

Multiple methods have been used to measure antibodies to polyomavirus virions. In order to have a common method for all polyomaviruses, we developed enzyme immunoassays (EIAs) using virus-like-particles (VLPs) produced in the baculovirus expression system. We tested serum samples from humans and rhesus macaques in VLP-based EIAs for the two human polyomaviruses, BK and JC virus, and two nonhuman primate polyomaviruses, simian virus 40 (SV40) and lymphotropic polyomavirus (LPV). Rhesus sera exhibited low level reactivity to BK and JC, and approximately 10 and 15% of human sera showed low level reactivity to SV40 and LPV, respectively. Competitive inhibition assays with VLP protein demonstrated that the reactivity of rhesus sera against BK and JC VLPs was blocked by both SV40 and the respective human polyomavirus, indicating that the BK and JC assays were detected cross-reacting antibodies Similarly, the reactivity of the majority of human sera to SV40 was blocked by both SV40 and BK or JC, demonstrating that the SV40 reactivity of human sera is largely due to cross reacting BK and JC antibodies. In contrast, the reactivity of human sera to LPV VLPs was blocked by LPV but not by BK or JC, providing serological evidence for an unknown human polyomavirus related to LPV. SV40 and LPV VLP-based EIAs and competitive inhibition assays with heterologous VLPs provide tools for seroepidemiological studies of possible SV40 and LPV-like infections of humans.

Introduction

Polyomaviruses are small nonenveloped DNA viruses. They are widely distributed in nature and have been described from humans, monkeys, cows, rabbits, mice, hamsters, chickens and parrots. The presently known human polyomaviruses are BK virus (BKV) and JC virus (JCV). Most primary infections with BKV and JCV occur in childhood and are asymptomatic. The viruses persist indefinitely as latent infections in the kidneys and B lymphocytes and can reactivate in times of immunological impairment. Reactivation of JCV may result in progressive multifocal leukoencephalopathy, a subacute demyelinating disease of the central nervous system.[1] BKV reactivation principally manifests in the kidneys as hemorrhagic cystitis or nephropathy.[2,3] Simian virus 40 (SV40) is a natural infection of some species of Asiatic macaques including the rhesus macaques of north India. Human exposure to SV40 occurred on a wide scale between 1955 and 1963 due to contamination of some lots of inactivated poliovaccines.[4] The recent detection of SV40 genomic sequences in human tumors has raised a question of SV40 infection in humans.[5-9] There is indirect evidence for human infection with another polyomavirus based on reactivity of human sera with a lymphotropic polyomavirus (LPV) of African green monkeys.[10,11]

Polyomaviruses and Human Diseases, edited by Nasimul Ahsan. ©2006 Eurekah.com and Springer Science+Business Media.

Hemagglutination inhibition (HI) assays have been the standard method for measurement of antibodies to BKV and JCV, and a virus infectivity neutralization assay has been the standard method for detection of SV40 antibodies.[12-16] There is no widely accepted standardized method for measurement of antibodies to LPV. Enzyme immunoassay (EIA) technology has become the preferred method for measurement of antiviral antibodies because EIA provides greater sensitivity and precision compared with HI and neutralization assays. EIA is also more economical for large-scale seroepidemiological studies. We recently established EIAs for BKV, JCV, SV40 and LPV using virus-like particles (VLPs) as antigens.[17] The capsid proteins of a wide range of viruses, when expressed in insect cells, yeast or *E. coli*, self assemble into empty particles that resemble native virions morphologically and antigenically. Polyomavirus capsids are composed of 72 capsomeres arranged on a T = 7 icosahedral lattice. The capsomers are pentamers of the VP1 major capsid protein, which forms the outer shell of the capsid. In addition to the 360 molecules of VP1, the native virion contains approximately 1 to 10 molecules of the minor capsid proteins VP2 and VP3. The VP1 proteins of several polyomaviruses have been expressed in yeast or insect cells and shown to self assemble into a capsid-like structure in the absence of the VP2 and VP3 proteins.[18-26] A 3D reconstruction of BKV-VLPs revealed a structure similar to that of native polyomaviruses.[26] VLPs have proven to be exceptionally good reagents for EIAs because they display surface conformational epitopes, which are often the immunodominant, type or species-specific and neutralizing epitopes. The availability of VLP-based EIAs for multiple polyomaviruses has made it possible to perform comparable serological assays for all the viruses and to evaluate cross-reactivity by adsorption studies. In this chapter we describe our detailed studies of serological cross reactivity between BKV, JCV, SV40 and LPV capsids using VLP-based EIAs.

Virus-Like Particle-Based Polyomavirus Enzyme Immunoassays

We obtained recombinant baculoviruses expressing the VP1 major capsid protein of BKV and JCV from Stephen Frye and Peter Jensen and constructed recombinant baculoviruses expressing the VP1 coding sequences of SV40, LPV and mouse polyomavirus (MPV) using the Bac-to-Bac baculovirus expression system. We purified VLPs from lysates of insect cells infected with the recombinant baculoviruses by CsCl density gradient ultracentrifugation and cation exchange or gel exclusion liquid chromatography.[17,27] SDS-PAGE analysis of purified VLPs of SV40, BKV and JCV showed a major protein band of about 40, 43 and 40 kDa, respectively, and electron microscopy of the VLP containing preparations revealed particles with a diameter of 45-50 nm, morphologically consistent with empty polyomavirus capsids (Fig. 1). The VP1 protein of LPV was approximately 40 kDa and formed 50 nm particles (data not shown). The optimum concentration of polyomavirus VLPs and serum dilution used in the EIA was determined by titration of positive and negative controls. As the assays are currently configured, wells of PolySorp microtiter plates (Nunc, Naperville, IL) are coated overnight at 4ºC with 20 to 30 nanograms of total protein per well and serum samples are tested at a 1:400 dilution. The plates are prepared the day before use and then blocked for 2 hours at room temperature with 0.5% (wt/vol) polyvinyl alcohol, MW 30,000-70,000 (Sigma, St Louis MO) in PBS (0.5% PVA). Serum samples are left to react for 1 h at 37ºC and antigen-bound immunoglobulin is detected with peroxidase-conjugated goat antibodies against human IgG (Zymed, San Francisco, CA), diluted 1:2000 in 0.5% PVA, 0.025% Tween 20, 0.8% (wt/vol) polyvinylpyrrolidone, MW 360,000 (Sigma) in PBS. After 30 min at 37ºC, color development is initiated by the addition of 2,2'-azino-di-(3-ethylbenzthiazoline-6-sulfonate) hydrogen peroxide solution (Kirkegaard and Perry, Gaithersburg, MD). The reaction is stopped after 20 min by addition of 1% dodecyl sulfate and absorbance is measured at 405 nm, with a reference wavelength of 490 nm, in an automated microtiter plate reader (Molecular Devices, Menlo Park, CA).

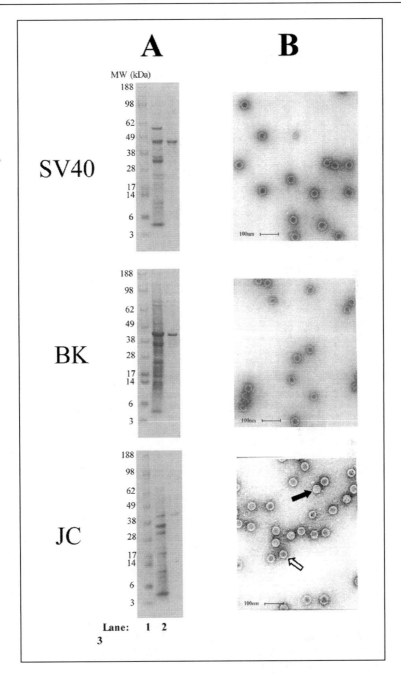

Figure 1. SDS-PAGE of lysates of insect cells infected with recombinant baculoviruses expressing SV40, BKV or JCV VP1 protein and of purified SV40, BKV and JCV VLPs (A) and transmission electron micrographs (x 105,000 magnification) of SV40, BKV, and JCV VLPs (B). In the electron micrograph, the open arrow points to an empty particle and the solid arrow to a full particle. From: Clin Diagn Lab Immunol 2003; 10(2):278-85, ©2003 American Society for Microbiology, with permission.

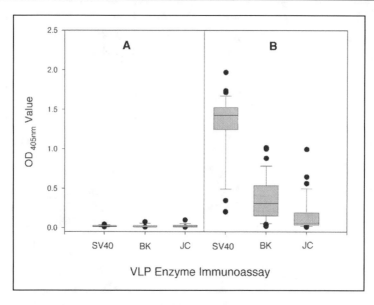

Figure 2. Reactivity of 17 SV40 neutralizing antibody negative (A) and 39 antibody positive (B) rhesus macaque sera in SV40, BKV and JCV VLP-based enzyme immunoassays. The length of the box corresponds to the 25-75% interquartile range. The horizontal line in the box indicates the median optical density value. The lines extending upward and downward from the box mark the 10th to 90th percentile range. Outlier values are shown as closed circles. From: Clin Diagn Lab Immunol 2003; 10(2):278-85, ©2003 American Society for Microbiology, with permission.

Reactivity of Rhesus Macaque Sera in VLP-Based Polyomavirus Enzyme Immunoassays

We tested rhesus sera known to be SV40 antibody–negative and antibody-positive by virus plaque neutralization tests for reactivity to SV40, BKV and JCV in the VLP EIAs (Fig. 2). The SV40 VLP EIA had 100% sensitivity and 100% specificity when compared with the reference standard of SV40 neutralization assay. The SV40-negative rhesus sera were nonreactive with all three VLPs, but the SV40 antibody-positive sera were clearly reactive with both BKV and JCV VLPs, but to a much lesser extent than with SV40 VLPS. It is unlikely that the reactivity is due to exposure of monkeys to BKV or JCV from human handlers because the BKV and JCV seroreactivity was not observed in SV40 antibody-negative sera, despite the fact that these macaques had the same risk of exposure to BKV and JCV. The most likely explanation for BKV and JCV reactivity of macaque sera is cross reacting antibodies elicited by SV40 infection. To further document cross reactivity, we developed competitive inhibition assays. Inhibition of seroreactivity to a particular VLP only with homologous VLP would be evidence of specific antibodies, whereas inhibition of seroreactivity to a particular VLP by a heterologous VLP would be evidence of cross reactivity. In preliminary experiments the reactivity of an SV40 antibody positive rhesus serum in the SV40 VLP-EIA was shown to decrease exponentially in the presence of increasing concentrations of SV40 VLPs in the diluent for the serum (Fig. 3). A concentration of 4 ug of SV40 VLP protein per ml resulted in near maximal inhibition of SV40 seroreactivity. Similar curves were obtained with other SV40 antibody positive rhesus sera (data not shown). We tested 34 SV40 antibody positive rhesus sera in the SV40 VLP EIA in the presence of 4 ug/ml of competing SV40, BKV, JCV, LPV or MPV VLP protein. The percent inhibition of SV40 reactivity by each VLP was calculated as $1 - OD_{competing\ VLP}/OD_{buffer\ control} \times 100$. In Figure 4, the percent inhibition by SV40 VLP protein is plotted versus percent inhibition by BKV VLP protein. SV40 seroreactivity was inhibited from 1.5%

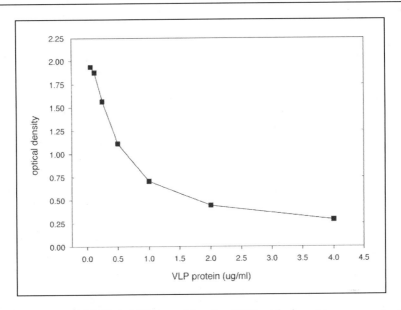

Figure 3. Competitive inhibition of SV40 reactivity of an SV40 antibody positive macaque serum by increasing concentrations of SV40 VLP protein. The serum sample was tested in the SV40-VLP EIA in the presence of serial 2-fold dilutions of SV40 VLP protein starting at a concentration of 4ug/ml. The assay was completed by the sequential addition of peroxidase-labeled goat anti-human IgG and ABTS substrate. The plate was read at 405 nm in an automated microtiter plate reader.

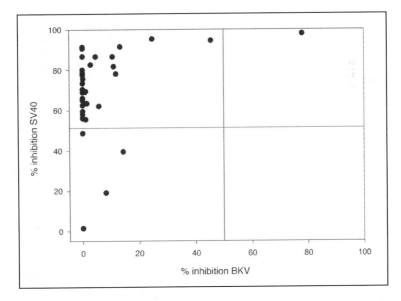

Figure 4. Scatter plot of percent competitive inhibition of SV40 reactivity of 34 macaque sera by SV40 and BKV VLP protein. Serum samples were tested in the SV40-VLP EIA in the presence of 4ug/ml of SV40 or BKV VLP protein. The assay was performed as described in the legend to Figure 3. Percent inhibition by each VLP was calculated as $1 - OD_{competing\ VLP}/OD_{buffer\ control}$ X 100. The percent inhibition by SV40 VLP protein (y-axis) is plotted versus percent inhibition by BKV VLP protein (x-axis). The horizontal and vertical lines mark 50% inhibition by SV40 and BKV VLP protein, respectively.

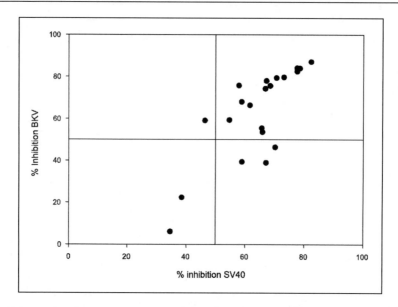

Figure 5. Scatter plot of percent competitive inhibition of BKV reactivity of 21 macaque sera by SV40 and BKV VLP protein. Serum samples were tested in the BKV or VLP EIA in the presence of 4ug/ml of SV40 or BKV VLP protein. The assay was performed as described in the legend to Figure 3 and percent inhibition was calculated as described in the legend to Figure 4. The percent inhibition by SV40 VLP protein (y-axis) is plotted versus percent inhibition by SV40 VLP protein (x-axis). The horizontal and vertical lines mark 50% inhibition by BKV and SV40 VLP protein, respectively.

to 98% by SV40 VLPs and from 0% to 78% by BKV VLPs. If horizontal and vertical reference lines are drawn at the 50% inhibition level for SV40 and BKV VLPs, respectively, the graph divides into four quadrants. We defined reactivity as SV40 specific if sera fell in the upper left quadrant (>50% inhibition by SV40 VLPs and <50% inhibition by BKV VLPs), as nonspecific if sera fell in the lower left or right quadrants (<50% inhibition by the SV40 VLPs), and cross reactive if sera fell in the upper right quadrant (>50% inhibition by SV40 and BKV VLPs). Based on these cut points, the reactivity of 29 (85%) of 34 SV40 antibody positive macaque sera was SV40 specific; the reactivity of 4 (12%) sera was nonspecific; and that of 1 (2.9%) serum sample was due to BKV cross reacting antibodies. In competitive inhibition assays with the other heterologous VLPS, we found that SV40 seroreactivity of macaque sera was never inhibited by more than 50% percent by JCV, LPV or MPV VLPs (data not shown). Thus, the data support the specificity of SV40 VLP reactivity of rhesus sera for SV40. When 21 rhesus sera reactive in the BKV VLP EIA were tested in competitive inhibition assays (Fig. 5), 15 sera were scored as cross reactive, 5 as nonspecific and one as BKV specific. The few sera that reacted to JCV VLPs were inhibited by both SV40 and JCV VLPs (data not shown). Thus, the antibodies in rhesus sera that react with BKV and JCV most likely are induced by SV40 infection and cross react with the human polyomaviruses.

Reactivity of Human Sera in VLP-Based Polyomavirus Enzyme Immunoassays

The detection of BKV and JCV cross reactive antibodies in sera of rhesus macaques infected with SV40 prompted us to test for the reciprocal response in human sera. We looked for evidence of cross reacting antibodies to SV40 in individuals infected with BKV or JCV. Infections with both BKV and JCV are common and occur early in life. The antibody prevalence to

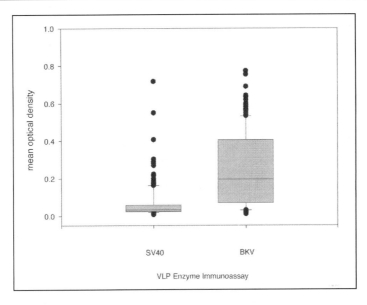

Figure 6. Comparison of reactivity of 586 human sera in BKV and SV40 VLP-based enzyme immunoassays. The control serum samples from a case-control study of lymphoma were tested for reactivity to SV40 and BKV. The length of the box corresponds to the 25-75% interquartile range. The horizontal line in the box indicates the median optical density value. The lines extending upward and downward from the box mark the 10th to 90th percentile range. Outlier values are shown as closed circles.

BKV reaches nearly 100% by the age of 10-11 years and then declines to around 70-80% in the older age groups. The antibody prevalence to JCV reaches a peak of about 75% by adult age.[13,28,29] Because of the controversy concerning human infection with SV40, a number of studies have examined the seroprevalence of SV40 in human populations. The reported prevalence of SV40-reactive antibodies in human sera by neutralization assay is between 3-10%.[16,30-35] The most comprehensive data are reported by Knowles et al[32] who examined over 2400 sera collected in England. The donors ranged in age from 1 to 69 years. The overall SV40 antibody prevalence was 3.2% and did not increase with age of the donor. More recently SV40 seroprevalence in human sera has been measured by VLP EIA. In a case-control study of lymphomas in Spain, we found 9.5% of 587 control sera reactive to SV40 in VLP EIA.[36] Sixty-five percent of the sera contained BKV antibodies. The levels of SV40 antibodies were low as compared to that of BKV antibodies (Fig. 6). In a population-based study of 415 adult sera from Washington State, Carter et al[37] reported 7.7% prevalence by SV40 VLP EIA. The origin of SV40 antibodies in humans is unclear since contact with macaques is rare in most human populations. It is possible that the antibodies reacting with SV40 are induced by the human polyomaviruses and cross-react with SV40 or that they result from infection of the human population with another virus or possibly SV40 from an unknown source.

We tested 67 human SV40 antibody positive sera in competitive inhibition assays to determine the specificity of the response. For 52 (78%) sera, greater than 50% of the SV40 reactivity was competitively inhibited by both SV40 VLP protein and either BKV or JCV VLP protein (Fig. 7). Four (6%) sera were inhibited by less than 50% by SV40 VLPs and were also weakly inhibited by BKV or JCV VLPs, suggesting that the reactivity is either nonspecific or the assay conditions were not optimal. Eleven (16%) sera gave a pattern of reactivity similar to that of SV40 antibody positive macaque sera, with greater than 50% inhibition by SV40 and less than 50% by BKV and JCV VLPs. There was no significant inhibition (>50%) of SV40

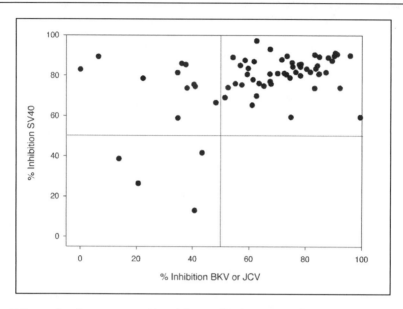

Figure 7. Scatter plot of percent competitive inhibition of SV40 reactivity of 67 human sera by SV40 and BKV or JCV VLP protein. Serum samples were tested in the SV40 VLP EIA in the presence of 4ug/ml of SV40, BKV or JCV VLP protein. The assay was performed as described in the legend to Figure 3 and percent inhibition was calculated as described in the legend to Figure 4. The percent inhibition by SV40 VLP protein (y-axis) is plotted versus maximal percent inhibition by BKV or JCV VLP protein (x-axis). The horizontal and vertical lines mark 50% inhibition by SV40 and BKV or JCV VLP protein, respectively.

seroreactivity by either LPV or MPV VLP protein (data not shown). The profile of reactivity of human sera to BKV and JCV VLPs in the competitive inhibition assays resembled that of macaque sera to SV40 VLPs. BKV seroreactivity was inhibited by BKV VLP protein but not by JCV VLP protein, and conversely, JCV seroreactivity was inhibited by JCV and not BKV VLP protein (Fig. 8). SV40, LPV, and MPV VLP proteins did not significantly inhibit either BKV or JCV seroreactivity (data not shown).

The question whether BKV or JCV antibodies cross react with SV40 has been addressed previously by comparing reactivity to SV40 and human polyomaviruses in serum samples from the same individual. Brown et al[38] examined this question for the first time in their study of 1500 sera from 28 isolated aboriginal populations that had no contact with monkeys and had not received polio vaccines. They found that 5% of 111 BKV-negative sera, and 35% of 40 BKV-positive sera (p<0.001) had low levels of neutralizing antibodies to SV40. They concluded that infection with BKV may account for the SV40 reactivity of their sera. In their study, Knowles et al[32] reported that 3.8% and 4.5% of human sera containing, respectively, BKV and JCV antibody, neutralized SV40 as compared to 0.9% and 2.5%, respectively, of BKV-negative and JCV-negative sera. These differences were highly significant. Only one of 79 sera with SV40 antibodies was negative for both BKV and JCV antibodies. Rollison et al[33] found that 11.9% of 96 BKV-positive and none of 20 BKV-negative sera neutralized SV40 (p=0.08). Using VLP-based assays, we found a correlation between BKV and SV40 antibioses (Spearman r = 0.60, p<0.001) and to a lesser extent, between JCV and SV40 antibodies (Spearman r = 0.18, p = 0.06).[17] In a population based sample of 415 adults sera tested by VLP EIA for all three viruses, Carter et al[37] reported a correlation between BKV and SV40 antibodies (Spearman r – 0.34, p < 0.001) and also between JCV and SV40 antibodies (Spearman r = 0.030, p < 0.001). Our competitive inhibition assays provide direct experimental evidence for cross reacting BKV and JCV antibodies as the explanation for the SV40 reactivity of most

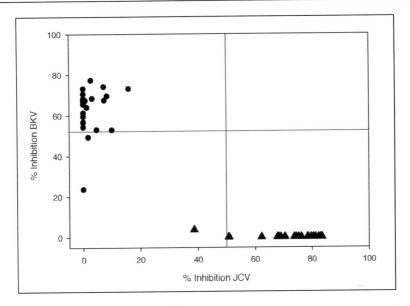

Figure 8. Scatter plot of percent competitive inhibition of BKV and JCV reactivity of 23 human sera by BKV and JCV VLP protein. Serum samples were tested in the BKV (circle) or JCV (triangle) VLP EIA in the presence of 4ug/ml of BKV or JCV VLP protein. The assay was performed as described in the legend to Figure 3 and percent inhibition was calculated as described in the legend to Figure 4. The percent inhibition by BKV VLP protein (y-axis) is plotted versus percent inhibition by JCV VLP protein (x-axis). The horizontal and vertical lines mark 50% inhibition by BKV and JCV VLP protein, respectively.

human sera. Carter et al.[37] also found that preadsorption of SV40-positive sera with BKV or JCV VLPs completely removed their SV40 reactivity.

Reactivity of Human Sera in LPV VLP-Based Enzyme Immunoassay

Lymphotropic polyomavirus was isolated from a B-lymphoblastoid cell line derived from an African green monkey.[39] Analysis of the complete genome sequence of LPV revealed conserved features of the polyomavirus genus and showed that LPV is only distantly related to SV40 and the human polyomaviruses.[40,41] Serological surveys have shown that approximately 30% of humans and all nonhuman primates surveyed, with the exception of baboons, have antibodies to LPV by either immunofluorescence, immunoprecipitation or neutralization assays.[10,11,42] We have detected LPV antibodies by VLP EIA in approximately 15% of human sera (unpublished data). In order to determine the specificity of LPV antibodies in human sera, we performed competitive inhibition assays on 42 LPV reactive human sera (Fig. 9). The LPV reactivity of 35 (83%) sera was inhibited by more than 50% by LPV VLPs and less than 50% by either BKV or JCV VLPs. Six (14%) sera were inhibited by more than 50% by LPV and BKV or JCV, and one serum sample (2%) was not inhibited by any VLP tested. These data indicate that LPV antibodies in human sera, unlike SV40 antibodies, cannot be attributed to cross reacting BKV or JCV antibodies.

Conclusions

We have demonstrated low levels of BKV and JCV antibodies in SV40 antibody positive macaques and low levels of SV40 antibodies in BKV or JCV antibody positive humans. In addition, we have shown that the BKV and JCV seroreactivity in macaques is competitively inhibited by the heterologous SV40 VLP and the SV40 seroreactivity in human sera is inhibited by heterologous BKV or JCV VLPs. Taken together the data suggest that SV40 infection

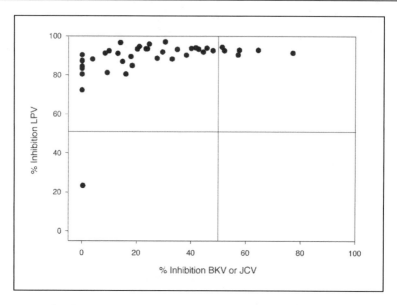

Figure 9. Scatter plot of percent competitive inhibition of LPV reactivity of 42 human sera by LPV and BKV or JCV VLP protein. Serum samples were tested in the LPV VLP EIA in the presence of 4ug/ml of LPV, BKV or JCV VLP protein. The assay was performed as described in the legend to Figure 3 and percent inhibition was calculated as described in the legend to Figure 4. The percent inhibition by LPV VLP protein (y-axis) is plotted versus maximal percent inhibition by BKV or JCV VLP protein (x-axis). The horizontal and vertical lines mark 50% inhibition by LPV and BKV or JCV VLP protein, respectively.

induces cross reacting antibodies to the human polyomaviruses and the human polyomaviruses, particularly BKV, induce cross reacting antibodies to SV40. The inhibition by a heterologous VLP cannot be explained by a shared antigen present in the VLP preparations because MPV and LPV VLPs did not inhibit the SV40 reactivity of human sera or the BKV and JCV reactivity of macaque sera. The serological cross reactivity is not surprising given the 77% amino acid identity between the JCV and SV40 VP1 proteins and the 83% identity between the BKV and SV40 VP1 proteins. However, JCV and BKV VP1 proteins, which share 80% amino acid identity, are antigenically distinct. Since BKV and JCV both infect humans, the most likely reason for the distinct antigenicity of their capsid proteins is positive selection for unique immunodominant surface epitopes, which allow one virus to replicate in the presence of immunity to the other. We identified a small number of SV40 antibody positive human sera that were inhibited by SV40 and not by BKV or JCV VLPs. Whether this reactivity is due to exposure of humans to SV40 needs to be addressed in carefully designed epidemiological studies and confirmed by detection of SV40 in biological samples from SV40 antibody positive subjects.

Lymphotropic polyomavirus was first described in 1979 and early serological studies using a variety of assay methods reported a seroprevalence of ~30% in human populations. Our studies with VLP-based assays confirm the presence of LPV reactive antibodies in a substantial proportion of human sera (~15%). Furthermore, competitive inhibition assays show that the reactivity is not the result of cross-reactivity with BKV or JCV antibodies. Although LPV was isolated from a B-lymphoblastoid cell line derived from an African green monkey, the host range of LPV is unknown. Takemoto et al[42] detected LPV antibodies in serum samples from humans and multiple species of nonhuman primates using an immunofluorescence assay. The highest seroprevalence was in gorillas (77%), Orangutans (58%), African green monkeys (48%) and squirrel monkeys (36%). In other species the seroprevalence ranged from 8-30% and in humans was 27%. The antibody titers were not reported. Given the host species specificity of other polyomaviruses it is unlikely that all these species are infected with the same virus. Serosurveys using VLP-based assays together with attempts to detect LPV viral sequences by PCR should be performed to determine the host species for LPV. Perhaps the LPV reactivity of human sera and that of some nonhuman primates is due to cross reacting antibodies induced by unknown LPV-related polyomaviruseses.

References

1. Berger JR, Major EO. Progressive multifocal leukoencephalopathy. Semin Neurol 1999; 19:193-200.
2. Reploeg MD, Storch GA, Clifford DB. Bk virus: A clinical review. Clin Infect Dis 2001; 33:191-202.
3. Hirsch HH. Polyomavirus BK nephropathy: A (re)emerging complication in renal transplantation. Am J Transplant 2002; 2:25-30.
4. Shah K, Nathanson N. Human exposure to SV40: Review and comment. Am J Epidemiol 1976; 103:1-12.
5. Strickler HD, Goedert JJ. Exposure to SV40-contaminated poliovirus vaccine and the risk of cancer- -a review of the epidemiological evidence. Dev Biol Stand 1998; 94:235-244.
6. Shah KV. Does SV40 infection contribute to the development of human cancers? Rev Med Virol 2000; 10:31-43.
7. Garcea RL, Imperiale MJ. Simian virus 40 infection of humans. J Virol 2003; 77:5039-5045.
8. Carbone M, Pass HI, Miele L et al. New developments about the association of SV40 with human mesothelioma Oncogene. 2003; 22:5173-5180.
9. Vilchez RA, Kozinetz CA, Arrington AS et al. Simian virus 40 in human cancers. Am J Med 2003; 114:675-684.
10. Takemoto KK, Segawa K. A new monkey lymphotropic papovavirus: Characterization of the virus and evidence of a related virus in humans. Prog Clin Biol Res 1983; 105:87-96.
11. Brade L, Muller-Lantzsch N, zur HH. B-lymphotropic papovavirus and possibility of infections in humans. J Med Virol 1981; 6:301-308.
12. Hamilton RS, Gravell M, Major EO. Comparison of antibody titers determined by hemagglutination inhibition and enzyme immunoassay for JC virus and BK virus. J Clin Microbiol 2000; 38:105-109.
13. Shah KV, Daniel RW, Warszawski RM. High prevalence of antibodies to BK virus, an SV40-related papovavirus, in residents of Maryland. J Infect Dis 1973; 128:784-787.
14. Padgett BL, Walker DL. Prevalence of antibodies in human sera against JC virus, an isolate from a case of progressive multifocal leukoencephalopathy. J Infect Dis 1973; 127:467-470.
15. Knowles WA, Gibson PE, Gardner SD. Serological typing scheme for BK-like isolates of human polyomavirus. J Med Virol 1989; 28:118-123.
16. Minor P, Pipkin P, Jarzebek Z et al. Studies of neutralising antibodies to SV40 in human sera. J Med Virol 2003; 70:490-495.
17. Viscidi RP, Rollison DE, Viscidi E et al. Serological cross-reactivities between antibodies to simian virus 40, BK virus, and JC virus assessed by virus-like-particle-based enzyme immunoassays. Clin Diagn Lab Immunol 2003; 10:278-285.
18. Chang D, Fung CY, Ou WC et al. Self-assembly of the JC virus major capsid protein, VP1, expressed in insect cells. J Gen Virol 1997; 78:435-1439.
19. Goldmann C, Petry H, Frye S et al. Molecular cloning and expression of major structural protein VP1 of the human polyomavirus JC virus: Formation of virus-like particles useful for immunological and therapeutic studies. J Virol 1999; 73:4465-4469.
20. Hale AD, Bartkeviciute D, Dargeviciune A et al. Expression and antigenic characterization of the major capsid proteins of human polyomaviruses BK and JC in Saccharomyces cerevisiae. J Virol Methods 2002; 104:93-98.
21. Kosukegawa A, Arisaka F, Takayama M et al. Purification and characterization of virus-like particles and pentamers produced by the expression of SV40 capsid proteins in insect cells. Biochim Biophys Acta 1996; 1290:37-45.
22. Sandalon Z, Oppenheim A. Self-assembly and protein-protein interactions between the SV40 capsid proteins produced in insect cells. Virology 1997; 237:414-421.
23. Sasnauskas K, Buzaite O, Vogel F et al. Yeast cells allow high-level expression and formation of polyomavirus-like particles. Biol Chem 1999; 380:381-386.
24. Pawlita M, Muller M, Oppenlander M et al. DNA encapsidation by viruslike particles assembled in insect cells from the major capsid protein VP1 of B-lymphotropic papovavirus. J Virol 1996; 70:7517-7526.

25. An K, Gillock ET, Sweat JA et al. Use of the baculovirus system to assemble polyomavirus capsid-like particles with different polyomavirus structural proteins: Analysis of the recombinant assembled capsid-like particles. J Gen Virol 1999; 80:1009-1016.
26. Li TC, Takeda N, Kato K et al. Characterization of self-assembled virus-like particles of human polyomavirus BK generated by recombinant baculoviruses. Virology 2003; 311:115-124.
27. Viscidi RP, Ahdieh-Grant L, Clayman B et al. Serum immunoglobulin G response to human papillomavirus type 16 virus- like particles in human immunodeficiency virus (HIV)-positive and risk- matched HIV-negative women. J Infect Dis 2003; 187:194-205.
28. Shah KV. Polyomaviruses. In: Fields BN, Knipe DM, Howley PM, eds. Fields Virology. 3rd ed. Philadelphia: Lippencott-Raven Publishers, 1996:2027-2043.
29. Stolt A, Sasnauskas K, Koskela P et al. Seroepidemiology of the human polyomaviruses. J Gen Virol 2003; 84:1499-1504.
30. Shah KV, McCrumb Jr FR, Daniel RW et al. Serologic evidence for a simian-virus-40-like infection of man. J Natl Cancer Inst 1972; 48:557-561.
31. Gerber P. Patterns of antibodies to SV40 in children following the last booster with inactivated poliomyelitis vaccines. Proc Soc Exp Biol Med 1967; 125:1284-1287.
32. Knowles WA, Pipkin P, Andrews N et al. Population-based study of antibody to the human polyomaviruses BKV and JCV and the simian polyomavirus SV40. J Med Virol 2003; 71:115-123.
33. Rollison DEM, Helzlsouer KJ, Alberg AJ et al. Serum antibodies to JC virus, BK virus, simian virus 40, and the risk of incident adult astrocytic brain tumors. Cancer Epidemiol Biomarkers Prev 2003; 12:460-463.
34. Jafar S, Rodriguez-Barradas M, Graham DY et al. Serological evidence of SV40 infections in HIV-infected and HIV- negative adults. J Med Virol 1998; 54:276-284.
35. Basetse HR, Lecatsas G, Gerber LJ. An investigation of the occurrence of SV40 antibodies in South Africa S Afr Med J 2002; 92:825-828.
36. de Sanjose S, Shah KV, Domingo-Domenech E et al. Lack of serological evidence for an association between simian virus 40 and lymphoma. Int J Cancer 2003; 104:522-524.
37. Carter JJ, Madeleine MM, Wipf GC et al. Lack of serologic evidence for prevalent simian virus 40 infection in humans. J Natl Cancer Inst 2003; 95:1522-1530.
38. Brown P, Tsai T, Gajdusek DC. Seroepidemiology of human papovaviruses. Discovery of virgin populations and some unusual patterns of antibody prevalence among remote peoples of the world. Am J Epidemiol 1975; 102:331-340.
39. zur HH, Gissmann L. Lymphotropic papovaviruses isolated from African green monkey and human cells. Med Microbiol Immunol 1979; 167:137-153.
40. Kanda T, Yoshiike K, Takemoto KK. Alignment of the genome of monkey B-lymphotropic papovavirus to the genomes of simian virus 40 and BK virus. J Virol 1983; 46:333-336.
41. Pawlita M, Clad A, zur HH. Complete DNA sequence of lymphotropic papovavirus: Prototype of a new species of the polyomavirus genus. Virology 1985; 143:196-211.
42. Takemoto KK, Furuno A, Kato K et al. Biological and biochemical studies of African green monkey lymphotropic papovavirus. J Virol 1982; 42:502-509.

CHAPTER 6

Molecular Genetics of the BK Virus

Christopher L. Cubitt

Abstract

The BK Virus (BKV) genome is a double-stranded, circular DNA molecule with genetic organization similar to other polyomaviruses, and high homology to JC Virus (JCV) and SV40. The archetypal form of BKV noncoding regulatory region (NCRR) is the infectious form of BKV that replicates in the urothelium and is excreted in the urine. Rearranged forms of the NCRR are found in kidney and other tissues often in association with disease. BKV strains can be assigned to genotype/serotype groups based on sequence variation in the VP1 gene. Sequencing of the complete genomes from patient samples will enhance BKV phylogenetic studies and identify genotypic differences and naturally occurring mutations in BKV that may correlate with incidence and/or severity of a disease. This chapter is a review of the molecular genetics of the BK virus in respect to BKV disease.

Introduction

BK virus (BKV) is the polyomavirus that, in the context of immunosuppression, is largely responsible for the diseases renal stenosis[1] and interstitial nephritis in kidney transplant patients (BK nephropathy, BKN) and hemorrhagic cystitis in bone marrow transplant patients.[2] First identified in 1970 by Gardner et al,[1] BKV is now known to be widespread in the human population. More than 80% of the world population is asymptomatically infected with the virus based on serological evidence and a recent study found that 38 out of 40 subjects (95%) had antibodies to BKV in the serum.[3]

BKV shares a 75% sequence identity with polyomavirus JC (JCV) and a 69% identity with SV40.[4,5] Like SV40 and JCV, BKV is a nonenveloped virus with 40.5-44 nm diameter icosahedral capsid. Also like the other primate polyomaviruses, the genome of BKV is a closed circular double-stranded molecule of DNA approximately 5 kb in length. Much of our knowledge pertaining to the molecular biology of BKV has been obtained from the two much more studied polyomaviruses, SV40 and JC virus. However, in recent years, there has been a renewed effort to study the BKV as this virus is increasingly recognized as a complicating infection following immunosuppressive medical procedures such as renal and bone marrow transplants. In this chapter I will review the current literature covering the molecular genetics of the BK virus in respect to BKV disease.

BKV Infection

BKV spread occurs human to human. The initial BKV infection is nearly always subclinical and typically occurs during childhood. BKV enters its new host by an oral route and it is thought that the tonsils may be the first site of BKV replication based upon studies which have detected BKV as well as JCV in tonsillar tissue.[6,7] It has been suggested by Chatterjee et al[3] that BKV enters the bloodstream by infecting PBMC as they circulate through the tonsillar tissue, therefore allowing the spread of the virus to secondary infection sites in the body including the

Polyomaviruses and Human Diseases, edited by Nasimul Ahsan. ©2006 Eurekah.com and Springer Science+Business Media.

kidneys. It is in the kidneys and urothelial cells where BKV usually remains in an asymptomatic state for the life of the host or until reactivation of BKV replication occurs during the third trimester of pregnancy[8,9] or other immunodeficient states.

At the cellular level, the pathway by which BKV enters the cell has historically been inferred from SV40 studies, however, recent studies have focused on the unique aspects of BKV infection.[10] It has been shown that a sialic-acid containing receptor is important for attachment of BK virions to the cell surface.[11] After binding to the surface of urothelial cells, BKV enters through specialized vesicles termed caveolae which normally function in the endocytosis of cholesterol.[10] After entering the cell by pinocytosis the caveolae have been observed to fuse with polymorphous membranous organelles that most likely transport the virus to the rough endoplasmic reticulum and eventually to the nucleus. However, it remains unclear whether BKV enters the nucleus as intact virions. This retrograde pathway to the rough endoplasmic reticulum protects the virus by avoiding lysosomal fusion.[12]

BKV Replication

Once in the nucleus, after viral disassembly, the BKV genome remains in an episomal state in humans. In contrast, the BKV genome has been found to integrate into the host genome when BKV is used to infect and/or transform rodent and rodent cell lines.[13-15] The genome of BKV consists of the genetically conserved early and late gene coding regions and the hyper-variable 300-500-bp noncoding regulatory region (NCRR) (see Fig. 1). Within the NCRR is the origin of replication as well as the binding sites for numerous regulatory factors involved in transcription and replication. BKV replication begins with the transcription of the early genes that encode the large T (TAg) and small t antigens (tAg) that are expressed soon after infection of the host cell. TAg and tAg are differentially translated by alternative splicing of the early mRNA transcript. Removal of the TAg intron splices the first exon with the next exon allowing translation of TAg. Alternatively, retention of the intron allows translation to reach a termination codon within the intron resulting in tAg. It is the production of the TAg that causes quiescent cells to reenter the cell cycle and thus begin replication of cellular DNA. As is the case for SV-40 and other polyomaviruses, TAg is a multifunctional transactivating factor necessary for regulating the transcription and replication of the viral genome (reviewed by Moens and Rekvig[16]). TAg autoregulates its own transcription[17] and is largely responsible for the cell transforming potential of BKV.[18] This transforming potential of TAg is attributed to its ability to bind and inhibit the function of host tumor suppressor proteins including p53 and p105RB1.[19-22] In permissive host cells, the T antigens act as regulatory proteins, directing the remaining events of viral replication that result in a productive infection.

Replication of the BKV genome occurs within the nucleus well after the transcription and translation of the early genes has begun. Replication begins at ori (Dunlop strain sequence[97]GAGGCA GAGGCG GCCTCG GCCTC[119]) within the NCRR and proceeds in both directions and is completed when the replication forks meet on the opposite side of the genome (Fig. 1).

The late genes, consisting of the structural proteins VP1, VP2 and VP3, and the agnoprotein genes, are predominately expressed after genomic replication has been initiated. VP2 and VP3 share coding sequence that is translated from the late transcript in the same reading frame while the VP1 gene is translated in a separate reading frame (Fig. 1). The completion of viral replication process concludes when the VP1, VP2 and VP3 proteins that will constitute the capsids are transported to the nucleus and the viral capsomeres assemble around the newly replicated genomes, forming stable virus particles. The replication rate of BKV in vivo is unknown, however, in vitro replication of BKV is efficient only in primary cultures of human fetal kidney or neuralgia cells[23,24] and requires 3 to 4 weeks to reach a maximum virus titer.[25,26]

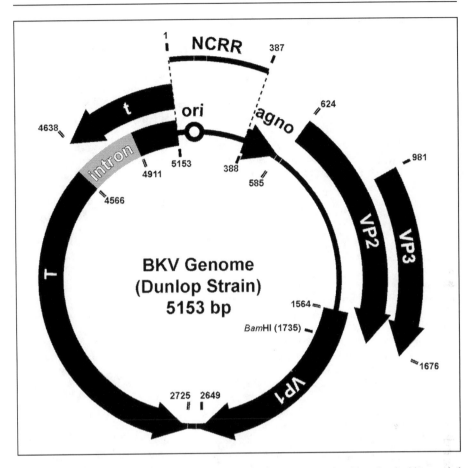

Figure 1. Genomic map of BK virus Dunlop strain. The BKV genome is a closed circular, double-stranded DNA molecule ~5-kb in size. The coding regions for the early genes, large and small T antigens (T and t), are transcribed in the counter-clockwise direction and the late genes, agnoprotein (agno) and VP1-3, are transcribed in the clockwise direction. The noncoding regulatory region (NCRR) is ~387-bp and includes the origin of replication (ori). Genomes of BKV contain a unique *Bam*H1 site located in VP1 that is useful for whole genome cloning. From Graft 2000; 5:528-535, with permission.

The NCRR of BKV and Its Rearrangements

The first NCRR DNA sequences of the BKV genome were obtained from virus preparations derived from urine and brain samples and propagated in cell cultures.[27] Because these virus stocks had replicated in vitro the sequence of the NCRR contained various deletions and duplications, typical features of some polyomaviruses grown in vitro. It was not until cloning techniques and direct PCR amplification became available for amplifying the NCRR from urine samples that the nonrearranged form of the NCRR was discovered.[28-30] It is this prearranged form (now termed the archetype) of the NCRR archetype form of BKV that predominates in the urine[30-33] and therefore is the transmissible or infectious form of the virus. A similar pattern has been found for JCV. When other tissues, such as the brain and kidneys, are screened for polyomavirus infection, JCV and BKV rearranged NCRR sequences predominate. It remains unclear how the archetype form of BKV is preferentially secreted in the urine even though both rearranged and archetype sequences can be found in the BKN kidney. This differential secretion pattern could be explained if the archetype form actively replicates in the tubular epithelial cells and rearranged forms are anatomically restricted to other parts of the kidney.

The archetype NCRR has been arbitrarily divided into regions O (142bp), P (68bp), Q (39bp), and R (63bp), based on the origin and regulatory binding sites and region S (63bp), the late leader sequence.[33,34] This scheme helps to visualize the archetype NCRR and its rearrangements. Figure 2 compares the NCRR from a rearranged strain originally isolated from peripheral blood from an immunocompetent individual (Dunlop strain, NCBI accession: PVBDUN) to a typical serotype I archetype sequence amplified from the urine of a renal transplant patient (Cubitt et al, manuscript in preparation). The archetype contains the full linear compliment of regions O, P, Q, R, and S. The rearrangement of the NCRR found in the Dunlop strain is designated O_{142}-P_{68}-P_{50}-P_{64}-S_{63} as demonstrated in Figure 2. The P region is triplicated and the entire Q and R regions are deleted. Rearrangement of most naturally occurring NCRRs involves duplication or triplication of the P region including portions of the neighboring O and Q regions. Likewise, deletions are found to occur anywhere within the P, Q, R, or S regions but frequently the deletion includes all or part of region R.

Both enhancement and suppression of transcription occurs through binding of cellular trans-activating factors. Jun/AP-1 binding to the TRE element located at the P-Q junction has been shown to have a role in regulating both early and late transcription.[34] Moens et al[35] have identified GRE/PRE binding sites in the NCRR S region which may confer regulation of transcription and replication through the presence of the steroidal hormones such as progesterone or estrogen (Fig. 2).

The mechanism and functional significance of BKV regulatory rearrangements remain unknown. However, it is believed that recombination occurs between the two newly synthesized daughter strands at nonhomologous points during replication (reviewed by Yoshiike and Takemoto[36]). It is known that archetype forms of BKV replicate poorly in cell cultures and NCRR rearrangements are necessary for efficient replication in vitro suggesting that NCRR rearrangement are an adaptation of the virus for growth in diverse cell types. Rearrangement of the NCRR can delete or add a number of binding sites for transcription factors. For example the triplication of the P region in Dunlop adds two more copies of the NF1 and CRE binding sites (Fig. 1). Kraus et al[37] have shown that binding of NF1 proteins to NF1 binding sites in the NCRR results in repression of the BKV major late promoter when template copy number is low and is relieved when template copy number is high. It is possible that through triplication of the NF1 binding sites free NF1 proteins are bound, reducing local free NF1 concentrations, and effectively mitigating NF1 repression of transcription.

Several clinical observations have demonstrated NCRR rearrangements that occur in association with disease. Boldorini et al[38] have identified both archetype and rearranged forms of BKV in renal biopsies taken from patients suspected of kidney allograft rejection.[39] Stoner et al have identified BKV DNA in a leukemia patient with tubulointersitial nephritis whose BKV disease led to a meningoencephalitis. The viral regulatory region in the PCR amplified urine sample was of the archetype form and was identical to the WWT strain. In the kidney several NCRR rearrangements were found that involved duplication followed by sequence deletion. However, in the brain and CSF, a single rearranged sequence dominated that contained a 94-bp deletion within each copy of a 71-bp tandem duplication indicating the deletion preceded the duplication. Only one clone of eight sequenced from brain and cerebrospinal fluid showed a rearrangement that differed from that of the direct PCR product. No archetype sequences were identified within the brain or CSF. A review of the BKV literature gives the impression that the NCRR of both BKV and JCV is progressively more rearranged with the progression of disease. Exactly which tissue(s) BKV rearrangement occurs in remains unknown, however, recent evidence by Chartterjee et al[3] suggests the rearrangement may occur outside the kidney. In that study, rearranged forms as well as the archetype form of BKV were found in PBL from healthy individuals.

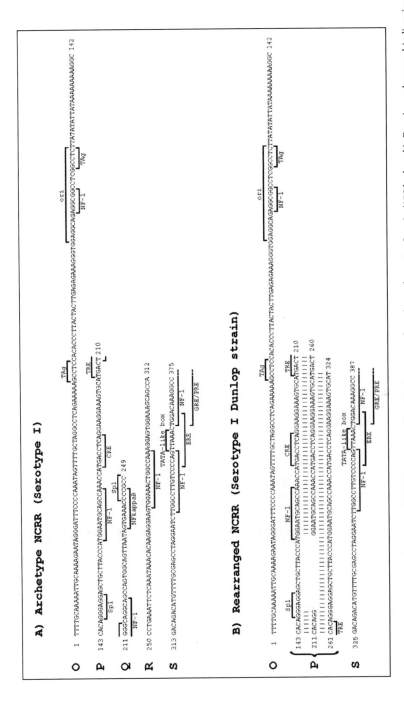

Figure 2. Comparison of archetype and rearranged NCRR sequences. Panel A. Sequence of a archetypal serotype I strain (375 bp length). Putative and proven binding sites for TAg and cellular transactivating factors are identified with brackets over or underneath the sequence. The structure is divided into regions O, P, Q, R, and S based on the boundaries of the duplications and deletions found in the rearranged form of BKV NCRR. Panel B. Sequence of a rearranged NCRR. The NCRR (387 bp length) of Dunlop strain of BKV (serotype I) is shown as an example of a rearranged regulatory region. Regions Q and R are deleted in this strain. The P region is repeated twice with an 18-bp deletion in the first repeat and a 4-bp deletion at the 3' end of the second repeat. Vertical lines represent sequence homology due to sequence duplication. From Graf 2000; 5:528-535, with permission.

Genotyping BKV

Currently, there are four known serotypes of BKV in the human population. Among the four serotypes there is nearly a 4% difference in sequence identity. Sequence variation within the VP1 gene accounts for the antigenic differences of the BKV serotypes.[40] Jin et al[41] have developed a method for determining the serotype of a BKV isolate based on the sequence and type-specific restriction endonuclease sites of a 327-bp PCR amplified region of VP1. VP1 sites which can be used to distinguish BKV genotypes are shown in Table I. Additional reliability in genotyping data could be used in conjunction with sequence data from the hyper-variable NCRR and the less conserved noncoding region between the 3' ends of VP1 and TAg (V-T intergenic region) to rapidly determine the genotype (and therefore the serotype) of clinical BKV isolates. Sequencing these two regions has proven to be invaluable for genotyping JCV and is likely to be helpful for typing and sub-typing BKV. It is interesting to note that there is only one serotype for JCV. This absence of multiple serotypes may be explained by the more highly conserved DNA sequence in JCV (approximately 1-2% difference between the eight known genotypes of JCV[42]). As progress is made in surveying BKV strains in the population, full genome sequence comparisons will be required for making accurate genotype assignments and for understanding the evolutionary relationships between them. Currently there are only three BKV strains with full genome sequences available; AS[43] (NCBI accession: M23122), Dunlop[27] (NCBI accession: PVBDUN), and MM[4] (NCBI accession: M23122)

Although considerable amounts of sequence data from the regulatory region can be found in the BKV literature, relatively little VP1 sequence data allowing genotype assignments has been published. A study by Jin et al[44] found that out of 41 BKV isolates, BKV Type I (63.4%) was the most frequently found genotype followed by Types II (21.9%), IV (9.8%), and III (4.9%). Interestingly, in this study, six out of eleven bone marrow transplant patients had Type II BKV followed by three of Type I and two of Type IV BKV. Baksh et al[45] identified BKV genotypes in the kidney tissues of 17 viral interstitial nephritis patients at the University of Pittsburgh Medical Center. Of these patients eleven were genotype I, one was type II, and five were type IV based on VP1 sequence.

Association of Mutations and Genotypes with Disease

The sequencing and genotyping of BKV in the urine of patients with a polyoma associated disease or healthy populations has the potential to provide information on type-specific disease incidence and prognosis. Several lines of evidence suggest that naturally occurring mutations in any of the BKV structural or regulatory proteins may enhance the ability of the virus to cause disease. Sequence variations may change the replication characteristics of the virus allowing the virus to grow unchecked in other organs and tissues or may help the virus to evade the host immune response. Bauer et al[46] have found that a single amino acid substitution in VP1 can affect binding of the LID strain of polyoma virus to its receptor and shorten the time to lethality by more than 3-fold in infected newborn C3H/Bi mice.

Koralnik et al[47] have identified a JCV VP1 epitope (amino acid sequence ILMWEAVTL) recognized by cytotoxic T-lymphocytes of PML patients. This epitope is semi-conserved in BKV (sequence LLMWEAVTV). Although this VP1 sequence has not been identified as an important epitote in BKV associated kidney diseases, it is conceivable that mutations in this region could alter the ability of the immune response to contain the BKV infection.

Genotyping of JCV DNA in the brain of PML patients and urine of a nonPML control group in the United States has suggested a correlation between genotype and risk of disease.[48] It was found that 19 out of 53 PML patients had JCV Type 2B compared to a matched control group in which only 7 out 119 people carried the Type 2B DNA sequence. This translates into an approximately 3-fold higher risk of developing PML for those with a Type 2B strain of JCV. One possible explanation for the observed differences in PML incidence is an amino acid change in TAg of Leu_{301} to Gln two residues away from the first coordinating cysteine in a DNA binding zinc finger.

Table 1. Representative typing sites for BKV

Serological Groups (strains)	Accession	1704	1716	1722	1744	1746	1747	1760	1766	1767	1768	1769	1770	1775	1780	1784	1787	1792	1793	1794	1809	1811	1824	1833	1848
I (DUN)	J02038	G	C	C	G	A	A	A	T	A	A	A	G	G	G	A	A	A	G	C	G	G	C	C	C
I (MM)	V01109	G	C	C	G	A	A	T	T	A	A	A	G	G	G	A	A	A	G	C	G	G	C	C	C
I (MT)	X56911	G	C	C	G	A	A	A	T	A	A	A	G	G	G	A	A	A	G	C	G	G	C	C	C
I (WW)	X56913	G	C	C	G	A	A	T	T	A	A	A	G	G	A	A	A	A	G	C	A	G	C	C	C
I (GS)	Z19537	G	C	C	G	A	A	A	T	A	A	A	G	G	G	A	A	A	G	C	A	G	C	C	C
I (Yale)	N/A	G	C	C	G	A	A	T	T	A	A	A	G	G	G	A	A	A	G	C	A	G	C	C	C
II (SB)	Z19536	G	T	C	G	T	A	A	A	G	C	A	C	C	G	A	C	G	A	A	C	A	T	T	A
III (AS)	M23122	G	T	C	G	T	G	A	A	A	A	C	A	G	G	C	C	G	A	G	C	G	G	T	A
IV (IV)	Z19535	A	T	T	A	T	G	G	T	A	A	G	A	C	G	C	C	G	A	G	C	G	C	C	A

A potentially more virulent strain of BKV (BKV(Cin)) has been identified in a AIDS patient in Cincinnati with severe tubulointerstitial nephritis.[49] BKV DNA was PCR amplified from the kidney of this patient and cloned. The sequenced NCRR of all clones were rearranged, the majority of which contained a 48-bp deletion and a 41-bp duplication. Sequencing of the TAg gene revealed a previously unidentified dinucletide mutation (TG to AA) that would result in a predicted amino acid change of a hydrophilic Gln_{169} to the hydrophobic Leu (the corresponding position is Ala in SV40). Based on SV40, this residue lies within the alpha-helical DNA binding domain of Tag.[50] Since Leu, Glu, Met, and Ala are known to be strong helix formers, this amino acid mutation could change the dynamics of protein folding or the DNA binding affinity of TAg. It is possible that a combination of both coding region mutations as well as regulatory region rearrangements as found in BKV(Cin) are important virological factors contributing to the pathogenicity of this and other BKV strains in the immunocompromised host. It is unknown whether this fatally virulent strain of BKV was generated anew in this patient or is circulating in the population. However, the same TAg mutation has recently been found in the urine of a renal transplant patient in conjunction with an archetypal regulatory region.[45]

BKV Molecular Genetics: Future Research

The first description of an archetypal regulatory region sequence in a polyomavirus can be credited to Rubinstein et al.[32] They described the regulatory region of BKV obtained from urine, and designated the structure the WW strain. The existence of an archetypal regulatory region in urinary JCV was first described by Yogo et al,[51] and the variant forms found were designated MY and CY. These genotypes were subsequently redefined on the basis of their coding regions. Numerous studies of the rearranged regulatory region in PML brain have confirmed that these structures are always constructed in a way that suggests derivation from the archetypal structure.[52-57] It now appears likely that the pattern in diseased tissue in BKV infection is much the same as for JCV. Individuals infected by strains with archetypal regulatory region sequences rearrange these in unknown tissues, apparently allowing selection of a more pathogenic viral variant. The progressive and pathogenic tissue infection occurring in PML or BKN is characterized by one or more extensive, but localized, regulatory rearrangements showing deletion and duplication of DNA sequence. These rearranged forms represent a dead-end infection. In neither virus do these rearrangements follow an easily identified pattern, in that no DNA sequence elements are regularly deleted or always duplicated.[52] However, it appears that the deletion step frequently precedes duplication, as the same deletion is often noted in both parts of a duplicated segment.

What can investigators of BKV pathogenesis in the kidney and other organs learn from the findings in the JCV field? Despite many studies, key questions remain unanswered. Nevertheless, five general principles regarding JCV rearrangements have emerged and are presented here as formulated in a review by Yogo et al:[58]

1. JCV with the archetype regulatory sequence is circulating in the human population.
2. The archetype regulatory sequence is highly conserved, in marked contrast to the hypervariable regulatory sequences of PML-derived isolates.
3. Each of the PML-type regulatory sequences is produced from the archetype by deletion and duplication or by deletion alone.
4. The shift of the regulatory region from archetype to PML type occurs during persistence in the host.
5. PML-type JCVs never return to the human population.

I suggest that analogous conclusions can be reached for BKV, for which rearrangement was originally thought be merely an artifact of in vitro virus culture.

In the case of JCV the original PML brain isolate, known as Mad-1,[59] was found to have 98-bp repeats[60] which were assumed to play a major role in the biology of the virus. However, these were absent from the archetypal regulatory region described by Yogo et al,[51] and have never been found in urine. Nor has the identical Mad-1 structure been obtained from another PML brain. This has raised questions about the distribution and significance of this prototype strain. On the other hand, the availability of both Mad-1 and the closely related Mad-4 from the American Type Culture Collection (ATCC) means that most labs studying JCV are contaminated with one or both of these strains, and tissue searches for JCV using super-sensitive PCR methods can easily be confounded by laboratory artifact. Reports of JCV Mad-1 or Mad-4 in human tumor tissues may be no more reliable that sightings of Bigfoot in the Pacific Northwest! To obviate this problem our lab has suggested the use of a Type 8 clone (pJCPNG-Ag, ATCC no. VRMC-24) obtained in Papua New Guinea.[61] DNA sequencing of the PCR product from reactions including this strain as a positive control can easily differentiate this laboratory strain from European, African, or other Asian genotypes likely to be present in infected or tumor tissues. Type 8 is unlikely to be found outside of Papua New Guinea and Melanesia in the Southwest Pacific. If similarly exotic strains of BKV can be identified for laboratory use, they would also be useful for ensuring the significance of BKV sequences amplified from infected or tumorous tissues, and transformed cells.

An additional PCR artifact associated with urine samples from PVAN patients results from the high degree of sequence similarity between SV-40 and BKV. Several commonly used SV-40 primers can amplify a DNA sequence from BKV bearing urine that when sequenced is found to be BKV DNA (personal observations). This finding reinforces the need to verify the identity of any PCR product amplified from polyomavirus containing samples.

The discoveries of BKV and JCV were originally reported in back-to-back papers in *The Lancet.*[62] These closely related persistent human viruses have much to contribute to each other for a fuller understanding of their potential for disease. Whether JCV contributes directly to polyomavirus nephropathy after transplantation is a different question that remains to be fully explored.[63]

References

1. Gardner SD, Field AM, Coleman DV et al. New human papovavirus (B.K.) isolated from urine after renal transplantation. Lancet 1971; i:1253-1257.
2. Hashida Y, Gaffney PC, Yunis EJ. Acute hemorrhagic cystitis of childhood and papova-like particles. J Pediatr 1976; 89:85-87.
3. Chatterjee M, Weyandt TB, Frisque RJ. Identification of archetype and rearranged forms of BK virus in leukocytes from healthy individuals. J Med Virol 2000; 60:353-362.
4. Yang RC, Wu R. BK virus DNA: Complete nucleotide sequence of a human tumor virus. Science 1979; 206:456-462.
5. Greenlee JE, Becker LE, Narayan O et al. Failure to demonstrate papovavirus tumor antigen in human cerebral neoplasms. Ann Neurol 1978; 3:479-481.
6. Monaco MCG, Jensen PN, Hou J et al. Detection of JC virus DNA in human tonsil tissue: Evidence for site of initial viral infection. J Virol 1998; 72:9918-9923.
7. Goudsmit J, Wertheim-van Dillen P, Van Strien A et al. The role of BK virus in acute respiratory tract disease and the presence of BKV DNA in tonsils. J Med Virol 1982; 10:91-99.
8. Bendiksen S, Rekvig OP, Van Ghelue M et al. VP1 DNA sequences of JC and BK viruses detected in urine of systemic lupus erythematosus patients reveal no differences from strains expressed in normal individuals. J Gen Virol 2000; 81:2625-2633.
9. Coleman DV, Wolfendale MR, Daniel RA et al. A prospective study of human polyomavirus infection in pregnancy. J Infect Dis 1980; 142:1-8.
10. Drachenberg CB, Papadimitriou JC, Wali R et al. BK polyoma virus allograft nephropathy: Ultrastructural features from viral cell entry to lysis. Am J Transplant 2003; 3:1383-1392.
11. Keppler OT, Stehling P, Herrmann M et al. Biosynthetic modulation of sialic acid-dependent virus-receptor interactions of two primate polyoma viruses. J Biol Chem 1995; 270:1308-1314.
12. Norkin LC, Anderson HA, Wolfrom SA et al. Caveolar endocytosis of simian virus 40 is followed by brefeldin A-sensitive transport to the endoplasmic reticulum, where the virus disassembles. J Virol 2002; 76:5156-5166.
13. Beth E, Giraldo G, Schmidt-Ullrich R et al. BK virus-transformed inbred hamster brain cells. I. Status of the viral DNA and the association of BK virus early antigens with purified plasma membranes. J Virol 1981; 40:276-284.

14. Chenciner N, Meneguzzi G, Corallini A et al. Integrated and free viral DNA in hamster tumors induced by BK virus. Proc Natl Acad Sci USA 1980; 77:975-979.
15. Meneguzzi G, Chenciner N, Corallini A et al. The arrangement of integrated viral DNA is different in BK virus- transformed mouse and hamster cells. Virology 1981; 111:139-153.
16. Moens U, Rekvig OP. Molecular biology of BK virus and clinical and basic aspects of BK virus renal infection. In: Khalili K, Stoner GL, eds. Human Polyomaviruses: Molecular and Clinical Perspectives 2001:359-408.
17. Deyerle KL, Subramani S. Human papovavirus BK early gene regulation in nonpermissive cells. Virology 1989; 169:385-396.
18. Corallini A, Tognon M, Negrini M et al. Evidence for BK virus as a human tumor virus. In: Khalili K, Stoner GL, eds. Human Polyomaviruses: Molecular and Clinical Perspectives 2001:431-60.
19. Harris KF, Christensen JB, Imperiale MJ. BK virus large T antigen: Interactions with the retinoblastoma family of tumor suppressor proteins and on cellular growth control. J Virol 1996; 70:2378-2386.
20. Shivakumar CV, Das GC. Interaction of human polyomavirus BK with the tumor-suppressor protein p53. Oncogene 1996; 13:323-332.
21. Dyson N, Bernards R, Friend SH et al. Large T antigens of many polyomaviruses are able to form complexes with the retinoblastoma protein. J Virol 1990; 64:1353-1356.
22. Kang S, Folk WR. Lymphotropic papovavirus transforms hamster cells without altering the amount or stability of p53. Virology 1992; 191:754-764.
23. Beckmann AM, Shah KV. Propagation and primary isolation of JCV and BKV in urinary epithelial cell cultures. Prog Clin Biol Res 1983; 105:3-14.
24. Takemoto KK, Mullarkey MF. Human papovavirus, BK strain: Biological studies including antigenic relationship to simian virus 40. J Virol 1973; 12:625-631.
25. Marshall WF, Telenti A, Proper J et al. Rapid detection of polyomavirus BK by a shell vial cell culture assay. J Clin Microbiol 1990; 28:1613-1615.
26. Seehafer J, Carpenter P, Downer DN et al. Observations on the growth and plaque assay of BK virus in cultured human and monkey cells. J Gen Virol 1978; 38:383-387.
27. Seif I, Khoury G, Dhar R. The genome of human papovavirus BKV. Cell 1979; 18:963-977.
28. Rubinstein R, Harley EH. BK virus DNA cloned directly from human urine confirms an archetypal structure for the transcriptional control region. Virus Genes 1988; 2:157-165.
29. Sundsfjord A, Johansen T, Flaegstad T et al. At least two types of control regions can be found among naturally occurring BK virus strains. J Virol 1990; 64:3864-3871.
30. Flaegstad T, Sundsfjord A, Arthur RR et al. Amplification and sequencing of the control regions of BK and JC virus from human urine by polymerase chain reaction. Virology 1991; 180:553-560.
31. Markowitz RB, Eaton BA, Kubik MF et al. BK virus and JC virus shed during pregnancy have predominantly archetypal regulatory regions. J Virol 1991; 65:4515-4519.
32. Rubinstein R, Pare N, Harley EH. Structure and function of the transcriptional control region of nonpassaged BK virus. J Virol 1987; 61:1747-1750.
33. Sundsfjord A, Flaegstad T, Flo R et al. BK and JC viruses in human immunodeficiency virus type 1- infected persons: Prevalence, excretion, viremia, and viral regulatory region. J Infect Dis 1994; 169:485-490.
34. Markowitz RB, Dynan WS. Binding of cellular proteins to the regulatory region of BK virus DNA. J Virol 1988; 62:3388-3398.
35. Moens U, Subramaniam N, Johansen B et al. A steroid hormone response unit in the late leader of the noncoding control region of the human polyomavirus BK confers enhanced host cell permissivity. J Virol 1994; 68:2398-2408.
36. Yoshiike K, Takemoto KK. Studies with BK virus and monkey lymphotropic papovavirus. In: Salzman NP, ed. The Papovaviridae, The Polyomaviruses. New York: Plenum Press, 1986; 1:295-326.
37. Kraus RJ, Shadley L, Mertz JE. Nuclear factor 1 family members mediate repression of the BK virus late promoter. Virology 2001; 287:89-104.
38. Boldorini R, Omodeo-Zorini E, Suno A et al. Molecular characterization and sequence analysis of polyomavirus strains isolated from needle biopsy specimens of kidney allograft recipients. Am J Clin Pathol 2001; 116:489-494.
39. Stoner GL, Alappan R, Jobes DV et al. BK virus regulatory region rearrangements in brain and cerebrospinal fluid from a leukemia patient with tubulointerstitial nephritis and meningoencephalitis. Am J Kidney Dis 2002; 39:1102-1112.
40. Knowles WA. The epidemiology of BK virus and the occurrence of antigenic and genomic subtypes. In: Khalili K, Stoner GL, eds. Human Polyomaviruses: Molecular and Clinical Perspectives. New York: Wiley-Liss, 2001:527-59.

41. Jin L. Molecular methods for identification and genotyping of BK virus. Methods Mol Biol 2001; 165:33-48.
42. Agostini HT, Jobes DV, Stoner GL. Molecular evolution and epidemiology of JC virus. In: Khalili K, Stoner GL, eds. Human Polyomaviruses: Molecular and Clinical Perspectives. New York: Wiley-Liss, 2001:491-526.
43. Tavis JE, Walker DL, Gardner SD et al. Nucleotide sequence of the human polyomavirus AS virus, an antigenic variant of BK virus. J Virol 1989; 63:901-911.
44. Jin L, Gibson PE, Knowles WA et al. BK virus antigenic variants: Sequence analysis within the capsid VP1 epitope. J Med Virol 1993; 39:50-56.
45. Baksh FK, Finkelstein SD, Swalsky PA et al. Molecular genotyping of BK and JC viruses in human polyomavirus-associated interstitial nephritis after renal transplantation. Am J Kidney Dis 2001; 38:354-365.
46. Bauer PH, Bronson RT, Fung SC et al. Genetic and structural analysis of a virulence determinant in polyomavirus VP1. J Virol 1995; 69:7925-7931.
47. Koralnik IJ, Du Pasquier RA, Kuroda MJ et al. Association of prolonged survival in HLA-A2$^+$ progressive multifocal leukoencephalopathy patients with a CTL response specific for a commonly recognized JC virus epitope. J Immunol 2002; 168:499-504.
48. Agostini HT, Ryschkewitsch CF, Singer EJ et al. JC Virus type 2B is found more frequently in brain tissue of progressive mulitifocal leukoencephalopathy patients than in urine from controls. J Hum Virol 1998; 1:200-206.
49. Smith RD, Galla JH, Skahan K et al. Tubulointerstitial nephritis due to a mutant polyomavirus BK strain, BKV (Cin), causing end-stage renal disease. J Clin Microbiol 1998; 36:1660-1665.
50. Simmons DT, Loeber G, Tegtmeyer P. Four major sequence elements of simian virus 40 large T antigen coordinate its specific and nonspecific DNA binding. J Virol 1990; 64:1973-1983.
51. Yogo Y, Kitamura T, Sugimoto C et al. Isolation of a possible archetypal JC virus DNA sequence from nonimmunocompromised individuals. J Virol 1990; 64:3139-3143.
52. Agostini HT, Ryschkewitsch CF, Singer EJ et al. JC virus regulatory region rearrangements and genotypes in progressive multifocal leukoencephalopathy: Two independent aspects of virus variation. J Gen Virol 1997; 78:659-664.
53. Ault GS, Stoner GL. Human polyomavirus JC promoter/enhancer rearrangement patterns from progressive multifocal leukoencephalopathy brain are unique derivatives of a single archetypal structure. J Gen Virol 1993; 74:1499-1507.
54. Pfister LA, Letvin NL, Koralnik IJ. JC virus regulatory region tandem repeats in plasma and central nervous system isolates correlate with poor clinical outcome in patients with progressive multifocal leukoencephalopathy. J Virol 2001; 75:5672-5676.
55. Vaz B, Cinque P, Pickhardt M et al. Analysis of the transcriptional control region in progressive multifocal leukoencephalopathy. J Neurovirol 2000; 6:398-409.
56. Yogo Y, Guo J, Iida T et al. Occurrence of multiple JC virus variants with distinctive regulatory sequences in the brain of a single patient with progressive multifocal leukoencephalopathy. Virus Genes 1994; 8:99-105.
57. Iida T, Kitamura T, Guo J et al. Origin of JC polyomavirus variants associated with progressive multifocal leukoencephalopathy. Proc Natl Acad Sci USA 1993; 90:5062-5065.
58. Yogo Y, Sugimoto C. The archetype concept and regulatory region rearrangement. In: Khalili K, Stoner GL, eds. Human Polyomaviruses: Molecular and Clinical Perspectives 2001:89-119.
59. Padgett BL, Walker DL, ZuRhein GM et al. Cultivation of papova-like virus from human brain with progressive multifocal leucoencephalopathy. Lancet 1971; 1:1257-1260.
60. Frisque RJ, Bream GL, Cannella MT. Human polyomavirus JC virus genome. J Virol 1984; 51:458-469.
61. Stoner GL, Hübner R. The human polyomaviruses: Past, present, and future. In: Khalili K, Stoner GL, eds. Human Polyomaviruses: Molecular and Clinical Perspectives. New York: Wiley-Liss, 2001:611-63.
62. Knowles WA. Serendipity - the fortuitous discovery of BK virus. In: Khalili K, Stoner GL, eds. Human Polyomaviruses: Molecular and Clinical Perspectives. New York: Wiley-Liss, 2001:45-71.
63. Randhawa P, Baksh F, Aoki N et al. JC virus infection in allograft kidneys - Analysis by polymerase chain reaction and immunohistochemistry. Transplantation 2001; 71:1300-1303.

CHAPTER 7

Serological Diagnosis of Human Polyomavirus Infection

Annika Lundstig and Joakim Dillner

Abstract

Measurement of antibody titres to the human polyomaviruses BK and JC has for many years had to rely on Hemagglutination inhibition. In recent years, viral serology based on virus-like particles (VLPs) in enzyme immunoassays (EIAs) has become widely used for a variety of viruses. We sought to establish a modern method for serological diagnosis of BK and JC viruses, by using purified VLPs containing the VP1 major capsid proteins. Antibody titres in assays based on VLPs of BKV (strain SB) showed no correlation to the titres in similar JCV assays. BKV (SB) seropositivity increases rapidly with increasing age of the children and reaches a 98 % seroprevalence at 7-9 years of age, whereas JCV seroprevalences increase more slowly with increasing age reaching 51% positivity among children 9-11 years of age. The antibody levels are almost identical in serial samples taken up to 5 years apart, suggesting that both BKV and JCV VLP seropositivitities are usually stable over time and can be used to measure cumulative exposure to these viruses.

Serology using SV40 VLPs showed strong cross-reactivity with human polyomaviruses, in particular with BKV strain AS, and establishing a specific VLP-based serology assay for SV40 required blocking with several hyperimmune sera to the human polyomaviruses. SV40-specific seropositivity also increased with increasing age of children, reaching 14% seroprevalence among children 7-9 years of age, but had limited stability over time in serial samples.

Introduction

Different serological methods have been used over the years to measure antibodies to the Polyomaviruses. Hemagglutination inhibition (HI) assay has been the standard method for this purpose because of the ease and rapidity with which it could be performed.[1] Neutralization test and plaque reduction assay, where cell culture is required as neutralization of virus infectivity has also been described for SV 40 and BKV antibody detection.[2,3]

In recent years enzyme immunoassays (EIAs) has become widely used. A modern EIA based on virus-like particles (VLPs) has been established to assess polyomavirus antibodies in serum samples.[4] The Polyoma VLPs are based on the major capsid protein, VP1 and produced in yeast cells from *Saccharomyces cerevisiae*.[5,6]

Four antigenic variants of BKV have been described: the BKV prototype, BKV AS, BKV SB and BKV IV.[7] These BKV strains were isolated from urine specimens from several patient groups.[8] Each strain has been characterized by nucleotide sequencing of the VP1 region, which encodes the major capsid protein of BKV. Specific variations correlate with serological typing by Hemagglutination inhibition.

Polyomaviruses and Human Diseases, edited by Nasimul Ahsan. ©2006 Eurekah.com and Springer Science+Business Media.

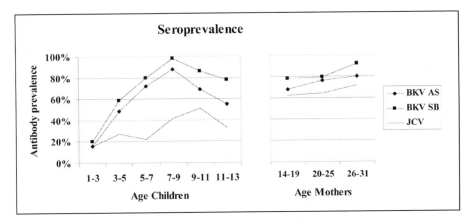

Figure 1. Prevalence of antibodies to the polyomaviruses BKV SB, BKV AS and JCV in children and pregnant women. Modification of a graph in reference 4.

Infection with BKV occurs at an earlier age than does JCV infection. In the United States antibodies to BKV are acquired by 50% of the children by the age of 3-4 years, whereas antibodies to JCV are acquired by 50% of the children by the age of 10-14 years. The antibody prevalence to BKV reaches nearly 100% by the age of 10-11 years and then declines to around 70-80% in older age groups. The antibody prevalence to JCV reaches a peak of about 75% by adult age.[9]

In a recent study, serum samples from 290 children and 150 pregnant women stratified by age of first pregnancy were analysed for antibodies to polyomaviruses in a VLP-based antibody assay. Samples from 290 Swedish children aged 1-13 years, stratified in age groups with 2 year intervals demonstrated that BKV seropositivity increased rapidly with increasing age of the children, reaching 98% seroprevalence at 7-9 years of age, followed by a minor decrease.[4,10]

JCV seroprevalence increased only slowly with increasing age and reached a 51 % positivity among children 9-11 years of age[4] (Fig. 1).

Simian Virus 40

Antibodies against SV40 have been reported to be present in about 5% of healthy individuals from the US and India. Most reactivities are low-titered, but occasionally humans with neutralizing antibody titers of very high magnitude are found (similar titers as in experimentally infected monkeys). In the few and limited surveys that have been performed, there has been no correlation of SV40 seroprevalences with history of poliovirus vaccination. This has been interpreted as showing that SV40 is now circulating in human populations.[11]

It is possible that the antibodies reacting with SV40 are induced by the human polyomaviruses and cross react with SV40. It is suggested that SV40 antibodies are cross-reactive BK antibodies and significant correlations have been reported between SV40 and BKV antibody levels, as well as with JCV antibody levels.[4,12] In our studies SV40 antibodies were most closely related to BKV strain AS antibodies (correlation coefficient = 0.70).[4] Sensitive and specific reagents for SV40 immune responses are needed to establish exposure to SV40 infection.[13] Only after blocking SV40 VLPs with high-titered hyperimmune sera against both BKV and JCV were we able to establish an SV40 serological assay devoid of cross-reactivity with BKV and JCV (unpublished observations). The SV40 seroprevalences increased with age of the children in a similar manner, as does BKV, with the peak being reached at 7-9 years of age with a 14% seroprevalence. SV40-specific antibodies appear to be less stable over time than BKV and JCV antibodies (unpublished observations).

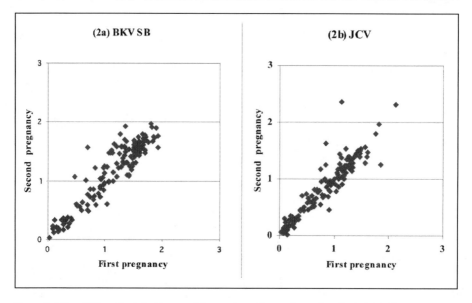

Figure 2. BK and JC antibody levels are stable over time. Comparison of antibody levels between 2 pregnancies, up to 5 years apart, using scatter plots of antibody levels. Panel a) BKV SB antibodies (r = 0.93). Panel b) JCV antibodies (r = 0.94). Modified from reference 4.

Antibody Stability

Polyomavirus seroprevalences appear to persist over time, but decrease slightly after early adulthood.[15,16] Similar seroprevalences could either reflect that antibody levels are generally stable on the individual level or may reflect that antibodies both come and go at similar rates. In our recent study 300 serum samples were taken from 150 women during their first and second pregnancy.[4] The sera were obtained from the population-based serologic screening program for congenital infections at the first trimester of pregnancy.[17,18] The 150 women were stratified by age of first pregnancy and had a second pregnancy during a 5-year follow up period. In the study, 50 women each were between 14-19 years, 20-25 years and 26-31 years of age at their first pregnancy.[4]

The BKV and JCV seropositivities were almost identical in both samples in the 5-year follow-up study. The correlation between the antibody titres in the first and second pregnancies was very high: the correlation coefficient was 0.93 for SB and 0.94 for JC (Fig. 2a,b).[4] For both BKV SB and JCV, there were no cases of seroconversion on follow-up and no cases of seroreversion (loss of seropositivity), suggesting low acquisition rates of these infections in adulthood.

Serological Methods

Hemagglutination inhibition (HI) has been the standard method for measurement of antibody titres to BKV and JCV. HI assays were used for this purpose because of the ease and rapidity with which they could be performed.[1] A lack of red blood cells agglutination means that antibodies are present and bind to viral antigen.[19] Both JC virus and BK virus have the ability to agglutinate human type O erythrocytes, unlike SV40. The major capsid protein VP1 is the predominant structural protein of the icosahedral virion particle and is responsible for attachment to cells and for erythrocyte agglutination.[20]

Many contemporary assays for measuring antibodies to viral and other antigens employ enzyme immunoassay (EIA) techniques because of their greater sensitivity and precision relative to

HI. Detection of JCV and BK virus (BKV) antigen in urine by antigen capture EIA was reported over a decade ago.[21] However, EIA for antigen capture or antibody detection did not become widely used because of the restricted range of cell types infectable by JCV, its lengthy growth cycle and poor replication capacity that made antigen preparation for use in EIAs labor intensive, time-consuming, and costly for testing large numbers of samples.[1]

A comparison of antibody titers to JC virus (JCV) or BK virus (BKV) was made by hemagglutination inhibition (HI) and enzyme immunoassay (EIA) with 114 human plasma samples. JCV was grown in SVG cells, a cell line established by immortalization of human fetal brain cells with an origin-defective mutant of SV40. BKV (Gardner strain) was grown in low-passage human embryonic kidney (HEK) cells.

The viruses were purified by density gradient ultracentrifugation and used in EIA. Antibody titers to JCV or BKV determined by HI were lower than those determined by EIA. Nevertheless, as HI titers increased so did EIA titers. When antibody data were compared by the Spearman rank correlation test, highly significant correlations were found between HI and EIA titers. The results, in agreement with those of others, suggest that humans infected by JCV or BKV produce antibodies to species-specific epitopes on their VP1 capsid protein, which is associated with hemagglutination and cellular binding.[1]

Plaque reduction assay using green monkey TC-7 cells has been described to detect SV40 serological reactivity. The plaque method is used for measuring viral infectivity and multiplication in cultured cells and whether antibodies have been able to neutralise this infectivity. Clear lysed areas or plaques develop as the viral particles are released from the infected cells.[3]

Examining presence of cytopathic effect (CPE) has also been used in neutralisation assays for both BKV and SV40.[2,3]

In recent years viral serology based on virus-like particles (VLPs) in enzyme immunoassays (EIAs) has become widely used in several viral systems,[22] including polyomavirus infections.[4] The polyoma EIA was based on yeast-expressed VLPs, containing the VP1 major capsid proteins of JC virus (JCV) and the AS and SB strains of BK virus (BKV).[23]

EIA Serological Method

The optimal concentration of polyomavirus VLPs and the serum dilutions used are determined by titration using positive and negative controls. Patients with PCR-detected BKV viruria usually have very high BKV antibody titres and serum samples from such patients are suitable as positive control reference samples. Samples from children of about 1 year of age rarely contain polyomavirus antibodies and are suitable negative control samples. We have used purified VLPs at a concentration of 6.25 ng per EIA well, coated in ice-cold PBS (pH 7.2). Half-area Costar 3690 EIA plates were incubated overnight at 4°C. After washing with 0.1% PBS/Tween, a blocking buffer consisting of 10% horse serum in PBS (HS-PBS) was added and incubated for 1 h at room temperature. The serum samples were diluted 1:40 in HS-PBS and incubated for 2 h at room temperature. The plates were washed five times with 150 ml PBS/Tween and an anti-human IgG mouse monoclonal antibody (Eurodiagnostica) diluted 1:800 was added and incubated for 90 min at room temperature. The plates were washed five times with 150 ul PBS/Tween and peroxidase-conjugated goat anti-mouse IgG (Southern Biotechnology) diluted 1:2000 in HS-PBS was added and incubated at room temperature for 60 min. Following another washing step, the peroxidase substrate ABTS was added and incubated for 30 min at room temperature and the absorbance measured at 415 nm.[4]

Preparation of Virus-Like Particles

Polyoma VLPs are based on the major capsid protein, VP1. The VP1 coding sequences were incorporated into the yeast expression vector pFX7 under the control of the galactose-inducible promoter. The pFX7- derived expression plasmids carrying the VP1 genes were transformed into the yeast *Saccharomyces cerevisiae* for cultivation. Polyoma VLPs from JCV, from the two antigenic variants of BKV (strains AS and SB) and from SV40 were produced in *S. cerevisiae*

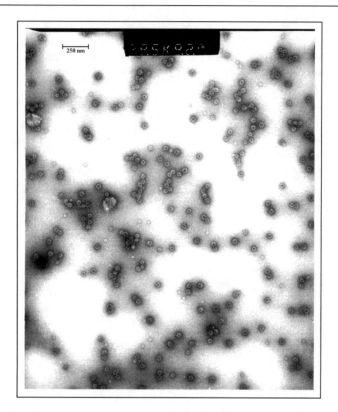

Figure 3. Negative-stain electron microscopy of BKV AS VLPs (x 28500) expressed in yeast (*S. cerevisiae*) cells.

cells. Yeast transformation, cultivation and recombinant protein purification were carried out as described previously.[5,6] Following disruption of yeast cells, lysate was centrifuged at 3000 g for 10 min at 4°C. Supernatants were then loaded on to a chilled 30% sucrose cushion and ultracentrifuged at 100 000 g for 3 h at 4°C. Resulting pellets were resuspended in 4 ml chilled disruption buffer and loaded on to CsCl gradients ranging from 1.23 to 1.38 g/ml and centrifuged at 100 000 g for 48 h. Fractions of 1 ml were collected and subjected to SDS-PAGE analysis. Fractions containing protein corresponding to a molecular mass of ~40-45 kDa were pooled, diluted with 1.31 g CsCl/ml and recentrifuged on a second CsCl gradient. Fractions were again collected and those containing VP1 were pooled and dialysed against PBS and analysed by SDS-PAGE, Western blot, electron microscopy (Fig. 3) and HI.[4,23]

Expression Systems

The expression of recombinant VP1 with spontaneous assembly into virus-like particles (VLPs) has been demonstrated for a number of polyomaviruses using both prokaryotic and baculovirus systems. VLPs of JCV have also been expressed in *Escherichia coli* and polyomavirus VP1 will also assemble into capsid-like particles in the nucleus of insect cells when expressed in the baculovirus system.[24,25] Yeast-derived recombinant VLPs offer many advantages over other expression systems in terms of protein yield, cost and ease of protein expression.[5,23]

The VLP-based assays are likely to be useful in determining past exposure to BKV and JCV in epidemiological studies and for serological diagnosis in patients at risk of polyomavirus-associated diseases or showing early signs of complications due to polyomavirus reactivation.[4]

References

1. Hamilton RS, Gravell M, Major EO. Comparison of antibody titers determined by hemagglutination inhibition and enzyme immunoassay for JC virus and BK virus. J Clin Microbiol 2000; 38(1):105-109.
2. Knowles WA, Pipkin P, Andrews N et al. Population-based study of antibody to the human polyomaviruses BKV and JCV and the simian polyomavirus SV40. J Med Virol 2003; 71(1):115-123.
3. Jafar S, Rodriguez-Barradas M, Graham DY et al. Serological evidence of SV40 infections in HIV-infected and HIV-negative adults. J Med Virol 1998; 54(4):276-284.
4. Stolt A, Sasnauskas K, Koskela P et al. Seroepidemiology of the human polyomaviruses. J Gen Virol 2003; 84(Pt 6):1499-1504.
5. Sasnauskas K, Buzaite O, Vogel F et al. Yeast cells allow high-level expression and formation of polyomavirus-like particles. Biol Chem 1999; 380(3):381-386.
6. Gedvilaite A, Frommel C, Sasnauskas K et al. Formation of immunogenic virus-like particles by inserting epitopes into surface-exposed regions of hamster polyomavirus major capsid protein. Virology 2000; 273(1):21-35.
7. Jin L, Gibson PE, Booth JC et al. Genomic typing of BK virus in clinical specimens by direct sequencing of polymerase chain reaction products. J Med Virol 1993; 41(1):11-17.
8. Jin L, Gibson PE, Knowles WA et al. BK virus antigenic variants: Sequence analysis within the capsid VP1 epitope. J Med Virol 1993; 39(1):50-56.
9. Shah KV. Polyomaviruses. 3rd ed. Philadelphia: Lipincott-Raven, 1996.
10. af Geijersstam V, Eklund C, Wang Z et al. A survey of seroprevalence of human papillomavirus types 16, 18 and 33 among children. Int J Cancer 1999; 80(4):489-493.
11. Butel JS, Lednicky JA. Cell and molecular biology of simian virus 40: Implications for human infections and disease. J Natl Cancer Inst 1999; 91(2):119-134.
12. Minor P, Pipkin P, Jarzebek Z et al. Studies of neutralising antibodies to SV40 in human sera. J Med Virol 2003; 70(3):490-495.
13. Vilchez RA, Kozinetz CA, Butel JS. Conventional epidemiology and the link between SV40 and human cancers. Lancet Oncol 2003; 4(3):188-191.
14. Padgett BL, al DLWe. Cultivation of papovalike virus from human brain with progressive multifocal leukoencephalopathy. Lancet 1971; 1:1257-1260.
15. Hogan TF, Padgett BL, Walker DL. Human polyomaviruses. In: Belshe RB, ed. Textbook of Human Virology, 1991.
16. af Geijersstam V, Kibur M, Wang Z et al. Stability over time of serum antibody levels to human papillomavirus type 16. J Infect Dis 1998; 177(6):1710-1714.
17. Kibur M, af Geijerstamm V, Pukkala E et al. Attack rates of human papillomavirus type 16 and cervical neoplasia in primiparous women and field trial designs for HPV16 vaccination. Sex Transm Infect 2000; 76(1):13-17.
18. Neel JV, Major EO, Awa AA et al. Hypothesis: "Rogue cell"-type chromosomal damage in lymphocytes is associated with infection with the JC human polyoma virus and has implications for oncopenesis. Proc Natl Acad Sci USA 1996; 93(7):2690-2695.
19. Tornatore C, Berger JR, Houff SA et al. Detection of JC virus DNA in peripheral lymphocytes from patients with and without progressive multifocal leukoencephalopathy. Ann Neurol 1992; 31(4):454-462.
20. Arthur RR, Shah KV, Yolken RH et al. Detection of human papovaviruses BKV and JCV in urines by ELISA. Prog Clin Biol Res 1983; 105:169-176.
21. Dillner J. The serological response to papillomaviruses. Semin Cancer Biol 1999; 9(6):423-430.
22. Hale AD, Bartkeviciute D, Dargeviciune A et al. Expression and antigenic characterization of the major capsid proteins of human polyomaviruses BK and JC in Saccharomyces cerevisiae. J Virol Methods 2002; 104(1):93-98.
23. Ou WC, Wang M, Fung CY et al. The major capsid protein, VP1, of human JC virus expressed in Escherichia coli is able to self-assemble into a capsid-like particle and deliver exogenous DNA into human kidney cells. J Gen Virol 1999; 80(Pt 1):39-46.
24. An K, Lovgren TR, Tilley MB et al. Use of the confocal microscope to determine polyomavirus recombinant capsid-like particle entry into mouse 3T6 cells. J Virol Methods 2000; 84(2):153-159.

CHAPTER 8

Human Polyomavirus JC and BK Persistent Infection

Kristina Doerries

Abstract

Primary contact with the human polyomaviruses (HPV) is followed by lifelong persistence of viral DNA in its host. The most prominent organs affected are the kidney, the Central Nervous System (CNS) and the hematopoietic system. Under impairment of immune competence limited activation of virus infection can be followed by prolonged virus multiplication, severe destruction of tissue and disease. The mechanisms responsible for activation episodes of the asymptomatic persistent infection are not understood and questions on cellular localization, routes of dissemination of HPV infection and its activation are controversially discussed. The type of interaction of HPVs with target organs and patients groups is highly differentiated. Organ-specific activation above basic level argues for strong dependence on the respective immune states of risk group patients. However, since immune impairment generally plays an important role in the activation of polyomavirus infection, amplification of virus deoxyribonucleic acid (DNA) and activation of virus replication is also a normal event that is probably subject to immunomodulation in the healthy individual. It also becomes clear that BKV and JCV infection is differentially regulated by mechanisms depending on the balance of immune control as well as on organ-specific signalling.

Introduction

The human polyomaviruses BKV and JCV are endemic worldwide with seroconversion rates of almost 90% by the age of 20 years. Primary infection, usually occurring during childhood or early in adulthood is followed by lifelong persistence of episomal viral genomes in target cells of infection. HPV infection regularly affects the urogenital tract, the central nervous system, lymphoid organs and as recently detected in the gastrointestinal tract. Viral persistence is characterized by the presence of genomic DNA and expression products in affected organs and body fluids (Fig. 1). Whereas infection in the immunocompetent individual is generally asymptomatic, under severe immune impairment virus infection can be highly activated, leading to destruction of tissue and disease. The most prominent underlying diseases are the acquired immune deficiency syndrome (AIDS), lymphoproliferative disorders and aggressive modern immunotherapies. These conditions are at the same time a prerequisite of activated asymptomatic virus growth. This indicates that besides immune impairment induced by the basic disorder, additional disease determining factors must come into effect in patients developing disease.

BKV most often is reported in urogenital tract diseases. Hemorrhagic cystitis can be a serious complication in bone marrow transplant (BMT) recipients and tubular nephritis with renal failure in renal transplantation (RT) patients. Rare cases of meningoencephalitis,

Polyomaviruses and Human Diseases, edited by Nasimul Ahsan. ©2006 Eurekah.com and Springer Science+Business Media.

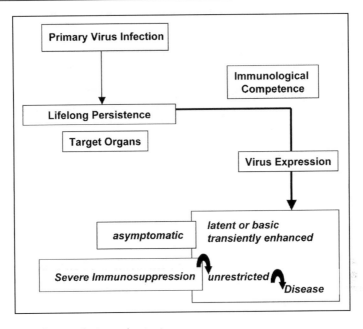

Figure 1. Course of HPV infection and activation.

pneumonitis, hemorrhagic cystitis, tubular nephritis and retinitis are described in immuno-suppressive patients and AIDS. The number of cases with highly active virus growth increased considerably with the introduction of new immunosuppressive therapeutic regimens thus confirming the dependence of virus growth on immunological control mechanisms.[1] In contrast, JCV is the cause for the demyelinating CNS disorder progressive multifocal leukoenphalopathy (PML).[2] The disease was described only in isolated cases in the pre-AIDS era, however, under the immunosuppressive state of infection with the human immune deficiency virus-1 (HIV-1) the number of PML cases increased considerably.

Although the characteristics of JCV associated PML are known for more than 30 years, the individual steps responsible for the progression from limited expression in the asymptomatic immunocompetent individual to highly active uncontrolled viral replication and disease are not yet resolved. Specifically, questions for the target cells affected in different states of infection and their possible pathogenetic role as well as for the routes of viral distribution in the host are not yet answered (Table 1). Much less is known on BKV pathogenesis, however, early studies on the BKV genome and the virus life cycle demonstrate not only genomic similarities among HPVs, but also related control mechanisms of persistence and activation. In addition, differences in viral cell specificity and transcriptional expression control are matched by common target organs of infection and close dependence on the hosts immune reactions and its signal pathways for activation of viral infection.

Virions can be repeatedly observed in target organs of infection and body fluids of persistently infected individuals (Fig. 2). It is not yet clear, whether asymptomatic persistent infection is generally in the latent state or might be continuously expressed at a low level. Recently, free virus DNA could be detected by polymerase chain reaction (PCR) in almost 100% of healthy individuals.[3] This indicates that basic HPV infection is rather characterized by a low level of expression than by a latent type of persistence. Basic infection in the immunocompetent host can be activated intermittently to a timely limited enhanced level of viral expression. It is of note that the virus load is generally very low in the persistent type of infection compared to that in polyomavirus associated diseases. Another difference is the

Table 1. Most prominent cell types involved in human Polyomavirus JC and BK infection in vivo

	Cell Types Affected*		
Organ	**JCV**	**BKV**	**HPV Disease**
Oropharynx			
tonsils	B-lymphocytes stromal cells	nd	none
Lung	no	pneumocytes fibrocytes endothelial cells smooth muscle cells	Interstitial Desquamative Pneumonitis
Urogenital system			Cystitis, Nephropathy
bladder	no	epithelial cells	
kidney	epithelial cells	epithelial cells	
sperm	sperm cells	sperm cells	
prostate	glandular epithelial cells	glandular epithelial cells	
Gastrointestinal tract			none
colon	mucosal epithelial cells	nd	
Lymphoid system			none
lymphnodes	nd	nd	
bone marrow	B lymphocytes precursor stem cells	nd	
circulating blood cells	B lymphocytes T lymphocytes granulocytes monocytes	nd	
CNS			PML BKV-related Subacute Meningoencephalitis
white matter	oligodendroglia	no	
cortex			
cerebellum	astroglia	astroglia	
	B lymphocytes	nd	
	mononuclear cells	mononuclear cells	
	no	epithelial cells	
	no	endothelial cells	
ventricular walls	no	ependymal cells	
leptomeninges	no	fibrocytes	
	no	endothelial cells	

* Methods of detection include Southern blot analysis, immunohistology, Cellseparation followed by molecular detection methods and PCR; nd celltype not determined; no not detected.

low number of cells affected in asymptomatic persistent infection compared to that in the diseased state. One important consequence for studies on the infection in immunocompetent individuals is the application of highly sensitive detection methods. This includes all molecular techniques, specifically highly sensitive PCR techniques for the detection of viral DNA and mRNA. Additionally, an important part to correlate presence of virus products with biological function is the intracellular localization of virus products by in situ hybridization and PCR techniques.

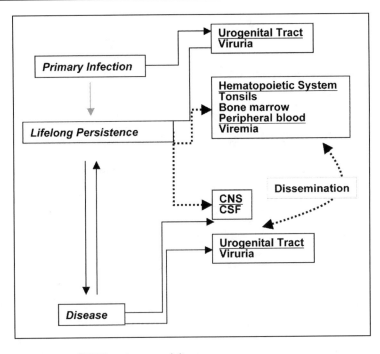

Figure 2. Target organs of HPV persistence and disease.

Urogenital Persistent BKV Infection

From the early beginnings, it was assumed that the urogenital tract is an important site of persistent BKV infection.[4] Analysis of urogenital infection revealed presence of BKV DNA at rates varying from 13% to more than 50% in asymptomatic kidney tissue in immunocompetent and deficient study groups. In these cases virus DNA was distributed in small foci throughout the kidney. This included cortex and medulla and affected surface transitional cells in ureter and bladder. Quantitative determination of renal BKV load after RT in asymptomatic kidneys revealed that the virus load is considerably lower than in BKV nephropathy predisease and disease stages. BKV DNA was also detected by PCR in asymptomatic prostate, cervical and vulvar tissue, in bladder and kidney at a rate of 50-80% of lymphoma and urinary tract carcinoma patients increasing to 87% of prostatic hyperplasia samples. Even the analysis of sperm gave an incidence of 95% for BKV DNA. In contrast to the high prevalence of BKV, lower rates of JCV were detected in cervical and vulvar tissue (5%), sperm (21%) and none in glandular tissue. Taken together, these findings confirm more pronounced tropism of BKV for urogenital tissue compared to that of JCV.[1]

Active BKV Infection in the Kidney

Dissemination of the virus to target sites and following establishment of persistence is discussed to occur at the time of primary infection and is then accompanied by limited phases of activation. However, whether all organs and cells carrying virus DNA are also able to support virus expression or may only serve as a shuttle for virus distribution is not yet clear. For the understanding of human polyomavirus/host interactions it is therefore not only important to characterize target tissues for DNA persistence, but also their potency to provide the background machinery for virus activation and shedding of virions into the surrounding compartment.[5]

BKV infection was originally detected by isolation of virions from urine and exfoliated cells. Later studies on the BKV specific humoral immune response indicated that viruria is rather due to an activation process than to primary infection or reinfection at later stages of life. The activating role of immune impairment for BK viruria became clear by studies on the influence of basic disorders at risk for polyomavirus disease on asymptomatic viruria. In HIV-1 patients viruria was detected at a rate of 44%. Subclassification according to total CD4+/CD8+ T-lymphocyte cell number and center for disease control (CDC) classification as an indicator of immunodeficiency status pointed to a correlation of immunodeficiency with BK viruria. In BMT patients asymptomatic viruria ranged to almost 100%, if multiple samples from one patient are analyzed. Intensive studies revealed that about 20% of patients with BK viruria develop microscopic hematuria. In most individuals these episodes are asymptomatic and self-limiting. It appears likely that asymptomatic viruria can progress to hematuria and with an increasing rate of tissue destruction to symptoms of cystitis. However, in about 20% of allogeneic BMT patients the activation process is not limited and proceeds to hemorrhagic cystitis. These findings indicate that persistent BKV infection is almost always activated after BMT to a level of molecular detection. It mostly remains asymptomatic and therefore seems to be a normal event comparable to the activation process in healthy individuals. Following activation to disease level is correlated with as yet unknown factors that may involve host genetics, individual competence of immunological defense, influences by the donor marrow or differences in therapeutic regimens.

In contrast to BMT, activation of BKV infection and viruria is not necessarily associated with RT. The prevalence of viruria is no more than 14%, although rates up to 43% were also reported. Most important, in RT patients a considerably lower virus load is observed in cases of asymptomatic activation compared to that after BMT. The course of virus excretion can be intermittent and highly variable in duration. Rather low rates of activation were also observed after cardiac transplantation. Apart from an influence of age and more aggressive underlying disease, the data resembled those on a group after RT. Whereas basic disease and therapeutic regimens appear to play a role in viruria after transplantation, in the autoimmune disease systemic lupus erythematosus (SLE) an elevated level of BK viruria was not influenced by immunosuppressive drugs. Thus indicating that under certain circumstances the basic immunological competence may have more impact on viruria than therapeutic intervention.

Pregnancy is the most common condition of reduced immunocompetence linked to polyomavirus activation. The onset of virus excretion occurs mostly late in the second trimester and continues intermittently often to term. Activation of infection had no clinical significance, but viruria was clearly related to the changes in the immunological control mechanisms. In contrast to BKV excretion rates of up to 47%, JC viruria appeared to be considerably lower in the same geographical regions. Immunocompetent individuals were often included as control groups in studies on polyomavirus excretion. Incidence of BKV excretion ranged from almost none to about 18%. Although one study found BKV excretion in 40% of immunocompetent patients, generally, the virus load was low, suggesting that asymptomatic BKV activation in immunocompetent adults is limited.

From these studies it appears likely that BKV activation in the urinary tract is correlated with immunological defense mechanisms that are specifically coined by a combination of the host's genetics, the respective disease and therapeutic regimens. The high variability of virus load as well as the limited number of diseased patients also suggests that additional functions must be involved in viral activation and virion production.

JCV in the Urogenital Tract

Detection of asymptomatic JCV infection in exfoliated urothelial cells of immunoimpaired patients and in pregnancy demonstrated interaction of JCV with renal cells. Direct evidence for the persistence of JCV in the kidney has been obtained by reports on the presence of episomal JCV genomes in kidney tissue. Renal JCV DNA is detectable at a rate that closely parallels the serological prevalence of JCV in randomly selected individuals and cancer patients. In contrast,

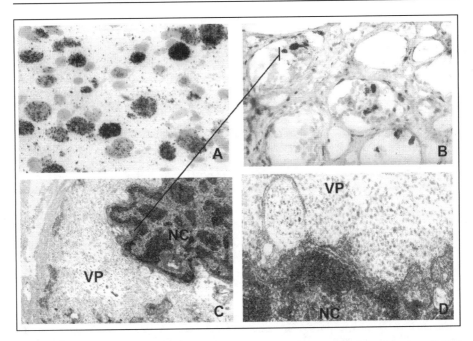

Figure 3. JCV infected cells in diseased brain and asymptomatic kidney tissue of a PML patient. A) JCV infected oligodendroglial cells at the rim of a PML focus. JCV DNA (black autoradiographic grains) was detected by in situ hybridization with a JCV-specific radioactive probe. B) Isolated JCV infected epithelial cells in the medulla of the kidney as demonstrated by ISH. C) Epithelial renal cell with vast areas of newly replicated virus. D) higher magnification of the nuclear membrane from the same renal cell. NC nucleus, VP virus particles.

the detection rate was almost 100% in PML patients with less sensitive methods, thus indicating a higher level of activation (Fig. 3). From these data it can be assumed that JCV infection in the kidney is either sensitive to activating factors mediated by basic disorders associated with PML, or the breakdown of the immune defense mechanisms commonly observed in those patients allows a higher rate of virus growth.

Activation of Urogenital JCV Infection

Provided disease specific factors have an influence on JCV expression activity in the urogenital tract, a higher level of viruria should occur in high risk patients.[4] Interestingly, under HIV-1 induced immune impairment incidence of excretion was in the range of 38%. This parallels findings in the normal population. In addition, the pattern of JCV shedding was not influenced by the AIDS status or aggressive chemotherapy. In contrast to BKV activation, excretion pattern were comparable to those of normal individuals. The frequency of excretion with increasing age did not differ significantly from that in HIV-1 negative individuals. Obviously, urogenital JCV activation is not essentially influenced by HIV-induced immune impairment or therapeutic intervention on the background of AIDS.[5]

In contrast to frequent BK viruria in BMT patients, the rate of JCV excretion was only around 7%. From the frequency of shedding, it appears likely that JCV persistent infection is not activated, but rather inhibited by BMT-associated immune impairment, either dependent on the basic disease or by therapy. In RT related interstitial nephropathies the dominant virus species is BKV. However, JCV was also detected and is occasionally coactivated at a low level. Altogether, the frequency of JC viruria is comparable to that in the normal host and the extent of BKV activation is more frequent and severe than that of JCV. In the attempt to analyze the role of CNS diseases other than PML on JCV renal activation, viruria was studied in a group of multiple sclerosis (MS) patients and a familarly related control group. The excretion rate of around 36% was comparable in both groups. Therefore an influence of disturbances in the CNS and related therapies on JCV renal infection appears to be rather unlikely. In combination with the findings on HIV-1 induced immune impairment or therapy on the background of AIDS, this is consistent with the 'rule' that PML patients must not have an enhanced incidence of JC viruria.[5,6]

JCV excretion in immunocompetent individuals demonstrated varying rates of renal activation ranging up to 52%. The extent and duration of excretion could be either stable or periodic, however incidence and virus load is clearly influenced by age. In summary, JCV activation followed by urinary excretion in the immunocompetent host is considerably higher than that of BKV. A low level of urinary coactivation demonstrates that shedding of BKV and JCV occurs independently. Excretion of the same JCV subtypes over long periods confirms that JC viruria in adults is regularly caused by the activation of a persistent virus and not by reinfection with new virus strains.

Taken together the influence of immunomodulation on BK viruria is obvious. The findings argue for a persistent BKV infection that is limited by the hosts defense mechanisms. If immunological control is impaired, infection is activated and may ultimately lead to extended disease. Interestingly, remaining immunological functions under treatment for transplantation are often able to limit infection to an extend that urogenital disease is self resolving. In contrast, JC viruria obviously occurs to a large extent in the immunocompetent host. Once polyomavirus infection is established, activation can be induced and virus multiplication may even continue throughout life on a low level. This points to a type of JCV persistence that is active at a basic level of expression in the urogenital tract under surveillance of an intact immune system.

Neurotropism of Human Polyomaviruses

BKV in the Central Nervous System

The first description of a BKV-associated CNS disease, a subacute meningoencephalitis in an AIDS patients included detection of virus DNA and virus proteins in situ as well as BK virion isolation from tissue and cerebrospinal fluid (CSF). This demonstrated that BKV can replicate in the CNS and argues for the long questioned interaction of BKV with other organs than the kidney. Most attempts to detect BKV in asymptomatic brain tissue in different groups of patients were not successful. However, when full length BKV genomes were isolated by cloning from brain tissue of immunocompetent patients without any amplification step, and nucleotide sequencing of new genomic BKV DNA subtypes confirmed the finding, presence of BKV had to be accepted. Whereas BKV and JCV has been often described together in the urogenital tract, detection of BKV DNA in the asymptomatic brain or in PML tissue is considerably less frequent than that of JCV.[1,5]

Cell free BKV DNA was detected in the CSF of patients with BKV-associated CNS disease. Therefore it can be assumed that positivity of the CSF is similarly indicative for an active BKV infection than in case of JCV infections. Studies on CSF of PML patients occasionally revealed the presence of BKV, although the patients did not suffer from BKV-typical disease. Coinfection of both polyomaviruses is widely accepted and although the data were mostly acquired on the high risk groups for PML, it can be anticipated that BKV dissemination to the CSF generally is rare event.

JCV in the Central Nervous System

JCV in PML and Asymptomatic Brain Tissue

PML is the only disease associated with JCV and occurs as a complication of preexisting chronic diseases altering immune reactivity. Several years of treatment regularly precede PML in lymphoproliferative diseases, rheumatoid arthritis, chronic asthma, sarcoidosis, chronic polymyositis or organ transplantation. All of these diseases as well as HIV-1 infection are also associated with JC viral activation in persistently infected individuals. The most important feature of PML is the cytolytically infected oligodendrocytes with JCV DNA and protein in the nucleus and the cytoplasm. In the center of PML plaques reactive astrocytes, occasionally contain JCV DNA and virus particles. At present, it is not decided whether astrocytes are permissive for JCV or may engulf infected cells. Whereas neurons were found to carry JCV in HIV/PML, involvement of ependymal cells was not reported and endothelial cell infection has not yet been confirmed by cell markers.[2,7,8]

The amount of JCV in PML tissue is very high and the virus can easily be detected (Fig. 3A). However, the pathogenic question whether PML is the result of either a cytolytic invasion of the tissue in the course of the basic disorders or a consequence of a preceding persistent infection is not yet solved. Attempts to detect JCV in nonPML tissue by less sensitive molecular techniques were unsuccessful. Even PCR analyses often give no evidence for polyomavirus persistence. However, several laboratories reported on presence of virus specific amplification or in situ hybridization in CNS tissue of randomly selected patients without PML with incidences ranging from over 30% to almost 70% (Table 2). In contrast to PML, JCV DNA sequences often were only detected in serial tissue samples, emphasizing the isolated localization of JCV positive cells (Fig. 4). Similar to the disseminated distribution of foci in PML, JCV

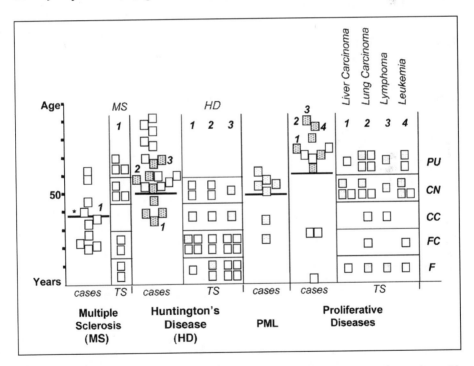

Figure 4. JCV DNA in different topographical areas of persistently infected brain tissue from patients with PML and huPyV-unrelated diseases. DNA was extracted from autopsy samples (TS) from putamen (PU), caudatus nucleus (CN), cerebellar cortex (CC), frontal cortex (FC) and frontal brain (F) of patients with Multiple Sclerosis, Huntington's disease, proliferative diseases and PML. Cases analysed were summarized and samples from PML patients were included as a positive control. All samples analysed were depicted in HD cases 1-3, MS case 1 and proliferative disease cases 1-4. DNA was subjected to Southern blot analysis with radioactive JCV-specific probes. Full length JCV genomes were cloned from cellular gene libraries: *mean value of age; open squares represent JCV-negative, shaded squares JCV-positive findings.

Table 2. Presence of JCV DNA in brain tissue of individuals without PML

Histopathological Diagnosis	Number of Cases	Age (yrs)	Presence of JCV Genomes*
Neurological diseases			
Multiple sclerosis	10	22-34	0/10
Huntington´s disease	24	20-90	9/24
Non-neurological diseases			
Malignant diseases	12	0-85	6/12
Systemic diseases	24	26-93	7/24
Total	70	0-93	22/70

* As determined by Southern blot analysis with a highly sensitive JCV-specific radioactive probe.

in asymptomatic, persistent infection has no preference for particular CNS segments. Morphologically intact, JCV-positive cells were characterized as oligodendrocytes in HIV-1 patients on the grounds of histochemical staining. However, it cannot be excluded that those patients suffered from an early stage PML. The state of full length JCV DNA was exclusively episomal with identical genetic complexity to that in the disease. The major difference between an asymptomatic and PML-type of infection is the virus load. Compared to thousands of genomes in PML foci the calculated amount of JCV DNA in asymptomatic individuals is in an estimated range of 1 to 100 genome equivalents per 20 cells. This most likely represents persistent infection and not early stages of disease.[5]

Activity of Asymptomatic JCV Infection in the CNS

The detection of persistent virus DNA is depending on the amount of DNA present and on the sensitivity of the detection system. Consequently, activation of infection with higher virus DNA load is leading to increasing detection rates. Remarkably, disorders at risk for PML including cancer, patients with AIDS, proliferative and inflammatory diseases are often associated with higher incidences of JCV DNA detection. An increased detection rate is also correlated with age. These findings demonstrate that immune impairment of basic diseases is not only a risk factor for the development of polyomavirus associated disease, but may also be responsible for a higher rate of asymptomatic activation in the CNS. Due to the asymptomatic state, the actual number of infected cells must be limited. Nevertheless, virus specific protein was detected in a limited number of oligodendrocytes and astrocytes in nonPML brain, supporting the thesis of an active expression of viral genes in JCV neuropersistence.

Similar to shedding of polyomavirus to the urine in urogenital disease, active CNS infection is strongly associated with the presence of JCV in CSF. Although not yet proven, whether virus in CSF originated from infected CNS cells or might rather be a marker for break down of the blood brain barrier and following JCV influx, the detection of JCV DNA in CSF may serve as an activation marker for increasing virus load in the CNS. Amplification of JCV DNA in CSF of nonPML patients with and without neurological symptoms is performed as control for the diagnosis of PML. Often JCV DNA is not detected in CSF of patients with high risk disorders or immunocompetent individuals with different neurological diseases, even if JCV DNA was present in corresponding CNS tissue samples. In other laboratories, JCV DNA was found in the CSF of patients with neurological symptoms and/or HIV-1 infection. This lead to highly divergent results (0.22% to 100%). Nevertheless, in the high risk groups of lymphoproliferative diseases and HIV/AIDS active infection appears to be more frequent than in immunocompetent individuals (Table 3). Although an influence of the immunosuppressive state as defined by the CD4+/CD8+ T lymphocyte ratio in AIDS patients was not found, the

Table 3. Presence of JCV DNA in cell-free cerebrospinal fluid of patients with PML and neurological symptoms unrelated to polyomavirus infection

Diagnosis	CSF Samples	JCV-Specific PCR Products[+]	Rate of JCV-Positive Samples (%)
PML	12	10/12	83
AIDS with neurological symptoms	92	45/92	48.9
HIV-1 infection with-out neurological symptoms	24	3/24	12.5
Immunocompetent with OND*	93	12/93	12.9

* Other neurological symptoms than PML. [+] Standard PCR followed by nested PCR and radioactive Southern blot analysis.

role of immune modulatory mechanisms for JCV activation was further supported by studies on multiple sclerosis (MS) patients with different types of disease. JCV DNA was detected at increasing rates in relapsing remitting courses (7.2%), in primary chronic progressive MS (CPMS) (16%) and in secondary CPMS (13%), all of which are exhibiting specific immunological response pattern. Studies on patients receiving different immunomodulatory or anti-inflammatory therapies[6] also suggested that those factors play a major role by exhibiting an activating effect on virus replication.

PCR based results on all groups of patients and materials are highly divergent. Without doubt, this is in part due to technical differences among laboratories. However, the heterogeneity of patients groups is high and epidemiological data are often not given, time of sampling in the course of disease and therapeutic regimens may also influence the activation of a persistent virus infection. Although specific conditions or factors cannot yet be pinned down, cloning and sequencing of new JCV subtypes from the CSF of nonPML individuals argues for JCV activation in persistently infected brain tissue.

Immune modulatory factors as introduced by basic diseases or therapy clearly influence JCV DNA detection rates in brain tissue and peripheral organs. JC virus persistent DNA in the CNS is similarly distributed as typically described in PML tissue. However, the amount of virus specific DNA is considerably lower, than that in the diseased state, confirming that activation of the infection must be a rare and probably transient event. Replication is probably severely restricted and thus remains limited to few isolated cells. In case of severe immunosuppression, however, it is likely that virus activation leads to an increasing number of infected cells as indicated by a higher incidence of polyomavirus DNA in multiple CNS specimens of patients with malignant diseases or higher frequency of activated JCV infection in the elderly. Whether this is followed by lifelong accumulation of JCV in the CNS that might eventually contribute to uncontrolled cytolytic virus growth and PML, can probably only be answered in an appropriate animal model. From these findings, it can be assumed that there is either intrathecal activation of JCV persistent infection or alternatively peripheral activation is associated with subclinical virus entry into the CNS, probably long before the induction of clinically overt PML.

Human Polyomaviruses in the Hematopoietic System

Persistent polyomavirus infection in peripheral organs and the central nervous system led to the question of possible routes of viral spread within the host. JCV foci in PML brain are often closely related to blood vessels and the description of polyomavirus particles in lymphocytes provided the background for discussions on an involvement of circulating hematopoietic cells in virus infection and hematogeneous spread of polyomaviruses.

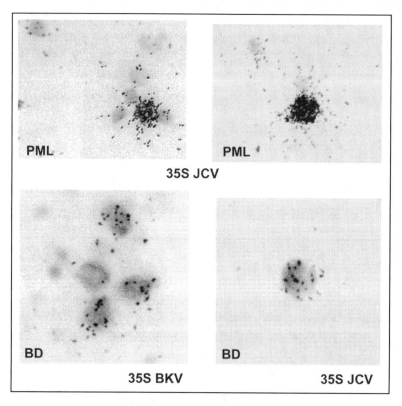

Figure 5. JCV DNA in infected hematopoietic cells of PML patients and healthy blood donors. Peripheral blood cells were purified by density gradient centrifugation and subjected to ISH with a JCV (35SJCV)- or BKV (35SBKV)-specific radioactive RNA probe. Black autoradiographic grains represent hybridized JCV DNA. Samples were collected from PML patients and healthy blood donors.

Association of BKV with Cells of the Immune System

First evidence for an interaction of BKV with hematopoietic cells was given by the report on a stimulatory effect of BKV infection on lymphocyte cultures and on BKV receptors on the surface of peripheral blood cells (PBCs). Interestingly, receptor-positive cells were described ultrastructurally as B-lymphocytes. In monocyte cultures protein expression remained negative after virus uptake indicating that monocytes might be involved in degradation rather than in virus multiplication. However, treatment of monocyte cultures with BKV-specific antisera was followed by virus replication and in mitogen-stimulated T-lymphocytes TAg expression was detected after infection. A more general role of lymphoid cells in polyomavirus infection was assumed after detection of BKV DNA in lymphoid tissue in the oropharynx including tonsils and by the demonstration of full length BKV DNA in PBCs (Fig. 5). Viral DNA was exclusively in the episomal state pointing to a persistent type of infection. PCR on PBCs from patients at risk for polyomavirus disease revealed that the incidence can increase to about 60% at later times after BMT, but following analyses remained discrepant. Similarly, in HIV-1 infected patients and immunocompetent individuals the rate of infection varied from none to almost 100%. Infection of PBCs became more likely by a study, asking for viral expression products in blood donors. Early BKV mRNA was detected by reverse transcription (RT) PCR in all samples that were positive by PCR for BKV DNA, thus providing evidence for an active expression of BKV in lymphoid cells.[9]

The divergence of studies on the tropism of BKV for circulating cells appears to be even higher than in other compartments of the host. Besides technical and study group differences, this can also be related to a possible individual susceptibility of blood cell subpopulations, to the half-life of an affected cell type or to the state of infection at the time of sampling. In addition, the sensitivity of the assays is crucial, as the amount of BKV DNA was estimated to be very low. Although a decision on the role of BKV infection in PBCs is rather difficult, with the localization of BKV specific DNA in PBCs by radioactive in situ hybridization, the detection of mRNA, and the indirect evidence for BKV susceptibility of monocytes, there is a body of evidence arguing for a regular blood cell tropism of BK virus in the host.

Studies on BKV DNA in plasma of RT patients with BKV associated viral nephropathy reported on free virus and stated that viremia and viruria is not always related quantitatively. Provided PBC infection contributes to BKV viremia, these findings argue for independent BKV activation at different sites of persistence. In contrast, in another group of patients BK virus load decreased not only in urine but also in plasma after successful therapy.[1] This rather indicates that activated BKV infection in the kidney is related to virus load in plasma and may therefore contribute to the circulating virus load. As therapeutic immune impairment could additionally be a modulating factor for BKV infection in the lymphoid compartment, at present factors and conditions influencing BKV hematopoietic infection cannot yet be defined.

JCV in Lymphoid Organs and Blood Cells

JCV infection in hematopoietic cells and their possible role as vectors for virus dissemination was already addressed in early studies, but lymphoid tissue was only occasionally found positive for JCV. The exception was a report on JCV DNA in 40% of spleen samples from HIV/PML patients suggesting that virus infection and following activation may be accompanied by accumulation of virus in lymphoid organs. Infected mononuclear cells were localized to Virchow-Robin spaces in the brain and infected glial cells adjacent to blood vessels pointed to a passage of infected circulating cells to the CNS. The idea of lymphocytes as a reservoir for JCV was also supported by the detection of tonsillar B-lymphocytes and stromal cells as target cells for JCV infection.[10] This argued for the involvement of circulating cells in persistent infection. Studies on PBCs by standard PCR analyses on immunocompetent and healthy individuals rendered highly variable results, but incidences of up to 80% were reported. If highly sensitive PCR techniques were combined with radioactive detection methods these rates even increased to almost 100%. The concentration of virus specific DNA was estimated to be less than one genome equivalent in 20 cells. This is on the borderline of detection and may explain the variable detection rates or even failure to amplify JCV DNA.

Several laboratories concentrated on the analysis of JCV DNA in blood cells of PML patients. JCV DNA was detected by in situ hybridization in 31% of mononuclear cells in bone marrow and PBCs. In following PCR studies it became clear that JCV DNA is consistently demonstrable in the cells. Irrespective of the underlying disease including HIV-1 infection, the affected cell type, the JCV burden or the number of infected cells the incidence of detection ranged from 30% to 100%. Quantification of virus DNA revealed a considerably higher virus load than in most normal persons, but copy number and immunodeficiency as determined by CD4/CD8+ T lymphocyte counts could not be correlated.[6]

Studies on PBCs of risk group patients addressed the question whether enhanced virus load in circulating cells may contribute to increased dissemination of virus to the effector organ prior to the induction of disease. In low risk groups including Multiple Sclerosis, Parkinson's disease and systemic lupus erythematosus (SLE) incidences well under 10% were reported. In high risk leukemia patients JCV DNA could be detected in almost all leukocyte samples from bone marrow and PBCs prior to conditioning for BMT. Interestingly, the incidence of JCV infection early after BMT dropped to 10-12%, whereas at 60 days after, an increase to almost 90% was reported. This confirms the assumption that immune modulatory treatment associated with transplantation also influences JCV infection.

An important step to further clarify the nature of viral interaction with hematopoietic cells was is the unequivocal characterization of the hematopoietic subpopulation involved. B-lymphocytes were the first target cells characterized in bone marrow, spleen and peripheral blood.[10] JCV specific DNA could be amplified in B-lymphocyte depleted PBCs from HIV-1 infected patients, in B- and T-lymphocyte cultures from bone marrow of leukemia patients (several observations) and in T-cells, B-cells, monocytes and granulocytes from peripheral blood.[11] The most prominent cell type affected regularly was the granulocytes and not cells of the lymphoid lineage. In each individual the affected cell types were individually distributed. In addition, unsorted cells from healthy persons often were negative for JCV, whereas in sorted populations JCV DNA was detectable in almost all individuals.[3] The finding of JCV in samples of the most prominent hematopoietic subpopulations combined with a highly variable DNA concentration in different subpopulations evidenced that the association of JCV DNA with circulating cells might be a rather nonspecific interaction or a combination of specific and nonspecific effects. Possible nonspecific interactions of JCV with circulating subpopulations could include phagocytosis or binding of virus to outer cellular membranes. This would lead to presence of virus in cytoplasm or attached to the cell.[12] In contrast, in persistent infection virus DNA would be expected within cellular nuclei or, in the productive state, in both compartments. Radioactive in situ hybridization implied a close association of JCV DNA with nuclei of PBCs and an increased number of positive cells under PML (Fig. 5). Recent unpublished findings of subcellular localization of JCV in PBC subpopulations by fluorescent in situ hybridization demonstrate that all three localization types can be found. Although not yet unequivocally clarified, this points to a differentiated interaction of JCV with PBCs that may include phagocytosis as well as persistence or an activated state of JCV infection.

Activation of JCV Infection in Hematopoietic Cells

The significance of JCV DNA in hematopoietic cells for persistence and pathogenesis depends not on the presence of viral DNA in subcellular compartments alone but rather on the functional activity in affected cells. Due to the low concentration of JCV DNA and the low number of cells affected, functional studies concentrated on transcription analyses. JCV expression was reported in B-lymphocytes and the nonB-lymphocyte fraction after magnetic separation of about 50% of diseased and healthy individuals, suggesting that JCV is continuously transcribed. Other studies detected mRNA in most PML patients, but no transcription in PBCs or B-lymphocytes of HIV-1 infected patients and healthy donors, implying a latent state of JCV infection in PBCs.

In cell culture infectious virus was produced by B-cell types and CD34+ hematopoietic progenitor cells. Interestingly, JCV susceptibility was lost in the CD34+ cells after differentiation to a macrophage-like cell. Activity was linked to varying expression levels of the transcription factor NF-1. This gives evidence that cellular differentiation and associated reorganization of cellular transcription pattern may be an important step for JCV persistence and activity in the hematopoietic compartment. In line with a very low level of JCV DNA amplification in circulating CD19+ B-cells of normal individuals, virus production in cell culture was restricted to about 2% of the B-lymphocytes.[12,13] This strengthens the idea that JCV infection might be associated with a specific cellular subset and adds further support to an infection of B-lymphocytes in vivo, which is inducible by the engagement of signal transduction pathways relevant for immune control mechanisms.

Besides the close association of JCV DNA with PBCs, virus DNA was also detected in cell free plasma. The rate of viremia varied from no virus present to 4% in SLE patients or control groups including healthy individuals. In HIV-1 infected patients rates from 4 to 23% were reported and in HIV/PML viremia was detected in about 32% of the patients. Although no correlation of virus presence and immunodeficiency could be observed, the incidence of detection appeared to be slightly higher under PML. Often presence of JCV DNA in PBCs and free circulating virus was not correlated (several observations), suggesting that either JCV carrying cells are quickly eliminated or there is another source for JCV in plasma than infected PBCs.

These findings shed a new light on the question, how the virus is disseminated from the periphery to the target organs. It can be hypothesized, that virus produced in any organ may find its way through intracellular spaces to the lymphoid compartment and can there be detectable as free circulating particle in the plasma. The question, how the virus may overcome the endothelial barrier in asymptomatic persistent infection is not yet answered. However, for BKV it was already shown that endothelial cells support virus replication, suggesting that these cells could also be involved in virus dissemination. Recently, both huPyVs were detected for the first time in arterial walls. Although the cell type involved is not yet identified, it is conceivable that either cells are actively infected or infected PBCs may carry the virus through vascular walls.

In summary, the discussion on a possible persistent JCV infection in PBCs remains controversial. However, the findings demonstrate that the amount of JCV DNA in PBCs is often limited and JCV DNA can only be detected after enrichment of PBC subtypes by cell separation techniques. In general, expression in PBCs appears to be suppressed, maintaining a level that cannot be detected by PCR on bulk DNA. It became clear that JCV is not only associated with blood cells, but also circulates freely in the host. The question, whether presence of JCV DNA in the samples is due to infection, to phagocytosis of virus by circulating cells, or is the consequence of unspecific binding to cellular membranes is not yet answered. Although detection of mRNA is a strong argument for an activated virus infection, the unequivocal localization of virus DNA to the nucleus of latently JCV infected lymphoid subtypes, is not yet achieved. Moreover, it can not be excluded that different types of virus cell interaction coexist in the host—each of them regulated by different mechanisms including cell specificity, hormonal changes or immune modulation. Besides the problems associated with PCR detection in blood, such a scenario would explain the extensive divergence of recent analyses from different laboratories all over the world. The enhanced virus load in PBCs of risk group patients and expression in hematopoietic precursor cells argues not only for infection of PBCs, but also suggests that virus interaction with circulating cells on a basic level might be affected by diseases at risk for PML. It is conceivable that immune modulatory stimuli mediate not only virus activation and repression but may also influence the susceptibility of blood cell subpopulations to JCV.

Acknowledgments

Work in the authors laboratory was supported by Graduate College 520 'Immunmodulation' of the Deutschen Forschungsgesellschaft and by Grant 99.061.1/2 of the Wilhelm Sander-Stiftung

References

1. Hirsch HH, Steiger J. Polyomavirus BK. Important review on BKV virology and pathogenesis. Lancet Infect Dis 2003; 3:611-623.
2. Walker DL, Padgett BL. The classical summary on PML. Progressive multifocal leukoencephalopathy. New York: Plenum Press, 1983; 18:161-193.
3. Doerries K, Sbiera S, Drews K et al. A study on JCV affected peripheral blood cell subopopulations emphasizing granulocytes as major affected cell type. Association of human polyomavirus JC with peripheral blood of immunoimpaired and healthy individuals. J Neurovirol 2003; 9(Suppl 1):81-87.
4. Arthur RR, Shah KV. Occurrence and significance of papovaviruses BK and JC in the urine. A summary of early studies of JCV and BKV viruria that remains a valuable source for the understanding of persistent huPyV infections. Prog Med Virol 1989; 36:42-61.
5. Doerries K. Latent and persistent human polyomavirus infection. Extensive review on persistent polyomavirus infection. In: Khalili K, Stoner GL, eds. Human Polyomaviruses. Molecular and clinical perspectives. New York: Wiley-Liss Inc. 2001:197-237.
6. Koralnik IJ, Boden D, Mai VX et al. JC virus DNA load in patients with and without progressive multifocal leukoencephalopathy. Important paper on the presence of JCV in different target compartments. Neurology 1999a; 52(2):253-260.
7. Du Pasquier RA, Corey S, Margolin DH et al. Productive infection of cerebellar granule cell neurons by JC virus in an HIV+ individual. The first report on the involvement of neurons in JCV infection. Neurology 2003; 61:775-782.

8. von Einsiedel RW, Samorei IW, Pawlita M et al. New JC virus infection patterns by in situ polymerase chain reaction in brains of acquired immunodeficiency syndrome patients with progressive multifocal leukoencephalopathy. Characterization of affected cell types and topography of PML lesions by modern molecular methods. J Neurovirol 2004; 10:1-11.

9. Doerries K. Human polyomaviruses in target cells of hematopoietic origin and mechanisms of activation in the course of infection. The review concentrates on interaction of huPyV with cells of hematopoietic origin. Current topics in Virology 1999b; 1:84-93.

10. Jensen PN, Major EO. Viral variant nucleotide sequences help expose leukocytic positioning in the JC virus pathway to the CNS. Concentrates on the possible role of JCV variants for viral dissemination. J Leukoc Biol 1999; 65:428-438.

11. Koralnik IJ, Schmitz JE, Lifton MA et al. Detection of JC virus DNA in peripheral blood cell subpopulations of HIV-1-infected individuals. Characterization of PBC subpopulations involved in JCV infection. J Neurovirol 1999b; 5:430-435.

12. Wei G, Liu CK, Atwood WJ. JC virus binds to primary human glial cells, tonsillar stromal cells, and B-lymphocytes, but not to T lymphocytes. Addresses the role of transcription factors and cell receptors for JCV infection. J Neurovirology 2000; 6:127-136.

13. Monaco MC, Sabath BF, Durham LC et al. JC virus multiplication in human hematopoietic progenitor cells requires the NF-1 class D transcription factor. Dependence of JCV replication on transcription factor family NF expression. J Virol 2001; 75:9687-9695.

CHAPTER 9

Immunity and Autoimmunity Induced by Polyomaviruses:
Clinical, Experimental and Theoretical Aspects

Ole Petter Rekvig, Signy Bendiksen and Ugo Moens

Abstract

In this chapter, polyomaviruses will be presented in an immunological context. Principal observations will be discussed to elucidate humoral and cellular immune responses to different species of the polyomaviruses and to individual viral structural and regulatory proteins. The role of immune responses towards the viruses or their proteins in context of protection against polyomavirus induced tumors will be described. One central aspect of this presentation is the ability of polyomaviruses, and particularly large T-antigen, to terminate immunological tolerance to nucleosomes, DNA and histones. Thus, in the present chapter we will focus on clinical, experimental and theoretical aspects of the immunity to polyomaviruses.

Introduction

Polyomaviruses are small naked viruses with an icosahedral capsid and a circular dsDNA genome. The name polyomavirus derives from early observations that these viruses may cause tumors when inoculated into newborn mice. Polyomaviruses are widespread among vertebrates, but the different species have a narrow host and cell range. Two polyomaviruses solely infecting humans were discovered in 1971 by two independent groups. Gardner et al[1] originally described BK virus (BKV) in the urine of a renal transplant patient, while JC virus (JCV) was isolated and partially characterized by Padgett et al[2] from the brain tissue of a patient with progressive multifocal leukencephalopathy. A third species, Simian virus 40 (SV40) was discovered already in 1960, and was originally discovered as a contaminant of inactivated Salk polio vaccine[3] that was distributed world-wide in the years between 1955 and 1963.[4]

The association between polyomavirus infection and immunity to the viral particles and their polypeptides has been determined in worldwide epidemiological surveys. This aspect has been studied extensively over the past 3-4 decades following the detection of BKV, JCV and SV40, the species dealt with in this chapter. These studies span from determination of humoral immunity against the virus in context of monitoring seroepidemiology, over humoral immunity of individual viral proteins, to T cell mediated immunity. A less known, but potentially important role of the polyomaviruses resides in the ability of polyomavirus encoded proteins to bind host autologous molecules and thereby induce antigen-selective autoimmunity to p53, histones and double-stranded (ds)DNA. This will be described in detail in the last part of this chapter.

Polyomaviruses and Human Diseases, edited by Nasimul Ahsan. ©2006 Eurekah.com and Springer Science+Business Media.

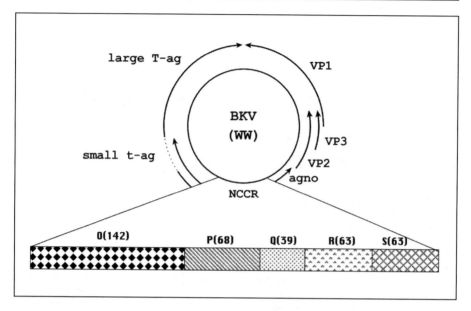

Figure 1. Organization of the archetypal BKV(WW) genome. The gene products encoded by the early region (large T-antigen and small t-antigen) and the late region (the agnoprotein, and the capsid proteins VP1, VP2, and VP3) are indicated. The noncoding control region, using the O-P-Q-R-S nomenclature[209,210] is shown. This region spans the origin of replication and the early and late promoter/enhancer sequences.

Polyomaviruses—Structure and Genomic Organization

To understand how polyomaviruses induce immunity and autoimmunity, a short description of the genomic and structural organization of the virus particle is essential.

BKV is a nonenveloped virus with an icosahedral capsid, and the virions are roughly made up of 88% proteins and 12% DNA. The viral genome consists of a single copy of a circular dsDNA molecule of approximately 5,300 base-pairs. The BKV genome shares 75% overall homology with JCV and 70% homology with the SV40 genome (reviewed in ref. 5). During virus replication, newly replicated viral DNA associates with host cell histones to form minichromosomes. Hence, in mature virions, viral DNA is complexed with the cellular histones to form a nucleosomal structure,[6,7] the core mononucleosome thus containing an octamer of histones H2A, H2B, H3 and H4, analogous with the structure of nucleosomes in mammals.[8-10] On the average, each polyomavirus genome contains 21 nucleosomes.[6]

The viral circular genome can be divided into three functional regions (Fig. 1): (i) the so-called early region encodes the regulatory proteins large tumor antigen (large T-antigen, in this chapter denoted T-ag) and small tumor antigen (small t-ag); (ii) the late region containing the genetic information for the structural (capsid) proteins VP1, VP2, VP3 and the agnoprotein; and (iii) the noncoding control region (NCCR) which harbor the origin of replication and the sequences involved in the transcriptional regulation of both the early and the late genes.

The early region is expressed at the initiation of the viral replication. T-ag is a multifunctional protein with distinct domains fulfilling different roles. Major crucial properties are its helicase activity and its ability to bind host cell regulatory proteins like the retinoblastoma protein family, p53 and others (for review, see refs. 5,11). These activities are important as they may control cell function and undermine the infected cell's destiny for apoptosis. Thus, T-ag controls both viral DNA replication, early and late gene transcription, and interferes with host cell transcription factors.[12]

The capsids are composed of 72 capsomers each consisting of the three major structural proteins, VP1, VP2 and VP3. For intact, infectious polyomaviruses, VP1 is the dominant solvent phase protein, and is the most redundant protein of the capsid and accounts for 70-80% of the total protein mass of the virus particle.[5] In fact, VP1 can self-assemble into virus-like particles in vitro.[13] Therefore, antibodies against this protein dominate immune responses to polyomaviruses, at least as detected in assays using intact virus particles as antigens, e.g., in hemagglutination inhibition assay (HI, an assay using antibodies to inhibit the potential for polyomaviruses BKV and JCV to agglutinate human blood group 0 erythrocytes), enzyme linked immunosorbent assay (ELISA), or immune electron microscopy. Important from an immunological point of view is the fact that the capsid proteins VP1-3 also bind DNA directly or indirectly. This is basically depending on two features of the polypeptides: i. due to nuclear localization signals present in the capsid proteins, and ii. to the fact that these proteins may associate directly with DNA structures or with other nucleosome/chromatin bound proteins like transcription factors.[5,14-17] In an immunological context, this information is important, as it may provide an explanation as to why and how polyomavirus infection may transform host cell nucleosomes immunogenic from a natural state of nonimmunogenicity of these structures.[18]

Serological studies have revealed that there exist several subtypes of BKV. The heterogeneity is due to differences in the sequences of the amino acids 61-83 of VP1.[19] The highest genetic diversity between different BKV isolates is, however, found in the NCCR. While the NCCR of the archetypal BKV strain WW has a linear arrangement of the transcription factor binding sequence blocks O-P-Q-R (Fig. 1), deletions, duplications and rearrangements have been reported in the NCCR of other BKV strains. It is generally believed that this polymorphism in the VP1 and NCCR may offer advantages to the virus in its host.[5]

Immunology of Polyomaviruses

Except for seroepidemiological studies and observations in polyomavirus large T-ag transgenic mice, there is little information about the role of innate and adaptive immunity related to these viruses. The main interest in this regard has been linked to humoral immune responses to trace the distribution of each of the polyomavirus species among human individuals, to try to establish the role of T cells in fighting the virus and to establish latent infection, and the role of virus-encoded proteins in the generation of autoimmunity to nucleosomes and DNA. Few studies describe how the innate immune system handle this virus, and which receptors on antigen-presenting cells (APC) bind this virus, and whether this interaction results in up-regulation of costimulatory signals necessary for full activation of the adaptive immune system. In the next sections, seroepidemiology of BKV, JCV and SV40, T cell recognition of virus-derived proteins and their role in initiating autoimmunity will be discussed.

Seroepidemiology of Polyomaviruses

Since these viruses were detected, their prevalence in the population has been thoroughly investigated. As all these viruses have been shown to inherit the potential to establish latent infections[20] and to induce tumors, at least in heterologous hosts (reviewed in ref. 21), it became important to study their prevalence in the human populations globally and locally to establish a base of information potentially important for studies of their clinical impact. Also, to perceive information of their distribution in the human population, an origin could be created to detect new possible diseases caused by such viruses based on cell tropism, cytopathogenic and oncogenic potential, and, as recently has been demonstrated, their potential to terminate immunological tolerance to DNA and to nucleosomes.[18,22-25]

Already the first studies demonstrated a high incidence of BKV and JCV in different populations,[26-29] although the incidence in remote areas could differ from this generalized picture.[30] There exist a large body of studies and literature covering this field (see e.g, refs. 13,19,31-33). In the context of this chapter, important aspects to understand the role of immunity to the polyomaviruses will be discussed.

Table 1. *Amino acid identity between the proteins of BKV (Dunlop strain, accession number V01108), JCV (CY strain, accession number AB038249) and SV40 (766 strain, accession number J02400)*

	BKV-JCV	BKV-SV40	JCV-SV40
VP1 (362/354/364)[a]	63%	80%	75%
VP2 (351/344/352)	80%	77%	73%
VP3 (232/225/234)	77%	72%	67%
Agno (66/71/62)	63%	58%	52%
Small t-ag (172/172/174)	78%	71%	68%
Large T-ag (695/688/708)	83%	75%	73%

[a]The numbers in parenthesis refer to the number of amino acids in the protein of BKV, JCV, or SV40, respectively.

Cross-Reactivity of Human Polyomavirus Antibodies

A high degree of amino acid sequence identity exists between the functional and structural proteins of the human polyomaviruses SV40, BKV, and JCV. Amino acid sequence identity varies between 58% up to 83% when comparing the different corresponding proteins of BKV (Dunlop), JCV (CY) and SV40 766 strains (see Table 1). Stretches of 10 consecutive or more identical amino acids were found in several regions of the distinct proteins (Fig. 2). Because of the high degree of identity between SV40, BKV, and JCV proteins, antibodies raised against polyomaviruses proteins have the potential to cross-react (reviewed in refs. 19,34). Results of seroepidemiological studies to determine the prevalence of antibodies against a certain species among human polyomaviruses should therefore be interpreted with care as serum antibodies can react with all three human polyomavirus species.

Seroepidemiology of BKV

Serological data obtained over 30 years demonstrate that infection with BKV is established in early childhood, and occurs globally with similar frequency in industrial and developing countries. Several immunology-based assays have been developed to monitor the infectivity of BKV. Of these, HI,[26,35] complement fixation,[26] indirect immunofluorescence (IIF),[36] RIA,[37] ELISA,[38,39] and western blot[40] have been the most widely used assays. These tests may have quite different sensitivities, and may detect different spectra of virus antibodies, a fact that could affect the interpretation of the prevalence determined in the different studies. Surprisingly, in light of the different assays used for antibody determination, and the technical development of sensitive assays for antibody detection over the last three decades, the observed prevalence for BKV in different populations is consistently high (see Table 2 for examples). Comparing two studies, one early of Gardner et al in 1973,[26] and one late of Stolt et al in 2003,[41] determining the prevalence for BKV antibodies in different age groups, the results are surprisingly consistent and comparable (Table 3), although performed with different assays (HI versus ELISA using recombinant viral proteins assembled into virus-like particles) to detect the antibodies, and timely distant from each other (30 years).

The prevalence of BKV varies in different studies between 40 and 95%. The overall differences between the reports cannot be explained by the use of different assay procedures, as results determined by HI spans from 40% (data published in 1976[42]) to 94% (1974[43]). These prevalences, obtained with HI, covers the figures obtained with most of the assays used in later studies. One explanation for this diversity may be that the cut off levels of the assays are not standardized internationally, and that exchange of sera for inter-laboratory standardization has not been performed or thoroughly documented. However, due to the nature of the study, one should expect differences in the prevalence of anti-BKV antibodies in different more or less well defined human populations. Analyzing the results collected over time, the discrepancies cannot be explained by improvements of the assays from early to late studies (see examples of data presented in Tables 2 and 3 collected over 30 years).

The antibodies recognizing the whole viral particle (presumable dominated by antibodies to the solution phased VP1, see above) seem to persist once the immune system is stimulated. This is strengthened by the fact that the detection of infectious particles has a much lower prevalence than that described above for anti-BKV antibodies (see Table 4). Antibodies to polyomavirus T-ag are relatively rare, although most individuals are infected with the virus, indicating that anti-T-ag antibodies are more closely linked to episodes of productive infections. In one situation we could directly trace this intimate and timely association between productive infection and transient humoral immune response to T-ag.[23] In that study, urinary secretion of polyomavirus DNA sequences was monitored weekly in 20 Systemic Lupus Erythematosus (SLE) patients over one year, and development of anti-T-ag antibodies was determined. There was an overall strong correlation between presence of anti-T-ag antibodies and productive infection as judged by BKV DNA PCR-positive urine samples. In one patient, the production of anti-T-ag antibodies coincided with the appearance of urinary BKV DNA sequences. As the BKV DNA sequences disappeared from the urine, the anti-T-ag antibody fainted over the next 6-8 weeks. This is consistent with the very low incidence of anti-T-ag antibodies in healthy individuals (<1%) we[44,45] and others[46] have detected. Thus, as VP antibodies seem to reflect an accumulative incidence of latent BKV infection, antibodies to T-ag seem to indicate present or recent productive infection with significant expression of T-ag as is essential for virus replication to take place.[5,11] Summarizing data on prevalence of antibodies to structural proteins and to T-ag, it is likely that antibodies to the structural proteins VP1-3 can be used to determine accumulated prevalence of the sum of active and latent polyomavirus infections, while antibodies to T-ag can potentially be used to trace prevalence of **productive** infection.

Seroepidemiology of JCV

As for BKV, seroepidemiology of JCV has been determined over the 3 decades since their detection. The first published study came from Padgett and Walker already in 1973,[27] two years after the original description of the virus. In this study, different age groups were examined (Table 3, data organized according to Walker and Padgett[47] from ref. 27) and the anti-JCV antibodies had roughly the same age-related profile as that seen for BKV antibodies (Table 3).[26,47] Stolt et al[41] determined the seroepidemiology of JCV using recombinant virus-like particles consisting of JCV VP1 as antigen in IgG-specific ELISA. In their study, antibodies to JCV peaked around the age of 9-11 years, and the accumulative incidence in humans aged 1-13 was 32% (Table 3), while in the early study of Padgett and Walker,[27,47] the accumulative incidence, using HI, in the age group 1-14 years was 28%. These results are strikingly consistent taken into account that the studies are performed with very different antibody assays (HI, versus VP1-specific ELISA, Table 3). and approximately 30 years apart. However, no attempts to ensure that the antibodies detected are specific for either BKV or JCV (or SV40 for that case) were undertaken.

That the frequency of the different polyomavirus species as determined by serological assays differs among humans is not an argument for species-specific virus antibodies, but may simply reflect the different distribution of the viruses. To ascertain that the antibodies indeed recognize one or another of the virus species, inhibition experiments should have been performed. In the work by Stolt et al, the authors describe different prevalence of BKV and JCV with lower frequency in the age groups of JCV in the same sera, indicating some species-specificity of the antibodies. Furthermore, in a report by Hogan et al,[48] where they investigated seroconversion in renal transplant patients, more of the patients seroconverted for JCV than for BKV. This directly demonstrated that at least in some individuals antibodies are produced that specifically recognize JCV.[48] Such results indicate presence of antibody subpopulations in the sera recognizing one single polyomavirus species, but do not rule out that antibodies may also recognize

```
                                            VP1
BKV:    M--APTKRKG  ECPGAAPKKP  KEPVQVPKLL  IKGGVEVLEV  KTGVDAITEV  ECFLNPEMGD
JCV:    M--APTKRKG  E-------R   KDPVQVPKLL  IRGGVEVLEV  KTGVDSITEV  ECFLTPEMGD
SV40:   MKMAPTKRKG  SCPGAAPKKP  KEPVQVPKLV  IKGGIEVLGV  KTGVDSFTEV  ECFLNPQMGN

BKV:    PDENLRGFSL  K-LSAENDFS  SDSPERK-ML  PCYSTARIPL  PNLNEDLTCG  NLLMWEAVTV
JCV:    PDEHLRGFS-  -SISISDTFE  SDSPN-KDML  PCYSVARIPL  PNLNEDLTCG  NILMWEAVTL
SV40:   PDEHQKGLS-  KSLAAEKQFT  DDSPD-KEQL  PCYSVARIPL  PNLNEDLTCG  NILMWEAVTV

BKV:    QTEVIGITSM  LNLHA---GS  QKVHEHGGGK  PIQGSNFHFF  AVGGEPLEMQ  GVLMNYRSKY
JCV:    KTEVLGVTTL  MNVHS---G   QATHDNGAGK  PVQGTSFHFF  SVGGEALELQ  GVVFNYRSKY
SV40:   KTEVIGVTAM  LNLHS---GT  QKTHENGAGK  PIQGSNFHFF  AVGGEPLELQ  GVLANYRTKY

BKV:    PDGTITPKNP  TAQSQVMNTD  HKAYLDKNNA  YPVECWVPDP  SRNENARYFG  TFTGGENVPP
JCV:    PDGTIFPKNA  TVQSQVMNTE  HKAYLDKNKA  YPVECWVPDP  TRNENTRYFG  TLTGGENVPP
SV40:   PAQTVTPKNA  TVDSQQMNTD  HKAVLDKDNA  YPVECWVPDP  SKNENTRYFG  TYTGGENVPP

BKV:    VLHVTNTATT  VLLDEQGVGP  LCKADSLYVS  AADICGLFTN  SSGTQQWRGL  ARYFKIRLRK
JCV:    VLHITNTATT  VLLDEFGVGP  LCKGDNLYLS  AVDVCGMFTN  RSGSQQWRGL  SRYFKVQLRK
SV40:   VLHITNTATT  VLLDEQGVGP  LCKADSLYVS  AVDICGLFTN  TSGTQQWKGL  PRYFKITLRK

BKV:    RSVKNPYPIS  FLLSDLINRR  TQRVDGQPMY  GMESQVEEVR  VFDGTERLPG  DPDMIRYIDK
JCV:    RRVKNPYPIS  FLLTDLINRR  TPRVDGQPMY  GMDAQVEEVR  VFEGTEELPG  DPDMMRYVDR
SV40:   RSVKNPYPIS  FLLSDLINRR  TQRVDGQPMI  GMSSQVEEVR  VYEDTEELPG  DPDMIRYIDE

BKV:    QGQLQTKML
JCV:    YGQLQTKML
SV40:   FGQTTTRMQ

                                          VP2/VP3
BKV:    MGAALALLGD  LVASVSEAAA  ATGFSVAEIA  AGEAAAAIEV  QIASLATVEG  ITSTSEAIAA
JCV:    MGAALALLGD  LVATVSEAAA  ATGFSVAEIA  AGEAAATIEV  EIASLATVEG  ITSTSEAIAA
SV40:   MGAALTLLGD  LIATVSEAAA  ATGFSVAEIA  AGEAAAAIEV  QLASVATVEG  LT-TSEAIAA
                                                                              ↓
BKV:    IGLTPQTYAV  IAGAPGAIAG  FAALIQTVSG  ISSLAQVGYK  FFDDWDHKVS  TVGLYQQSGM
JCV:    IGLTPETYAV  ITGAPGAVAG  FAALVQTVTG  GSAIAQLGYR  FFADWDHKVS  TVGLFQQPAM
SV40:   IGLTPQAYAV  ISGAPAAIAG  FAALLQTVTG  VSAVAQVGYR  FFSDWDHKVS  TVGLYQQPGM

BKV:    ALELFNPDEY  YDILFPGVNT  FVNNIQYLDP  RHWGPSLFAT  ISQALWHVIR  DDIPSITSQE
JCV:    ALQLFNPEDY  YDILFPGVNA  FVNNIHYLDP  RHWGPSLFST  ISQAFWNLVR  DDLPSLTSQE
SV40:   AVDLYRPDDY  YDILFPGVQT  FVHSVQYLDP  RHWGPTLFNA  ISQAFWRVIQ  NDIPRLTSQE

BKV:    LQRRTERFFR  DSLARFLEET  TWTIVNAPIN  FYNYIQQYYS  DLSPIRPSMV  RQVAEREGTR
JCV:    IQRRTQKLFV  ESLARFLEET  TWAIVNSPVN  LYNYISDYYS  RLSPVRPSMV  RQVAQREGTY
SV40:   LERRTQRYLR  DSLARFLEET  TWTVINAPVN  WYNSLQDYYS  TLSPIRPTMV  RQVANREGLQ

BKV:    VHFGHTY--S  IDDADSIEEV  TQRMDLRNQQ  S--VHSGEFI  EKTIAPGGAN  QRTAPQWMLP
JCV:    ISFGHSYTQS  IDDADSIQEV  TQRLDLKT--  -PNVQSGEFI  EKSIAPGGAN  QRSAPQWMLP
SV40:   ISFGHTY-DN  IDEADSIQQV  TERWEAQS-Q  SPNVQSGEFI  EKFEAPGGAN  QRTAPQWMLP

BKV:    LLLGLYGTVT  PALEAYEDGP  NQKKRRVSRG  SSQKAKGTRA  SAKTTNKRRS  RSSRS
JCV:    LLLGLYGTVT  PALEAYEDGP  NKKKRR----  ---K-EGPRA  SSKTSYKRRS  RSSRS
SV40:   LLLGLYGSVT  SALKAYEDGP  NKKKRKLSRG  SSQKTKGTSA  SAKARHKRRN  RSSRS

                                       Agnoprotein
BKV:    MVLRQLSRQA  SVKVGKTWTG  TKKRAQRIFI  FILELLLEFC  RGEDSVDGKN  KSTT------
JCV:    MVLRQLSRKA  SVKVSKTWSG  TKKRAQRILI  FLLEFLLDFC  TGEDSVDGKK  RQKHSGLTEQ
SV40:   MVLRRLSRQA  SVKVRRSWTE  SKKTAQRLFV  FVLELLLQFC  EGEDTVDGKR  KKPER-LTEK

BKV:    ---ALPAVKD  SVKDS
JCV:    RYSALPEPKA  T
SV40:   -----PES
```

Figure 2. Proteins encoded by polyomavirus BKV, JCV and SV40 share amino acid sequence homologies. Alignment of the primary amino acid sequence of the structural proteins VP1, VP2, VP3, the agnoprotein, and the functional proteins large T- and small t-antigen of BKV (Dunlop), JCV (CY), and SV40 (strain 766) identify high degree of homology regions with impact on serological crossreactions and thereby on seroepidemiology of the individual polyomavirus strains. Identical amino acids are shown in black, while different amino acids are gray (shown in red in online version). Arrow indicates start of the VP3 sequence. Figure continued on next page.

```
                                 Large T-antigen

    BKV:    MDKVLNREES MELMDLLGLE RAAWGNLPLM RKAYLRKCKE FHPDKGGDED KMKRMNTLYK
    JCV:    MDKVLNREES MELMDLLGLD RSAWGNIPVM RKAYLKKCKE LHPDKGGDED KMKRMNFLYK
    SV40:   MDKVLNREES LQLMDLLGLE RSAWGNIPLM RKAYLKKCKE FHPDKGGDEE KMKKMNTLYK

    BKV:    KMEQDVKVAH QPDFGT-WSS SEVPTYGTEE WESWWSSFNE KWDEDLFCHE DMFASDEEAT
    JCV:    KMEQGVKVAH QPDFGT-WNS SEVPTYGTDE WESWWNTFNE KWDEDLFCHE EMFASDDENT
    SV40:   KMEDGVKYAH QPDFGGFWDA TEIPTYGTDE WEQWWNAFNE ---ENLFCSE EMPSSDDEAT

    BKV:    ADSQHSTPPK KKRKVEDPKD FPSDLHQFLS QAVFSNRTLA CFAVYTTKEK AQILYKKLME
    JCV:    G-SQHSTPPK KKKKVEDPKD FPVDLHAFLS QAVFSNRTVA SFAVYTTKEK AQILYKKLME
    SV40:   ADSQHSTPPK KKRKVEDPKD FPSELLSFLS HAVFSNRTLA CFAIYTTKEK AALLYKKIME

    BKV:    KYSVTFISRH MCAGHNIIFF LTPHRHRVSA INNFCQKLCT FSFLICKGVN KEYLLYSALT
    JCV:    KYSVTFISRH GFGGHNILFF LTPHRHRVSA INNYCQKLCT FSFLICKGVN KEYLFYSALC
    SV40:   KYSVTFISRH NSYNHNILFF LTPHRHRVSA INNYAQKLCT FSFLICKGVN KEYLMYSALT

    BKV:    RDPYHTIEES IQGGLKEHDF SPEEPEETKQ VSWKLITEYA VETKCEDVFL LLGMYLEFQY
    JCV:    RDPFSVIEES LPGGLKEHDF NPEEAEETKQ VSWKLVTEYA METKCDDVLL LLGMYLEFQY

    BKV:    NVEECKKCQK KDQPYHFKYH EKHFANAIIF AESKNQKSIC QQAVDTVLAK KRVDTLHMTR
    JCV:    NPLQCKKCEK KDQPNHFNHH EKHYYNAQIF ADSKNQKSIC QQAVDTVAAK QRVDSLHMTR
    SV40:   SFEMCLKCIK KEQPSHYKYH EKHYANAAIF ADSKNQKTIC QQAVDTVLAK KRVDSLQLTR

    BKV:    EEMLTERFNH ILDKMDLIFG AHGNAVLEQY MAGVAWLHCL LPKMDSVIFD FLHCIVFNVP
    JCV:    EEMLVERFNF LLDKMDLIFG AHGNAVLEQY MAGVAWIHCL LPQMDIVIYE FLKCIVLNIP
    SV40:   EQMLTNRFND LLDRMDIMFG STGSADIEEW MAGVAWLHCL LPKMDSVVYD FLKCMVYNIP

    BKV:    KRRYWLFKGP IDSGKTTLAA GLLDLCGGKA LNVNLPMERL TFELGVAIDQ YMVVFEDVKG
    JCV:    KKRYWLFKGP IDSGKTTLAA ALLDLCGGKS LNVNMPLERL NFELGVGIDQ FMVVFEDVKG
    SV40:   KKRYWLFKGP IDSGKTTLAA ALLELCGGKA LNVNLPLDRL NFELGVAIDQ FLVVFEDVKG

    BKV:    TGAESKDLPS GHGINNLDSL RDYLDGSVKV NLEKKHLNKR TQIFPPGLVT MNEYPVPKTL
    JCV:    TGAESRDLPS GHGISNLDCL RDYLDGSVKV NLERKHQNKR TQVFPPGIVT MNEYSVPRTL
    SV40:   TGGESRDLPS GQGINNLDNL RDYLDGSVKV NLEKKHLNKR TQIFPPGIVT MNEYSVPKTL


    BKV:    QARFVRQIDF RPKIYLRKSL QNSEFLLEKR ILQSGMTLLL LLIWFRPVAD FATDIQSRIV
    JCV:    QARFVRQIDF RPKAYLRKSL SCSEYLLEKR ILQSGMTLLL LLIWFRPVAD FAAAIHERIV
    SV40:   QARFVKQIDF RPKDYLKHCL ERSEFLLEKR IIQSGIALLL MLIWYRPVAE FAQSIQSRIV

    BKV:    EWKERLDSEI SMYTFSRMKY NICMGKCILD ITREEDSETE DSGHGSSTE- ----------
    JCV:    QWKERLDLEI SMYTFSTMKA NVGMGRPILD FPREEDSEAE DSGHGSSTE- ----------
    SV40:   EWKERLDKEF SLSVYQKMKF NVAMGIGVLD WLRNSDDDDE DSQENADKNE DGGEKNMEDS

    BKV:    -------SQS QCSSQVSDTS -APAEDSQRS DPHSQELHLC KGFQCFKRPK TPPPK
    JCV:    -------SQS QCSSQVSEAS GADTQ----- -EH-CTYHIC KGFQCFKKPK TPPPK
    SV40:   GHETGIDSQS QGSFQ----- -AP-QSSQSV HDHNQPYHIC RGFTCFKKPP TPPPEPET


                                 Small t-antigen

    BKV:    MDKVLNREES MELMDLLGLE RAAWGNLPLM RKAYLRKCKE FHPDKGGDED KMKRMNTLYK
    JCV:    MDKVLNREES MELMDLLGLD RSAWGNIPVM RKAYLKKCKE LHPDKGGDED KMKRMNFLYK
    SV40:   MDKVLNREES LQLMDLLGLE RSAWGNIPLM RKAYLKKCKE FHPDKGGDEE KMKKMNTLYK

    BKV:    KMEQDVKVAH QPDFG-TWSS SEVCADFPLC P--DTLYCKE WPICSKKPSV HCPCMLCQLR
    JCV:    KMEQGVKVAH QPDFG-TWNS SEVGCDFPPN S--DTLYCKE WPNCATNPSV HCPCLMCMLK
    SV40:   KMEDGVKYAH QPDFGGFWDA TEVFASS-LN PGVDAMYCKQ WPECAKKMSA NCICLLC-L-

    BKV:    LR--HLNRKF LRKEPLVWID CYCIDCFTQW FGLDLTEETL QWWVQIIGET PFRDLKL
    JCV:    LR--HRNRKF LRSSPLVWID CYCFDCFRQW FGCDLTQEAL HCWEKVLGDT PYRDLKL
    SV40:   LRMKHENRKL YRKDPLVWVD CYCFDCFRMW FGLDLCEGTL LLWCDIIGQT TYRDLKL
```

Figure 2. Continued.

Table 2. Examples of data on prevalence of BK virus in the human population. Data are selected that compare techniques and time for antibody detection

Assay	Age Range	Frequency (%)		Year	References
HI	8-20 (control sera)	21/30	(70)	1972	(183)
HI	2-70	117/203	(58)	1973	(29)
HI	>14	44/66	(67)	1977	(35)
HI	newborn->50	254/409	(62)	1973	(26)
CF	newborn->50	276/508	(54)	1973	(26)
IFA	newborn-65	197/311	(63)	1974	(36)
IgG ELISA*	newborn-80	340/461	(74)	1986	(38)
IgG ELISA	1-80	218/320	(68)	1989	(39)
IgG ELISA VP1**	1-13	206/288	(72)**	2003	(41)

* BKV particles purified from Vero cell cultures were used as solid phase antigens. ** ELISA using purified yeast-expressed virus-like particles containing the VP1 major capsid protein of AS and SB strains of BKV. In this table data combining the results using both strain's VP1 is presented. Table modified from reference 28.

determinants shared by the different viruses. In one study, Taguchi et al[49] determined the prevalence and age of acquisition of antibodies against JCV and BKV. About 50% of the children in this study acquired antibodies against BKV by 3 years of age and against JCV by 6 years of age. These results indicate that dual latent infections with both viruses are common,

Table 3. Comparison of age dependent prevalence of antibodies to BKV and JCV using hemagglutination inhibition (26) or ELISA using virus-like particle (VLP) containing recombinant BKV or JCV VP1 (41)

Virus	HI,CF or IIF*		VP1 ELISA**	
	Age Groups	Frequency (%)	Age Groups	Frequency (%)
BKV	1-5	17/46(37)	1-3	10/50 (20)
	6-10	43/52(83)	3-5	31/49 (63)
	11-17	33/40(83)	5-7	40/50 (80)
	18-25	27/34(79)	7-9	49/50 (98)
	>50	26/49(53)	9-11	45/49 (92)
	11-13	31/40 (78)		
All	1->50	146/221 (66)	1-13	206/288 (72)
JCV	0-4	2/20(10)	1-3	8/50(16)
	5-9	16/69(23)	3-5	13/49(27)
	10-14	13/20(65)	5-7	11/50(22)
	15-19	10/20(50)	7-9	21/50(42)
	>50	120/157(76)	9-11	25/49(51)
	11-13	13/40(33)		
All	0->50	61/286(56)	1-13	91/288 (32)

* HI: Hemagglutination inhibition assay based on the ability of BKV to agglutinate red blood cells; CF: Complement fixation test; IIF, indirect immunofluorescence test; ** ELISA using BKV- or JCV-like VP1 containing particles as antigen.

Table 4. Prevalence of human polyomavirus replication in healthy individuals as determined by the presence of viral proteins, DNA sequences or virions in urine samples[a]

Virus	Number of Positive Samples/ Number of Tested (%)	References
BKV	191/19,845 (0.96)	67,184-200
JCV	303/870 (34.8)	48,67,184,187,197, 198,201-207
SV40	1/100 (1)	197,208

[a]Viral sequences, proteins or virions were detected by hybridisation, PCR, ELISA, indirect immunofluorescence, hemagglutination inhibition test, light microscopy ('Decoy' cells), or electron microscopy.

and that antibodies can be used to determine seroconversion of either of the viruses.[49] More work is, however, needed to determine whether polyomavirus antibodies cross-react over the species barriers, as recently discussed by Knowles.[34] This information is important to exactly determine the prevalence of each individual polyomavirus in the human population.

Seroepidemiology of SV40

Although originally described as a natural habitant of Asiatic macaques, SV40 can infect humans.[50-52] Recovery of infectious SV40 virions indicates an established infection and implies that humans may function as a natural host for this polyomavirus. For almost a decade (1955-1963), millions of children worldwide were administered SV40-contaminated poliovirus vaccines and therefore it is not surprising that antibodies against SV40 could be present in the human population. However, seropositive individuals are also found amongst those that never received contaminated poliovirus vaccines.

Recent seroepidemiological studies using different detection methods by different groups revealed that approximately 10% (range 0-12%) of sera obtained from individuals around the world have low titer antibodies to SV40. No significant differences were found in the seropositive prevalence of sera obtained from individuals that most probably had received contaminated vaccine compared to those that were vaccinated with SV40-free vaccines.[13,53-61] These results are in good agreement with older studies on SV40 seropositivity (3-13%) in individuals that had never received contaminated vaccines (see ref. 60).

These antibody titers may be low due to either limited viral replication in the human host or failure of the human system to recognize and respond robustly to SV40 infections.[62] Alternatively, the low titers and low prevalence of SV40 antibodies may be due to cross-reactivation with the other human polyomaviruses BKV and JCV. Indeed, the study by Carter and colleges detected SV40 antibodies in 46 out of 699 serum samples tested using a virus particle-like ELISA. However, all these samples were also positive for BKV and JCV and in fact these antibodies were cross-reacting with these other polyomaviruses.[57] Of a total of 3669 serum samples tested by Minor and collaborators, 187 were SV40 seropositive, but just one serum had only antibodies against SV40, suggesting that most seropositive individuals have cross-reactive antibodies generated by infection with human polyomaviruses BKV and/or JCV. However, this only positive sample argues against that all SV40 seropositive individuals are the result of cross reactivity.[61] Because of these problems, results of serological studies should be interpreted carefully and be supplemented with data on the presence of SV40 DNA as an evidence of the presence of this virus in the normal human population. The low prevalence of SV40 viruria in this population (1%, see Table 4). reflects the low SV40 seropositive rates and argues against frequent presence of current SV40 infection in healthy individuals.

The origin of antibodies to SV40 remains to be explained but data from several groups suggest that these antibodies do not solely arise from exposure to SV40-contaminated poliovirus vaccines.[54,60,61] A highly specific serological assay for SV40 is required for unambiguous assessment of SV40 prevalence in the human population.

Epidemiology of Productive Polyomavirus Infection in Healthy Individuals

After primary infection in early child-hood, BKV establishes a life-long latent infection in immunocompetent individuals. This latent infection in healthy individuals is supported by the low prevalence (3.6%, n=300) of BKV IgM antibodies in healthy adult blood donors[63] and the low prevalence of BKV viral proteins, virions, or viral nucleic acid sequences in urine samples of immunocompetent individuals. BKV replication as evidence for reactivation has been monitored by the presence of virions as determined by electron microscopy or by Decoy cells (i.e., polyomavirus-laden uroepithelial cells), which are hallmarks of BK virus replication, or by propagation of urine samples on permissive cell cultures. In recent years, PCR has been applied to detect BKV nucleic acid sequences (reviewed in ref. 64). Using these methods, about 1% of healthy controls (n = 19,845) showed signs of BKV productive infection (Table 4). JCV IgM antibodies were detected in 15% of healthy blood donors in England[65] and there was a positive association between JCV seropositivity and age.[34] Thus JCV immunity may be boosted throughout life by persistent infection, reactivation or reinfection. The higher prevalence of JCV IgM antibodies in immunocompetent individuals corresponds well with higher prevalence of JCV viruria in this human population. Almost 35% (n=870) of normal individuals showed PCR-based signs of JCV viruria, and there was a higher incidence of urinary JCV excretion in older individuals.[66] The prevalence of SV40 seropositive individuals in healthy blood donors varied between 1.3-5% throughout all age groups examined.[34] In accordance, urinary SV40 was detected in 1% (n = 100) in immunocompetent persons (Table 4). All the epidemiological data taken together (seroepidemiology and epidemiology of productive infection) indicate that most human individuals are latently infected with polyomaviruses, while productive infection is rare among healthy individuals, and that antibodies to T-ag have an incidence similar to that of productive infection. This points at two phenomenona: anti-polyomavirus antibodies (presumably against VP1-3) are stable and long-lasting, while anti-T-ag antibodies seem to faint, as the productive infection is terminated, consistent with observations described above.[23,44,67]

Polyomaviruses and T Cell Responses

Antigen Processing and Viral Infection

To establish relevant and protective immune responses to a viral infection, peptides derived from viral proteins need to be presented to two main effector T cell populations, CD8+ and CD4+ T cells. The former are meant to kill virus-infected cells, while the latter provide help for B cells to produce anti-viral antibodies. Both systems are important in defense against viral infections.

The critical event in antigen recognition by T cells is the way antigenic peptides are presented and thus recognized by the T cell receptor (TCR). The central molecules in this presentation are the foreign antigen peptide and MHC molecules with two distinct classes: MHC class I and MHC class II. These two MHC classes deliver peptides to the cell surface from two different intracellular compartments reflecting the origins of the antigens that are processed; either intracellular, or taken up from the outside of the cell. MHC molecules are glycoproteins that localize to the cell surface. These two classes of MHC molecules differ both in function, structure and cell distribution. While MHC class I is present on all nucleated cells, MHC class II are present mainly on specialized antigen-presenting cells.

The peptides that bind to MHC class I molecules classically derive from virus-encoded proteins. Such proteins are generated by translation in the cytosol and transported to the endoplasmic reticulum (ER) by transporter proteins called Transporters associated with antigen Processing-1 and 2 (TAP1 and TAP2),[68,69] where they associate with MHC class I complex. At this stage, the fully folded MHC class I-peptide complex is released from the TAP complex in the ER and is transported to the plasma membrane, where the peptides are presented to appropriate CD8+ T cells.

The antigen peptides that bind to MHC class II enter the cell by endocytosis and are arrested in the endosomes. This occurs in specialized APC, although not exclusively as e.g., nonprofessional APC may also present peptides in context of MHC class II molecules (see below). Endosomal and lysosomal proteases are activated by low pH, and thereby degrade the proteins into peptides, which now are ready to be bound by MHC class II molecules.[70] Due to presence of peptides in this compartment that are not generated from (antigenic) proteins taken up by the cell, the peptide-binding cleft of the folded MHC class II molecules is protected from binding unwanted peptides through transient binding of the invariant chain (Ii). The Ii binds noncovalently to MHC class II[71] and prevents binding of irrelevant (autologous) peptides. A second function of the invariant chain is to target the MHC class II-invariant chain complex to the endosomal compartment where the invariant chain is degraded by acidic proteases in successive steps and replaced by the peptides that will be presented at the cell surface (see refs. 70,72 for more details).

Thus, MHC class I-peptide complexes activate CD8+ T cells committed to kill e.g., virus-infected cells, while MHC class II-peptide complexes activate CD4+ T cells aimed at activating macrophages (Th1 cells) or B cells (Th2 cells). Both these arms of antigen presentation are operational in context of polyomavirus infections.

Role of T Cells in Polyomavirus Infection

From the nature of the immune system and its activation, both the innate and the adaptive immune systems are engaged in defense against virus infection. The innate system is important for proper presentation of antigenic peptides, and to provide appropriate costimulatory molecules to ensure activation of T cells recognizing the infectious-derived peptides. Costimulation is necessary for both CD4+ and CD8+ T cells. According to Janeway and Medzhitov,[73-77] polyomaviruses belong to the group of infectious nonself agens delivering pathogen-associated molecular patterns (PAMP) that are recognized by cell surface pattern recognition receptors (PRR) on APC.[78] Interaction between PAMP and PRR may be required for up-regulation of costimulatory molecules like CD80 and CD86. It is, however, not known by which pattern polyomaviruses may increase expression of these molecules on APC. However, one study may be relevant. Velupillay et al[79] investigated the role of the innate immune system using the PERA/Ei mouse strain (PE mice), which is highly susceptible to tumor induction by polyomavirus. This susceptibility can be transmitted in a dominant manner in crosses with resistant C57BR/cdJ mice (BR mice). The authors demonstrated that PE and F[1] mice infected by polyomavirus responded by increased costimulatory molecule B7.2 (CD86) expression on APC, whereas BR mice responded with increased expression of B7.1 (CD80) molecules.[79] A system like this may, if pursued, provide information about the underlying processes determining if CD80 or CD86 are increasingly expressed.

T cell immunity to polyomaviruses has been studied in quite different natural and experimental conditions. Most of these studies focus on T-ag, and investigations of T cell responses to other virus-encoded proteins are rare. T-ag is, however, suitable to examine, as it is highly immunogenic and induces T cell as well as B cell responses.[22,23,33,80-83] We have characterized T cell responses to T-ag in randomly selected healthy humans and in SLE patients. By stimulating peripheral blood mononuclear cells (PBMC) from these with purified SV40 T-ag, virtually all responded by T cell proliferation, and T cell lines could be established by T-ag and nucleosome-T-ag complexes.[45,82,84] Since T-ag from BKV, JCV and SV40 demonstrate 73%-83% amino acid homology (see above), the data obtained using SV40 T-ag probably do not reflect a high incidence of SV40 infected individuals, but more likely that most individuals have cross-reactive T-ag-specific memory T cells. The T cell responses in this system were dominated by CD4+ T cells, as demonstrated by a substantial decrease in proliferation when adding anti-human CD4 antibodies to the cultures prior to antigenic stimulation. Using anti-CD8 antibodies in this system resulted in a weak reduction of T cell proliferation. Similar results were observed in mice immunized with SV40 T-ag.[83] The CD4+ T cell lines established had the potential to induce weak anti-T-ag antibody production in vitro when cocultured with highly purified autologous B cells.[82] Drummond et al[85] found that all of healthy seropositive individuals had T cells proliferating in vitro in response to antigens prepared from BKV-infected fibroblasts. Seronegative individuals did not harbor such reactive T cells. Although not definitively established, some of these T cells may be CD4+, since they correlated with presence of antibodies to BKV.[85]

In one artificial study by Bates et al,[86] the role of CD8+ T cells in abrogating SV40 infectious cycle in vitro has been the focus. In that study, they showed that SV40-encoded T-ag translocated into the cell membrane in addition to the nucleus of SV40-infected permissive monkey cells. The surface T-ag in SV40-transformed mouse cells provided a target for the cytotoxic T lymphocytes (CTL) which recognized SV40 T-ag in association with experimentally transfected murine K/D, (MHC) class I H-2 antigens. Treatment of SV40-infected TC-7/H-2Db and TC-7/H-2Kb with T-ag specific CD8+ T cell clones abrogated the virus lytic cycle. This opened for the possibility that this could take place also in vivo, and that CD8+ T cells could remove polyomavirus-infected cells.[86]

Additional studies have been performed in determining T cell mediated immunity against T-antigen induced tumors. This field has recently been extensively reviewed by Tevethia and Schell,[33] and principal observations only will be summarized here. It has been known for a long time that polyomaviruses and T-ag of these viruses can induce tumors. Early evidence that SV40 encoded antigens could serve as a tumor specific antigen was provided by Tevethia et al in 1980, as they demonstrated that prior immunization of hamsters with SV40 particles, or SV40 transformed cells induced T cell-mediated resistance to a subsequent tumor challenge (reviewed in ref. 33). Interestingly, in constitutive T-ag transgenic mice, this protection against tumorogenesis was not obtained. While T-ag has the potential to induce tumors in diverse organs relative to the organ-specificity of the promoters introduced, T cell immunity to T-ag does not develop in these mice. This is most probably due to tolerance development, either central or peripheral.

An interesting demonstration of this was provided in our laboratory when developing T-ag transgenic mice under the control of a tetracycline-responsive transcriptional activator (tTA). We tested two opposite tetracycline-dependent transgenic systems, i. gene activation in the absence of tetracycline (tet-off), and ii. activation in the presence of tetracycline (tet-on). In control experiments, we examined the tendency for leakage of the T-ag gene by direct visualization of T-ag under nonexpressing conditions, and tested T cell responses after turning the gene on. In the tet-on system, spontaneous expression was observed in absence of tetracycline, as determined by RT-PCR and immune electron microscopy, and these mice did not respond to immunization with T-ag. The tet-off system was tight, and in the nonexpressing situation, the mice responded to T-ag immunization by producing antibodies to T-ag, and T cells responded in vitro to T-ag by vivid proliferation (manuscript in preparation).

Thus, tumorogenesis in constitutively expressing T-ag transgenic mice cannot be inhibited by the immunity to T-ag in such mice, simply due to tolerance development. In an interesting study by Ye et al[87] a correlate to this observation was done in unconditioned T-ag transgenic mice. If the promoter used to control T-ag expression (the RIPI T-ag2 mouse) allowed expression in embryonic life, T cell tolerance developed. If another promoter was selected (the RIPI T-ag4 mouse), this situation changed as expression started several weeks after birth. These mice were immunologically responsive to T-ag. Furthermore, immunization of these mice with T-ag by SV40 infection delayed the T-ag induced tumor growth by up to one year. When the tumors in such mice appeared, the T cell responses to T-ag had fainted.[87] In RT3 mice, expressing T-ag as a transgene controlled by the insulin promoter, crossed with H2-K^k-restricted TCR transgenic mice, CD8+ T cells developed normally, and did not possess tolerance, even after several months of observations.[88,89] As above, this may be due to the prolonged delay after birth for the transgene to be expressed. Extrapolating from these data, T cells may become autoantigenic to determinants expressed a substantial (not exactly defined) time interval after birth.[89] These few examples demonstrate that tumors induced by polyomavirus T-ag may be suppressed if CD8+ T cells specific for T-ag are not rendered tolerant. This may occur through expression of T-ag before immune competency is reached, i.e., during fetal life. From this, one may speculate whether acquired latent infection with potentially oncogenic polyomaviruses may perpetuate T cell mediated immunity to e.g., T-ag that may protect against tumor development in the infected organism. This may actually explain why it is so difficult to equivocally prove the oncogenic potential of polyomaviruses in (at least healthy) humans.[90]

The role of CD4+ T lymphocytes in immunity to SV40 induced tumors has been less studied, but is thought to provide help for MHC class I-restricted CD8+ cytotoxic (anti-tumor) T lymphocytes. These latter T cells, according to e.g., observations referred to above, seem to serve as the predominant effector cell in killing tumor cells. In a recent study, Kennedy et al[91] evaluated the role of T lymphocyte subsets in tumor immunity induced by recombinant SV40 T-ag within an experimental murine pulmonary metastasis model of SV40 T-ag-expressing tumors. By depleting BALB/c mice of either CD4+ or CD8+ T cells in the induction phase of the immune response to SV40 T-ag, indications were found that CD4+ T cells but not CD8+ T cells were critical in the production of antibodies to SV40 T-ag and in tumor immunity after SV40 T-ag immunization. Among the anti-T-ag antibodies, IgG1 was the dominating IgG subclass, indicating that Th2 type T helper cells were involved. Those results suggested that CD4+ T cells, along with antibody responses, indeed may play a role in the induction of tumor immunity to e.g., an SV40 encoded tumor antigen.

In another polyomavirus-mediated disease, JCV can reactivate and cause progressive multifocal leukencephalopathy (PML), a fatal demyelinating disease of the central nervous system. For this to develop, deficit of cell-mediated immunity must occur, which seems to be the case in acquired immunodeficiency syndrome (AIDS), malignancies or in organ transplant recipients. The humoral immune response, measured by the presence of JCV-specific IgG antibodies in the blood or intrathecally, as detected in the cerebrospinal fluid, is inversely related to progression of PML. Consistent with the underlying immunosuppression, the proliferative response of CD4+ T lymphocytes to mitogens or JCV antigens is reduced in PML patients.[92] CD8+ cytotoxic T lymphocytes recognize intracellularly synthesized viral proteins in context of MHC class I molecules (see above). One JCV peptide, the VP1(p100) ILMWEAVTL, has been characterized as a cytotoxic T cell epitope in HLA-A *0201 positive PML survivors. Studies demonstrated that VP1(p100)-stimulated peripheral blood mononuclear cells from 5 out of 7 PML survivors had JCV-specific cytotoxic T cells, versus none of 6 PML progressors. The cellular immune response against the VP1(p100) peptide may therefore be crucial in the prevention of PML disease progression (reviewed in[92]).

In another recent study, Gasnault et al[93] confirmed these results by demonstrating that all of nine healthy donors and seven of thirteen nonPML HIV-infected patients with urinary JCV excretion had positive JCV-specific CD4+ T cell responses. No significant response was found in 14 patients with active PML, while nine of 10 PML **survivors** had positive responses. A restoration of JCV-specific CD4+ T cell responses was associated with JCV clearance from the cerebrospinal fluid. Thus, JCV-specific CD4+ T cell responses appeared also in this study to play a critical role in the control of cerebral JCV infection, preventing PML development. Such responses can be restored in PML survivors possibly following effective and prolonged antiretroviral therapy.

From these few examples, it may be clear that both CD4+ and CD8+ T cells are important in establishing control of polyomavirus induced tumor progression and metastasis, and in controlling other consequences of productive polyomavirus infection like PML. A possible link between latent polyomavirus infection and protective immunity controlling tumorogenesis is important to establish. To eventually settle this, well planned prospective studies must be performed particularly comparing seropositive healthy individuals that acquire immune deficiencies with normal seropositive healthy controls. T cells operational in context of polyomavirus-related induction of autoimmunity to DNA and nucleosomes will be discussed in relevant sections below.

Polyomaviruses, SLE and Autoimmunity to Nucleosomes and dsDNA

Systemic Lupus Erythematosus (SLE) and Anti-dsDNA Antibodies

SLE, the prototype of a systemic rheumatic syndrome, is characterized by production of a wide array of autoantibodies.[94] Dominant proportions among these are antibodies directed against nuclear constituents[95] (antinuclear antibodies, ANA). Aside from their diagnostic importance, subpopulations of ANA, especially those binding dsDNA may have the additional effect as initiators of glomerulonephritis typical for this autoimmune syndrome.[96-103] Not all anti-dsDNA antibodies are involved in SLE nephritis, but those that are nephritogenic seem to recognize mammalian dsDNA, although some reports indicate that antibodies specific for nucleosomes also may have nephritogenic potential.[99,104-106]

The ethiology of SLE is, although the disease has been described for at least 15 centuries ago,[107] an unresolved matter. One may, according to the pleotropic picture of the disease, question whether SLE represents one disease entity, or represents a continuous overlap of individual, etiologically unrelated, organ manifestations (discussed in ref. 25). Hence, the term SLE may theoretically represent a heading for a wide variety of intrinsically unrelated disease manifestations, explaining the highly diverse picture of the disorder,[108] and may therefore principally be meaningless to use to define a single disease entity. On this background, it is important to try to understand at least the molecular and cellular origin of one of the major pathogenic and disease modifying factors characterizing this disease, namely antibodies to dsDNA. In this section, the cellular and molecular impact of polyomaviruses and polyomavirus-encoded DNA binding proteins on production of anti-DNA antibodies will be discussed in terms of their direct and measurable effect on initiation and sustained production of this antibody population. We have during recent years continuously developed in vivo and in vitro experimental systems employing intact BKV or SV40 T-ag to describe processes that have shed light on this enigmatic autoimmune response (reviewed in refs. 22,24,25,109,110).

B Cells Specific for dsDNA Can Be Activated by Polyomaviruses— The Phenomenon

This research program was initiated in 1986 based on an unintended observation done by Christie and colleagues in their attempts to induce antibodies to BKV in rabbits.[40] Their main focus was to develop an ELISA to trace polyomavirus antibodies in humans. After deliberate immunization of rabbits with purified, infectious BKV particles, development of serum antibodies were assayed by several detection methods, including western blots. As expected, they observed antibodies to capsid proteins, in addition to several low molecular weight polypeptides.[40] These were assumed to be host cell histones, which are used by viral DNA to form minichromosomes.[6,7] Extrapolating from these data, we reconsidered an old idea to explain how autoimmunity to DNA and nucleosomes could be initiated. This idea originated from early studies on immunogenicity of haptens, defined as molecules that could bind antibodies, but not by themselves stimulate to antibody production. In other words, they were nonimmunogenic. For haptens to gain immunogenic potential there is a need (i) for B cells to recognize that particular hapten, and (ii) for the hapten to be coupled to a carrier protein in order for cognate interacting T cells to be stimulated and thereby to provide help for hapten-specific B cells.

The Hapten-Carrier System—Formal Requirements

The first prerequisite relevant to use a hapten-carrier system to explain how polyomaviruses may initiate autoimmunity to DNA is the presence of B cells specific for dsDNA. The B cell receptors for antigens are generated by several stochastic events during somatic maturation of the B cells to ensure generation of all for the organism necessary antibody specificities. These events include (i) random recombination of one each of a large repertoire of V, D, and J genes for the immunoglobulin heavy chains and V and J genes for the light ones, (ii) insertion of nontemplate nucleotides between the variable region genes, and (iii) the use of full length, truncated or inverted D genes in all three reading frames.[111] Combination of heavy and light chains to constitute intact immunoglobulin molecules adds to this manifold of specificities.[72] Such random processes generate large arrays of immunoglobulin specificities, including specificity for autologous constituents. Provided naïve DNA-specific B cells have high affinity receptors for the autoantigen, they may be deleted, preferentially in the bone marrow,[112] or their receptors may be revised, a process called receptor editing, implying that the B cell substitute one light chain by another, thus changing its antigenic specificity.[113] However, due to the adaptive nature of the B cell receptor, antigen stimulation of low-affinity B cells may through somatic mutations linked to progression of the immune response, result in higher affinity for that given antigen.[114] Deletion of high-affinity B cells specific for autoantigens is therefore not a guarantee against development of high-affinity autoantibodies.

Secondly, for B cells to be stimulated, they need cognate interacting T helper cells.[115] T cells specific for autologous ligands may be physically or functionally inactivated in the thymus,[72] or rendered nonresponsive in the periphery (see e.g., refs. 25,73). Thus, although B cells may recognize autologous ligands, they still will not be activated by a given autoantigen due to the lack of sufficient T cell help. This may be circumvented if an autoantigen form complexes in vivo with a nonself antigen. In this situation, a scenario may be created that fulfill all demands to activate autoimmune B cells, provided the auto-specific B cell process and present peptides derived from the complexed nonself ligand. In other words, this model is in harmony with the hapten-carrier system to induce anti-hapten antibodies by otherwise nonimmunogenic haptens.[116,117] In this context, the autoantigen is analogous to the (nonimmunogenic) hapten, while the nonself complexed ligand represents the carrier protein. The conceptual framework for the research program described here for polyomavirus dependent termination of tolerance to DNA, histones and nucleosomes relied on this hapten-carrier model.

The Hapten-Carrier System for Induction of Anti-dsDNA Antibodies— Experimental Systems and Clinical Observations

In a prospective set of experiments, the first series of evidences that polyomaviruses had the potential to induce antibodies to the major components of nucleosomes, DNA and histones, were provided.[118] That this immunization regime resulted in antibodies recognizing mammalian dsDNA in both ELISA and the *Crithidia luciliae* assay, regarded as specific for SLE,[119] was important as the current view at that time was that mammalian dsDNA was nonimmunogenic.[120-123] In subsequent experiments we verified this observation,[124,125] and unequivocally proved that the antibodies bound different forms of DNA; mammalian ssDNA and dsDNA, and different synthetic single-stranded and double-stranded analogous of DNA.[126,127] In the latter experiments, the induced antibodies possessed DNA specificities reflecting the DNA used for immunization. If polyomavirus DNA complexed with methylated bovine serum albumin (mBSA) was used as immunogen, the emerging antibodies were mainly specific for that DNA, and did not crossreact with mammalian DNA, similar to what had been observed in other experimental systems.[121-123] However, if experimental animals were primed with viral DNA-carrier protein complexes, they responded to subsequent immunization using calf thymus (CT) dsDNA-mBSA by producing antibodies cross-reacting with mammalian dsDNA including human and CT dsDNA.[127]

In a next set of experiments, we tested whether natural infection with BKV resulted in similar sets of anti-nucleosomal antibodies. In that study we demonstrated that the earlier described anti-dsDNA responses to BKV in experimental animals also appeared during natural BKV infection in man.[128] Fifty-nine children were examined over time for serological signs (development of IgG and IgM anti-VP antibodies) of primary BKV infection. Of eight children found to undergo primary infection with BKV, anti-BKV-dsDNA specific antibodies appeared in all. In 4 of the 8 patients the antibodies cross-reacted significantly with mammalian dsDNA, and weak antibody binding to mammalian dsDNA was also noted in at least three other patients.[128] The antibodies resembled those induced in the experimental model with regard to their high relative affinity for BK dsDNA, and somewhat lower, but definitive, affinity for mammalian dsDNA. In contrast, most, but not all, anti-dsDNA antibodies from 10 SLE patients cross-reacted extensively with dsDNA from viral and mammalian origin. Thus, a dsDNA virus like BKV may provoke immunological intolerance to mammalian dsDNA, with features similar to those encountered in SLE. Furthermore, these observations demonstrated that induction of anti-dsDNA antibodies was not restricted to experimental immunization of animals, but did also take place in humans during naturally acquired BKV infection.

A logic question following these observations was how autoimmune (e.g., (NZB/NZW)F1 mice) mice responded to polyomaviruses compared to responses in normal mice. After inoculation with polyomavirus or polyomavirus-dsDNA complexed with mBSA, the normal Balb/C mice responded by producing anti-DNA antibodies mostly recognizing polyomavirus ssDNA and dsDNA, while the autoimmune mice readily produced nephritogenic anti-mammalian dsDNA antibodies.[129] Highly relevant, and similar to our results, Gilkeson et al[130] compared anti-DNA antibody responses in normal and (NZBxNZW)F1 mice after immunization with bacterial DNA-mBSA complexes. Whereas the immunologically normal mice produced antibodies that were specific for the immunizing bacterial DNA, (NZBxNZW)F1 mice produced antibodies that also bound CT dsDNA. Furthermore, the induced antibodies resembled lupus anti-DNA antibodies in their fine specificity for synthetic analogous of ss/dsDNA or *Crithidia luciliae* kinetoplast DNA.[130]

All together, these data demonstrated that ubiquitous human viruses like polyomaviruses, when activated in vivo, had the potential to induce the production of pathogenic anti-DNA antibodies in disposed individuals. In a subsequent study, we generated anti-dsDNA producing B cell hybridomas from mice hyper-immunized with polyomavirus BK. The structure and gene usage of the variable regions of heavy and light chains of these induced anti-dsDNA antibodies were determined in order to compare the structural features of the induced antibodies with those characterized in murine SLE[131-141] This study revealed that the polyomavirus induced anti-dsDNA antibodies were highly similar to potentially pathogenic anti-DNA antibodies produced in context of murine SLE, particularly with respect to the presence of the basic amino acid arginine at amino acid positions 99-101 in the heavy chain variable regions.[142] Thus, both polyomavirus and bacterial DNA, when complexed with an immunogenic carrier protein, had the potential to induce pathogenic anti-dsDNA antibodies with variable regions structures similar to those described in SLE.[118,129,130]

These results were all in agreement with the hapten-carrier model, and opened for aimed studies to determine the origin and nature of the carrier protein involved in the immune response to DNA. It became important to search for the origin of in vivo-produced proteins that **rendered** DNA immunogenic, instead of searching for **immunogenic** DNA.

Polyomavirus T-ag: A Natural Carrier Protein for dsDNA

Since polyomaviruses obviously had the potential to induce the production of anti-dsDNA antibodies in experimental animals,[118,129,142] this pointed at virus-encoded proteins as potential carrier molecules rendering DNA immunogenic. As described above, e.g., VP1 has both nuclear localization signals (NLS) and potential to bind DNA directly and indirectly through interaction with DNA bound proteins.[5,14-17] On the other hand, in the permissive host another virus encoded protein could be more relevant, as it is required for viral transcription and replication, and binds both viral and host DNA—polyomavirus large T-ag.[5] Thus, T-ag could represent a nonself DNA-bound protein that served as the T cell determinant. This assumed process would require that DNA-specific B cells indeed had the potential to present T-ag-derived peptides in context of sufficient costimulatory signals, and that T cells were primed by T-ag presented by conventional antigen-presenting cells.

In two different experimental systems these presumptions were verified. The first was based on immunizations with plasmids encoding T-ag under control of eukaryotic promoters[22] Immunologically normal mice inoculated with plasmids encoding wild-type, DNA-binding T-ag produced antibodies to this protein. These antibodies were kinetically linked to significant production of antibodies to dsDNA, histones, and to certain transcription factors, deduced to be produced according to the basic idea of the model: all autologous ligands linked to T-ag could theoretically be rendered immunogenic provided the presence of a (functional) repertoire of B cells.[22] Injection of plasmids expressing irrelevant nonDNA-binding proteins like luciferase, or plasmids containing T-ag sequences but lacking a promoter, did not result in such antibodies,[22] indicating that plasmid DNA itself was nonimmunogenic. In the second experimental approach,[23] we could directly demonstrate i. that SLE patients were highly susceptible to persistent productive polyomavirus infections, or recurrent virus reactivation, as opposed to normal individuals; and ii. that linked to virus expression, antibodies to T-ag, DNA and to transcription factors like TBP and CREB, but not to other nonnucleosomal autoantigens, were produced. Interestingly, antibodies to mammalian dsDNA correlated with persistent infection in the SLE patients.[23,109] These studies[22,23] have resulted in novel knowledge about a possible source of these antibodies and about a process that may explain how antibodies to dsDNA can be generated.

The SLE-Related Polyomaviruses Belong to Wild-Type Strains

As polyomaviruses demonstrated a strong tendency to productive infection in SLE,[23,67] but not in normal individuals, nor in rheumatoid arthritis patients, it was important to assess whether these viruses differed from those latently infecting normal individuals. A detailed characterization of the NCCR of the virus genome containing the promoter/enhancer region,[67] and the gene encoding the main capsid protein VP1,[143] potentially important for binding to, and thereby infecting, cells was therefore undertaken. However, for both genomic regions mostly sequences were detected identical to strains circulating in the healthy human population, demonstrating that such regions probably were not responsible for the strong tendency for productive infection in SLE patients.[67,143] A provisional explanation is therefore that SLE patients have lost their ability to control this virus, as described for e.g., immune deficient individuals.[5,11]

Virus-Induced Anti-dsDNA Antibodies—A Model Not Restricted to Polyomaviruses

Collectively, the data generated so far demonstrate that in vivo expression of the polyomavirus DNA-binding T-ag resulted in generation of IgG antibodies to T-ag and nucleosomal ligands like DNA, histones and transcription factors, but not to other autoantigens not linked to nucleosomes, indicating an antigen-selective T cell dependent B cell response. Complexes formed in vivo and in vitro of T-ag and nucleosomes created a molecular basis for antigen-selective interaction of T-ag specific T cells and nucleosome (DNA) specific B cells.[82] In harmony with this, B cells cocultured with T-ag specific T cells and stimulated with T-ag or nucleosome-T-ag complex, could present T-ag-derived peptides to T cells and produce antibodies with specificity reflecting the nature of the stimulating antigens, e.g., against T-ag or DNA.[82] Thus, T-ag may both initiate and maintain an autoantibody response to e.g., DNA in situations where T-ag is actively expressed.

This hapten-carrier model has been proven valid in other, but not all, studies of termination of immunological tolerance to DNA by viruses. Whether human cytomegalovirus (HCMV) was expressed in SLE and correlated with development of autoimmunity was examined in our laboratory using the same biological material as in the foregoing studies.[23,143] The result of this study was that HCMV did not correlate with autoimmunity, as active infection was not detected in these patients as judged from lack of both viruria and lack of increased IgM and IgG anti-HCMV antibody titers.[144] These data, however, do by no means rule out that other viruses, and even HCMV, may participate in generating autoimmunity to nucleosomal antigens.

Immunization of immunologically normal mice with complexes of the DNA-binding domain of the human papillomavirus E2 protein and a DNA fragment encompassing the E2-binding site resulted in antibodies against the E2 protein and dsDNA. The latter antibodies reacted with free and E2-bound dsDNA but not with the protein.[145] Similar to data discussed above,[22] mice inoculated with a vector expressing the single DNA-binding protein EBNA-1 of the Epstein-Barr virus, generated autoantibodies to both dsDNA and the Sm antigen,[146] probably in context of a carrier function of the EBNA-1 antigen. Similarly, a recent case report presented evidence that a 22-year old woman developed SLE following infection with Epstein- Barr virus. Antibodies to dsDNA and EBNA-1 characterized the antibody profile of this patient.[147]

In a study by Dong et al[148] high titer antibodies specific for the p53 tumor suppressor protein were induced in mice immunized with purified complexes of murine p53 and the SV40 T-ag, but not in mice immunized with either protein separately. The autoantibodies to p53 in these mice were primarily of the IgG1 isotype and were not cross-reactive with T-ag. The high levels of autoantibodies to p53 in mice immunized with p53-T-ag complexes were transient, similar to the induced anti-dsDNA antibodies described above, but low levels of the anti-p53 antibodies persisted. The latter may have been maintained by the self antigen, since the anti-p53, but not the anti-T-ag response could be restimulated with murine p53. One explanation for their results may be that antigen processing of the complex of T-ag and p53 could activate both T-ag-specific and autoreactive p53-specific T helper cells, thus driving anti-p53 autoantibody production. The induction of autoantibodies during the course of an immune response directed against this naturally occurring complex of self and nonself antigens may therefore be relevant to the generation of specific autoantibodies in context of viral infections, irrespective whether the individual suffers from SLE or not.

In the interpretation of their data, Reeves and Dong et al[148,149] indicated that humoral autoimmunity can be initiated by a "hit and run" mechanism in which the binding of a viral antigen to a self protein triggers an immune response that subsequently can be perpetuated by self antigen. For this to occur, however, autoimmune T cells must also be engaged in context of the viral infection, and not be rendered tolerant once the infection (and production of autoantigen-binding viral proteins) is terminated. This has been an important focus in advancing our studies on polyomavirus-induced tolerance to autoantigens, and experiments described below explain how T cell tolerance to nucleosomes may be terminated in context of stimulation with nucleosome-T-ag complexes. The results so far have provided us with a carrier protein, large T-ag, that has the potential to render DNA/nucleosomes immunogenic, and which may be constitutively expressed in vivo in SLE patients, but transiently and rarely in normal individuals. This insight opened for the study of determinant spreading, or better: the consequence of linked presentation of self nucleosomal peptides and nonself T-ag derived peptides to activate dormant autoimmune T cells.

Indirect Activation of Nucleosome-Specific T Cells through Determinant Spreading Requires Complex Formation of T-ag and Nucleosomes

Based on results described above, regulation of T cell tolerance to nucleosomes became important, as T cells in SLE, but not in healthy humans, are intolerant to this complex.[45,82,84,150-152] Central in this perspective was to test whether autoimmune, nucleosome-specific T cells are physically eliminated in the thymus through deletion, or whether such cells are entering the periphery where they may receive stimuli that result either in activation, anergy or in deletion. We approached these problems by testing whether T-ag expression also could have the potential to terminate histone-specific T cell anergy as a consequence of linked presentation by APC of histones and T-ag. This was likely to occur in vivo, as we succeeded in determining and characterizing this process in vitro.[45] Thus, by stimulating PBMC with nucleosome-T-ag complexes, but not with nucleosomes **or** T-ag, such T cell cultures could functionally be restimulated in the next round by nucleosomes or histones.[45] This would be in accordance with a model that implies APC-mediated linked presentation of nonself T-ag and (self) histone peptides. In this situation, responder T-ag-specific T cells may, through secretion of IL-2, activate nonselectively autoimmune, histone-specific T cells present in the microenvironment.[153,154] Subsequently, these T cells may clonally expand provided that histone-derived peptides are presented by APC in context of HLA class II, and that sufficient costimulatory signals are available.[155-159] The full picture of this model, including activation of autoimmune, histone-specific T cells and initiation of autoimmune DNA-specific B cells is outlined in Figure 3.

The results obtained using T cells from healthy human individuals and human SLE were reproduced experimentally in mice immunized with nucleosomes and nucleosome-T-ag complexes.[83] Only mice immunized with nucleosome-T-ag complexes harbored T cells that subsequently responded to pure nucleosomes or histones, presumably due to a linked presentation of nucleosomal peptides and T-antigen derived peptides by the same APC in vivo.[83] Thus, in this latter study, we obtained experimental results mimicking those described for the human system.[44,45,82] These results therefore strongly indicate that all individuals may harbor autoimmune nucleosome-specific T cells similar to those detected in active SLE.

In a recent study, the complementary determining region 3 (CDR3) structures of the TCR V(α) and/or V(β) chains were determined.[84] Histone- and T-ag- specific T cells were generated by stimulation of PBMCs with nucleosome-T-ag complexes and subsequently maintained by pure histones. T-ag-specific T cell clones were initiated and maintained by T-ag. The frequencies of circulating histone- or T-ag-specific T cells were determined in healthy individuals and in SLE patients by limiting dilution of PBMCs, and TCR gene usage and variable-region structures were determined by complementary DNA sequencing. These sequences were compared between T-ag- and histone-specific T cells and between normal individuals and SLE patients for each specificity. Individual in vitro-expanded histone-specific T cells from normal individuals displayed identical TCR V(α) and/or V(β) CDR3 regions sequences, indicating that they were clonally expanded in vivo. Essentially the same was observed for T-ag-specific T cells. The frequencies of in vitro antigen-responsive T-ag- or histone-specific T cells from normal individuals were similar to those from SLE patients. Although heterogeneous for variable-region structure and gene usage, histone- specific T cells from healthy individuals and SLE patients selected the acidic amino acids aspartic and/or glutamic acids at positions 99 and/or 100 in the V(β) CDR3 regions which may be important in recognizing basic amino acids within histone polypeptides. Thus, autoimmune T cells from healthy individuals can be activated by nucleosome- T-ag complexes and maintained by histones in vitro and in vivo. Such T cells possessed TCR structures similar to those from SLE patients, demonstrating that T cell autoimmunity to nucleosomes may be an inherent property of the normal immune system. This is further strengthened by the fact that such autoimmune T cells were clonally expanded in vivo, although nonresponsive at the time they were isolated.[84]

Thus, complexes formed by virus-encoded DNA-binding T-ag and host cell nucleosomes are directly immunogenic to DNA-specific B cells,[22,23] and indirectly to autoimmune, histone- or nucleosome-specific T cells through linked presentation of nonself and self peptides in context of HLA II molecules.[45,83,84]

Precedence for this model relates to diversification of T cell responses to include responses to determinants between different polypeptides contained within molecular complexes or within mixtures of solitaire molecules, provided that T cells are present which are able to respond to one of the components.[160,161] For example, Lin et al[161] observed that autologous cytochrome C was nonimmunogenic with regard to T cell proliferation. However, T cells purified from mice that were immunized with self and nonself cytochrome C subsequently proliferated to isolated self cytochrome C. Similar results have been obtained after immunization of normal mice with self/nonself snRNP.[162]

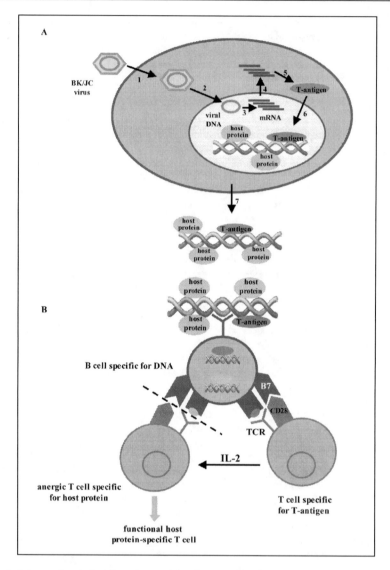

Figure 3. Polyomavirus induced autoimmunity to DNA and nucleosomes—a Hapten-Carrier model. Model for how a viral, nonself molecule like polyomavirus T-ag may initiate production of antibodies to DNA, and also to terminate histone-specific T cell anergy through a linked presentation of T-ag and histones by autologous B cells. A) After infection of a host cell (1), the viral genome is released (2), is replicated and transcribed in the nucleus (3). Viral transcripts are transported to the cytoplasm (4) and are translated into viral proteins (5). One of these proteins, large T-antigen enters the nucleus (6) and bind to cellular chromatin. Large T-antigen-chromatin complexes may be released (7) upon virus-induced lysis of the infected cell, or if virus-infected cells are killed by CD8+ T cells. B) When T-ag-nucleosome complexes become accessible, they may be bound by DNA-specific B cells, which subsequently process and present peptides derived from both T-ag and e.g., histones. This may be sufficient to transform B cells to anti-DNA antibody-producing plasma cells, and to terminate histone-specific T cell anergy. The latter phenomenon may be explained by activation of T-ag-specific CD4+ T cells, which start to secrete IL-2 into the microenvironment. IL-2 may then induce proliferation of histone-specific T cells, which may terminate the anergic state of these autoimmune T cells.[153,154]

Why Is a Nonself Viral Protein Necessary for Induction of B Cell and T Cell Autoimmunity to Nucleosomes?

There may be several reasons why pure autologous nucleosomes may not be immunogenic although B cells specific for e.g., dsDNA, histones or transcription factors are present in the body and amenable to antigenic stimulation.[22,163] First, T cells specific for nucleosomes or nucleosome-derived peptides may be sorted out in the thymus, one of the places in the body where nucleosomes must be generated in large amounts due to clonal deletion of autoreactive T cells.[164-166] Whether the T cells specific for nucleosomes or histones, as those described above, have escaped clonal deletion due to low affinity for their autologous ligands remains to be established. Alternatively, autoimmune T cells may have escaped deletion merely based on stochastic events—for them a fortunate event, for the body, however, an unlucky one as they now can participate in unwanted potentially pathogenic autoimmune responses. In the periphery, on the other hand, several control mechanisms may be involved to control autoimmune T cells that have escaped clonal deletion in the thymus. These mechanisms are linked to both the innate and the adaptive immune system.

In this sense, we must differentiate between infectious pathogens and autologous molecules or complexes of these. Invading antigens in the form of e.g., infectious agens are mostly drained into the lymph nodes, where antigens can be processed and presented properly by professional APCs delivering appropriate costimulatory signals and activation signals for antigen-selective T cells. This may initiate meaningful immune responses with the elimination of the infectious agens as the intended goal. In certain situations, a potentially pathogenic side effect of this process is, however, that (in our context) nucleosomes may be rendered immunogenic both for B cells and T cells along pathways described above (see Fig. 3 for details). Thus, viral infections may induce potentially pathogenic autoimmunity. Subsequently, pure nucleosomes devoid of nonself polypeptides could theoretically stimulate and expand this autoimmune response further, provided that such T cells are not functionally down-regulated. This may, however, actually be achieved by APCs not providing costimulatory signals or by MHC class II expressing cells of nonlymphoid organs. For example, stimulation of Toll-like receptors by infectious ligands seems to trigger dendritic cells to maturate, subsequently resulting in up-regulation of costimulatory molecules and increased antigen-presenting capacity for T cells.[75-77,167] Lack of stimulation of these receptors may result in lack of expression of costimulatory molecules. This may be the case for e.g., antigens like human autologous nucleosomes/chromatin that may lack PAMPs recognized by cell surface PRR (see above, and ref. 76). In situations where autologous nucleosomes are available to e.g., dendritic cells, nucleosomes may therefore tolerate T cells by presenting e.g., nucleosome-derived peptides rather than activating them.

Furthermore, nonlymphoid cells like endothelial or epithelial cells may have the capacity to present peptides in context of HLA class II,[168-170] but without providing costimulatory signals mediated by CD80/86.[171-173] This is, however, controversial, as others have detected also costimulatory signal molecules on e.g., endothelial cells.[174-176] In situations where APCs present autologous peptides in context of HLA class II but lacking costimulation, T cells will not respond properly,[156,177] and may instead be antigen-selectively anergized.[155,178]

If this holds to be true, evolution has responded immensely meaningfully to an unexpected threat exerted by e.g., viruses aside from their cytopathogenic effects. These may directly be able to initiate autoimmunity, as complexes formed by autoantigens (here: nucleosomes) and viral proteins (like polyomavirus T-ag) may be drained from the focus of the infection into lymph nodes. Following this, germinal centers may be established, with autoimmune responses as a result (Fig. 3). However, once such autoimmune T cells receive their stimuli, they proliferate and recirculate. During this latter process, they may encounter the same nucleosomal peptides in the periphery, now presented by inappropriate APCs like immature dendritic cells or HLA II expressing nonlymphoid cells lacking costimulatory molecules, thus bringing the active (functional) state of the T cells back to a state of tolerance.

Is a Protein Like the DNA-Binding Polyomavirus Encoded T-ag Essential for Terminating Immune Nonresponsiveness to Nucleosomes?

Apoptosis is an event that characterizes the living organism, and must represent a heavy load of work for the phagocytic system. As all the apoptotic material will be accessible to cells capable of ingesting it, evolution must have developed control mechanisms protecting the body against autoimmunity to such material and against development of autoimmune disorders. Since it is quite obvious that autoimmune B cells and antigen-related T cells exist in the periphery, and since they can be activated antigen-selectively, the determination whether the immune system shall respond or not cannot rely solely on these cells. The intriguing ideas of Janeway and Medzhitov, describing PAMPs and PRRs as systems to differentiate between infectious nonself and noninfectious self,[73,77] directly point at the innate immune system as a main control station to prevent autoimmunity. Although not yet clearly established, one may assume, also from the logic of evolution, that the receptors of cells of the innate system (e.g., dendritic cells), such as Toll like receptors (the membrane bound version of the PRR) do not recognize for example autologous nucleosomes, dsDNA or histones, as they simply do not have PAMPs. This is in contrast to e.g., bacterial DNA that differs from autologous DNA by having substantially more of PAMPs like CpG. From this, one may speculate whether the innate immune system may protect against immune responses to autoantigens like those present on chromatin.

As tolerance to nucleosomes is maintained in a healthy body it must be effectively controlled by the innate and/or the adaptive immune system. There are, however, several problems that need to be solved. For example, in DNAse 1[179] or Nrf2[180] knock-out mice, autoimmunity to dsDNA spontaneously develops, followed by antibody deposition in kidneys and development of nephritis. In the normal counterpart of these mice, this does not take place. One potential explanation for this is that e.g., DNAse 1 may be important for degradation and elimination of nucleosomes. DNAse1 deficiency may correlate to decreased degradation, decreased elimination and increased extra-cellular storage of nucleosomes. This, according to others,[100,181] may result in **altered** degradation of chromatin, resulting in presentation of cryptic or altered self-determinants not present in the normal organism.[181,182] If such neo-antigens can stimulate e.g., dendritic cells to up-regulate costimulatory molecules is not, however, established. Nevertheless, if true, such altered determinants may, due to increased extra-cellular amounts, also be processed and presented globally in the organism, and thereby potentially also by nonprofessional APCs. These may, provided they do not up-regulate costimulatory molecules, reverse the activated state of the T cells to a state of anergy. Thus, although results from the DNAse 1 knock out mouse indicate that autologous nucleosomes may stimulate the immune system to produce anti-DNA antibodies, a concise and direct experimental system confirming this model is still missing. This problem, whether pure self (in context of apoptosis, altered self may also be self) can induce anti-self, needs, in light of the problems discussed here, further studies.

Irrespective Whether Self-Derived or Infectious-Derived Proteins Serve as Carrier Proteins for (Nucleosomal) DNA, Stimulation of DNA-Specific May Be the Net Result

The development of the induced anti-DNA antibodies, and their qualities, is described in Figure 4. If stimulated properly, the immune system produces antibodies to dsDNA that may develop from two principally different sources. One may be somatic mutation of variable regions of antibodies to ssDNA, with introduction of highly basic amino acids (particularly arginines) at distinct positions, yielding specificity for dsDNA.[139,144,146,148] The other may be represented by stimulation of B cells with an inherent (initial) specificity for dsDNA normally deleted in the bone marrow[112] If such B cells escape deletion, they may be adequately stimulated by dsDNA, and clonally expanded, provided it is complexed with an immunogenic carrier protein.

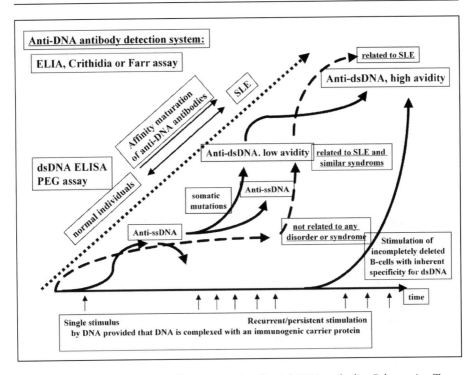

Figure 4. Kinetic development and affinity maturation of anti-dsDNA antibodies. Polyomavirus T-ag as an immunogenic carrier protein may in individual SLE patients play a role in induction of anti-DNA antibodies and influence the fine balance between generation of antibodies to ssDNA and dsDNA by forming complexes with nucleosomes (see Fig. 3). Antibodies against dsDNA are regarded as clinically important to settle the diagnosis SLE, and may be important in developing nephritis. This antibody sub-population can develop from two sources. As a consequence of somatic mutations of anti-ssDNA antibody variable regions, anti-dsDNA antibodies may progress from early anti-ssDNA secondary to continuous stimulation of DNA-specific B cell clones. The second source may be the result of stimulation of B cell clones with an inherent specificity for dsDNA. Such clones are normally deleted, but may escape deletion, and rather proliferate provided immunogenic DNA (i.e., for example DNA complexed with T-ag) is available for clonal B cell stimulation. (This figure is modified from ref. 5.) Anti-dsDNA antibody assays suitable for detection of antibodies with different affinities and their clinical impact are indicated.

Concluding Remarks

Polyomaviruses are strong stimulators of the immune system. The immune responses that evolve have all the characteristics of a secondary, adaptive, T cell dependent response. This is also true for the autoimmune responses against chromatin constituents induced through the involvement of polyomavirus-encoded ligands. These principally dual responses, anti-self and anti-nonself, reflect the Janus face of polyomaviruses, in the healthy body they are dormant and try to hide without irritating the immune system, but in situations where they are activated, they may initiate autoimmunity, and even induce tumors after prolonged productive infection.

References

1. Gardner SD, Field AM, Coleman DV et al. New human papovavirus (B.K.) isolated from urine after renal transplantation. Lancet 1971; 1(712):1253-1257.
2. Padgett BL, Walker DL, ZuRhein GM et al. Cultivation of papova-like virus from human brain with progressive multifocal leucoencephalopathy. Lancet 1971; 1(7712):1257-1260.

3. Sweet BH, Hilleman MR. The vacuolating virus, S.V. 40. Proc Soc Exp Biol Med 1960; 105:420-427.
4. Shah K, Nathanson N. Human exposure to SV40: Review and comment. Am J Epidemiol 1976; 103(1):1-12.
5. Moens U, Rekvig OP. Molecular biology of BK virus and clinical and basic aspects of BK virus renal infection. In: Khalili K, Stoner GL, eds. Human Polyomaviruses. Molecular and Clinical Perspectives. New York: Wiley-Liss Inc., 2001:359-408.
6. Meneguzzi G, Pignatti PF, Barbanti-Brodano G et al. Minichromosome from BK virus as a template for transcription in vitro. Proc Natl Acad Sci USA 1978; 75(3):1126-1130.
7. Varshavsky A, Levinger L, Sundin O et al. Cellular and SV40 chromatin: Replication, segregation, ubiquitination, nuclease-hypersensitive sites, HMG-containing nucleosomes, and heterochromatin-specific protein. Cold Spring Harb Symp Quant Biol 1983; 47(Pt 1):511-528.
8. Kornberg RD. Structure of chromatin. Annu Rev Biochem 1977; 46:931-954.
9. McGhee JD, Felsenfeld G. Nucleosome structure. Annu Rev Biochem 1980; 49:1115-1156.
10. Kornberg RD, Lorch Y. Twenty-five years of the nucleosome, fundamental particle of the eukaryote chromosome. Cell 1999; 98(3):285-294.
11. Moens U, Seternes OM, Johansen B et al. Mechanisms of transcriptional regulation of cellular genes by SV40 large T- and small t-antigens. Virus Genes 1997; 15(2):135-154.
12. Cole CN. Polyomaviruses: The viruses and their replication. In: Fields BN, Knipe DM, Howley PM, eds. Fields Virology. Philadelphia: Lippincot-Raven Publishers, 1996:1997-2025.
13. Viscidi RP, Rollison DE, Viscidi E et al. Serological cross-reactivities between antibodies to simian virus 40, BK virus, and JC virus assessed by virus-like-particle-based enzyme immunoassays. Clin Diagn Lab Immunol 2003; 10(2):278-285.
14. Wychowski C, Benichou D, Girard M. The intranuclear location of simian virus 40 polypeptides VP2 and VP3 depends on a specific amino acid sequence. J Virol 1987; 61(12):3862-3869.
15. Wychowski C, Benichou D, Girard M. A domain of SV40 capsid polypeptide VP1 that specifies migration into the cell nucleus. EMBO J 1986; 5(10):2569-2576.
16. Gharakhanian E, Kasamats H. Two independent signals, a nuclear localization signal and a Vp1-interactive signal, reside within the carboxy-35 amino acids of SV40 Vp3. Virology 1990; 178(1):62-71.
17. Gharakhanian E, Takahashi J, Clever J et al. In vitro assay for protein-protein interaction: Carboxyl-terminal 40 residues of simian virus 40 structural protein VP3 contain a determinant for interaction with VP1. Proc Natl Acad Sci USA 1988; 85(18):6607-6611.
18. Rekvig OP, Moens U, Fredriksen K et al. Human polyomavirus BK and immunogenicity of mammalian DNA: A conceptual framework. Methods 1997; 11(1):44-54.
19. Knowles WA. The epidemiology of BK virus and the occurence of antigenic and genomic subtypes. In: Khalili K, Stoner GL, eds. Human Polyomaviruses. Molecular and Clinical Perspectives. New York: Wiley-Liss, 2001:527-559.
20. Dorries K. Latent and persistant polyomavirus infection. In: Khalili K, Stoner GL, eds. Human Polyomaviruses. Molecular and Clinical Perspectives. New York: Wiley-Liss Inc., 2001:197-235.
21. Tooze J. DNA tumor viruses. Molecular biology of tumor viruses. Cold Spring Harbor: Cold Spring Harbor Laboratory, 1980.
22. Moens U, Seternes OM, Hey AW et al. In vivo expression of a single viral DNA-binding protein generates systemic lupus erythematosus-related autoimmunity to double-stranded DNA and histones. Proc Natl Acad Sci USA 1995; 92(26):12393-12397.
23. Rekvig OP, Moens U, Sundsfjord A et al. Experimental expression in mice and spontaneous expression in human SLE of polyomavirus T-antigen. A molecular basis for induction of antibodies to DNA and eukaryotic transcription factors. J Clin Invest 1997; 99(8):2045-2054.
24. Van Ghelue M, Moens U, Bendiksen S et al. Autoimmunity to nucleosomes related to viral infection: A focus on hapten-carrier complex formation. J Autoimmun 2003; 20(2):171-182.
25. Rekvig OP, Nossent JC. Anti-double-stranded DNA antibodies, nucleosomes, and systemic lupus erythematosus: A time for new paradigms? Arthritis Rheum 2003; 48(2):300-312.
26. Gardner SD. Prevalence in England of antibody to human polyomavirus (B.K.). BMJ 1973; i:77-78.
27. Padgett BL, Walker DL. Prevalence of antibodies in human sera against JC virus, an isolate from a case of progressive multifocal leukoencephalopathy. J Infect Dis 1973; 127(4):467-470.
28. Shah KV, Daniel RW, Wazawski RM. High prevalence of antibodies to BK virus, an SV40-related papovavirus, in residents of Maryland. J Infect Dis 1973; 128(6):784-787.
29. Mantyjarvi RA, Meurman OH, Vihma L et al. A human papovavirus (B.K.), biological properties and seroepidemiology. Ann Clin Res 1973; 5(5):283-287.

30. Brown P, Tsai T, Gajdusek DC. Seroepidemiology of human papovaviruses. Discovery of virgin populations and some unusual patterns of antibody prevalence among remote peoples of the world. Am J Epidemiol 1975; 102(4):331-340.
31. Rollison DEM, Shah KV. The epidemiology of SV40 infection due to contaminated polio vaccines: Relation of the virus to human cancer. In: Khalili K, Stoner GL, eds. Human Polyomaviruses. Molecular and Clinical Perspectives. New York: Wiley-Liss, 2001:561-584.
32. Agostini HT, Jobes DV, Stoner GL. Molecular evolution and epidemiology of JC virus. In: Khalili K, Stoner GL, eds. Human Polyomaviruses. Molecular and Clinical Perspectives. New York: Wiley-Liss, 2001:491-526.
33. Tevethia SS, Schell TD. The immune response to SV40, JCV, and BKV. In: Khalili K, Stoner GL, eds. Human Polyomaviruses. Molecular and Clinical Perspectives. New York: Wiley-Liss, 2001:585-610.
34. Knowles WA, Pipkin P, Andrews N et al. Population-based study of antibody to the human polyomaviruses BKV and JCV and the simian polyomavirus SV40. J Med Virol 2003; 71(1):115-123.
35. Flower AJ, Banatvala JE, Chrystie IL. BK antibody and virus-specific IgM responses in renal transplant recipients, patients with malignant disease, and healthy people. Br Med J 1977; 2(6081):220-223.
36. Portolani M, Marzocchi A, Barbanti Brodano G et al. Prevalence in Italy of antibodies to a new human papovavirus (BK virus). J Med Microbiol 1974; 7(4):543-546.
37. Zapata M, Mahony JB, Chernesky MA. Measurement of BK papovavirus IgG and IgM by radioimmunoassay (RIA). J Med Virol 1984; 14(2):101-114.
38. Flaegstad T, Traavik T, Kristiansen BE. Age-dependent prevalence of BK virus IgG and IgM antibodies measured by enzyme-linked immunosorbent assays (ELISA). J Hyg Lond 1986; 96(3):523-528.
39. Flaegstad T, Ronne K, Filipe AR et al. Prevalence of anti BK virus antibody in Portugal and Norway. Scand J Infect Dis 1989; 21(2):145-147.
40. Christie KE, Flaegstad T, Traavik T. Characterization of BK virus-specific antibodies in human sera by Western immunoblotting: Use of a zwitterionic detergent for restoring the antibody-binding capacity of electroblotted proteins. J Med Virol 1988; 24(2):183-190.
41. Stolt A, Sasnauskas K, Koskela P et al. Seroepidemiology of the human polyomaviruses. J Gen Virol 2003; 84(Pt 6):1499-1504.
42. Corallini A, Barbanti-Brodano G, Portolani M et al. Antibodies to BK virus structural and tumor antigens in human sera from normal persons and from patients with various diseases, including neoplasia. Infect Immun 1976; 13(6):1684-1691.
43. Dougherty RM, Distefano HS. Isolation and characterization of a papovavirus from human urine. Proc Soc Exp Biol Med 1974; 146(2):481-487.
44. Bredholt G, Olaussen E, Moens U et al. Linked production of antibodies to mammalian DNA and to human polyomavirus large T antigen: Footprints of a common molecular and cellular process? Arthritis Rheum 1999; 42(12):2583-2592. [published erratum appears in Arthritis Rheum 2000; 43(4):929].
45. Andreassen K, Moens U, Nossent H et al. Termination of human T cell tolerance to histones by presentation of histones and polyomavirus T antigen provided that T antigen is complexed with nucleosomes. Arthritis Rheum 1999; 42(11):2449-2460.
46. Takemoto KK. Human polyomaviruses: Evaluation of their possible involvement in human cancer. In: Essex M, Todaro G, zur Hausen M, eds. Viruses in Naturally Occuring Cancers. Cold Spring Harbor, New York: Cold Spring Harbor Conference on cell proliferation, 1980:7:311-318.
47. Walker DL, Padgett BL. The epidemiology of human polyomaviruses. Prog Clin Biol Res 1983; 105:99-106.
48. Hogan TF, Borden EC, McBain JA et al. Human polyomavirus infections with JC virus and BK virus in renal transplant patients. Ann Intern Med 1980; 92(3):373-378.
49. Taguchi F, Kajioka J, Miyamura T. Prevalence rate and age of acquisition of antibodies against JC virus and BK virus in human sera. Microbiol Immunol 1982; 26(11):1057-1064.
50. Kravetz HM, Knight V, Chanock RM et al. Respiratory syncytial virus. III. Production of illness and clinical observations in adult volunteers. JAMA 1961; 176:657-663.
51. Morris JA, Johnson KM, Aulisio CG et al. Clinical and serologic responses in volunteers given vacuolating virus (SV-40) by respiratory route. Proc Soc Exp Biol Med 1961; 108:56-59.
52. Melnick JL, Stinebaugh S. Excretion of vacuolating SV-40 virus (papova virus group) after ingestion as a contaminant of oral poliovaccine. Proc Soc Exp Biol Med 1962; 109:965-968.
53. Basetse HR, Lecatsas G, Gerber LJ. An investigation of the occurrence of SV40 antibodies in South Africa. S Afr Med J 2002; 92(10):825-828.

54. Butel JS, Wong C, Vilchez RA et al. Detection of antibodies to polyomavirus SV40 in two central European countries. Cent Eur J Public Health 2003; 11(1):3-8.

55. Butel JS, Arrington AS, Wong C et al. Molecular evidence of simian virus 40 infections in children. J Infect Dis 1999; 180(3):884-887.

56. Rollison DE, Helzlsouer KJ, Alberg AJ et al. Serum antibodies to JC virus, BK virus, simian virus 40, and the risk of incident adult astrocytic brain tumors. Cancer Epidemiol Biomarkers Prev 2003; 12(5):460-463.

57. Carter JJ, Madeleine MM, Wipf GC et al. Lack of serologic evidence for prevalent simian virus 40 infection in humans. J Natl Cancer Inst 2003; 95(20):1522-1530.

58. De Sanjose S, Shah K, Engels EA et al. Lack of serological evidence for an association between simian virus 40 and lymphoma. Int J Cancer 2003; 107(3):507-508.

59. Hamilton RS, Gravell M, Major EO. Comparison of antibody titers determined by hemagglutination inhibition and enzyme immunoassay for JC virus and BK virus. J Clin Microbiol 2000; 38(1):105-109.

60. Jafar S, Rodriguez-Barradas M, Graham DY et al. Serological evidence of SV40 infections in HIV-infected and HIV-negative adults. J Med Virol 1998; 54(4):276-284.

61. Minor P, Pipkin P, Jarzebek Z et al. Studies of neutralising antibodies to SV40 in human sera. J Med Virol 2003; 70(3):490-495.

62. Vilchez RA, Butel JS. Polyomavirus SV40 infection and lymphomas in Spain. Int J Cancer 2003; 107(3):505-506.

63. Brown DW, Gardner SD, Gibson PE et al. BK virus specific IgM responses in cord sera, young children and healthy adults detected by RIA. Arch Virol 1984; 82(3-4):149-160.

64. Hirsch HH, Steiger J. Polyomavirus BK. Lancet Infect Dis 2003; 3(10):611-623.

65. Knowles WA, Gibson PE, Hand JF et al. An M-antibody capture radioimmunoassay (MACRIA) for detection of JC virus-specific IgM. J Virol Methods 1992; 40(1):95-105.

66. Kitamura T, Aso Y, Kuniyoshi N et al. High incidence of urinary JC virus excretion in nonimmunosuppressed older patients. J Infect Dis 1990; 161(6):1128-1133.

67. Sundsfjord A, Osei A, Rosenqvist H et al. BK and JC viruses in patients with systemic lupus erythematosus: Prevalent and persistent BK viruria, sequence stability of the viral regulatory regions, and nondetectable viremia. J Infect Dis 1999; 180(1):1-9.

68. Song R, Harding CV. Roles of proteasomes, transporter for antigen presentation (TAP), and beta 2-microglobulin in the processing of bacterial or particulate antigens via an alternate class I MHC processing pathway. J Immunol 1996; 156(11):4182-4190.

69. Uebel S, Tampe R. Specificity of the proteasome and the TAP transporter. Curr Opin Immunol 1999; 11(2):203-208.

70. Pieters J. MHC class II-restricted antigen processing and presentation. Adv Immunol 2000; 75:159-208.

71. Brachet V, Raposo G, Amigorena S et al. Ii chain controls the transport of major histocompatibility complex class II molecules to and from lysosomes. J Cell Biol 1997; 137(1):51-65.

72. Janeway CA, Travers P, Walport M et al. Immunobiology. The immune system in health and disease. 5th ed. New York: Churchill Livingstone, 2003.

73. Janeway Jr CA. The immune system evolved to discriminate infectious nonself from noninfectious self. Immunol Today 1992; 13(1):11-16.

74. Janeway Jr CA, Bottomly K. Signals and signs for lymphocyte responses. Cell 1994; 76(2):275-285.

75. Janeway Jr CA, Medzhitov R. Innate immune recognition. Annu Rev Immunol 2002; 20:197-216.

76. Medzhitov R, Janeway Jr CA. Decoding the patterns of self and nonself by the innate immune system. Science 2002; 296(5566):298-300.

77. Medzhitov R, Janeway Jr CA. How does the immune system distinguish self from nonself? Semin Immunol 2000; 12(3):185-188.

78. Perniok A, Wedekind F, Herrmann M et al. High levels of circulating early apoptic peripheral blood mononuclear cells in systemic lupus erythematosus. Lupus 1998; 7(2):113-118.

79. Velupillai P, Carroll JP, Benjamin TL. Susceptibility to polyomavirus-induced tumors in inbred mice: Role of innate immune responses. J Virol 2002; 76(19):9657-9663.

80. Tevethia SS, Flyer DC, Tjian R. Biology of simian virus 40 (SV40) transplantation antigen (TrAg). VI. Mechanism of induction of SV40 transplantation immunity in mice by purified SV40 T antigen (D2 protein). Virology 1980; 107(1):13-23.

81. Tevethia SS, Lewis M, Tanaka Y et al. Dissection of H-2Db-restricted cytotoxic T-lymphocyte epitopes on simian virus 40 T antigen by the use of synthetic peptides and H-2Dbm mutants. J Virol 1990; 64(3):1192-1200.

82. Andreassen K, Bredholt G, Moens U et al. T cell lines specific for polyomavirus T-antigen recognize T- antigen complexed with nucleosomes: A molecular basis for anti- DNA antibody production. Eur J Immunol 1999; 29(9):2715-2728.
83. Bredholt G, Rekvig OP, Andreassen K et al. Differences in the reactivity of CD4+ T-cell lines generated against free versus nucleosome-bound SV40 large T antigen. Scand J Immunol 2001; 53(4):372-380.
84. Andreassen K, Bendiksen S, Kjeldsen E et al. T cell autoimmunity to histones and nucleosomes is a latent property of the normal immune system. Arthritis Rheum 2002; 46(5):1270-1281.
85. Drummond JE, Shah KV, Donnenberg AD. Cell-mediated immune responses to BK virus in normal individuals. J Med Virol 1985; 17(3):237-247.
86. Bates MP, Jennings SR, Tanaka Y et al. Recognition of simian virus 40 T antigen synthesized during viral lytic cycle in monkey kidney cells expressing mouse H-2Kb- and H-2Db-transfected genes by SV40-specific cytotoxic T lymphocytes leads to the abrogation of virus lytic cycle. Virology 1988; 162(1):197-205.
87. Ye X, McCarrick J, Jewett L et al. Timely immunization subverts the development of peripheral nonresponsiveness and suppresses tumor development in simian virus 40 tumor antigen-transgenic mice. Proc Natl Acad Sci USA 1994; 91(9):3916-3920.
88. Geiger T, Soldevila G, Flavell RA. T cells are responsive to the simian virus 40 large tumor antigen transgenically expressed in pancreatic islets. J Immunol 1993; 151(12):7030-7037.
89. Geiger T, Gooding LR, Flavell RA. T-cell responsiveness to an oncogenic peripheral protein and spontaneous autoimmunity in transgenic mice. Proc Natl Acad Sci USA 1992; 89(7):2985-2989.
90. Arrington AS, Butel JS. SV40 and human tumors. In: Khalili K, Stoner GL, eds. Human Polyomaviruses. Molecular and Clinical Perspectives. New York: Wiley-Liss, 2001:461-489.
91. Kennedy RC, Shearer MH, Watts AM et al. CD4+ T lymphocytes play a critical role in antibody production and tumor immunity against simian virus 40 large tumor antigen. Cancer Res 2003; 63(5):1040-1045.
92. Koralnik IJ. Overview of the cellular immunity against JC virus in progressive multifocal leukoencephalopathy. J Neurovirol 2002; 8(Suppl 2):59-65.
93. Gasnault J, Kahraman M, de Goer de Herve MG et al. Critical role of JC virus-specific CD4 T-cell responses in preventing progressive multifocal leukoencephalopathy. AIDS 2003; 17(10):1443-1449.
94. Amital H, Shoenfeld Y. Autoimmunity and autoimmune diseases such as Systemic lupus erythematosus. In: Lahita RG, ed. Systemic Lupus Erythematosus. San Diego, London, Boston, New York, Sidney, Tokio, Totonto: Academic Press, 1999:1-16.
95. Reeves WH, Satoh M, Richards HB. Origins of antinuclear antibodies. In: Lahita RG, ed. Systemic Lupus Erythematosus. San Diego, London, Boston, New York, Sidney, Tokio, Toronto: Academic Press, 1999:293-317.
96. Raz E, Brezis M, Rosenmann E et al. Anti-DNA antibodies bind directly to renal antigens and induce kidney dysfunction in the isolated perfused rat kidney. J Immunol 1989; 142(9):3076-3082.
97. Van Bruggen MC, Kramers C, Berden JH. Autoimmunity against nucleosomes and lupus nephritis. Ann Med Interne Paris 1996; 147(7):485-489.
98. Van Bruggen MC, Walgreen B, Rijke TP et al. Antigen specificity of anti-nuclear antibodies complexed to nucleosomes determines glomerular basement membrane binding in vivo. Eur J Immunol 1997; 27(6):1564-1569.
99. Kramers C, Hylkema MN, Van Bruggen MC et al. Anti-nucleosome antibodies complexed to nucleosomal antigens show anti-DNA reactivity and bind to rat glomerular basement membrane in vivo. J Clin Invest 1994; 94(2):568-577.
100. Berden JH, Licht R, Van Bruggen MC et al. Role of nucleosomes for induction and glomerular binding of autoantibodies in lupus nephritis. Curr Opin Nephrol Hypertens 1999; 8(3):299-306.
101. Vlahakos DV, Foster MH, Adams S et al. Anti-DNA antibodies form immune deposits at distinct glomerular and vascular sites. Kidney Int 1992; 41(6):1690-1700.
102. Madaio MP, Shlomchik MJ. Emerging concepts regarding B cells and autoantibodies in murine lupus nephritis. B cells have multiple roles; all autoantibodies are not equal [editorial]. J Am Soc Nephrol 1996; 7(3):387-396.
103. D'Andrea DM, Coupaye Gerard B, Kleyman TR et al. Lupus autoantibodies interact directly with distinct glomerular and vascular cell surface antigens. Kidney Int 1996; 49(5):1214-1221.
104. Amoura Z, Piette JC, Bach JF et al. The key role of nucleosomes in lupus. Arthritis Rheum 1999; 42(5):833-843.
105. Amoura Z, Koutouzov S, Chabre H et al. Presence of antinucleosome autoantibodies in a restricted set of connective tissue diseases: Antinucleosome antibodies of the IgG3 subclass are markers of renal pathogenicity in systemic lupus erythematosus. Arthritis Rheum 2000; 43(1):76-84.

106. Cervera R, Vinas O, Ramos-Casals M et al. Anti-chromatin antibodies in systemic lupus erythematosus: A useful marker for lupus nephropathy. Ann Rheum Dis 2003; 62(5):431-434.
107. Benedek TG. Historical background of discoid and systemic lupus erythematosus. In: Wallace DJ, Hahn BH, eds. Dubois' Lupus Erythematosus. Baltimore, Philadelphia, London, Paris, Bangkok, Buenos Aires, Hong Kong, Munich, Sydney, Tokio, Wroclaw: Williams & Wilkins, 1997:3-16.
108. Lahita RG. Systemic Lupus Erythematosus. 3th ed. New York: Academic Press, 1999.
109. Rekvig OP. Polyoma induced autoimmunity to DNA; experimental systems and clinical observations in human SLE. Lupus 1997; 6(3):325-326.
110. Rekvig OP, Andreassen K, Moens U. Antibodies to DNA-towards an understanding of their origin and pathophysiological impact in systemic lupus erythematosus [editorial]. Scand J Rheumatol 1998; 27(1):1-6.
111. Max EE. Immunoglobulins: Molecular Genetics. In: Paul WE, ed. Fundamental Immunology. New York: Lippincott, Williams & Wilkins, 1999:111-182.
112. Chen C, Nagy Z, Radic MZ et al. The site and stage of anti-DNA B-cell deletion. Nature 1995; 373(6511):252-255.
113. Chen C, Prak EL, Weigert M. Editing disease-associated autoantibodies. Immunity 1997; 6(1):97-105.
114. Wagner SD, Neuberger MS. Somatic hypermutation of immunoglobulin genes. Annu Rev Immunol 1996; 14:441-457.
115. Parker DC. T cell-dependent B cell activation. Annu Rev Immunol 1993; 11:331-360.
116. Benacerraf B, Paul WE, Green I. Hapten-carrier relationships. Ann NY Acad Sci 1970; 169(1):93-104.
117. Goodman JW. Antigenic determinants and antibody combining sites. In: Sela M, ed. The Antigens. New York: Academic Press, 1975:127-187.
118. Flaegstad T, Fredriksen K, Dahl B et al. Inoculation with BK virus may break immunological tolerance to histone and DNA antigens. Proc Natl Acad Sci USA 1988; 85(21):8171-8175.
119. Aarden LA, de Groot ER, Feltkamp TE. Immunology of DNA. III. Crithidia luciliae, a simple substrate for the determination of anti-dsDNA with the immunofluorescence technique.
120. Madaio MP, Hodder S, Schwartz RS et al. Responsiveness of autoimmune and normal mice to nucleic acid antigens. J Immunol 1984; 132(2):872-876.
121. Schwartz RS, Stollar BD. Origins of anti-DNA autoantibodies. J Clin Invest 1985; 75(2):321-327.
122. Stollar BD. Antibodies to DNA. CRC Crit Rev Biochem 1986; 20(1):1-36.
123. Stollar BD. Immunochemistry of DNA. Int Rev Immunol 1989; 5(1):1-22.
124. Rekvig OP, Flaegstad T, Fredriksen K et al. Stimulation of clones specific for dsDNA or idiotypes of anti-dsDNA as a consequence of BK virus inoculation. Immunol Invest 1989; 18(5):657-669.
125. Fredriksen K, Traavik T, Flaegstad T et al. BK virus terminates tolerance to dsDNA and histone antigens in vivo. Immunol Invest 1990; 19(2):133-151.
126. Fredriksen K, Traavik T, Rekvig OP. Anti-DNA antibodies induced by BK virus inoculations. Demonstration of the specificities for eukaryotic dsDNA and synthetic polynucleotides. Scand J Immunol 1990; 32(2):197-203.
127. Fredriksen K, Brannsether B, Traavik T et al. Antibodies to viral and mammalian native DNA in response to BK virus inoculation and subsequent immunization with calf thymus DNA. Scand J Immunol 1991; 34(1):109-119.
128. Fredriksen K, Skogsholm A, Flaegstad T et al. Antibodies to dsDNA are produced during primary BK virus infection in man, indicating that anti-dsDNA antibodies may be related to virus replication in vivo. Scand J Immunol 1993; 38(4):401-406.
129. Fredriksen K, Osei A, Sundsfjord A et al. On the biological origin of anti-double-stranded (ds) DNA antibodies: Systemic lupus erythematosus-related anti-dsDNA antibodies are induced by polyomavirus BK in lupus-prone (NZBxNZW) F1 hybrids, but not in normal mice. Eur J Immunol 1994; 24(1):66-70.
130. Gilkeson GS, Pippen AM, Pisetsky DS. Induction of cross-reactive anti-dsDNA antibodies in preautoimmune NZB/NZW mice by immunization with bacterial DNA. J Clin Invest 1995; 95(3):1398-1402.
131. Marion TN, Tillman DM, Jou NT. Interclonal and intraclonal diversity among anti-DNA antibodies from an (NZB x NZW)F1 mouse. J Immunol 1990; 145(7):2322-2332.
132. Marion TN, Krishnan MR, Desai DD et al. Monoclonal anti-DNA antibodies: Structure, specificity, and biology. Methods 1997; 11(1):3-11.
133. Marion TN, Tillman DM, Jou NT et al. Selection of immunoglobulin variable regions in autoimmunity to DNA. Immunol Rev 1992; 128:123-149.
134. Krishnan MR, Marion TN. Structural similarity of antibody variable regions from immune and autoimmune anti-DNA antibodies. J Immunol 1993; 150(11):4948-4957.

135. Krishnan MR, Marion TN. Comparison of the frequencies of arginines in heavy chain CDR3 of antibodies expressed in the primary B-cell repertoires of autoimmune-prone and normal mice. Scand J Immunol 1998; 48(3):223-232.
136. Krishnan MR, Jou NT, Marion TN. Correlation between the amino acid position of arginine in VH- CDR3 and specificity for native DNA among autoimmune antibodies. J Immunol 1996; 157(6):2430-2439.
137. Radic MZ, Mascelli MA, Erikson J et al. Structural patterns in anti-DNA antibodies from MRL/lpr mice. Cold Spring Harb Symp Quant Biol 1989; 54(Pt 2):933-946.
138. Radic MZ, Weigert M. Genetic and structural evidence for antigen selection of anti- DNA antibodies. Annu Rev Immunol 1994; 12:487-520.
139. Radic MZ, Mackle J, Erikson J et al. Residues that mediate DNA binding of autoimmune antibodies. J Immunol 1993; 150(11):4966-4977.
140. Shlomchik MJ, Marshak-Rothstein A, Wolfowicz CB et al. The role of clonal selection and somatic mutation in autoimmunity. Nature 1987; 328(6133):805-811.
141. Shlomchik MJ, Aucoin AH, Pisetsky DS et al. Structure and function of anti-DNA autoantibodies derived from a single autoimmune mouse. Proc Natl Acad Sci USA 1987; 84(24):9150-9154.
142. Rekvig OP, Fredriksen K, Hokland K et al. Molecular analyses of anti-DNA antibodies induced by polyomavirus BK in BALB/c mice. Scand J Immunol 1995; 41(6):593-602. [published erratum appears in Scand J Immunol 1995 Aug;42(2):286].
143. Bendiksen S, Rekvig OP, Van Ghelue M et al. VP1 DNA sequences of JC and BK viruses detected in urine of systemic lupus erythematosus patients reveal no differences from strains expressed in normal individuals. J Gen Virol 2000; 81(Pt 11):2625-2633.
144. Bendiksen S, Van Ghelue M, Rekvig OP et al. A longitudinal study of human cytomegalovirus serology and viruria fails to detect active viral infection in 20 systemic lupus erythematosus patients. Lupus 2000; 9(2):120-126.
145. Cerutti ML, Centeno JM, Goldbaum FA et al. Generation of sequence-specific, high affinity anti-DNA antibodies. J Biol Chem 2001; 276(16):12769-12773.
146. Sundar K, Jaques S, Spatz L et al. Mice immunized with Epstein-Barr nuclear antigen-1 expressing plasmids secrete antibodies to EBNA-1, dsDNA and Sm. Faseb J 2001; 15:A 1058.
147. Verdolini R, Bugatti L, Giangiacomi M et al. Systemic lupus erythematosus induced by Epstein-Barr virus infection. Br J Dermatol 2002; 146(5):877-881.
148. Dong X, Hamilton KJ, Satoh M et al. Initiation of autoimmunity to the p53 tumor suppressor protein by complexes of p53 and SV40 large T antigen. J Exp Med 1994; 179(4):1243-1252.
149. Reeves WH, Dong X, Wang J et al. Initiation of autoimmunity to self-proteins complexed with viral antigens. Ann NY Acad Sci 1997; 815:139-154.
150. Mohan C, Adams S, Stanik V et al. Nucleosome: A major immunogen for pathogenic autoantibody- inducing T cells of lupus. J Exp Med 1993; 177(5):1367-1381.
151. Datta SK, Kaliyaperumal A. Nucleosome-driven autoimmune response in lupus. Pathogenic T helper cell epitopes and costimulatory signals. Ann NY Acad Sci 1997; 815:155-170.
152. Voll RE, Roth EA, Girkontaite I et al. Histone-specific Th0 and Th1 clones derived from systemic lupus erythematosus patients induce double-stranded DNA antibody production. Arthritis Rheum 1997; 40(12):2162-2171.
153. Beverly B, Kang SM, Lenardo MJ et al. Reversal of in vitro T cell clonal anergy by IL-2 stimulation. Int Immunol 1992; 4(6):661-671.
154. Jenkins MK. The role of cell division in the induction of clonal anergy. Immunol Today 1992; 13(2):69-73.
155. Lenschow DJ, Walunas TL, Bluestone JA. CD28/B7 system of T cell costimulation. Annu Rev Immunol 1996; 14:233-258.
156. Gimmi CD, Freeman GJ, Gribben JG et al. Human T-cell clonal anergy is induced by antigen presentation in the absence of B7 costimulation. Proc Natl Acad Sci USA 1993; 90(14):6586-6590.
157. Schwartz RH. Costimulation of T lymphocytes: The role of CD28, CTLA-4, and B7/BB1 in interleukin-2 production and immunotherapy. Cell 1992; 71(7):1065-1068.
158. Mueller DL, Jenkins MK, Schwartz RH. Clonal expansion versus functional clonal inactivation: A costimulatory signalling pathway determines the outcome of T cell antigen receptor occupancy. Annu Rev Immunol 1989; 7:445-480.
159. Schwartz RH. T cell anergy. Annu Rev Immunol 2003; 21:305-334.
160. Mamula MJ, Lin RH, Janeway Jr CA et al. Breaking T cell tolerance with foreign and self coimmunogens. A study of autoimmune B and T cell epitopes of cytochrome c. J Immunol 1992; 149(3):789-795.
161. Lin RH, Mamula MJ, Hardin JA et al. Induction of autoreactive B cells allows priming of autoreactive T cells. J Exp Med 1991; 173(6):1433-1439.

162. Mamula MJ, Fatenejad S, Craft J. B cells process and present lupus autoantigens that initiate autoimmune T cell responses. J Immunol 1994; 152(3):1453-1461.
163. Desai DD, Krishnan MR, Swindle JT et al. Antigen-specific induction of antibodies against native mammalian DNA in nonautoimmune mice. J Immunol 1993; 151(3):1614-1626.
164. Kisielow P, von Boehmer H. Development and selection of T cells: Facts and puzzles. Adv Immunol 1995; 58:87-209.
165. Sprent J, Kishimoto H, Cai Z et al. The thymus and T cell death. Adv Exp Med Biol 1996; 406:191-198.
166. Surh CD, Sprent J. T-cell apoptosis detected in situ during positive and negative selection in the thymus. Nature 1994; 372(6501):100-103.
167. Liu Y, Janeway Jr CA. Microbial induction of costimulatory activity for CD4 T-cell growth. Int Immunol 1991; 3(4):323-332.
168. Collins T, Korman AJ, Wake CT et al. Immune interferon activates multiple class II major histocompatibility complex genes and the associated invariant chain gene in human endothelial cells and dermal fibroblasts. Proc Natl Acad Sci USA 1984; 81(15):4917-4921.
169. Page C, Rose M, Yacoub M et al. Antigenic heterogeneity of vascular endothelium. Am J Pathol 1992; 141(3):673-683.
170. Marelli Berg FM, Hargreaves RE, Carmichael P et al. Major histocompatibility complex class II-expressing endothelial cells induce allospecific nonresponsiveness in naïve. T cells. J Exp Med 1996; 183(4):1603-1612.
171. Marelli-Berg FM, Frasca L, Imami N et al. Lack of T cell proliferation without induction of nonresponsiveness after antigen presentation by endothelial cells. Transplantation 1999; 68(2):280-287.
172. Corrigall VM, Solau-Gervais E, Panayi GS. Lack of CD80 expression by fibroblast-like synoviocytes leading to anergy in T lymphocytes. Arthritis Rheum 2000; 43(7):1606-1615.
173. Byrne B, Madrigal-Estebas L, McEvoy A et al. Human duodenal epithelial cells constitutively express molecular components of antigen presentation but not costimulatory molecules. Hum Immunol 2002; 63(11):977-986.
174. Lohse AW, Knolle PA, Bilo K et al. Antigen-presenting function and B7 expression of murine sinusoidal endothelial cells and Kupffer cells. Gastroenterology 1996; 110(4):1175-1181.
175. Murray AG, Khodadoust MM, Pober JS et al. Porcine aortic endothelial cells activate human T cells: Direct presentation of MHC antigens and costimulation by ligands for human CD2 and CD28. Immunity 1994; 1(1):57-63.
176. Denton MD, Geehan CS, Alexander SI et al. Endothelial cells modify the costimulatory capacity of transmigrating leukocytes and promote CD28-mediated CD4(+) T cell alloactivation. J Exp Med 1999; 190(4):555-566.
177. June CH, Ledbetter JA, Linsley PS et al. Role of the CD28 receptor in T-cell activation. Immunol Today 1990; 11(6):211-216.
178. Marelli-Berg FM, Lechler RI. Antigen presentation by parenchymal cells: A route to peripheral tolerance? Immunol Rev 1999; 172:297-314.
179. Napirei M, Karsunky H, Zevnik B et al. Features of systemic lupus erythematosus in Dnase1-deficient mice. Nat Genet 2000; 25(2):177-181.
180. Yoh K, Itoh K, Enomoto A et al. Nrf2-deficient female mice develop lupus-like autoimmune nephritis. Kidney Int 2001; 60(4):1343-1353.
181. Herrmann M, Zoller OM, Hagenhofer M et al. What triggers anti-dsDNA antibodies? Mol Biol Rep 1996; 23(3-4):265-267.
182. Berden JH, Grootscholten C, Jurgen WC et al. Lupus nephritis: A nucleosome waste disposal defect? J Nephrol 2002; 15(Suppl 6):S1-10.
183. Meurman OH, Mantyjarvi RA, Salmi AA et al. Prevalence of antibodies to a human papova virus (BK virus) in subacute sclerosing panencephalitis and multiple sclerosis patients. Z Neurol 1972; 203(2):191-194.
184. Arthur RR, Dagostin S, Shah KV. Detection of BK virus and JC virus in urine and brain tissue by the polymerase chain reaction. J Clin Microbiol 1989; 27(6):1174-1179.
185. Arthur RR, Shah KV. Occurrence and significance of papovaviruses BK and JC in the urine. Prog Med Virol 1989; 36:42-61.
186. Azzi A, Cesaro S, Laszlo D et al. Human polyomavirus BK (BKV) load and haemorrhagic cystitis in bone marrow transplantation patients. J Clin Virol 1999; 14(2):79-86.
187. Azzi A, De Santis R, Ciappi S et al. Human polyomaviruses DNA detection in peripheral blood leukocytes from immunocompetent and immunocompromised individuals. J Neurovirol 1996; 2(6):411-416.

188. Biel SS, Held TK, Landt O et al. Rapid quantification and differentiation of human polyomavirus DNA in undiluted urine from patients after bone marrow transplantation. J Clin Microbiol 2000; 38(10):3689-3695.

189. Degener AM, Pietropaolo V, Di Taranto C et al. Identification of a new control region in the genome of the DDP strain of BK virus isolated from PBMC. J Med Virol 1999; 58(4):413-419.

190. Degener AM, Pietropaolo V, Di Taranto C et al. Detection of JC and BK viral genome in specimens of HIV-1 infected subjects. New Microbiol 1997; 20(2):115-122.

191. Di Taranto C, Pietropaolo V, Orsi GB et al. Detection of BK polyomavirus genotypes in healthy and HIV-positive children. Eur J Epidemiol 1997; 13(6):653-657.

192. Itoh S, Irie K, Nakamura Y et al. Cytologic and genetic study of polyomavirus-infected or polyomavirus-activated cells in human urine. Arch Pathol Lab Med 1998; 122(4):333-337.

193. Jin L, Pietropaolo V, Booth JC et al. Prevalence and distribution of BK virus subtypes in healthy people and immunocompromised patients detected by PCR-restriction enzyme analysis. Clin Diagn Virol 1995; 3:285-295.

194. Jin L. Rapid genomic typing of BK virus directly from clinical specimens. Mol Cell probes 1993; 7:331-334.

195. Leung AY, Suen CK, Lie AK et al. Quantification of polyoma BK viruria in hemorrhagic cystitis complicating bone marrow transplantation. Blood 2001; 98(6):1971-1978.

196. Reese JM, Reissing M, Daniel RW et al. Occurrence of BK virus and BK virus-specific antibodies in the urine of patients receiving chemotherapy for malignancy. Infect Immun 1975; 11(6):1375-1381.

197. Shah KV, Daniel RW, Strickler HD et al. Investigation of human urine for genomic sequences of the primate polyomaviruses simian virus 40, BK virus, and JC virus. J Infect Dis 1997; 176(6):1618-1621.

198. Tsai RT, Wang M, Ou WC et al. Incidence of JC viruria is higher than that of BK viruria in Taiwan. J Med Virol 1997; 52(3):253-257.

199. Ling PD, Lednicky JA, Keitel WA et al. The dynamics of herpesvirus and polyomavirus reactivation and shedding in healthy adults: A 14-month longitudinal study. J Infect Dis 2003; 187(10):1571-1580.

200. Ding R, Medeiros M, Dadhania D et al. Noninvasive diagnosis of BK virus nephritis by measurement of messenger RNA for BK virus VP1 in urine. Transplantation 2002; 74(7):987-994.

201. Hogan TF, Padgett BL, Walker DL et al. Survey of human polyomavirus (JCV, BKV) infections in 139 patients with lung cancer, breast cancer, melanoma, or lymphoma. Prog Clin Biol Res 1983; 105:311-324.

202. Stoner GL, Agostini HT, Ryschkewitsch CF et al. JC virus excreted by multiple sclerosis patients and paired controls from Hungary. Mult Scler 1998; 4(2):45-48.

203. Pagani E, Delbue S, Mancuso R et al. Molecular analysis of JC virus genotypes circulating among the Italian healthy population. J Neurovirol 2003; 9(5):559-566.

204. Chima SC, Ryschkewitsch CF, Stoner GL. Molecular epidemiology of human polyomavirus JC in the Biaka Pygmies and Bantu of Central Africa. Mem Inst Oswaldo Cruz 1998; 93(5):615-623.

205. Ryschkewitsch CF, Friedlaender JS, Mgone CS et al. Human polyomavirus JC variants in Papua New Guinea and Guam reflect ancient population settlement and viral evolution. Microbes Infect 2000; 2(9):987-996.

206. Miranda JJ, Sugimoto C, Paraguison R et al. Genetic diversity of JC virus in the modern Filipino population: Implications for the peopling of the Philippines. Am J Phys Anthropol 2003; 120(2):125-132.

207. Koralnik IJ, Boden D, Mai VX et al. JC virus DNA load in patients with and without progressive multifocal leukoencephalopathy. Neurology 1999; 52(2):253-260.

208. Li RM, Branton MH, Tanawattanacharoen S et al. Molecular identification of SV40 infection in human subjects and possible association with kidney disease. J Am Soc Nephrol 2002; 13(9):2320-2330.

209. Markowitz RB, Dynan WS. Binding of cellular proteins to the regulatory region of BK virus DNA. J Virol 1988; 62(9):3.388-3398.

210. Moens U, Johansen T, Johnsen JI et al. Noncoding control region of naturally occurring BK virus variants: Sequence comparison and functional analysis. Virus Genes 1995; 10(3):261-275.

The Pathobiology of Polyomavirus Infection in Man

Parmjeet Randhawa, Abhay Vats and Ron Shapiro

Abstract

This article traces the discovery of polyomaviruses and outlines investigations, which shed light on potential modes of transmission of this increasingly important group of human pathogens. The pathobiology of the virus is summarized with particular reference to interactions with host cell receptors, cell entry, cytoplasmic trafficking, and targeting of the viral genome to the nucleus. This is followed by a discussion of sites of viral latency and factors leading to viral reactivation. Finally, we present biochemical mechanisms that could potentially explain several key elements of tissue pathology characteristic of BKV mediated damage to human kidney.

Biology of Polyomaviruses

Polyomaviruses (PV) are 45nm sized particles with a 5 kb genome.[1,2] The viral genome is comprised of double-stranded, circular, supercoiled DNA. The viral genome is typically arranged in three general regions: non-coding control region (NCCR), the early coding region coding for the small and large T antigens, and the late coding region coding for the viral capsid proteins (VP-1, VP-2, VP-3) and agnoprotein. The direction of early and late transcription is divergent, with opposite DNA strands participating in these processes.[3] The NCCR contains (a) the origin of replication (ori), and (b) regulatory regions containing enhancer elements that are important activators of viral transcription.[4] There is clinical and laboratory evidence that NCCR variants determine host cell permissivity and rate of viral replication.[5,6] The T antigens bind to tumor suppressor proteins Rb and p53 and stimulate host cell entry into the cell cycle.[7,8] This observation provides a theoretical basis for multiple lines of accumulating evidence that PV may be carcinogenic in man, as discussed elsewhere in this book. The viral capsid proteins VP-1, VP-2, and VP-3 are structural proteins required for the assembly of complete virions. The viral capsid coding regions display considerable genetic heterogeneity, and this feature has been used to divide polyomavirus BK (BKV) into distinct genotypes I, II, III, and IV,[9-13] and polyomavirus JC (JCV) into Types 1, 2A, 2B, and 3-8.[14-20] In mice, specific mutations in the viral capsid protein VP-1 region have been associated with increased viral pathogenicity.[21,22] The existence of potential relationships between viral genotype and clinical virulence is illustrated by the observation that progressive multifocal leucoencephalopathy is associated primarily with JCV Type 2B infection. Agnoprotein protein localizes primarily to the cytoplasmic and perinuclear regions of the host cell. This distribution has led to the suggestion that agnoprotein may promote virion release from cell.[23] Other proposed roles for this protein include participation in host cell lysis, enhanced nuclear localization of viral capsid protein VP-1, and help in viral capsid assembly.[24] Cultured cells infected with agnogene mutants show a 17-100 fold reduction in

Polyomaviruses and Human Diseases, edited by Nasimul Ahsan. ©2006 Eurekah.com and Springer Science+Business Media.

virion burst size.[25] A detailed discussion of the molecular biology of the polyomaviruses is presented elsewhere in this book.

Historical Aspects

The polyomavirus species most relevant to human disease are BKV, JCV, and simian virus 40 (SV40).[3] SV40 was first discovered in 1960 as a contaminant of poliovirus vaccines prepared in monkey kidney cell lines.[26] Millions of human subjects developed iatrogenic infection as a result of mass vaccinations programs carried out in the late 1950s and early 1960s. These individuals did not develop any acute sequelae, nor any definitely proven long term effects, although the potential role of SV40 in some human neoplasms is currently an area of active investigation. BKV was discovered in 1970 by Dr. Sylvia Gardner while examining a urine specimen from a Sudanese kidney transplantation recipient with a ureteric stricture. This specimen was found to contain numerous cells bearing viral inclusions.[27] Electron microscopy demonstrated viral particles that resembled papillomavirus. However, inoculation of the urine into secondary rhesus monkey kidney cells and human embryonic kidney cells produced a viral cytopathic effect indicating that the virus was different from papillomavirus. Hence, this microbe was identified as a new virus and named BKV after the initials of the patient from whom it was isolated. Subsequently, BKV was shown to be distinct from polyomavirus JC (JCV), a virus cultured from a patient with progressive multifocal encephalopathy. Electron microscopic evidence suggesting that this disease is viral in etiology was published by two independent laboratories in 1964.[28,29] However, the medical community remained unconvinced until isolation of JCV from a patient with progressive multifocal encephalopathy in 1971. Interestingly, this finding was reported in the same issue of The Lancet, which reported the discovery of BKV.[30]

Following these discoveries extensive epidemiological studies showed that up to 90% of some human populations become exposed to polyomaviruses BKV or JCV by adulthood.[1] After transplantation, 10-60% of renal allograft recipients were noted to excrete virus in the urine. However, infection was typically asymptomatic or associated with only transient graft dysfunction. There were only rare reports of viral inclusions being present in specimens examined following nephrectomy or at autopsy. Sporadic cases of virus-induced kidney damage were also observed in the setting of congenital immunodeficiency[31] and human immunodeficiency virus infection.[32] A new era in the study of polyomavirus infections after renal transplantation was ushered in by a patient with full blown BKV nephropathy diagnosed by a needle biopsy of the allograft kidney. This case, which was diagnosed in 1993 at the University of Pittsburgh, but published in 1996,[33] led to a flurry of additional cases reported from virtually all major kidney transplant centers around the world.[34-36] The emergence of BKV nephropathy in the 1990s is generally attributed to the widespread use of potent immunosuppressive drugs such as tacrolimus, mycophenolate mofetil, and sirolimus.

Modes of Natural Transmission

Primary polyomavirus infection occurs typically in childhood. Adult levels of seroprevalence, on the order of 65-90% in most studies, are reached between 5 and 10 years of age. This high incidence of polyomavirus infection raises obvious questions about the mode of transmission from one individual to another. Given the known latency of the virus in the kidney, urine would appear to be a natural vehicle for spread within and between families. A variety of laboratory techniques have accordingly been used to assess the prevalence of viruria in the pediatric age group. Urine cytology investigations show viral inclusions in 0-1.2% of children. Viral cultures give a similarly low yield varying from 0-1%. Higher rates of viruria can be detected using PCR, but the results vary in different studies ranging from 4% to 26.7%, with all but one study in children reporting values <5%.[12] In adults, viral DNA has been amplified from 0-40% of urine samples, with a tendency to higher values in older subjects. Viral DNA concentrations reported have varied from <3 fg/ml to 5 pg/ml. Other body fluids may also be involved in viral transmission. Thus, BKV DNA has been amplified in 1% of nasopharyngeal aspirates obtained from hospitalized infants with serious respiratory infections.[37] The possibility of feco-oral transmission has been recently raised by the demonstration of viral DNA in urban sewage.[38] Blood, semen, genital tissues, and normal skin biopsies have also been shown to contain BKV.[39,40] Hence, it is possible that the virus may be transmitted by intimate contact with infected individuals.

Transplacental transmission of polyomaviruses from mother to fetus is controversial. BKV specific IgM antibodies were demonstrated in three of six infants whose mothers seroconverted during pregnancy.[41,42] On the other hand, Shah et al[43] could not detect anti-BKV IgM antibodies in the cord blood of 387 infants. Admittedly, only three of the mothers evaluated in the latter study had anti-BKV IgM antibodies in the serum. Coleman et al[44] studied 309 mothers, 39 of whom excreted viral inclusion bearing cells in the urine during pregnancy. Neonatal and cord blood samples drawn from the offspring consistently tested negative for BKV-specific IgM. Transplacental transmission of polyomavirus has been demonstrated in mice,[45] and it is conceivable that the same could occur in man.

Transmission of Polyomavirus via Organ Transplantation

Given that polyomavirus is latent in the kidney, it is reasonable to believe that the donor kidney will be the source of infection in a proportion of transplant recipients. Attempts to determine the frequency with which this occurs have relied on serologic analysis of pre-transplant donor and post-transplant recipient sera. Gardner et al[46] found 6 of 48 (12%) kidney transplant patients to be seronegative for BKV at the time of transplantation. Two of these six (33%) patients subsequently developed seroconversion indicative of primary BKV infection, and one patient developed viruria. The incidence of primary and secondary JCV infection in this study was 23% and 46% respectively.[46]

Noss detected anti-BKV antibodies in103/168 (61.3%) of renal transplant recipients using indirect immunofluorescence or virus neutralization assays. In an analysis of 62 paired donor and recipient sera, it was determined that primary infection occurred in 18 (29%) patients, typically within 3 months of transplantation. The remaining 44 patients developed presumed reactivation infection, usually after 3 months following transplantation.[47]

Andrews et al[48] conducted a serological study of 496 renal transplant recipients and donors for BKV and JCV infections. They found that a seropositive donor increased the risk of primary and reactivated infections with BKV and of primary infection with JCV. Specifically, a donor seropositive and recipient seronegative combination was associated with a 43% incidence of primary infection defined by serologic methods. In comparison, a 10% incidence of reactivation infection was observed in seropositive recipients of seropositive organs.[2]

In a more recent study, BKV specific hemagglutination inhibition antibodies were found in 59/78 (77%) serum samples collected before transplantation.[49] Of 23 patients with post-transplant decoy cell shedding, 18 (78%) were seropositive and 5 (22%) seronegative prior to receiving the donor organ. It was observed that 3 of 5 seronegative patients developed BK viremia, and one went on to develop nephropathy

Viral Interactions with Host Cell Receptors

Defining the cellular mechanism of BK infection is important, because this may lead to the identification of biochemical molecules that could be targeted in drug discovery studies. Viral receptor interactions are believed to be important determinants of host range and tissue tropism. The primary receptor binding determinant on all polyomaviruses is the VP-1 molecule, which is arranged in the form of icosahedrally symmetric pentamers. Despite the fact that BKV, JCV, and SV40 are related viruses, there is growing evidence that these microorganisms use distinct mechanisms to target their host cells.

The mouse polyomavirus has small and large plaque strains, which recognize a cell surface associated N-linked glycoprotein containing terminal α (2-3)-linked sialic acid.[50] The small plaque strain also recognizes a branched disialyl structure containing α (2-3)- and α (2-6)-linked sialic acids. The ability of the small and large plaque strains to distinguish between these two sialic acid configurations has been attributed to a single amino acid polymorphism at position 92 in the VP-1 protein.[51] Specifically, the replacement of a negatively charged glutamic acid by glycine at this position correlates with the increased in-vitro pathogenicity of the large plaque strain. Recently $\alpha 4\beta 1$ integrins have been found to act as cell receptor for murine polyomavirus.[52] Treatment with blocking antibodies before and after virus adsorption indicate that the effect on cell permissivity is at the post-attachment level. Binding of virus to $\alpha 4\beta 1$ is mediated by integrin binding motifs located in the DE and EF loops of the VP-1 protein. These motifs were not found in a BKV AS strain and a JCV ML-6 strain analyzed by the authors. The mouse lymphotropic papovavirus interacts with a O-linked glycoprotein containing terminal α (2-6)-linked sialic acid. This receptor is restricted to B-cells, and accounts for the limited tissue tropism of this virus.

The simian virus SV40 is unlike other polyomaviruses in that cell entry is independent of surface sialic acids. Instead, SV40 VP-1 interacts with major histocompatibility class I proteins and O-linked glycan molecules. Accordingly, anti-MHC class I antibodies inhibit infection of glial cells by SV40 but not JCV.[50] SV40 does not compete with sialic acid dependent polyomaviruses for binding to host cells.

Considerable work has been done on characterization of receptors for the human virus JCV. Receptors on the surface of glial cells and B-cells have been shown to bear a N-linked glycoprotein containing terminal α (2-3)- and α (2-6)-linked sialic acids.[53] Treatment of cultured glial cells with proteases, phospholipases, and neuraminidases inhibits viral binding, indicating that virus can bind to a wide variety of cell surface ligands. However, only neuraminidase inhibits infectivity, and this has been attributed to the ability of this enzyme to cleave both α (2-3) and α (2-6)-linked sialic acids from the cell surface. A recombinant neuraminidase that specifically cleaves the α (2-3) linkage of sialic acid has no effect on either virus binding or infection. Competitive binding assays with sialic acid specific lectins also support the notion that viral interaction is primarily with α (2-6)-linked sialic acids.[50] Indirect overlay assays have demonstrated that virus like particles (VLP) comprised of recombinant VP-1 can bind to a number of sialoglycoproteins, including $\alpha 1$-acid glycoprotein, ferritin and transferrin receptor. Binding was also demonstrated to glycolipids, such as lactosylceramide, and gangliosides, including GM3, GD2, GD3, GD1b, GT1b, and GQ1b. VLP bound weakly to GD1a, but did not bind to GM1a, GM2, or galactocerebroside. Furthermore, a chemically synthesized neoglycoprotein containing the terminal α 2-6-linked sialic acid and the ganglioside GT1b inhibited JCV infection in the susceptible cell line IMR-32. These results suggest that the oligosaccharides of glycoproteins and glycolipids work as JCV receptors and may be appropriate targets in the quest to develop effective anti-JCV drugs.[54]

There is very limited information available about the early steps of BKV binding to the host cell. Digestion of human red blood cells by Vibiro cholerae neuraminidase inhibits virus induced hemagglutination activity suggesting a role for α (2-3)-linked sialic acid residues.[55] However, the chemical nature of the associated receptors has not been described. The presence of glycolipids has been impicated based on phospholipases digestion experiments.[56] Unfortunately, such studies cannot distinguish between specific and non-specific interactions with cell surface ligands, unless parallel investigations are performed to determine if actual entry of the virus into the cell is also affected.

Entry of Virus into Host Cells

The mechanism of polyomavirus intra-cellular entry is species dependent. Thus, JCV enters the cell by clathrin dependent endocytosis, which is believed to be a constitutive process, and unlike SV40 entry, does not depend on a virus dependent extracellular signal. Clathrin facilitated endocytosis can be blocked by chlorpromazine and clozapine.[57] Clathrin dependent endosomes have an acidic milieu, which induces conformational changes in viral glycoproteins, thereby promoting uncoating of viruses.[58] Viruses that enter by endocytosis generally disassemble in the endosomes. Neutralization of endosomal pH by ammonium chloride or bafilomycin A2 inhibits viral infection of host cells.

In contrast to JCV, SV40 viral entry is a caveolae dependent endocytosis susceptible to nystatin, rather than chlorpromazine.[59] The sequence of events begins with the virus binding to MHC class 1 molecules in the plasma membrane. At this point, the virus transmits an extracellular signal that promotes virus enclosure in caveolae with in 30 minutes of surface binding.[60] This signal activates the tyrosine kinase and calcium independent protein kinase pathways, as evidenced by upregulation of c-myc, c-jun, and c-sis.[61] There is no activation of the Raf or mitogen activated protein kinase (MAP/ERK1). Caveosomes are 'pH neutral' organelles (i.e., their function is not affected by intra-cellular pH), and do not contain markers for endosomes, lysosomes, golgi complex or endoplasmic reticulum. In passing, it should be noted that caveolae are also involved in the intracellular trafficking of mouse polyomavirus virions,[62] human immunodeficiency virus, *Toxoplasma gondii*, *Plasmdium falciparum* and *Campylobacter jejuni*.[63]

Little published information is available about the mechanisms used by BKV for intracytoplasmic transport, but electron microscopic observations on human biopsy material show that the virus is associated with non-clathrin coated vesicles, which may represent caveolae.[64]

Cytoplasmic Trafficking

It is now well recognized that, following receptor mediated cell entry, the transport of viral particles in the cytoplasm is not a matter of simple diffusion. Rather, it is an active process mediated by interactions between virus containing vesicles and the cellular cytoskeleton. Detailed studies of the interactions between virus particle containing vesicles and the host cytoskeleton have been carried out for the mouse polyomavirus. It appears that this virus moves predominantly along microfilaments.[62] Actin filaments are involved in the early stage of infection, when the viral VP-1 protein colocalizes with disorganized actin microfilaments. In later stages of infection, VP-1 is associated with microtubules. Colocalization of VP-1 and tubulin can be detected around the nuclei, in mitotic spindles, and in centromeres. Lack of free viral particles in this location, however, led one group of investigators to speculate that the microtubular compartment might be involved in viral disassembly. In apparent conflict with this interpretation, it has been observed that the microfilament destroying agent cytochalasin D has no effect on viral infectivity, while the microtubule disrupting agent nocodazole inhibits viral transport efficiently.[65] These discrepant results could mean that there are two different trafficking mechanisms, the relative importance of which depends on the experimental conditions.

Cytoplasmic trafficking of SV40 virions resembles the mouse polyomavirus in being susceptible to nocodazole, but not cytochalasin.[66] Video enhanced live fluorescence microscopy has demonstrated a two-step vesicular transport pathway to the endoplasmic reticulum. The first step consists of SV40 entry into caveolin rich vesicles, which subsequently direct virions to a caveolin-free microtubules. Microtubules in turn target the virus to a syntaxin 17-positive smooth endoplasmic reticulum compartment.[67] During its transport to the endoplasmic reticulum, SV40 passes thru an intermediate compartment containing b-COP, a protein best known for its association with Golgi cisternae and their derivative budding vesicles. b-COP is believed to be involved in the Golgi to endoplasmic reticulum recycling pathway. An unusual feature of caveola-mediated SV40 entry is that the virus bypasses the endosomal compartment, and is transported to the endoplasmic reticulum.[63] More commonly, endocytic cargo is channelized to the endosomal-lysosomal pathway. Microfilaments are not required for early entry steps of SV40, but do facilitate viral trafficking following entry of the virus into caveolae.[58]

JCV has a complex intra-cellular transport mechanism involving sequential involvement of several classes of cytoskeletal elements. Unlike SV40 transport, which is inhibited only by nocodazole, JCV transport is inhibited by nocodazole, cytochalasin B, as well as acrylamide, indicating that microtubules, microfilaments, and intermediate filaments all play a role in intra-cellular trafficking. Actin polymerization facilitates clathrin-mediated endocytosis. The plasma membrane is intimately linked to the underlying cytoskeleton, and surface events such as vesicle budding require remodeling of the actin framework. The microtubular system, with its microtubule organizing center located close to the nucleus, is anatomically well suited for the intra-cellular transport of viruses that replicate within the intranuclear compartment. The role of intermediate filaments in viral trafficking is not yet well understood. The mechanisms of endocytosis and intra-cellular trafficking utilized by BKV have not been investigated to date.

Nuclear Targeting

Viral entry into the cytoplasm does not in itself ensure subsequent transport to the nucleus. Thus, synthetic virus like particles composed of VP-1 protein (with no enclosed viral DNA) can enter the cytoplasm, but fail to enter the intranuclear compartment, where viral replication normally occurs.[62] Instead, empty viral particles are internalized in large vesicles prior to undergoing degradation.

The mechanism by which polyomavirus traverses the nuclear envelope to enter the nucleus is controversial. Monoclonal antibodies to nucleoporin (a protein associated with the nuclear pore complex) have been shown to block the entry of SV40 into the nucleus of 3T3 cells. However, this observation needs to be reconciled with the fact that the maximal diameter of a particle that can pass through the nuclear pore is 23 nm,[68] whereas the diameter of the encapsidated polyomavirus particle is approximately 50nm. Observations on human biopsy material suggest that fully assembled viral particles tend to accumulate in the nucleus as large crystalline arrays until complete cell lysis. This may be due to fibrils attached to the nuclear pore, which prevent egress of SV40 particles from the infected nucleus.[69]

The uncoating process of polyomaviruses has been stated to occur after the virions have entered the cell nuclei. However, Richterova et al[62] found no convincing VP-1 signal in the nuclei of fibroblasts infected with the mouse polyomavirus. Norkin et al[63] showed viral capsid proteins VP-2 and VP-3 overlapping the endoplasmic reticulum within 5 hours of infection. Since these antigens are normally not exposed on the surface of the viral capsid, this finding implies that SV40 disassembly can occur in the endoplasmic reticulum. VP-2 and VP-3 normally insert into the axial cavity of the VP-1 pentamer by hairpin-like loops anchored by strong hydrophobic interactions. Dissociation of these high affinity interactions is likely facilitated by molecular chaperones, one of which may be the viral T-antigen. Interestingly, VP-2 and VP-3 contain a nuclear transport signal and also have a non-specific DNA binding domain[70] These latter properties provide the functions required for the nuclear delivery of the viral minichromosome. Consistent with this concept, injection of antibodies to VP-2 and VP-3 in the cytoplasm blocks the transport of viral DNA to the intranuclear compartment.[71]

Clinical Sequelae of Primary Infection in Man

No systematic clinical observations have been made in individuals undergoing polyomavirus seroconversion. When recorded the most frequent symptom is an upper respiratory infection. Unfortunately, some of the reported cases also had concurrent infections with other known respiratory viruses, making it difficult to attribute the observed symptoms entirely to primary polyomavirus infection.[37,72] Sporadic case reports of children presenting with cystitis, with or without hematuria, are also on record.[73-75] Unusual clinical manifestations associated with BKV seroconversion include Guillane-Barre syndrome and encephalitis.[76,77]

Sites of Viral Latency

After primary infection has resolved the virus enters a latent phase. It appears that viral latency can be maintained in a number of different sites:
1. Viral DNA is detected most often in the urogenital tract including the kidneys, urinary bladder, prostate, cervix, vulva, and semen.[78]
2. Peripheral blood mononuclear cells are the second most important site of polyomavirus latency. In healthy individuals rates of detection vary from 0-94%.[79] JCV has a particular propensity for B-lymphocytes. Limited BKV infection has been shown in T-cells and B-cells maintained in culture. In one study, monocytes showed BKV attachment and penetration,

but no viral replication, unless the cells were treated with anti-macrophage antiserum.[80] BKV mRNA has been detected in circulating mononuclear cells of healthy donors by RT-PCR and in-situ hybridization.[81,82]

3. Mucosa-associated lymphoid tissue is a potential site of latency, since BKV DNA has been demonstrated in throat washings and tonsil tissue obtained from children.[37,83]
4. Other proposed sites of viral latency include the brain,[84] normal bone, and bone tumors.[81]

Reactivation of Latent Virus

Activation of latent virus has been reported in a variety of clinical settings summarized below:

1. Asymptomatic viruria can occur in old age, pregnancy, and diabetes mellitus, presumably as a result of hormonal effects on anti-viral immunity.[78]
2. Co-infection with other viruses has been proposed to be one of the mechanisms of polyomavirus reactivation. Thus, there is evidence that polyomavirus JCV reactivation can be triggered by infection with herpesvirus 6 (HHV6).[85] Human immunodeficiency virus encoded HIV-1 Tat protein can transactivate polyomavirus JCV by induction of the JCV promoter.[86, 87]
3. Immunosuppression is a well-known risk factor for viral reactivation. This likely reflects interference with the normal cell mediated immune mechanisms that keep viral replication in check. Accordingly, BK viruria has been reported in 20-44% of HIV infected individuals, 22-100% of bone marrow transplant recipients, 10-60% of kidney transplant recipients, and 50% of heart transplant recipients.[79] A small proportion of viruric patients go on to develop BKV nephropathy, ureteric stricture, or hemorrhagic cystitis. Progressive multifocal encephalopathy is well known complication of JCV infection in HIV infected patients. In recent years, SV40 DNA has been documented in allograft kidneys, native kidneys with glomerular disease, and in a variety of neoplasms, particularly mesotheliomas, brain tumors, and non-Hodgkin lymphomas. A detailed discussion of polyomavirus associated clinical syndromes is provided elsewhere in the book.

Pathogenesis of Tissue Damage in Polyomavirus Infected Tissues

Our understanding of the actual metabolic pathways utilized by polyomavirus to initiate and sustain tissue damage is rudimentary. Using Affymetrix HG-U133 DNA microarray analysis of BKV infected WI-38 cells, our laboratory has obtained data indicating that viral infection causes up-regulation of several major groups of intra-cellular mRNA's.[88] These virus-induced changes in host gene expression offer potential insights into the pathogenesis of BK virus allograft nephropathy, as summarized below:

1. Cell cycle proteins were by far the largest group of proteins that were upregulated following BKV infection. Initiation of the host cell cycle is an important event because polyomavirus is dependent upon host cellular factors for replication, and the required cellular factors are not present in quiescent host cells
2. Several pro-inflammatory cytokines were up regulated, including molecules participating in both the early (IL-1 and TNF induced proteins) and late (IL-6, IL-11) phases of the inflammatory response. It is pertinent to note that IL-1 is known to be induced by nearly all microbes. It initiates a febrile response and stimulates IL-6 and IL-11. IL-6 and IL-11 share the gp130 signaling pathway and are capable of further intensifying the acute phase response associated with viral infection.[89]
3. There was increased expression of cytokine receptors IL-4R, IL-13R, and TNF soluble factor 15. IL-4 has a biological role in antibody production. It is significant that increased B-cells and plasma cells have been noted in human biopsy material with BKV nephropathy.[90] IL-13 is a cytokine that is similar to IL-4 in its anti-inflammatory properties and ability to enhance antibody production by B-cells.[91]

4. The chemokines RANTES (regulated on activation T-cell secreted chemokine) and IL-8 were found to be stimulated by viral infection. RANTES is known to be expressed by tubular epithelium in inflammatory disease states such as acute cellular rejection. IL-8 facilitates influx of polymorphonuclear cells and offers a plausible explanation for the presence of polymorphonuclear cells in biopsies with viral interstitial nephritis.[92]

5. BKV infection led to increased mRNA for the intercellular adhesion molecule ICAM-1 (CD54). ICAM-1 is expressed by tubular epithelial cells and is believed to play a role in the pathogenesis of interstitial inflammation in the kidney.[92]

6. There was enhanced transcription for three groups of major histocompatibility complex class I molecules (HLA-B, HLA-C, and HLA-F) in BKV infected cultured cells. Occurrence of the same phenomenon in the transplanted kidney would put the graft at increased risk for acute cellular rejection. This would explain why the pathology of BKV nephropathy overlaps with acute cellular rejection.

7. Increased mRNA was demonstrated for Collagen VII and extracellular matrix protein 1. Collagen type VII is the major component of the anchoring fibrils at the dermal-epidermal junction. It is usually not present in normal glomeruli, but has recently been shown to be actively synthesized in areas of glomerular and/or tubular scarring in many kidney diseases.[93] Viral induced synthesis of collagen VII may contribute to the progressive scarring that can accompany BKV nephropathy.

8. Expression of vascular endothelial growth factor (VEGF) mRNA was increased. There is evidence that VEGF participates in the pathogenesis of chronic renal allograft rejection.[94] This raises the possibility that BKV may accelerate this process in the transplanted kidney by a similar mechanism.

The participation of interleukins, cytokines and cellular adhesion molecules in the pathogenesis of BKV nephropathy raises the possibility of using pharmacological means of ameliorating virus mediated allograft injury. Such intervention may be particularly indicated in patients with progressive interstitial nephritis, who do not respond to reduction of immunosuppression and cidofovir therapy. Several molecules shown to be up regulated by BKV infection are targets for currently ongoing efforts to devise anti-inflammatory therapy using cytokine antagonists. For example: (a) anti-IL-4 antibody has potential utility in the treatment of rheumatoid arthritis,[95] (b) IL-1 receptor inhibitors are being developed and investigated in the setting of rheumatoid arthritis, septic shock and steroid resistant graft versus host disease, (c) Patients with Crohn's disease and refractory rheumatoid arthritis are being treated with anti-TNF antibody (Infliximab, Remicade), anti-IL-8 (Abgenix), and anti-IL-6 antibodies, and (d) anti-ICAM-1 monoclonal antibody (enlimomab) has been used for the prevention of acute rejection in cadaveric renal transplantation.[96-98] Proof of concept studies showing the applicability of these treatment modalities to viral disease are yet to be performed. We do not know whether abolishing the inflammatory response will have a deleterious or beneficial effect on the natural history of BKV nephropathy. It is also possible that cytokine redundancy may make the use of single pharmacologic agents ineffective.

Concluding Remarks

There is increasing recognition of the importance of polyomavirus infections in clinical medicine. The spectrum of human disease caused by polyomaviruses BK, JC, and SV40 has expanded considerably as a result of investigations in the past two decades. A frustrating issue is our currently limited ability to treat these diseases by effective drug therapy. Further progress in this field would require more intensive investigations into the mechanisms of virus mediated tissue injury. There is also an urgent need for high throughput assays capable of screening currently available libraries of chemical compounds for anti-polyomavirus activity.

References

1. Demeter LM. JC, BK, and other polyomaviruses; progressive multifocal leukoencephalopathy. In: Mandel GL, Bennett JE, Dolin R, eds. Principles and Practice of Infectious Diseases. New York: Churchill Livingstone, 1995:1400-1406.
2. Shah KV. Human polyomavirus BKV and renal disease. Nephrol Dial Transpl 2000; 15:754-755.
3. Lednicky JA, Butel JS. Polyomaviruses and human tumors: a brief review of current concepts and interpretations. Front Biosci 1999; 4:D153-164.
4. Moens U, Johansen T, Johnsen JI et al. Noncoding control region of naturally occurring BK virus variants: sequence comparison and functional analysis. Virus Genes 1995; 10:261-275.
5. Johnsen JI, Seternes OM, Johansen T et al. Subpopulations of non-coding control region variants within a cell culture-passaged stock of BK virus: sequence comparisons and biological characteristics. J Gen Virol 1995; 76(Pt 7):1571-1581.
6. Daniel AM, Swenson JJ, Mayreddy RP et al. Sequences within the early and late promoters of archetype JC virus restrict viral DNA replication and infectivity. Virology 1996; 216:90-101.
7. Carbone M, Rizzo P, Grimley PM et al. Simian virus-40 large-T antigen binds p53 in human mesotheliomas. Nat Med 1997; 3:908-912.
8. De Luca A, Baldi A, Esposito V et al. The retinoblastoma gene family pRb/p105, p107, pRb2/p130 and simian virus-40 large T-antigen in human mesotheliomas. Nat Med 1997; 3:913-916.
9. Jin L. Rapid genomic typing of BK virus directly from clinical specimens. Molecular & Cellular Probes 1993; 7:331-334.
10. Jin L, Gibson PE. Genomic function and variation of human polyomavirus BK (BKV). Rev Med Virol 1996; 6:201-214.
11. Jin L, Gibson PE, Booth JC et al. Genomic typing of BK virus in clinical specimens by direct sequencing of polymerase chain reaction products. J Med Virol 1993; 41:11-17.
12. Knowles WA. The epidemiology of BK virus and the occurrence of antigenic and genomic subtypes. In: Khalili K, Stoner GL, eds. Human Polyomaviruses: Molecular and Clinical Perspectives New York: Wiley-Liss, 2001:527-560.
13. Knowles WA, Gibson PE, Gardner SD. Serological typing scheme for BK-like isolates of human polyomavirus. J Med Virol 1989; 28:118-123.
14. Agostini HT, Ryschkewitsch CF, Baumhefner RW et al. Influence of JC virus coding region genotype on risk of multiple sclerosis and progressive multifocal leukoencephalopathy. J Neurovirol 2000; 6 Suppl 2:S101-108.
15. Agostini HT, Ryschkewitsch CF, Mory R et al. JC virus (JCV) genotypes in brain tissue from patients with progressive multifocal leukoencephalopathy (PML) and in urine from controls without PML: Increased frequency of JCV type 2 in PML. J Infect Dis 1997; 176:1-8.
16. Agostini HT, Ryschkewitsch CF, Stoner GL. Genotype profile of human polyomavirus JC excreted in urine of immunocompetent individuals. J Clin Microbiol 1996; 34:159-164.
17. Agostini HT, Ryschkewitsch CF, Stoner GL. Complete genome of a JC virus genotype type 6 from the brain of an African American with progressive multifocal leukoencephalopathy. J Hum Virol 1998; 1:267-272.
18. Agostini HT, Shishidohara Y, Baumhefner RW et al. Jc Virus Type 2—Definition of subtypes based on DNA sequence analysis of ten complete genomes. J Gen Virol 1998; 79(Part 5):1143-1151.
19. Agostini HT, Yanagihara R, Davis V et al. Asian genotypes of JC virus in native americans and in a pacific island population—Markers of viral evolution and human migration. Proc Natl Acad Sci USA 1997; 94:14542-14546.
20. Jobe DV, Friedlaender JS, Mgone CS et al. New JC virus (JCV) genotypes from papua new guinea and micronesia (type 8 and type 2E) and evolutionary analysis of 32 complete JCV genomes. Arch Virol 2001; 146:2097-2113.
21. Bauer PH, Bronson RT, Fung SC et al. Genetic and structural analysis of a virulence determinant in polyomavirus VP1. J Virol 1995; 69:7925-7931.
22. Mannova P, Liebl D, Krauzewicz N et al. Analysis of mouse polyomavirus mutants with lesions in the minor capsid proteins. J Gen Virol 2002; 83(Pt 9):2309-2319.
23. Resnick J, Shenk T. Simian virus 40 agnoprotein facilitates normal nuclear location of the major capsid polypeptide and cell-to-cell spread of virus. J Virol 1986; 60:1098-1106.
24. Carswell S, Alwine JC. Simian virus 40 agnoprotein facilitates perinuclear-nuclear localization of VP1, the major capsid protein. J Virol 1986; 60:1055-1061.
25. Ng SC, Mertz JE, Sanden-Will S et al. Simian virus 40 maturation in cells harboring mutants deleted in the agnogene. J Biol Chem 1985; 260:1127-1132.
26. Sweet BH, Hilleman MR. The vacuolating virus. Proc Soc Exp Biol Med 1960; 105:420-427.

27. Gardner SD, Field AM, Coleman DV et al. New human papovavirus (B.K.) isolated from urine after renal transplantation. Lancet. 1971; 1:1253-1257.

28. Astrom KE. Progressive multifocal leukoencephalopathy: the discovery of a neurologic disease. In: Khalili K, Stoner GL, eds. Human Polyomaviruses: Molecular and Clinical Perspectives. New York: Wiley-Liss, 2001:1-10.

29. ZuRhein GM. Papova virions in progressive multifocal leukoencephalopathy: A discovery at the interface of neuropathology, virology, and oncology. In: Khalili K, Stoner GL, eds. Human Polyomaviruses: Molecular and Clinical Perspectives. New York: Wiley-Liss, 2001:11-24.

30. Padgett BL, Walker DL, ZuRhein GM et al. Cultivation of papova-like virus from human brain with progressive multifocal leucoencephalopathy. Lancet 1971; 1:1257-1260.

31. Rosen S, Harmon W, Krensky AM et al. Tubulo-interstitial nephritis associated with polyomavirus (BK type) infection. N Engl J Med 1983; 308:1192-1196.

32. Smith RD, Galla JH, Skahan K et al. Tubulointerstitial nephritis due to a mutant polyomavirus BK virus strain, BKV(Cin), causing end-stage renal disease. J Clin Microbiol 1998; 36:1660-1665.

33. Pappo O, Demetris AJ, Raikow RB et al. Human polyoma virus infection of renal allografts: Histopathologic diagnosis, clinical significance, and literature review. Mod Pathol 1996; 9:105-109.

34. Nickeleit V, Hirsch HH, Binet IF et al. Polyomavirus infection of renal allograft recipients: From latent infection to manifest disease. J Am Soc Nephrol 1999; 10:1080-1089.

35. Drachenberg CB, Beskow CO, Cangro CB et al. Human polyoma virus in renal allograft biopsies: Morphological findings and correlation with urine cytology. Human Pathology 1999; 30:970-977.

36. Howell DN, Smith SR, Butterly DW et al. Diagnosis and management of BK polyomavirus interstitial nephritis in renal transplant recipients. Transplantation 1999; 68:1279-1288.

37. Sundsfjord A, Spein AR, Lucht E et al. Detection of BK virus DNA in nasopharyngeal aspirates from children with respiratory infections but not in saliva from immunodeficient and immunocompetent adult patients. J Clin Microbiol 1994; 32:1390-1394.

38. Bofill-Mas S, Pina S, Girones R. Documenting the epidemiologic patterns of polyomaviruses in human populations by studying their presence in urban sewage. Appl Environ Microbiol 2000; 66:238-245.

39. Chatterjee M, Weyandt TB, Frisque RJ. Identification of archetype and rearranged forms of BK virus in leukocytes from healthy individuals. J Med Virol 2000; 60:353-362.

40. Monini P, Rotola A, de Lellis L et al. Latent BK virus infection and Kaposi's sarcoma pathogenesis. Int J Cancer 1996; 66:717-722.

41. Taguchi F, Nagaki D, Saito M et al. Transplacental transmission of BK virus in human. Jpn J Microbiol 1975; 19:395-398.

42. Pietropaolo V, Di Taranto C, Degener AM et al. Transplacental transmission of human polyomavirus BK. J MedVirol 1998; 56:372-376.

43. Shah K, Daniel R, Madden D et al. Serological investigation of BK papovavirus infection in pregnant women and their offspring. Infect Immun 1980; 30:29-35.

44. Coleman DV, Wolfendale MR, Daniel RA et al. A prospective study of human polyomavirus infection in pregnancy. J Infect Dis 1980; 142:1-8.

45. McCance DJ, Mims CA. Transplacental transmission of polyoma virus in mice. Infect Immun 1977; 18:196-202.

46. Gardner SD, MacKenzie EF, Smith C et al. Prospective study of the human polyomaviruses BK and JC and cytomegalovirus in renal transplant recipients. J Clin Pathol 1984; 37:578-586.

47. Noss G. Human polyoma virus type BK infection and T antibody response in renal transplant recipients. Zentralbl Bakteriol Mikrobiol Hyg [A] 1987; 266:567-574.

48. Andrews CA, Shah KV, Daniel RW et al. A serological investigation of BK virus and JC virus infections in recipients of renal allografts. J Infect Dis 1988; 158:176-181.

49. Hirsch HH, Knowles W, Dickenmann M et al. Prospective study of polyomavirus type BK replication and nephropathy in renal-transplant recipients. N Engl J Med 2002; 347:488-496.

50. Liu CK, Wei G, Atwood WJ. Infection of glial cells by the human polyomavirus JC is mediated by an N-linked glycoprotein containing terminal alpha(2-6)-linked sialic acids. J Virol 1998; 72:4643-4649.

51. Freund R, Garcea RL, Sahli R et al. A single-amino-acid substitution in polyomavirus VP1 correlates with plaque size and hemagglutination behavior. J Virol 1991; 65:350-355.

52. Caruso M, Cavaldesi M, Gentile M et al. Role of sialic acid-containing molecules and the alpha4beta1 integrin receptor in the early steps of polyomavirus infection. J Gen Virol 2003; 84(Pt 11):2927-2936.

53. Atwood WJ. Cellular receptors for the polyomaviruses. In: Khalili K, Stoner GL, eds. Human Polyomaviruses: Molecular and Clinical Perspectives. New York: Wiley-Liss, 2001:179-196.

54. Komagome R, Sawa H, Suzuki T et al. Oligosaccharides as receptors for JC virus. J Virol 2002; 76:12992-13000.
55. Seganti L, Mastromarino P, Superti F et al. Receptors for BK virus on human erythrocytes. Acta Virol 1981; 25:177-181.
56. Sinibaldi L, Goldoni P, Pietropaolo V et al. Role of phospholipids in BK virus infection and haemagglutination. Microbiologica 1992; 15:337-344.
57. Atwood WJ. A combination of low-dose chlorpromazine and neutralizing antibodies inhibits the spread of JC virus (JCV) in a tissue culture model: Implications for prophylactic and therapeutic treatment of progressive multifocal leukencephalopathy. J Neurovirol 2001; 7:307-310.
58. Ashok A, Atwood WJ. Contrasting roles of endosomal pH and the cytoskeleton in infection of human glial cells by JC virus and simian virus 40. J Virol 2003; 77:1347-1356.
59. Atwood WJ, Norkin LC. Class I major histocompatibility proteins as cell surface receptors for simian virus 40. J Virol 1989; 63:4474-4477.
60. Chen Y, Norkin LC. Extracellular simian virus 40 transmits a signal that promotes virus enclosure within caveolae. Exp Cell Res 1999; 246:83-90.
61. Dangoria NS, Breau WC, Anderson HA et al. Extracellular simian virus 40 induces an ERK/MAP kinase-independent signalling pathway that activates primary response genes and promotes virus entry. J Gen Virol 1996; 77(Pt 9):2173-2182.
62. Richterova Z, Liebl D, Horak M et al. Caveolae are involved in the trafficking of mouse polyomavirus virions and artificial VP1 pseudocapsids toward cell nuclei. J Virol 2001; 75:10880-10891.
63. Norkin LC, Anderson HA, Wolfrom SA et al. Caveolar endocytosis of simian virus 40 is followed by brefeldin A-sensitive transport to the endoplasmic reticulum, where the virus disassembles. J Virol 2002; 76:5156-5166.
64. Drachenberg CB, Papadimitriou JC, Wali R et al. BK polyoma virus allograft nephropathy: Ultrastructural features from viral cell entry to lysis. Am J Transplant 2003; 3:1383-1392.
65. Krauzewicz N, Stokrova J, Jenkins C et al. Virus-like gene transfer into cells mediated by polyoma virus pseudocapsids. Gene Ther 2000; 7:2122-2131.
66. Shimura H, Umeno Y, Kimura G. Effects of inhibitors of the cytoplasmic structures and functions on the early phase of infection of cultured cells with simian virus 40. Virology 1987; 158:34-43.
67. Pelkmans L, Kartenbeck J, Helenius A. Caveolar endocytosis of simian virus 40 reveals a new two-step vesicular-transport pathway to the ER. Nat Cell Biol 2001; 3:473-483.
68. Dworetzky SI, Feldherr CM. Translocation of RNA-coated gold particles through the nuclear pores of oocytes. J Cell Biol 1988; 106:575-584.
69. Maul GG. Fibrils attached to the nuclear pore prevent egress of SV40 particles from the infected nucleus. J Cell Biol 1976; 70:714-719.
70. Clever J, Dean DA, Kasamatsu H. Identification of a DNA binding domain in simian virus 40 capsid proteins Vp2 and Vp3. J Biol Chem 1993; 268:20877-20883.
71. Nakanishi A, Clever J, Yamada M et al. Association with capsid proteins promotes nuclear targeting of simian virus 40 DNA. Proc Natl Acad Sci USA 1996; 93:96-100.
72. Goudsmit J, Wertheim-van Dillen P, van Strien A et al. The role of BK virus in acute respiratory tract disease and the presence of BKV DNA in tonsils. J Med Virol 1982; 10:91-99.
73. Hashida Y, Gaffney PC, Yunis EJ. Acute hemorrhagic cystitis of childhood and papovavirus-like particles. J Pediatr 1976; 89:85-87.
74. Saitoh K, Sugae N, Koike N et al. Diagnosis of childhood BK virus cystitis by electron microscopy and PCR. J Clin Pathol 1993; 46:773-775.
75. Mininberg DT, Watson C, Desquitado M. Viral cystitis with transient secondary vesicoureteral reflux. J Urol 1982; 127:983-985.
76. van der Noordaa J, Sol CJ, Schuurman R. Bovine polyomavirus, a frequent contaminant of calf sera. Developments in Biological Standardization 1999; 99:45-47.
77. Voltz R, Jager G, Seelos K et al. BK virus encephalitis in an immunocompetent patient. Arch Neurol 1996; 53:101-103.
78. Randhawa PS, Vats A, Shapiro R et al. BK virus: Discovery, epidemiology, and biology. Graft 2002; 5(supplement):S19-27.
79. Dorries K. Latent and persistent polyomavirus infection. In: Khalili K, Stoner GL, eds. Human Polyomaviruses: Molecular and Clinical Perspectives. New York: Wiley-Liss, 2001:197-236.
80. Traavik T, Uhlin-Hansen L, Flaegstad T et al. Antibody-mediated enhancement of BK virus infection in human monocytes and a human macrophage-like cell line. J Med Virol 1988; 24:283-297.
81. De Mattei M, Martini F, Corallini A et al. High incidence of BK virus large-T-antigen-coding sequences in normal human tissues and tumors of different histotypes. Int J Cancer 1995; 61:756-760.

82. Dorries K, Vogel E, Gunther S et al. Infection of human polyomaviruses JC and BK in peripheral blood leukocytes from immunocompetent individuals. Virology 1994; 198:59-70.

83. Mantyjarvi RA, Meurman OH, Vihma L et al. A human papovavirus (B.K.), biological properties and seroepidemiology. Ann Clin Res 1973; 5:283-287.

84. Elsner C, Dorries K. Evidence of human polyomavirus BK and JC infection in normal brain tissue. Virology 1992; 191:72-80.

85. Blumberg BM, Mock DJ, Powers JM et al. The HHV6 paradox: ubiquitous commensal or insidious pathogen? A two-step in situ PCR approach. J Clin Virol 2000; 16:159-178.

86. Remenick J, Radonovich MF, Brady JN. Human immunodeficiency virus Tat transactivation: induction of a tissue-specific enhancer in a nonpermissive cell line. J Virol 1991; 65:5641-5646.

87. Valle LD, Croul S, Morgello S et al. Detection of HIV-1 Tat and JCV capsid protein, VP1, in AIDS brain with progressive multifocal leukoencephalopathy. J Neurovirol 2000; 6:221-228.

88. Randhawa P, Luo J, Zygmunt D et al. Induction of host gene expression in BK virus in cultured WI-38 cells: Implications for the pathogenesis of BK virus nephropathy. Modern Pathol 2003; 16:1224A.

89. Jacobsen SE. Interleukin-11. In: Thomson AW, ed. The Cytokine Handbook. New York: Academic Press, 1998:365-390.

90. Ahuja M, Cohen EP, Dayer AM et al. Polyoma virus infection after renal transplantation. Use of immunostaining as a guide to diagnosis. Transplantation 2001; 71:896-899.

91. Malefyt RW, Vries JEd. Interleukin-13. In: Thomson AW, ed. The Cytokine Handbook. New York: Academic Press, 1998:427-442.

92. Segerer S. The role of chemokines and chemokine receptors in progressive renal diseases. Am J Kidney Dis 2003; 41(3 Suppl 1):S15-18.

93. Onetti Muda A, Ruzzi L, Bernardini S et al. Collagen VII expression in glomerular sclerosis. J Pathol 2001; 195:383-390.

94. Pilmore HL, Eris JM, Painter DM et al. Vascular endothelial growth factor expression in human chronic renal allograft rejection. Transplantation. 1999; 67:929-933.

95. Frieri M, Agarwal K, Datar A et al. Increased interleukin-4 production in response to mast cell mediators and human type I collagen in patients with rheumatoid arthritis. Ann Allergy 1994; 72:360-367.

96. Game X, Malavaud B, Alric L et al. Infliximab treatment of Crohn disease ileovesical fistula. Scand J Gastroenterol 2003; 38:1097-1098.

97. Yang XD, Corvalan JR, Wang P et al. Fully human anti-interleukin-8 monoclonal antibodies: potential therapeutics for the treatment of inflammatory disease states. J Leukoc Biol 1999; 66:401-410.

98. Salmela K, Wramner L, Ekberg H et al. A randomized multicenter trial of the anti-ICAM-1 monoclonal antibody (enlimomab) for the prevention of acute rejection and delayed onset of graft function in cadaveric renal transplantation: A report of the European Anti-ICAM-1 Renal Transplant Study Group. Transplantation 1999; 67:729-736.

CHAPTER 11

Polyomavirus-Associated Nephropathy in Renal Transplantation:
Critical Issues of Screening and Management

Hans H. Hirsch, Cinthia B. Drachenberg, Juerg Steiger and Emilio Ramos

Abstract

P olyomavirus-associated nephropathy (PVAN) is an emerging disease in renal transplant patients with variable prevalence of 1-10% and graft loss up to 80%. BK virus (BKV) is the primary etiologic agent, but JC virus (JCV) and possibly simian virus SV40 may account for some cases. Intense immunosuppression is viewed as the most important risk factor. However, the preferential manifestation in renal transplants as compared to other allografts or to autologous kidneys of other organ transplants suggests that organ determinants and immunologic factors synergize: Renal tubular epithelial cells and their compensatory proliferation to restore tubular integrity after immunologic, ischemic or toxic injury may provide the critical cellular milieu supporting polyomavirus replication while immune control is impaired due to maintenance immunosuppression, anti-rejection treatment and HLA-mismatches. Patient determinants (older age, male gender, seronegative recipient), and viral factors (genotype, serotype) may have a contributory role. The definitive diagnosis of PVAN requires allograft biopsy which is, however, challenged by (i) limited sensitivity due to (multi-)focal involvement (sampling errors); (ii) varying presentations with cytopathic-inflammatory and/or fibrotic/scarring patterns; (iii) coexisting acute rejection which is difficult to differentiate, but impacts on intervention strategies. Screening for polyomavirus replication in the urine and in the plasma complements allograft biopsy by high sensitivity and allows for noninvasive monitoring. Thus, we suggest a terminology similar to invasive fungal diseases where viruria ("decoy cells") defines patients at risk ("possible PVAN") who should be evaluated for plasma viral load. Increasing BK viremia (>10,000 copies/mL) or urine VP-1 mRNA ($>6.5\times10^5$ copies/ng total RNA) load defines "presumptive PVAN" for which an intervention of reducing immunosuppression should be considered even if the diagnosis could not be confirmed by allograft biopsy ("definitive PVAN"). The response to intervention should be monitored using plasma DNA or urine mRNA load.

Introduction

The human polyomaviruses type 1 and type 2 were isolated in the early 1970s and named after the initials B.K and J.C. of the respective patients.[1,2] However, the medical and scientific context was significantly different. For JC virus (JCV), the isolation was driven by a clear link to disease which followed the electron microscopic visualization of polyomavirus particles half a decade earlier in brain tissues from patients with progressive multifocal leucoencephalopathy (PML).[2] In contrast, the discovery of BKV is more reminiscent of

Polyomaviruses and Human Diseases, edited by Nasimul Ahsan. ©2006 Eurekah.com and Springer Science+Business Media.

"chance favoring a prepared mind" when particles of polyomavirus-like morphology were noted in cytopathically altered urinary cells of a renal transplant patient with ureteric stenosis.[1] The pathogenic role of BKV remained elusive, to the point that BKV was declared an orphan virus in search of a human disease. However, 25 years later, the salient feature of the initial isolation, namely "decoy cells" in the urine of a renal transplant patient has become a paradigm in the emerging PVAN.[3-5] Less well known is the fact that four of todays cardinal features of PVAN in renal transplants have been published as early as 1978 by Mackenzie and coworkers, namely the shedding of decoy cells, the presence of viral inclusions in tubular epithelial cells in allograft biopsies, the erroneous interpretation of allograft dysfunction with infiltrates as acute rejection and the role of intense immunosuppression and its reduction, all of which can be gathered from the paper entitled "Human polyoma virus—a significant pathogen in renal transplantation" and the appended discussion protocol.[6,7] Subsequently, sporadic cases of PVAN in patients with complex immunodeficiencies or advanced HIV-disease were reported.[8,9] Thus, the appearance of PVAN is remarkable after decades of virtual nondiagnosis in renal transplantation.[3,4,10-12] Given the presumed coevolution of human polyomaviruses with humans and the basically unchanged seroepidemiology,[13] the recent surge of PVAN points to new risk factors and critical, but as yet ill-understood, changes in our transplantation protocols.

Infection, Replication and Disease

The virological aspects of BKV, JCV and SV40 have been described in detail (see Chapters 1, 6, 20). BKV and JCV are specific for the human host and despite a high degree of genetic homology of >70% are independently transmitted from one another.[13,14] Epidemiologic, clinical and virologic aspects suggest coevolutionary adaptation resulting from a long-standing virus-host interaction:[9]

1. High prevalence of infection reaching 70-90% among adults;
2. Low morbidity of primary infection;
3. Latency in the renourinary tract as the epidemiologically most relevant site;
4. Asymptomatic reactivation and shedding into the urine;
5. Extensive dependence on host cell functions for viral gene expression and replication;
6. Chimeric nucleosomes consisting of host cell histones and viral DNA which are even packaged into virions;
7. Linkage of polyomavirus subtypes to defined human populations and their historic migration patterns across continents.[9]

Thus, polyomavirus genomes resemble (mini-)chromosomes, yet without access to their hosts' germline remain dependent on a minimal set of functions to reach out and colonize to the next generation by infection. In contrast, human exposure to the simian virus SV40 resulted accidentally from contaminated polio- and adenovirus vaccines in the 1960s. Significant spread of SV40 among humans is not supported by serological data, but a role in disease has been put forward by some.[15] Possibly, accidental exposure may be ongoing in areas with significant contacts to macaques e.g., in animal parks in rural areas of developing countries.

Polyomaviruses are small nonenveloped viruses of 45nm diameter and establish a state of nonreplicative infection termed latency in urogenital epithelial cells. Switching to the replicative mode requires viral regulatory functions, most notably the large T-antigen encoded in the early gene region. The large T-antigen is a multifunctional protein which governs viral transcription and replication in concert with cellular factors by cross-talking to host cell proteins including transcription and replication factors, cell cycle proteins and DNA binding proteins (see Chapter 9). After replication of the viral double-stranded DNA genome of 5300 bp, the late genes encoding the viral capsid proteins VP1, VP2, and VP3 are expressed and transported to the nucleus for virion assembly. The agnoprotein may play a role in the early and in the late phase of viral replication and virion assembly. Release of infectious progeny requires host cell

Table 1. Patterns of polyomavirus-associated disease

Disease Pattern	Principle	Prototypic Example
Cytopathic	Predominant polyomavirus replication	PML[1] by JCV in AIDS
Cytopathic – inflammatory	Replication plus inflammatory infiltrate	PVAN[2] pattern B (interstitial nephritis) in renal transplantation
Immune reconstituting	Predominant inflammatory immune response subsequent to replication	PML by JCV in AIDS[3] following initiation of HAART[4] Hemorrhagic cystitis by BKV in stem cell transplantation
Autoimmune	Pathologic immune response triggered by previous replication Antigenic complexes - viral DNA: host cell histones - large T-antigen:host cell DNA - viral capsid: host cell DNA	Systemic lupus by BKV?
Transforming	Uncoupling of cell proliferation from lytic replication	Urothelial carcinoma by BKV Lymphoma by JCV, SV40?

[1] PML, progressive mulitfocal leucoencephalopathy; [2] PVAN, polyomavirus-associated nephropathy; [3] AIDS, acquired immunodeficiency syndrome; [4] HAART, highly active antiretroviral therapy.

lysis. Thus, despite being relatively slowly replicating as compared to e.g., herpes simplex virus in epithelial cells, significant polyomavirus replication is lytic and hence cytopathic. Host cell lysis releasing viral and cellular constitutents may elicit nonspecific inflammatory responses and depending on the state of the immune system, a specific cellular and humoral immune response. Of note, polyomavirus infections have been associated with diverse disease pattern which involve either cytopathic, inflammatory, immunological or oncogenic pathologies (Table 1). The underlying mechanisms are not well understood, but may reflect differences in the time and load of infection, in the infected cell types and their state of differentiation as well as different individual immunogenetic background and/or their modification by inherited, acquired or therapeutic immune dysfunction.[9]

Thus, *polyomavirus infection* is defined as serological or virological evidence of virus exposure without distinguishing between replicating, latent or transforming patterns.[9] *Polyomavirus replication* is defined as evidence for ongoing virus multiplication (synonymous with lytic infection) by detecting: infectious virus by cell culture; polyomavirus particles by electron microscopy; polyomavirus structural proteins by immunohistochemistry; messenger RNA expression of late genes (e.g., VP1); polyomavirus DNA in nonlatency sites (e.g., in plasma); cytological (e.g., decoy cells) or histological evidence for polyomavirus replication.[9] If detected in a seronegative or a seropositive individual, polyomavirus replication is termed primary or secondary, respectively. *Polyomavirus disease* corresponds to histological evidence of polyomavirus-mediated organ pathology. Conceptually, cytopathic, cytopathic-inflammatory or immune reconstitution patterns are closely linked to significant polyomavirus replication which is most likely in patients lacking at one time specific immune effector cells e.g., in seronegative individuals or in patients with inherited, acquired or therapeutically induced immune dysfunction.[9,16] In autoimmune disease, a pathologic immune response is triggered at some point by prior replication, but has become independently thereof.[17] In oncogenic transformation, the replicative state of the host cell is uncoupled from virus induced host cell lysis.[9,18] As discussed in more detail below, PVAN may present as cytopathic, cytopathic-inflammatory or immune reconstitution patterns.

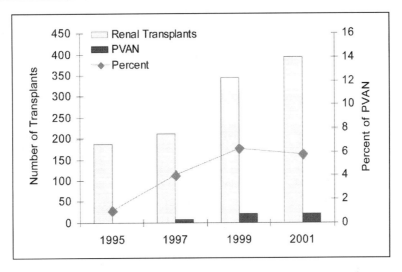

Figure 1. Increasing prevalence of PVAN from year 1995 to 2001 (data from ref. 19).

Epidemiology

Following the inaugurating report by Randhawa and coworkers in 1995,[3] a stepwise increase in PVAN has been observed from 1% in 1995 to 5% in 2001 (Fig. 1).[19,20] Other reports from 2002-2004 identified PVAN in 1% to 10% of renal transplant patients (mean 5.1%, median 4.5%, Table 2) which correspond well to Kaplan-Meier estimates of 8% for the incidence of PVAN (95% confidence interval 1% - 15%) described in a prospective study.[21] The majority of cases occur within the first year posttransplantation, but approximately a quarter of cases are diagnosed later (Fig. 2).[9,21,31] Loss of renal allograft ranges from 10% - >80% of cases

Table 2. PVAN prevalence, drug use and outcome in reports 2002-2004

Study	Prevalence (%)	Tacrolimus (%)	Mycophenolate Mofetil (%)	Graft Loss (%)
Mengel et al 2003 (22)	1.1	57	87	71
Trofe et al 2003 (23)	2.1	77	54	54
Buehrig et al 2003 (20)	2.7	100	89	38
Ginevri et al 2003 (24)	3.0	66	66	33
Rahaminov et al 2003 (25)	3.8	100	87	14
Kang et al 2003 (26)	3.9	100	33	100
Ramos et al 2002(27)	5.1	91	97	82 (30)*
Hirsch et al 2002 (21)	6.0	60	40	0
Li et al 2002 (28)	7.0	100	50	33
Maiza et al 2002 (29)	7.1	50	50	50
Sachdeva et al 2004 (55)	9.3	0	0	Not reported
Moriyama et al 2003 (30)	10.3	36	n.a.**	22
Mean	5.1	70	60	46.2
(median/range)	(4.5/1.1-10.3)	(70/0-100)	(70/0-89)	(44/0-100)

* Graft loss over 60 months (12 months) of follow-up. ** Not available.

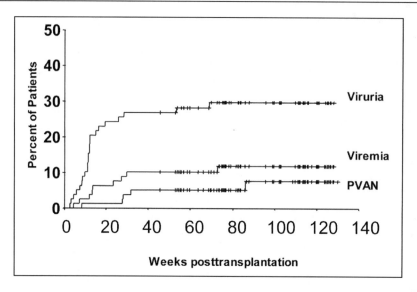

Figure 2. Kaplan-Meier estimates of the incidence of polyomavirus replication (decoy-cell shedding), BK viremia and polyomavirus-associated nephropathy (PVAN) in renal transplant recipients. From: Hirsch HH, Knowles W, Dickenmann M et al. N Engl J Med 2002; 347:488-496, ©2002 Massachusetts Medical Society, with permission.[21]

(Table 2).[4,9,12,27,32] In transplant centers screening for polyomavirus replication in the urine, plasma or in protocol biopsies, the rate of graft loss seems to be lower.[20,21,31,33-36]

Molecular studies indicate that most cases of PVAN are caused by BKV.[21,30,33,34,37-40] A role for JCV and the simian virus SV40 has been suggested which may either act alone[41-44] or in concert with BKV,[28,45] and should be investigated further.

Risk Factors

The risk factors for PVAN in renal transplantation are still only incompletely understood. Appropriately sized prospective multi-center studies are lacking and the results of hitherto published reports are often contradictory. Most likely, PVAN results from multiple, partly complementing factors including determinants of the patient (age >50 years, male gender, negative BKV serostatus of recipient prior to transplantation, impaired BKV specific T-cell response, white ethnicity, cytomegalovirus coinfection, diabetes mellitus), of the allograft (HLA mismatches, prior episodes of acute rejection, calcineurin-inhibitor toxicity) and of the virus (new BKV serotypes, adaptive changes in immune and replicative control regions with presumably increased viral fitness) (Table 3). It is conceivable that these factors are modulated by immunosuppression, inflammatory response patterns, antiviral and antiproliferative activities e.g., cidofovir, immunoglobulins, and/or coinfections e.g., cytomegalovirus, JCV, SV40 (Fig. 3).[9] There is, however, general consensus that immunosuppression is the *conditio sine qua non* for PVAN. It has been noted[4] that the emergence of PVAN coincided with the widespread use of tacrolimus (TAC) and mycophenolate mofetil (MMF).[53] However, a proof of causality is lacking. Their different mode of action suggests that the intensity of immunosuppression rather than the specific agent is the most relevant factor.[4,7,11,47,54] The role of the net state of immunosuppression is underscored by the fact that reducing, switching or discontinuing components of maintenance therapy represents currently the primary mode of intervention (see below). As a note of caution, this argument does not exclude drug-specific mechanisms promoting polyomavirus replication which act at different, yet synergizing levels and would be expected to respond also to this intervention. Almost all diagnoses of PVAN were made in patients receiving a triple therapy of four drug classes

Table 3. Presumed risk factors for polyomavirus-associatedd nephropathy

Risk Factor	Increased with	Refs.
Immunosuppression		
Triple combinations	Tacrolimus, Mycophenolate mofetil, Prednisone	4,22,35
Drug levels	Tacrolimus trough levels >8 ng/mL	22
Drug dosing	Mycophenolate mofetil ≥2 g/day	22
	Prednisone	46
Anti-rejection treatment	Anti-lymphocyte globulin	21
	Methylprednisolone pulses	21
Patient determinants		
Age	>50 years	27
Gender	Male > female	23,27
Race	White > other	19,23
BKV seropositivity	Antibody titer < 1:40	24
BKV-specific T-cells	Interferon-γ production	48,49
	Polymorphism linked to low interferon-γ expression	50
Co-morbidity	Diabetes mellitus	12,23
	Cytomegalovirus infection	20,51
Organ determinants		
Immunologic injury	HLA-mismatches	21
	Prior acute rejections	21,22,37
Drug toxicity	Tacrolimus ?	23
Viral determinants		
Non-coding control region	Rearrangements ?	52
	Point mutations in GM-CSF response element ?	
Viral capsid protein-1	Mutations in serotype domain ?	39

(calcineurin inhibitors, anti-metabolites, mTOR inhibitors and corticosteroids). In approximately 90% of patients reported to date, these triple combinations contained TAC or MMF (Table 2)[9] which were used concurrently in >50% of the cases. Conversely, <10% of all reported cases of PVAN received triple immunosuppressive regimens that did not contain TAC or MMF.[9] Of note, a recent retrospective histopathology study from India described 30 cases of PVAN in patients treated with triple combinations of cyclosporine (CyA), azathioprine (AZA) and prednisone (PRE).[55] Yet, the type of polyomavirus involved and impact on allograft function is not known at present. Taken together, it is clear that PVAN can arise in patients not treated with TAC or MMF although less frequently,[7,9] while an increased risk for sustained BKV viruria or for PVAN was reported for patients treated with triple combinations of TAC, MMF and PRE[22,35] or with TAC trough levels higher than >8ng/mL.[22]

Using antilymphocyte preparations for induction was not significantly associated with BKV viruria, viremia or PVAN,[4,21,56] or with histologically more severe PVAN.[20] In this way, replication of polyomavirus and cytomegalovirus differ possibly reflecting viral differences in propensity to reactivate, in sites of latency and in immunological control. In contrast, antilymphocyte preparations were associated with an increased risk for polyomavirus replication when administered for the treatment of acute rejection episodes in patients receiving combination of TAC-AZA and/or CyA-MMF.[4,21] The differential effect of antilymphocyte preparations for PVAN suggests a cofactorial role of tubular epithelial cell injury and regeneration, similar to animal models.[7,16,57]

Steroids may also increase the risk of polyomavirus replication when given as part of a triple combination[46,58] or as intravenous bolus to treat rejection as long as maintenance immunosuppression is continued or intensified.[4,12,21,59] This effect of steroids synergizes with the intensity

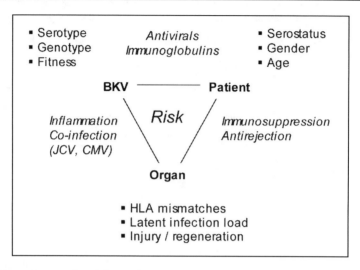

Figure 3. Determinants and modulators of PVAN.

of the maintenance immunosuppression and is potentially less relevant if coupled to decreased or modified maintenance immunosuppression.[21,51,59] Of note, glucocorticoid response elements have been reported in the regulatory region of polyomaviruses[60] suggesting a molecular explanation for an increased risk of replication in concert with immunosuppression.

Diagnosis

The diagnosis of PVAN requires the demonstration of polyomavirus induced cytopathic changes in tubular or glomerular epithelial cells (see Chapters 14, 15). The histopathological changes of PVAN are fairly characteristic, but should be confirmed with ancillary tests such as immunohistochemical detection of the large T-antigen which is most commonly used (see Chapter 14). The sensitivity and specificity of the histological diagnosis of PVAN is complicated by (i) the focality of renal involvement, particularly early in the disease (pattern A); (ii) a wide spectrum of associated changes, in particular inflammatory infiltrates which may be unspecifically elicited by tubular cell necrosis or result from virus-specific cellular immune responses and are difficult to differentiate from acute rejection (pattern B); (iii) by pronounced tubular atrophy and fibrosis of late stages (pattern C) where only few viral cytopathic changes are seen to the point where they may even be undetectable (false negative).[31,37,61,62] Given the diverse determinants (Fig. 3) and presentations of PVAN and confounding concurrent pathologies, hands-on stratification can be achieved by searching for BKV replication in urine. Because of its high negative predictive value, lack of detectable BKV replication in the urine practically excludes PVAN. Conversely, if BKV replication is detectable, the risk for PVAN is increased and further diagnostic studies are warranted. Thus, the hallmark of PVAN is that ongoing polyomavirus replication is detectable as BKV viremia, viruria and decoy cell shedding in all of these presentations.[4,5,21,31,35,63] The limited sensitivity of allograft biopsy is also critical for the definition of "resolved PVAN" as the goal of any intervention. Therefore, resolution of PVAN not only requires the disappearance of the histological signs of active disease (e.g., viral replication, inclusions, necrosis, inflammatory infiltrates) and negative immunohistochemistry, but should also include negative results of the surrogate replication markers such as BKV viremia and viruria. Thus, we suggest a terminology similar to invasive fungal diseases where viruria ("decoy cells") defines patients at risk ("possible" PVAN) who should be evaluated for plasma viral load. BKV replication above thresholds such as increasing BK viremia (>10,000 copies/mL) (Fig. 4) defines "presumptive" PVAN for which an intervention of reducing immunosuppression should be

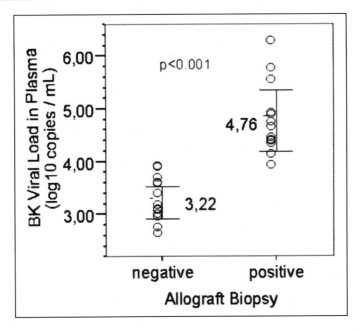

Figure 4. BKV load in plasma of patients with PVAN-negative n=13) and positive (n=16) allograft biopsies (H.H. Hirsch, unpublished).

considered, preferably with, but, due to the limited sensitivity, not dependent on prior histological confirmation ("definitive PVAN") (Table 4). In summary, surrogate markers of polyomavirus replication complement the limited sensitivity of PVAN biopsy and allows for noninvasive monitoring.

Polyomavirus replication can be demonstrated by several methods such as urine cytology (decoy cells), quantification of urinary BKV DNA or VP1 mRNA load,[4,5,21,33,63] or electron microscopy for polyomavirus particles.[5,64] The different screening methods have not been compared, but are assumed to be equivalent given sufficient local expertise. Because self-limiting

Table 4. Polyomavirus replication and PVAN diagnosis in renal transplantation

	PVAN			Acute Rejection	
	Possible	Presumptive	Definitive	Yes	no
Screening test	+	+	+		
Adjunct test	–	+	+	(+?)	(–)
Biopsy	–	–	+	+	–
			Pattern A-C	Banff'97	
Intervention indicated	No	(?)	Yes	Yes	No

Screening tests for polyomavirus replication are the presence of decoy cells in urine cytology, of BKV DNA or RNA or polyomavirus particle in urine. Positive adjunct testing corresponds BKV VP1 mRNA (6.5×10^5 copies/ng total RNA) in urine or BKV DNA in plasma (10^4 copies/mL; see text for details).

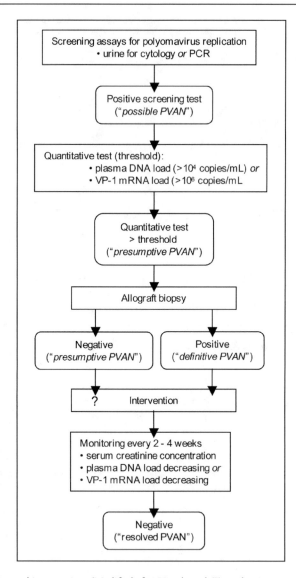

Figure 5. Screening and intervention. (Modified after Hirsch et al. Transplantation 2005; in press.)

(transient) polyomavirus replication has been observed in renal transplant patients,[21,31,62] it is recommended that positive screening results are confirmed within four weeks, followed by adjunct quantitative diagnostic assays such as quantification of BKV DNA load in plasma (Fig. 5)[21,65,66] or VP1 mRNA load in urine.[33] Detecting higher levels of BKV replication above empirically defined thresholds may provide specificity and specificity of >93% such as BKV VP-1 mRNA 6.5×10^5 copies/ng total RNA[33] or BKV DNA load in plasma ≥10'000 copies/mL (Figs. 4, 5).[21,65] To monitor the course of disease, quantitative polyomavirus testing should be performed every 2-4 weeks until viral replication drops below the threshold or is no longer detectable. However, further interlaboratory and clinical validation of threshold values in plasma and urine is needed.

Table 5. Modification of maintenance immunosuppression in renal transplant patients with PVAN

Strategy	Intervention	Comment	Refs.
Switching			
TAC → CYA	Trough levels 100-150 ng/mL	Consider in patients on TAC-MMF-PRE combinations due to MMF lowering effect of CYA	(11,21,28,51)
MMF → AZA	Dosing ≤100 mg/day	Consider in patients on TAC-MMF-PRE with prior rejections	(21)
TAC → SIR	Trough levels <6 ng/mL	Consider in patients with calcineurin inhibitor toxicity	(67)
MMF → LEF	Trough levels >30 ng/mL	Consider in patients with concurrent cytomegalovirus infection	(68)
Decreasing			
TAC	Trough levels <6 ng/mL	Consider in patients with limited early disease or "presumptive PVAN"	(12,32)
MMF	Dosing ≤1 g/day	Consider in patients with limited early disease or "presumptive PVAN"	(23,27,32)
CYA	Trough levels 100 ng/mL	Consider in patients with limited early disease or "presumptive PVAN"	(21,32)
Stopping			
	Continue dual	Consider in patients with presumptive PVAN,	(19,69,70)
TAC	therapy	with stable graft function during the second	
or	TAC-PRE	year posttransplant without prior acute	
MMF	CYA-PRE	rejection episodes	
or	MMF-PRE		
CYA	SIR-PRE		

TAC, tacrolimus; CYA, cyclosporine; MMF, mycophenolate mofetil; LEF, leflunomide; PRE, prednisone; SIR, sirolimus.

Intervention

At the present time, there is no approved treatment for PVAN. In the absence of safe, specific and efficacious antivirals, the current mainstay of intervention resides in the judicious reduction of immunosuppression similar to cytomegalovirus infection in the era before ganciclovir. As indicated above, most cases diagnosed with PVAN to date are on triple immunosuppressive maintenance combinations containing calcineurin inhibitors (TAC, CyA), antiproliferative agents (MMF, AZA), and corticosteroids (PRE), or more recently sirolimus (SIR).[28,65] However, there are no prospective randomized trials evaluating the efficacy and safety of the different interventions. In principle, three different, but not exclusive modes have been reported which include reducing, switching and stopping immunosuppressive drugs (Table 5). It should be noted that these experiences are anecdotal and reflect individualized approaches to patients and cannot be generalized. More recently, switching to leflunomide, an inhibitor of pyrimidine synthesis and protein tyrosine kinase, or the newer derivative FK778 has been proposed as these immunosuppressive drugs have also anti-viral activity in vitro.[68]

A critical issue with regard to management is the diagnosis of acute rejection concurrently with PVAN. Although PVAN is generally considered a complication of intense immunosuppression, both disease entities may start focally and show different kinetics which may lead to concurrence. In addition, reconstitution of BKV-specific cellular immunity may be difficult to distinguish from, and in fact, trigger acute rejection.[9] Given a *bona fide* diagnosis of PVAN and concurrent rejection, there is controversy regarding the use of antirejection treatment with steroids in this situation. Based on the initital experience it is clear that PVAN progression is frequently observed when anti-rejection treatment is administered and the maintenance immunosuppression is maintained or intensified.[4,12,21,59] However, in some centers, a two-step protocol of antirejection treatment coupled to a reduction of maintenance immunosuppression has been successful.[21,71] The sole reduction of maintenance immunosuppression in this situation seems to be particularly risky as it might precipitate severe rejection and premature graft loss. In general, the response to reduced immunosuppression seems to better when PVAN is diagnosed early, with only limited involvement[20,21,25,31,36] which most likely also applies to the concurrence of PVAN and rejection.

Several drugs have polyomavirus-inhibitory activity in vitro, including cidofovir, leflunomide, and certain quinolone antibiotics. In the clinical situation, the use of these drugs was combined with reduced immunosuppression which limits the evaluation of their efficacy. Amantidine has been used in the treatment of PVAN without discernable effect.[23,72] Cidofovir has a significant in vitro effect inhibiting nonhuman polyomaviruses. However, the pronounced nephrotoxicity limits its use particularly in renal transplantation. A number of patients have been treated with a combination of low-dose Cidofovir and reduced immunosuppression with variable results. In most published reports, its use was associated with a decrease in viremia, but viruria often persisted for prolonged times.[73-75] Some patients have gone on to develop end-stage renal disease which may, however, be multifactorial. This off-label use of cidofovir is at a low dose of 0.25 mg/kg, administered every two weeks. The patients are usually premedicated, with increased intravenous fluids.[73-75] Chandraker et al[76] have shown that the quinolones also have anti- polyomavirus activity in vitro, and observed resolution of BKV replication in vivo in some of 10 prospectively studied patients. Although the efficacy is less than requested for an antipolyomaviral agent, these data suggest that the BKV encoded helicase activity may represent a significant drug target for further development.

Retransplantation

There is only limited experience with regard to retransplantation of patients who have lost a previous graft due to PVAN. Based on the 15 cases reported to date, the recurrence may be more frequent compared to that seen in primary transplants (13% versus 8%).[49,72,77-79] Although conclusive evidence is lacking, persistent polyomavirus replication in the urine and/or in the plasma in a patient undergoing retransplantation is viewed as increased risk for recurrence of PVAN. In these patients, reduction or discontinuation of immunosuppression should be considered unless this option is limited by other coexisting grafts (often pancreas). In patients on hemodialysis, administration of antiviral drugs (e.g., cidofovir) may be considered prior to retransplantation. Although tansplant nephroureterectomy does not appear to be required prior to retransplantation, this intervention should be considered in patients with persisting polyomavirus replication. Following retransplantation, the question arises whether or not the same immunosuppressive drugs and combinations can be used as for the primary graft. The data compiled in a multicenter survey by Ramos et at[79] suggest that the same drugs can be used, but that intense immunosuppression should be avoided. Recommendations for screening and treatment of polyomavirus are the same as for patients with a first renal allograft.

Conclusion

The association of BKV with PVAN in renal transplant recipients emphasizes the role of allo-situation in addition to immunosuppression. Most likely, patient, organ and virus specific determinants interact in a complementary fashion and are subject to dose- and magnitude dependent modulators (e.g., immunosuppression). BKV screening of renal transplant patients is warranted to enable early diagnosis of "possible", "presumptive" or "definitive" PVAN as well as of "resolved" PVAN after appropriate intervention. The detection of a plasma BKV DNA load or VP1 mRNA in the urine above thresholds should trigger allograft biopsy to confirm PVAN and exclude acute rejection. Antivirals or immunosuppressants with antiviral activity are interesting new avenues that remain to be explored. Large prospective studies are needed to identify risk factors and to evaluate intervention strategies for PVAN.

Acknowledgement

This work was supported in part by the Swiss National Fonds Grant 3200-62021 to HHH.

References

1. Gardner SD, Field AM, Coleman DV et al. New human papovavirus (B.K.) isolated from urine after transplantation. Lancet 1971; i:1253-1257.
2. Padgett BL, Walker DL, Zu Rhein GM et al. Cultivation of papova-like virus from human brain with progressive multifocal leucoencephalopathy. Lancet 1971; i:1257-1260.
3. Purighalla R, Shapiro R, McCauley J et al. BK virus infection in a kidney allograft diagnosed by needle biopsy. Am J Kidney Dis 1995; 26:671-673.
4. Binet I, Nickeleit V, Hirsch HH et al. Polyomavirus disease under new immunosuppressive drugs: A cause of renal graft dysfunction and graft loss. Transplantation 1999; 67:918-922.
5. Drachenberg CB, Beskow CO, Cangro CB et al. Human polyoma virus in renal allograft biopsies: Morphological findings and correlation with urine cytology. Hum Pathol 1999; 30:970-977.
6. Mackenzie EF, Poulding JM, Harrison PR et al. Human polyoma virus (HPV)-a significant pathogen in renal transplantation. Proc Eur Dial Transplant Assoc 1978; 15:352-360.
7. Hirsch HH. Polyomavirus BK nephropathy: A (re)emerging complication in renal transplantation. Am J Transplant 2002; 2:25-30.
8. Rosen S, Harmon W, Krensky AM et al. Tubulo-interstitial nephritis associated with polyomavirus (BK type) infection. N Engl J Med 1983; 308:1192-1196.
9. Hirsch HH, Steiger J. Polyomavirus BK. Lancet Infect Dis 2003; 3:611-623.
10. Pappo O, Demetris AJ, Raikow RB et al. Human polyoma virus infection of renal allografts: Histopathologic diagnosis, clinical significance, and literature review. Mod Pathol 1996; 9:105-109.
11. Mathur VS, Olson JL, Darragh TM et al. Polyomavirus-induced interstitial nephritis in two renal transplant recipients: Case reports and review of the literature. Am J Kidney Dis 1997; 29:754-758.
12. Randhawa PS, Finkelstein S, Scantlebury V et al. Human polyoma virus-associated interstitial nephritis in the allograft kidney. Transplantation 1999; 67:103-109.
13. Knowles WA, Pipkin P, Andrews N et al. Population-based study of antibody to the human polyomaviruses BKV and JCV and the simian polyomavirus SV40. J Med Virol 2003; 71:115-123.
14. Shah KV, Daniel R, Warszawski R. High prevalence of antibodies to BK virus, an SV40-related papovavirus, in residents of Maryland. J Infect Dis 1973; 128:784-787.
15. zur Hausen H. SV40 in human cancers—an endless tale? Int J Cancer 2003; 107:687.
16. Fishman JA. BK virus nephropathy—polyomavirus adding insult to injury. N Engl J Med 2002; 347:527-530.
17. Moens U, Rekvig OP. Molecular biology of BK virus and clinical and basic aspectes of BK virus renal infection. In: Khalili K, Stoner GL, eds. Human Polyomaviruses: Molecular and clinical perspectives. New York: Wiley-Liss, 2001:215-226.
18. Tognon M, Corallini A, Martini F et al. Oncogenic transformation by BK virus and association with human tumors. Oncogene 2003; 22:5192-5200.
19. Ramos E, Drachenberg CB, Portocarrero M et al. BK virus nephropathy diagnosis and treatment: Experience at the University of Maryland Renal Transplant Program. Clin Transpl 2002:143-153.
20. Buehrig CK, Lager DJ, Stegall MD et al. Influence of surveillance renal allograft biopsy on diagnosis and prognosis of polyomavirus-associated nephropathy. Kidney Int 2003; 64:665-673.
21. Hirsch HH, Knowles W, Dickenmann M et al. Prospective study of polyomavirus type BK replication and nephropathy in renal-transplant recipients. N Engl J Med 2002; 347:488-496.
22. Mengel M, Marwedel M, Radermacher J et al. Incidence of polyomavirus-nephropathy in renal allografts: Influence of modern immunosuppressive drugs. Nephrol Dial Transplant 2003; 18:1190-1196.
23. Trofe J, Gaber LW, Stratta RJ et al. Polyomavirus in kidney and kidney-pancreas transplant recipients. Transpl Infect Dis 2003; 5:21-28.
24. Ginevri F, De Santis R, Comoli P et al. Polyomavirus BK infection in pediatric kidney-allograft recipients: A single-center analysis of incidence, risk factors, and novel therapeutic approaches. Transplantation 2003; 75:1266-1270.
25. Rahamimov R, Lustig S, Tovar A et al. BK polyoma virus nephropathy in kidney transplant recipient: The role of new immunosuppressive agents. Transplant Proc 2003; 35:604-605.

26. Kang YN, Han SM, Park KK et al. BK virus infection in renal allograft recipients. Transplant Proc 2003; 35:275-277.
27. Ramos E, Drachenberg CB, Papadimitriou JC et al. Clinical course of polyoma virus nephropathy in 67 renal transplant patients. J Am Soc Nephrol 2002; 13:2145-2151.
28. Li RM, Mannon RB, Kleiner D et al. BK virus and SV40 coinfection in polyomavirus nephropathy. Transplantation 2002; 74:1497-1504.
29. Maiza H, Fontaniere B, Dijoud F et al. Graft dysfunction and polyomavirus infection in renal allograft recipients. Transplant Proc 2002; 34:809-811.
30. Moriyama T, Namba Y, Kyo M et al. Prevalence and characteristics of biopsy-proven BK virus nephropathy in Japanese renal transplant patients: Analysis in Protocol, NonEpisode and Episode Biopsies. J Am Soc Nephrol 2003; 14:F-PO571.
31. Drachenberg CB, Papadimitriou JC, Hirsch HH et al. Histological patterns of polyomavirus nephropathy: Correlation with graft outcome and viral load. Am J Transplantation 2004; 4:2082-2092.
32. Trofe J, Cavallo T, First M et al. Polyomavirus in kidney and kidney-pancreas transplantation: A defined protocol for immunosuppression reduction and histologic monitoring. Transplant Proc 2002; 34:1788-1789.
33. Ding R, Medeiros M, Dadhania D et al. Noninvasive diagnosis of BK virus nephritis by measurement of messenger RNA for BK virus VP1 in urine. Transplantation 2002; 74:987-994.
34. Ramos ER, Drachenberg CB, Papadimitriou JC et al. Impact of prospective urine cytology on graft function (GF) for earlier diagnosis of polyoma virus nephropathy. J Am Soc Nephrol 2003; 13:378A (Abstract #561).
35. Agha I, Brennan DC. BK virus and current immunosuppressive therapy. Graft 2002; 5:S65-S72-.
36. Drachenberg CB, Papadimitriou JC, Wali R et al. Improved outcome of polyoma virus allograft nephropathy with early biopsy. Transplant Proc 2004; 36:758-759.
37. Nickeleit V, Hirsch HH, Binet IF et al. Polyomavirus infection of renal allograft recipients: From latent infection to manifest disease. J Am Soc Nephrol 1999; 10:1080-1089.
38. Nickeleit V, Klimkait T, Binet IF et al. Testing for polyomavirus type BK DNA in plasma to identify renal-allograft recipients with viral nephropathy. N Engl J Med 2000; 342:1309-1315.
39. Randhawa PS, Khaleel-Ur-Rehman K, Swalsky PA et al. DNA sequencing of viral capsid protein VP-1 region in patients with BK virus interstitial nephritis. Transplantation 2002; 73:1090.
40. Randhawa PS, Vats A, Zygmunt D et al. Quantitation of viral DNA in renal allograft tissue from patients with BK virus nephropathy. Transplantation 2002; 74:485-488.
41. Wen MC, Wang CL, Wang M et al. Association of JC virus with tubulointerstitial nephritis in a renal allograft recipient. J Med Virol 2004; 72:675-678.
42. Kazory A, Ducloux D, Chalopin JM et al. The first case of JC virus allograft nephropathy. Transplantation 2003; 76:1653-1655.
43. Hurault de Ligny B, Etienne I, Francois A et al. Polyomavirus-induced acute tubulo-interstitial nephritis in renal allograft recipients. Transplant Proc 2000; 32:2760-2761.
44. Milstone A, Vilchez RA, Geiger X et al. Polyomavirus simian virus 40 infection associated with nephropathy in a lung-transplant recipient. Transplantation 2004; 77:1019-1024.
45. Baksh FK, Finkelstein SD, Swalsky PA et al. Molecular genotyping of BK and JC viruses in human polyomavirus-associated interstitial nephritis after renal transplantation. Am J Kidney Dis 2001; 38:354-365.
46. Trofe J, Roy-Chaudhury P, Gordon J et al. Early cessation/avoidance regimens are associated with lower incidence of polyomavirus nephropathy. Am J Transplantation 2003; 3:371 (Abstract).
47. Hirsch HH, Steiger J, Mihatsch MJ. Immunosuppression and BKV Nephropathy. N Engl J Med 2002; 347:2079-2080.
48. Comoli P, Basso S, Azzi A et al. Dendritic cells pulsed with polyomavirus BK antigen induce ex vivo polyoma BK virus-specific cytotoxic T-cell lines in seropositive healthy individuals and renal transplant recipients. J Am Soc Nephrol 2003; 14(12):3197-3204.
49. Ginevri F, Pastorino N, De Santis R et al. Retransplantation after kidney graft loss due to polyoma BK virus nephropathy: Successful outcome without original allograft nephrectomy. Am J Kidney Dis 2003; 42:821-825.
50. Vaz B, Swarup S, Randhawa PS et al. Cytokine gene polymorphism is associated with BK virus nephropathy in renal transplantation. J Am Soc Nephrol 2003; 13:(Abstract) [SA-FC191].
51. Barri YM, Ahmad I, Ketel BL et al. Polyoma viral infection in renal transplantation: The role of immunosuppressive therapy. Clin Transplant 2001; 15:240-246.
52. Randhawa P, Zygmunt D, Shapiro R et al. Viral regulatory region sequence variations in kidney tissue obtained from patients with BK virus nephropathy. Kidney Int 2003; 64:743-747.
53. Helderman JH, Bennett WM, Cibrik DM et al. Immunosuppression: Practice and trends. Am J Transplantation 2003; 3(S4):41-52.

54. Hodur DM, Mandelbrot D. Immunosuppression and BKV Nephropathy. N Engl J Med 2002; 347:2079.
55. Sachdeva MS, Nada R, Jha V et al. The high incidence of BK polyoma virus infection among renal transplant recipients in India. Transplantation 2004; 77:429-431.
56. Wong W, Hirsch HH, Pascual MDMT et al. BK virus replication in kidney transplant recipients who received thymoglobulin induction. J Am Soc Nephrol 2003; 14:(Abstract) [SU-PO539].
57. Atencio IA, Shadan FF, Zhou XJ et al. Adult mouse kidneys become permissive to acute polyomavirus infection and reactivate persistent infections in response to cellular damage and regeneration. J Virol 1993; 67:1424-1432.
58. Dadhania D, Muthukumar T, Snopkowski C et al. Epidemiology of BK virus replication in renal allograft recipients and identification of corticosteroid maintenance therapy as an independent risk factor. Am J Transplantation 2004; 4:S198 (Abstract #144).
59. Celik B, Shapiro R, Vats A et al. Polyomavirus allograft nephropathy: Sequential assessment of histologic viral load, tubulitis, and graft function following changes in immunosuppression. Am J Transplant 2003; 3:1378-1382.
60. Moens U, Subramaniam N, Johansen B et al. A steroid hormone response unit in the late leader of the noncoding control region of the human polyomavirus BK confers enhanced host cell permissivity. J Virol 1994; 68:2398-2408.
61. Drachenberg RC, Drachenberg CB, Papadimitriou JC et al. Morphological spectrum of polyoma virus disease in renal allografts: Diagnostic accuracy of urine cytology. Am J Transplant 2001; 1:373-381.
62. Nickeleit V, Steiger J, Mihatsch MJ. BK virus infection after kidney transplantation. Graft 2003; 5:S46-S57.
63. Nickeleit V, Hirsch HH, Zeiler M et al. BK-virus nephropathy in renal transplants-tubular necrosis, MHC-class II expression and rejection in a puzzling game. Nephrol Dial Transplant 2000; 15:324-332.
64. Howell DN, Smith SR, Butterly DW et al. Diagnosis and management of BK polyomavirus interstitial nephritis in renal transplant recipients. Transplantation 1999; 68:1279-1288.
65. Hirsch HH, Mohaupt M, Klimkait T. Prospective monitoring of BK virus load after discontinuing sirolimus treatment in a renal transplant patient with BK virus nephropathy. J Infect Dis 2001; 184:1494-1495.
66. Limaye AP, Jerome KR, Kuhr CS et al. Quantitation of BK virus load in serum for the diagnosis of BK virus-associated nephropathy in renal transplant recipients. J Infect Dis 2001; 183:1669-1672.
67. Wali R, Drachenberg CB, Hirsch HH et al. Early detection of BK virus-nephropathy in renal allograft recipients and modification of immunosuppressive therapy to combinations with sirolimus and prednisone is associated with a reduction in BK viremia and improvement of allograft function. Transplantation 2004; 78:1069-1073.
68. Josephson M, Javaid B, Robert H et al. Polyoma nephropathy: Leflunomide blood levels needed for control of this infection. Am J Transplantation 2004; 4:S587 (Abstract #1563).
69. Brennan DC, Agha I, Bohl DL et al. Incidence of BK with tacrolimus versus cyclosporine and impact of presumptive immunosuppression reduction. Am J Transplant 2005; 5:in press.
70. Ramos E, Drachenberg CB, Portocarrero M et al. Effects of type of immunosuppression reduction in patients with BK allograft nephropathy. Am J Transplantation. 2003; 561:(Abstract #1596).
71. Mayr M, Nickeleit V, Hirsch HH et al. Polyomavirus BK nephropathy in a kidney transplant recipient: Critical Issues of Diagnosis and Management. Am J Kidney Dis 2001; 38:13E.
72. Al Jedai AH, Honaker MR, Trofe J et al. Renal allograft loss as the result of polyomavirus interstitial nephritis after simultaneous kidney-pancreas transplantation: Results with kidney retransplantation. Transplantation 2003; 75:490-494.
73. Kadambi PV, Josephson MA, Williams J et al. Treatment of refractory BK virus-associated nephropathy with cidofovir. Am J Transplant 2003; 3:186-191.
74. Vats A, Shapiro R, Randhawa PS et al. BK virus associated nephropathy and cidofovir: Long term experience. Am J Transplantion 2003; 190:(Abstract #148).
75. Vats A, Shapiro R, Singh RP et al. Quantitative viral load monitoring and cidofovir therapy for the management of BK virus-associated nephropathy in children and adults. Transplantation 2003; 75:105-112.
76. Chandraker A, Ali S, Drachenberg C et al. Use of fluorochinolones to treat BK infection in renal transplant recipients. Am J Transplantation 2004; 4:587 (Abstract #1564).
77. Boucek P, Voska L, Saudek F. Successful retransplantation after renal allograft loss to polyoma virus interstitial nephritis. Transplantation 2002; 74:1478.
78. Poduval RD, Meehan SM, Woodle ES et al. Successful retransplantation after renal allograft loss to polyoma virus interstitial nephritis. Transplantation 2002; 73:1166-1163.
79. Ramos E, Vincenti F, Lu WX et al. Retransplantation in patients with graft loss caused by polyoma virus nephropathy. Transplantation 2004; 77:131-133.

CHAPTER 12

BK Virus and Immunosuppressive Agents

Irfan Agha and Daniel C. Brennan

Abstract

The last decade has witnessed the introduction of several potent immunosuppressive agents in the field of transplant medicine. Contemporaneously, infection with BK virus (BKV) has emerged as an important complication of immunosuppression and an important cause of allograft loss after kidney transplantation. Rhandhawa et al reported the first case of BKV associated nephropathy (BKVN) in the modern era of transplantation, in 1995. Since then there has been a resurgence of interest in the epidemiology, biology and pathogenic associations of BKV especially in transplant medicine. Up to 90% of adults have serologic evidence of exposure to BKV. However, only 1-5% of normal healthy adults excrete the virus in the urine (asymptomatic viruria). Thus, for a vast majority of the population, the virus remains perfectly latent and this state of latency is of no obvious consequence. Almost all instances of disease by the BKV have been seen in immunocompromised patients. In recent years, BKV has been associated with nephropathy (BKVN) in about 5% of renal transplant patients. Once established, the disease may result in allograft loss in 45-70% of patients. Although not proven by any prospective study, BKVN causing allograft failure has been linked to immunosuppressive regimens containing tacrolimus or mycophenolate mofetil. This is noteworthy, as both these agents have been used increasingly as the primary maintenance immunotherapy in solid organ transplantation since their introduction around 1990. In addition to the immunosuppressed state, other factors like allograft injury have been thought to be involved in the pathogenesis of the disease. We believe that reactivation of the BKV from its latent state crucially depends on an immunocompromised state but more factors than one dictate precipitation of clinical end organ disease.

In this Chapter, we will discuss the clinical aspects of BKV infection in the renal transplant recipient. We will focus on the role of immunosuppression as a seminal factor allowing replication of the virus. Not all patients who have replicating BKV go on to develop nephropathy: we will discuss other host factors that may constitute a 'second hit' allowing replicating BKV to precipitate BKVN. Results of our recently concluded prospective study on the issue of current immunosuppressive agents in the development of BKVN will be discussed. Finally, based on our experience, we will provide some guidelines for early diagnosis and management of this disease.

Biology of BKV Infection: From Primary Infection to Manifest Disease

The life cycle of BKV has been discussed elsewhere in this book. Briefly, almost everyone is exposed to the virus as a child.[1-4] The primary infection is either completely asymptomatic or takes the form of a mild respiratory illness, cystitis, or occasionally encephalitis.[5,6-8] After the primary infection, virus becomes latent in the kidney. Renal tubular cells, the parietal epithelial layer of Bowman's capsule as well as transitional epithelium have been known to harbor the virus.[9] BK virions enter the renal tubular cell in smooth (noncoated) mono-pinocytotic vesicles that are morphologically consistent with caveolae.[10] Virion assembly in the nucleus follows.

Polyomaviruses and Human Diseases, edited by Nasimul Ahsan. ©2006 Eurekah.com and Springer Science+Business Media.

This can be seen as viral inclusions on kidney biopsy or as sheets of crystalline intra nuclear particles on electron microscopy of infected cells. The immune system is very effective in suppressing BKV replication and the virus seldom reactivates in the immune competent host. Hence, virus replication and host cell damage does not happen during the state of latency and virus inclusions, mRNA or DNA is not demonstrable in the urine of a patient with latent virus. However, even subtle changes in the status of the immune system like pregnancy,[11-13] diabetes[14] and old age[15] may allow reactivation. Nevertheless, clinically important reactivation (and progression to disease) is seen only in states of severe immune deficiency due to hereditary or acquired cause.[16-23] Tubular cells actively infected with BK virus demonstrate massive virally induced necrosis, dissolution of basement membranes and spillage of virions into the intertubular space. The virions thus get into the peritubular interstitial space. Destruction of intertubular capillary walls may potentially breach the urine-blood barrier of sorts, gaining access for the virus into the blood stream.[10,24] This is manifested as viremia.

The "Second Hit" Hypothesis

Thus far, two important factors i.e., failure of immune surveillance and aggressive virus replication, appear to result in a high virus burden in the urine and blood. However, there are other factors that affect the final outcome. The BKV has a strong tropism for the urogenital tract. Importantly, the disease spectrum noted with the virus varies significantly and predictably depending on the patient subgroup. In the bone marrow transplant patient, hemorrhagic cystitis is the end-organ disease manifestation most usually seen. In the kidney transplant patient however, the virus causes BKVN or ureteral stenosis. This suggests that in addition to an immunosuppressed state leading to virus replication, a "second hit" is required, probably in some form of tissue damage.[25,26] This would explain the specific tissue tropisms described above. Immunologic injury like clinical or subclinical rejection may make the transplanted kidney vulnerable to BKVN.[26] BKVN is characterized by extensive tubular necrosis.[27] Intriguingly, generalized damage of apparently noninfected cells has been observed in addition to necrosis of infected cells in biopsy samples of patients with BKVN.[10] This damage to noninfected cells may actually have been pharmacologically induced from immunosuppressive agent

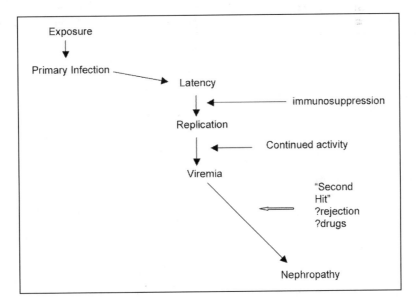

Figure 1. From primary infection to nephropathy.

toxicity or immunologically induced from clinical or sub-clinical rejection. In any case, injury may have predisposed the allograft to invasion by the BKV.[27,28] The analogy holds in other clinical circumstances as well. In the case of bone marrow transplant patients, damage to the bladder by cyclophosphamide may explain BKV tropism for the bladder and clustering of BKV hemorrhagic cystitis in this population.[29] Surgical or stent trauma sustained by the ureter may make it susceptible to BKV invasion accounting for BKV associated ureteral stenosis.[30] However, in spite of severe renal injuries sustained during other solid organ transplantation such as heart and liver, there appears to be paucity of BKVN in these patients, disputing the second hit hypothesis. The paradigm is outlined in Figure 1.

Clinical Correlates of BKV Infection in Renal Transplant Recipients

Based on the above paradigm, the following clinical stages of the infection may be teased out.

Latency

BKV DNA may be demonstrated in kidney tissue (or perhaps peripheral blood lymphocytes) but there is no active viral replication. Over 98% of the general population will maintain this status indefinitely.

Replication

The virus (or evidence of viral cytopathic effects) can be detected in the urine in the form decoy cells or demonstration of viral DNA by PCR. This stage signifies a state of active virus replication, which has not progressed to organ system disease.

Viremia

Occurs during a high state of viral replication resulting in viral access to the blood stream (with lytic effect of replication on tubular cells and disruption of the urine-blood barrier) with an imminent threat of precipitation of BKVN.

Disease

The virus now causes renal parenchymal damage. The renal function may remain steady for some time despite ongoing parenchymal damage but starts to deteriorate once BKVN has firmly established. The patient will have coexisting viruria and viremia. The various histological features of BKVN have been discussed in great detail elsewhere in this book.

Impact of Immunosuppression: Net State or Asymmetric Predisposition?

Since the first case of BKVN in the modern era was reported in 1995[31] an increased incidence of BKVN has been noted in the literature. There is a bias towards suspecting and diagnosing the disease early given heightened awareness. However, this bias does not completely explain the increased incidence. Several centers have carried out extensive retrospective reviews of the transplant kidney biopsy archives. Nickeleit et al[26] reviewed kidney biopsies of 616 patients transplanted from 1985-1995 on cyclosporine-azathioprine based immunosuppression and found no cases of BKVN. However, on review of patients from 1996-1999 (tacrolimus-MMF based immunosuppression), eleven cases of BKVN were identified. This is consistent with other observations and a true rise in the incidence of BKVN is accepted. As indicated previously, BKV replication can occur in states of relative immune deficiency such as pregnancy, diabetes mellitus or old age. However, in these states, the immune deficit is not critical enough to allow a complete breakthrough of the virus. Thus, in these conditions, all we see is asymptomatic viruria, if at all. Actual end organ damage resulting in BKV disease occurs only with more severe forms of immune suppression (like HIV or with solid organ transplantation). The increased incidence of BKV infection in the modern era coincides with introduction of new immunosuppression agents. As incidence with cyclosporine and azathioprine was low, attention was immediately focused on the two agents, tacrolimus and mycophenolate mofetil (MMF), which were introduced into clinical transplantation in the early 1990s. An obvious explanation is the increased net state of immunosuppression exposes the patient to the risk of BKV infection. A slightly different (but not mutually exclusive) explanation is that of asymmetric predisposition to develop BKVN disease due to use of a particular agent.

Tacrolimus has been implicated as the drug with the greatest potential to cause BKV reactivation. In a retrospective study by Nickeleit et al,[32] 8 out of 11 (73%) patients with BKVN were on tacrolimus. Interestingly, 10/11 patients had suffered a rejection episode in the weeks to months prior to the diagnosis of BKVN and the tacrolimus trough levels were frequently over 15 ng/ml as part of immunologic rescue protocols. Similarly, 20/22 (91%) of patients with BKVN in a study by the Pittsburgh Group received tacrolimus as the primary calcineurin inhibitor in use. Again, many patients with BKVN had suffered steroid responsive rejection episodes prior to the diagnosis.[33] Similarly, MMF may also play a role. Barri et al[34] reviewed 8 consecutive patients with BKVN: all 8 were on MMF and 7 out of 8 were on tacrolimus. Importantly, 75% of the patients had been treated for rejection while 63% had more than 1 rejection episode prior to the diagnosis of BKVN. The use of anti-rejection therapy after histological diagnosis of BKV infection was not associated with improvement of renal function despite a histological appearance suggestive of acute rejection. A review of BKVN from 1995 to 1998 at the Duke University Medical Center identified 7 cases of BKVN. It was noted that 6/7 patients were on MMF with cyclosporine and steroids.[35] A role of MMF in this infection was thus suggested.[34,35] Recently, reports implicating Sirolimus in renal transplant recipients have been published as well.[36]

Thus, based on retrospective data, most cases of BKVN have been associated with use either tacrolimus or MMF or the combination. It is apparent that many of these patients were treated for acute rejection episodes prior to precipitation of BKVN. Based on our paradigm of pathogenesis, this represents the perfect set up for BKVN: an intense milieu of immunosuppression and ongoing or recent immunologic injury, providing the "two hits". But these data still do not indicate if this is from a high state of immunosuppression alone or if any of these agents or combinations may have a predisposing role to play.

Another observation sheds some light on this issue. In one study, patients diagnosed with BKVN and on a dual immunosuppressive regimen (steroid plus FK506, Cyclosporine, sirolimus or MMF) had less graft loss and higher viral clearance in comparison to those patients who were on triple immunosuppression drugs (steroid plus FK506, Cyclosporine or sirolimus and MMF) at the time of diagnosis.[37] This seemed to suggest that the combined immunosuppressive effect was perhaps more important than any individual agent.

BKVN was poorly understood a few years ago. The evolution of clinical protocols at various transplant centers to deal with this problem lends some instructive insights into the nature of this infection. Initially, many cases of BKVN were histologically confused with rejection or read as rejection with coexisting BKVN. Therefore, these patients were treated with intensification of immunosuppression, with disastrous results. BKVN progressed rapidly leading to adverse outcomes. Astute clinicians caught on to this and started refraining from intensification strategies and reduced immunosuppression instead.[24,33] Randhawa et al[38] subsequently published outcomes of BKVN based on prompt versus delayed reduction of immunosuppression. Fifty percent of the patients whose immunosuppression was not reduced showed a persistently high viral load and 80% had persistent or worsened cytopathic effects on repeat biopsy. Conversely, early reduction of immunosuppression led to viral clearance in 70% of the patients. Thus, even with manifest disease, it seemed that reduction in the net state of immunosuppression provided the only chance to control the disease and stabilize allograft function. Timing was a vital factor. Results of immunosuppression decrease were best when this was instituted early in the course, as observed above. Another study elaborates this key point: BKVN was studied prospectively using protocol biopsies: BKVN was identified in two clinical settings: on surveillance biopsies as part of the protocol (when it was not clinically associated with allograft dysfunction), or on a for-cause biopsy when BKVN was causing allograft dysfunction. Patients diagnosed when clinically silent (implying early stage disease) responded better to decrease in immunosuppression compared to patients who had manifest allograft dysfunction.[39]

A few assumptions emerge from the foregoing:

1. BKV infection is a problem of immunocompromised patients.
2. The net state of immunosuppression impacts the incidence of the disease.
3. Newer immunosuppressive agents have increased the incidence of the disease either due to more potent immunosuppression or an asymmetric predilection of a particular agent(s) to cause BKVN.
4. The disease has a severe course especially if immunosuppression is not decreased.

Prospective Look at BKVN: Role of Immunosuppression

Our current understanding of the interplay between immunosuppressive regimens and BKV disease were founded on studies outlined above. They are remarkable in the insights they provide into this quite complex problem. However, they do have the disadvantage of being retrospective in their design.

To settle the issue of the role these newer and more potent immunosuppressive agents may play in asymmetrically predisposing to BKV, we have recently concluded a prospective, randomized trial of adult renal transplant patients. Patients received either tacrolimus or cyclosporine A in addition to other immunosuppression as per our protocol. BKV was detected using a modified light-cycler based real time PCR technique. All patients were screened for the virus in urine (those not anuric) and plasma prior to transplant. After transplant, the urine and plasma were screened weekly for 16 weeks, then at months 5, 6, 9 and 12. The results of the PCR were available in real time allowing for therapeutic interventions. All positive specimens were quantified to establish viral loads in urine and blood. This design allowed us prospectively to follow the course of a patient before and after detection of virus replication. Early on in the course of the study, we discovered that viremia never occurred without concomitant viruria. In most cases, viruria preceded viremia by several weeks. Thus, viruria identified a group of patients at risk for viremia. Viremia, however, is the most pivotal feature of BKV infection. Previous observations have suggested viremia to be strongly associated with nephropathy. In one study all 9 patients with evidence of BKVN on histopathology had positive blood BKV PCR that had turned positive 16-33 weeks prior to clinical declaration of BKVN.[40] Similarly, in another retrospective study all 4 patients with histologic evidence of BKVN had positive blood BKV PCRs while none of the 16 controls had a positive test (p<0.0001); blood BKV PCR turned positive at a median of 32 weeks before the diagnosis of BKVN. Interestingly, blood BKV titers decreased after reduction of immunosuppression in 3 of the 4 patients.[41] We therefore believe patients with viremia are in imminent danger of developing BKVN. As immunosuppression is a cardinal requirement for progression of the infection process, we believed viremia was a significant enough stage to take action in this respect: built into the study was a protocol for graduated responses to viremia. At the first positive blood PCR, the antimetabolite component of the immunosuppressive regimen (azathioprine or MMF) was withdrawn. If viremia failed to clear, the calcineurin inhibitor was tapered to minimum acceptable levels (typically targeting trough cyclosporine A [CyA] levels around 100-200 ng/ml and tacrolimus [FK] levels of 3-5 ng/ml). The obvious aim of this approach was to lower immunosuppression at this critical time, allowing for immune surveillance to recover enough to stop the infection from progressing. The major risk was of course going too far and lowering immunosuppression to an extent to allow breakthrough rejection.

All patients who developed an unexplained elevation of the serum creatinine underwent a kidney biopsy interpreted by a pathologist blinded to the treatment arms. All biopsies were evaluated for the BKV with light and electron microscopy as well as immunoperoxidase stain employing the mc3 antibody to the large T-antigen of SV40 virus. Additionally, biopsies were sent out to an independent pathologist blinded to treatment arms or BKV status. A total of 200 patients were enrolled. Preliminary results of the first 100 patients shall be discussed here.

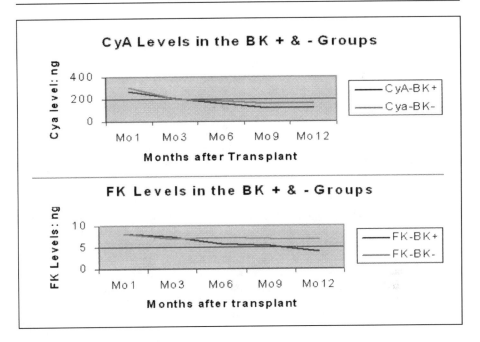

Figure 2. Calcineurin inhibitor levels in the BK positive and negative patients.

Of the 100 patients enrolled, 34 were in the CyA arm and 66 in the FK arm. The minimum follow-up period was 12 months. Baseline recipient or donor characteristics were not dissimilar. BK viruria was detected in 36 (36%) of the patients, 12/34 (35%) in the CyA group and 24/66 (36%) in the FK group (p = 0.90). Viremia was noted in 11 (11%), with 3/34 (9%) in the CyA arm and 8/66 (12%) (P = 0.87). Viruria always preceded viremia. FK or CyA levels were not different in the viruric and nonviruric patients early on. Later however, the FK and CyA levels of the viruric patients trended down due to the intentional decrease in immunosuppression in the viremic patients. As the study was not blinded, it is possible that immunosuppression was reduced in the viruric patients as a result of bias. This is shown in Figure 2.

Twelve of 36 (33%) viruric patients were on CyA-azathioprine (AZA), 12 on FK-AZA and 12 on FK- mycophenolate mofetil (MMF). No patient on CyA-MMF developed viruria in this cohort of 100 patients. Of the viremic patients, 6/36 were on FK-AZA, 3/36 were on CyA-AZA while 2 were on FK-MMF. The impact of immunosuppression subgroup was not statistically significant (p = 0.18). Again none of the patients on CyA-MMF developed viremia. The mean time of onset of viruria was 54 days post transplantation. Timing of the onset of viruria had an important impact on subsequent behavior of the virus: Of all viruric patients, 27/36 (75%) demonstrated replication early (within the first 16 weeks after transplantation). Of note, all 11 patients progressing to viremia activated the virus early. None of the late onset viruric patients progressed to viremia. The mean virus titer in the urine for patients with early viruria was 6.56 ± 2.08 log 10 copies /ml compared to 4.17 ± 1.58 log 10 copies /ml for the late viruric patients (p = 0.003). Thus, it appears that early and robust replication of BKV signifies a higher likelihood of progression to viremia.

The mean virus titer in the urine of patients who had viremia was significantly higher than those demonstrating viruria only (7.59 ± 1.57 vs. 5.42 ± 2.08 log 10 copies/ml, p = 0.003). The onset of viruria was also earlier among patients who subsequently developed viremia (44 ± 29 days) compared to those who were only viruric (126 ± 139 days) (p = 0.06). This again underscores the importance of the magnitude of replication on subsequent behavior of the virus: the higher the degree of replication, the higher is the chance of progression. However, a high urine titer independently did not predict the risk of viremia. The specificity of even quite high urine titers for viremia remained unsatisfactory. This dictates the need for checking a blood PCR to stratify risk of BKVN in patients with positive urine PCR.

Viremia triggered immunosuppression modulation per protocol. All viremic patients cleared viremia during the course of the study follow up, with no evidence of BKVN developing in any case. This reduction in immunosuppression did not result in an increased rate of rejection: At 12 months post-transplant, one patient in CyA arm (3%) and two patients in the FK arm (3%) had an acute rejection episode (p = *ns*). Only one patient (in the FK group) suffered a rejection directly due to protocol driven reduction of immunosuppression. This patient had developed viremia and was asked to decrease his FK dose as his viremia persisted despite discontinuing his adjuvant agent. He suffered a Banff IB rejection but responded to pulsed steroids and treatment with intravenous immunoglobulin. He stabilized on an FK-sirolimus combination with a creatinine of 1.8 mg/dl at the end of the study. Another patient was asked to reduce the dose of FK because of persistent viremia. He stopped taking immunosuppression altogether and suffered a Banff II acute cellular rejection. He was successfully treated with intravenous immunoglobulin and a steroid pulse. His serum creatinine stabilized at 2.5 mg/dl. Both patients had cleared BK-viremia before the rejection episode and remained viremia-free at the end of the study. In this particular group of patients, kidney function in the BK positive patients was significantly reduced at the end of one year (mean creatinine levels of 1.6 ± 0.4 mg/dl while that of BK negative patients was 1.3 ± 0.4 mg/dl, p = 0.006). Of note, though, on analysis of the full cohort (200 patients), this effect was no longer statistically significant. It therefore represents a type II error.

Graft survival was similar at one year between the two groups (CyA 100% versus FK 92%, P = NS). No patients suffered graft loss in the CyA arm and 5 patients suffered graft loss in the FK arm. Three of the FK-treated graft losses were due to early graft thrombosis, one due to noncompliance and one due to death with a functioning graft.

At one year patient survival was 100% in the CyA arm and 97% in the FK arm, P = NS. Two patients in the FK group died; one patient expired from central nervous system post-transplant lymphoproliferative disorder (PTLD) at post-operative day 136 and one patient expired at post-operative day 48 due to liver carcinoma.

Reflections on the Biologic Behavior of the Virus

Taken together the above observations suggest that the initial site of reactivation is the urinary tract and the first manifestation of viral reactivation is asymptomatic excretion of the virus in the urine. This is reinforced by the observation that positive urine PCR preceded positive blood PCR in all cases. In a few cases, the urine and blood were detected to be positive on simultaneously obtained samples. In no case was blood positive prior to demonstrated urine positivity. Also, in patients being managed with immunosuppression reduction, the blood always cleared before the urine.

After reactivation, the virus can potentially take three routes: it can clear spontaneously; persist in the urine or progress to viremia as depicted in Figure 3. At lower levels of replication, the virus is probably contained by the immune system. It is either completely cleared or persists at low levels. As discussed earlier, the cytopathic effect is probably not severe enough and the viral load not high enough to effectively breach the urine-blood barrier. At higher levels of replication, arguably achieved due to more intense immunosuppression, the barrier is breached and viremia occurs. BK viremia thus may serve as a de-facto in-vivo bioassay marker betraying a state of over-immunosuppression. Patients with high titer persistent viruria are at prime risk to develop viremia.

Almost all studies have identified viremia as a key feature vis-à-vis diagnosis of BKVN.[28,40,41] However, positive blood PCR is not synonymous with BKVN. A variable period of sustained viremia is required for BKVN to set in, as observed by Nickeleit et al[40] as well as Limaye et al.[41]

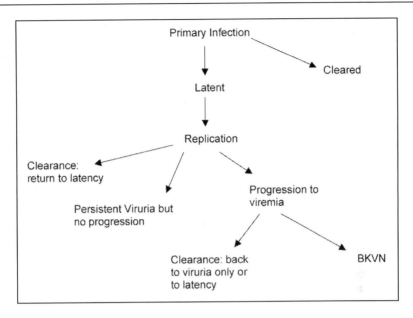

Figure 3. Possible outcomes of BKV infection.

Thus, viremia indicates a high rate of BKV replication and if persistent, a high likelihood of progression to BKVN. It is a key bridge that links asymptomatic viruria to BKVN.

Therefore, viremia indicates the need for action. The risk of BKVN can be averted should viremia reverse itself. In practice, this can be achieved by timely modification in the intensity of immunosuppression. We have noted a decrease in virus titers in the blood after decrease in immunosuppression to a point where the PCR becomes negative. Similar changes are also seen in virus titers in the urine. The fact that we did not see any cases of BKVN and that viremia resolved in all cases during the course of this study was quite remarkable and underscores the effectiveness and safety of careful reduction of immunosuppression to prevent BKVN in patients demonstrating BK viremia.

Risks of Alteration of Immunosuppression

Our data support that the best approach for management of BKVN probably is active surveillance for reactivation and preemptive decrease in immunosuppression to prevent progression from viremia to disease. The obvious risk associated with this approach is under-immunosuppression and risk of rejection. Nickeleit et al have attempted to study the relationship of BKV and rejection. Unlike CMV, BKV does not seem to increase acute rejection. However, this issue remains of paramount concern and deserves extreme caution and close follows up of patients. In our study population, despite active preemptive reduction of immunosuppression after detection of a positive blood BKV PCR, the acute rejection rate remained <5%. This study was a short-term study, though. It remains to be seen if there will be a higher incidence of chronic rejection in these patients and ultimate long-term outcomes are yet to be determined. It must also be kept in mind that our institution uses near universal induction with Thymoglobulin, which serves as a protective umbrella of sorts during various immunosuppression modulations.

Immunosuppression Management for BKV Infection

The most sensitive marker for BKV reactivation is viruria. Therefore, urine PCR or other reliably sensitive tests like the decoy cell preparation, where available are reasonable methods to

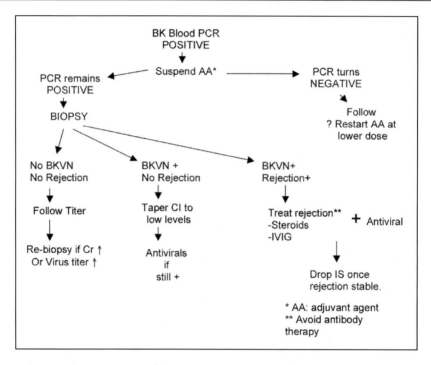

Figure 4. Approach to management of BKVN.

screen for virus reactivation. However, though extremely sensitive, the specificity of positive urine PCR (or decoy cell) remains low for viremia as well as BKVN. In most cases, it needs to be confirmed with repeat urine tests and ultimately followed up with a blood PCR. Thus, we now believe that the best test to screen for BKVN is viremia. This directly isolates a group of patients at the highest risk of nephropathy in a single step and provides a clear decision point for subsequent action.

1. Once a patient declares viremia it is reasonable to suspend the adjuvant agent. The patient's virus titer should be monitored at 2-4 weeks interval.

2. If viremia fails to clear after one to two months or if allograft dysfunction develops, allograft biopsy is recommended before decreasing immunosuppression further. This is important to establish histologic abnormalities consistent with BKVN and to exclude rejection.

3. Further decisions are made in light of histopathologic changes. Following are the possibilities, as shown in Figure 4.

No BKVN Seen

This defines the preclinical stage of BKV infection where viremia has not yet precipitated histologically manifest disease. These patients need to be monitored closely. Quantitative PCR can be a useful tool in this situation. Followed at 2-4 week intervals, another biopsy may be prompted should the virus titer increase abruptly or if renal dysfunction precipitates.

BKVN Is Observed without Concomitant Rejection

If histologic evidence of BKVN is seen, tapering of the calcineurin inhibitor to lower levels is justified given the likelihood of progressive renal dysfunction and high rates of graft loss associated with the disease.[42,43]

BKVN Is Observed with Coexisting Rejection

This is a very tricky situation. We advocate treating the rejection but avoiding the 'big guns" like monoclonal or polyclonal antibodies. We have had success with steroid pulses and/or IVIG in this scenario. As soon as the rejection is stabilized, immunosuppression is carefully reduced to allow recovery from the virus infection. Use of cidofovir may be considered in such a situation.

Our data do not suggest an asymmetric predisposition to develop BKVN with use of tacrolimus or MMF independently. It appears that the intensity of overall immunosuppression is a key factor in predisposing to BKVN. The choice of the immunosuppressive agents currently used probably does not play a determining role in the development of BK viruria or viremia. Rather, each patient appears to be his own "in-vivo bioassay" for determination of what could be considered over immunosuppression as manifested by the development of BK viruria and progression to viremia. Our findings indicate that active surveillance and preemptive reduction in immunosuppression are effective management strategies to deal with BKV in renal transplant patients to obviate clinically significant nephropathy.

References

1. Shah KV. Polyomaviruses. In: Fields BN, Knipe DM, Howley PM, eds. Fields Virology. 3rd ed. Philadelphia: Lippincott-Raven, 1996:2027-2043.
2. Gardner SD. Prevalence in England of antibody to human polyoma virus (BK). Br Med J 1973; 1:77-8.
3. Shah KV, Daniel RW, Warszawski RM. High prevalence of antibodies to BK virus, an SV 40 related papovavirus, in residents of Maryland. J Infect Dis 1973; 128:784-7.
4. Portolani M, Marzocchi A, Barbanti-Brodano G et al. Prevalence in Italy of antibodies to a new human papova virus (BK Virus). J Med Microbiol 1974; 7:543-6.
5. Goudsmid J, Van Dillen WP, van Strein A et al. The role of BK virus in acute respiratory tract disease and the presence of BKV DNA in tonsils. J Med Virol 1982; 10:91-9.
6. Hashida Y, Gaffney PC, Younis EJ. Acute hemorrhagic cystitis of childhood and and papova-like particles. J Paedriatics 1976; 89:85-7.
7. Saitoh K, Sugae N, Koike N et al. Diagnosis of childhood BK virus cystitis by electron microscopy and PCR. J Clin Path 1993; 46:773-5.
8. Voltz R, Jager G, Seelos K et al. BK virus encephalitis in an immunocompetent patient. Arch Neurol 1996; 53:101-3.
9. Howell DN, Smith SR, Butterly DW et al. Diagnosis and management of BK polyomavirus interstitial nephritis in renal transplant recipients. Transplantation 1999; 68(9):1279-88.
10. Drachenberg CB, Papadimitriou JC, Wali R et al. Polyoma virus allograft nephropathy: Ultrastructural features from viral cell entry to lysis. Am J of Transplantation 2003; 3:1383.
11. Hirsch HH. Polyoma BK nephropathy: A (Re) emerging complication in renal transplantation. Am J of Transplantation 2002; 2:25-30.
12. Chang D, Wang M, Ou WC et al. Genotypes of human polyomaviruses in urine samples of pregnant women in Taiwan. J Med Virol 1996; 48(1):95-101.
13. Coleman DV, Gardner SD, Mulholland C et al. Human polyomavirus in pregnancy. A model for the study of defense mechanisms to virus reactivation. Clin Exp Immunol 1983; 53(2):289-96.
14. Borgatti M, Costanzo F, Portolani M et al. Evidence for reactivation of persistent infection during pregnancy and lack of congenital transmission of BK virus, a human papovavirus. Microbiologica 1979; 2:173-8.
15. Kahan AV, Coleman DV, Koss LG. Activation of human polyomavirus infection-detection by cytologic techniques. Am J Clin Pathol 1980; 74(3):326-32.
16. Kitamura T, Aso Y, Kuniyoshi N et al. High incidence of urinary JC virus excretion in nonimmunosuppressed older patients. J Infect Dis 1990; 161(6):1128-33.
17. Azzi A, Ciappi S, De Santis R et al. Hemorrhagic cystitis associated with BKV in patients with refractory acute lymphoblastic leukemia. Am J Hematol 1996; 52(2):121-2.
18. De Silva LM, Bale P, de Courcy J et al. Renal failure due to BK virus infection in an immunodeficient child. J Med Virol 1995; 45(2):192-6.
19. Rosen S, Harmon W, Krensky AM et al. Tubulo-interstitial nephritis associated with polyomavirus (BK type) infection. N Engl J Med 1983; 308(20):1192-6.

20. Boldorini R, Zorini EO, Viagano P et al. Cytologic and biomolecular diagnosis of polyoma virus infection in urine specimens of HIV-positive patients. Acta Cytologica 2000; 44(2):205-10.
21. Smith RD, Galla JH, Skahan K et al. Tubulointerstitial nephritis due to a mutant polyomavirus BK virus strain, BKV (Cin), causing end-stage renal disease. J Clin Microbiol 1998; 36(6):1660-5.
22. Vallbracht A, Lohler J, Gossmann J et al. Disseminated BK type polyomavirus infection in an AIDS patient associated with central nervous system disease. Am J Pathol 1993; 143(1):29-39.
23. Nebuloni M, Tosoni A, Boldorini R et al. BK virus renal infection in a patient with the acquired immunodeficiency syndrome. Arch Pathol Lab Med 1999; 123(9):807-11.
24. Nickeleit V, Hirsch HH, Zeiler M et al. BK-virus nephropathy in renal transplants-tubular necrosis, MHC-class II expression and rejection in a puzzling game. Nephrol Dial Transplant 2000; 15(3):324-32.
25. Atencio IA, Shadan FF, Zhou XJ et al. Adult mouse kidneys become permissive to acute polyomavirus infection and reactivate persistent infections in response to cellular damage and regeneration. J Virol 1993; 67(3):1424-32.
26. Nickeleit V, Hirsch H, Binet I et al. Polyomavirus infection of renal allograft recipients: From latent infection to manifest disease. J Am Soc Nephrol 1999; 10:1080-1089.
27. Drachenberg RC, Drachenberg CB, Papadimitriou JC et al. Morphological spectrum of polyoma virus disease in renal allografts: Diagnostic accuracy of urine cytology. Am J Transplant 2001; 1:378-381.
28. Hirsch HH, Knowles W, Dickenmann M et al. Prospective study of polyomavirus type BK replication and nephropathy in renal transplant recipients. N Engl J Med 2002; 347:488-496.
29. Bedi A, Miller CB, Hanson JL et al. Association of BK virus with failure of prophylaxis against hemorrhagic cystitis following bone marrow transplantation. J Clin Oncol 1995; 13(5):1103-9.
30. Coleman DV, Mackenzie EF, Gardner SD et al. Human polyomavirus (BK) infection and ureteric stenosis in renal allograft recipients. J Clin Pathol 1978; 31(4):338-347.
31. Purighalla R, Shapiro R, McCauley J et al. BK Virus infection in a kidney allograft diagnosed by needle biopsy. Am J Kidney Dis 1995; 26:671-673.
32. Binet I, Nickeleit V, Hirsch HH et al. Polyomavirus disease under new immunosuppressive drugs: A cause of renal graft dysfunction and graft loss. Transplantation 1999; 67(6):918-922.
33. Randhawa PS, Finkelstein S, Scantlebury V et al. Human polyomavirus-associated interstitial nephritis in the allograft kidney. Transplantation 1999; 67(1):103-109.
34. Barri YM, Ahmad I, Ketel BL et al. Polyoma viral infection in renal transplantation: The role of immunosuppressive therapy. Clin Transplant 2001; 15(4):240-246.
35. Howell DN, Smith SR, Butterly DW et al. Diagnosis and management of BK polyomavirus interstitial nephritis in renal transplant recipients. Transplantation 1999; 68(9):1279-1288.
36. Hirsch HH, Mohaupt M, Klimkait T. Prospective monitoring of BK virus load after discontinuing sirolimus treatment in a renal transplant patient with BK virus nephropathy. J Infect Dis 2001; 184:1494.
37. Ramos E, Drachenberg CB, Portocarrero M et al. BK virus nephropathy diagnosis and treatment: Experience at the University of Maryland renal transplant program. Clin Transpl 2002; 143-153.
38. Celik B, Shapiro R, Vats A et al. Polyomavirus allograft nephropathy: Sequential assessment of histologic viral load, tubulitis and graft function following changes in immunosuppression. Am J Transplantation 2003; 3:1378-1382.
39. Buehrig CK, Lager DJ, Stegall MD et al. Influence of surveillance renal allograft biopsy on diagnosis and prognosis of polyomavirus-associated nephropathy. Kidney Int 2003; 64(2):665-673.
40. Nickeleit V, Klimkait T, Binet IF et al. Testing for polyomavirus type BK DNA in plasma to identify renal-allograft recipients with viral nephropathy. N Engl J Med 2000; 342(18):1309-1315.
41. Limaye AP, Jerome KR, Kuhr CS et al. Quantitation of BK virus load in serum for the diagnosis of BK virus-associated nephropathy in renal transplant recipients. J Infect Dis 2001; 183(11):1669-1672.
42. Randhawa PS, Demetris AJ. Nephropathy due to polyomavirus type BK. N Engl J Med 2000; 342(18):1309-1915.
43. Ahuja M, Cohen EP, Dayer AM et al. Polyoma virus infection after renal transplantation. Use of immunostaining as a guide to diagnosis. Transplantation 2001; 71(7):896-899.

BK Virus Infection
after Non-Renal Transplantation

Martha Pavlakis, Abdolreza Haririan and David K. Klassen

Abstract

Infection with BK virus (BKV), a member of the Polyomavirus (PV) family, is ubiquitous, with the virus remaining in a latent form in the kidney and urinary tract.[1,2] This infection is usually asymptomatic, but with impairment of the cellular immune system the virus can reactivate and lead to tissue damage. In recipients of bone marrow and solid organ transplants, PV reactivation can be associated with disease in urinary tract and kidneys. BKV was first discovered in 1971 from the urine of a kidney transplant recipient who had developed ureteral stenosis 4 months after transplantation. While much of the subsequent research focuses on patients after renal transplantation, we will review PV impact in patients after bone marrow transplant (BMT) and those with non-renal solid organ transplants.

BKV-BMT-Hemorrhagic Cystitis

PV primary infection occurs during childhood in 60-100% of general population.[3] Virus is likely acquired through a respiratory or oral route. While the primary infection is usually asymptomatic, the virus seeds the urinary system and brain and remains in a latent form.[4,5] It is not clear if lymphocytes are a site of persistence of the virus, or just a target site of reactivation. Extensive experience over the past two decades has shown the prevalence and clinical importance of PV reactivation in patients with bone marrow and solid organ transplantation.

The first evidence of PV in BMT was reported in 1981, with the detection of BKV in the urine of 13 patients, 1 to 6 weeks after transplantation.[6] Appearance of BK viruria was associated with transient hepatic dysfunction in these BMT recipients. While no direct link to clinical disease could be made from this evidence, it represents the first successful attempt to find this virus in BMT recipients.

BK infection is associated with the condition of hemorrhagic cystitis (HC) in BMT patients. HC results from damage to the bladder urothelium and blood vessels by toxins, irradiation, viruses and drugs, such as cyclophosphamide. Recipients of autologous bone marrow transplant (BMT) are at a particularly high risk for hemorrhagic cystitis, with an incidence of approximately 30 percent.[7,8] HC episodes can vary in severity and often prolong hospitalization, require use of blood products and can result in impairment of bladder and kidney function. Unlike recipients with kidney transplantation, renal parenchymal involvement associated with BKV reactivation has not yet been reported after BMT. Renal dysfunction with BKV-associated hemorrhagic cystitis (HC) has been attributed to obstructive nephropathy secondary to clot formation in the bladder. Detection of virus in the urine can be hampered by the use of intravesical saline irrigation, a treatment modality for HC. The method of detection of BKV in the urine of patients with HC is variable and may be confounded by the presence of viremia

Polyomaviruses and Human Diseases, edited by Nasimul Ahsan. ©2006 Eurekah.com and Springer Science+Business Media.

and subsequent bleeding into the bladder. Blood containing BKV can contaminate urinary specimens and mislead investigators as to its source.

The first clinical link between BKV reactivation and clinically important events after BMT was found in the association between the presence of BKV in the urine (by ELISA and DNA hybridization assays) and hemorrhagic cystitis lasting more than 7 days.[9] In this study, excretion of BKV in urine was demonstrated in almost half of the patients studied, but occurred more frequently in those with significant hemorrhagic cystitis. Subsequent reports have observed that up to 90% of allogenic bone marrow transplant recipients shed BKV in the urine.[10] Prolonged cystitis was observed more commonly in recipients of allogeneic BMT than in those of autologous or syngeneic BMT. Subsequent reports confirmed this finding, using culture and electron microscopy to detect the virus.[11] One group reported a preponderance of microscopic, but not gross, hematuria in BMT recipients who were shedding BKV in their urine.[12] However, other studies failed to confirm a temporal association of PV shedding with hemorrhagic cystitis, as in some BMT recipients, gross hematuria began prior to the detection of BKV in the urine.

The most convincing evidence to date of a causal association between BKV in the urine and HC in BMT patients was demonstrated by Bedi et al.[13] They studied 95 consecutive BMT patients for evidence of BK virus excretion in the urine by PCR. BK virus was found in at least one urine specimen of over half of the recipients and 40% had persistent viruria. Viral excretion began 2 to 15 weeks after transplantation. All of the recipients with BK viruria post-BMT were seropositive prior to transplantation, suggesting reactivation, rather than primary infection, was the source of viral replication. In this study, the incidence of BK viruria was independent of the marrow source (allogeneic vs. autologous). Fifty percent of the patients with persistent BK viruria developed hemorrhagic cystitis, while none of those without viruria experienced this complication. This study showed that, despite prophylaxis with mesna or forced diuresis, virtually every patient with HC had associated BK viruria. Since HC associated with BK virus was often delayed until several weeks following BMT at the time of hematologic recovery and discontinuation of immunosuppressive therapy, they suggested that development of HC associated with BK viral reactivation may require immunocompetent T lymphocytes.

Other groups have not seen a tight association of BK shedding in the urine after BMT and HC.[14-17] In one small study, Azzi et al[17a] looked for BK viruria by DNA detection methods in 52 unselected BMT recipients. While BK viruria was demonstrated before the onset and during the bleeding episodes in only half the cases of HC, BK viruria was noted in more than three fourths of BMT recipients without HC. This suggests that BK viruria is not necessary for HC to occur, nor is it always associated with HC.

The presence of BKV shedding in the urine is not, in of itself, diagnostic of an active disease. It is known that immunocompetent individuals can shed BKV in the urine without any associated hematuria or other bladder disease. Some groups have noted that quantitation of viruria in normal people and in BMT recipients without HC is lower than that seen in BMT recipients with HC.[10] Leung et al[18] noted healthy controls had BK viruria in levels comparable to BMT recipients without HC. They hypothesized that immunosuppression leads to increased BKV reactivation. When the viral replication exceeds a certain level, cytopathic effects of BKV contribute to the disruption of bladder mucosa and in hematuria. It is also possible that the immunologic response to viral activity leads to more intense cellular damage, and thereby more severe hematuria. The difference between clinical syndromes of BK reactivation in bone marrow transplant recipients as compared to renal transplant recipients may hold a clue as to the sequence of events leading to injury. Renal transplantation is associated with varying degrees of ischemic injury to the allografted kidney. Although ureteral complications have been reported in association with BKV, the most common syndrome in renal allograft patients is an interstitial nephritis and viral particles detected by EM in the swollen nuclei of tubular epithelial cells. It is possible that this initial ischemic injury to the kidney (and ureter) or injury from an alloimmune response is the "first hit" in a series of events leading to tissue injury. The reactivation of BKV in these damaged tissues, facilitated by immunosuppression, could provide a

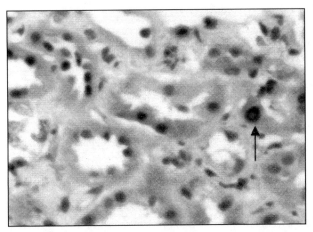

Figure 1. Hematoxylin and eosin staining of this patient's biopsy shows a tubular epithelial cell with characteristic cytopathic changes due to PV reactivation (arrow). There is minimal interstitial fibrosis.

second hit, leading to a clinically apparent injury. In this model, radiation and chemotherapy induced damage to the bladder mucosa is the first hit in BMT recipients, who are more likely to develop HC if they have BKV reactivation.

An alternate explanation was forwarded by Akiyama and coworkers,[19] who studied 45 BMT recipients who had developed HC for evidence of adenovirus and BK activity. Based on the results of PCR screening of the urine samples, they suggested that increased BK viral shedding is secondary to HC, and reported a strong correlation between adenovirus excretion in the urine and post-BMT HC. It is possible that disruption in mucosal immunity caused by either adenovirus or HC itself, is responsible for BK reactivation.

Given that BK viruia is not a specific predictor for HC in BMT patients, Priftakis and colleagues[17] studied 25 BMT patients with BK viruria and analyzed the presence of a mutation in the transcription factor Sp1 binding site in the non-coding control region of the BKV genome. Sixteen of the 25 patients had HC. They found the mutation was present in 43% of the patients with HC, but none in those without HC. The biological significance of this mutation is unclear, but they hypothesized that these point mutations increase the binding capacity of the transcription factor Sp1, that leads to enhanced viral replication and more cytopathic effects.

There is no proven effective therapy for BKV associated HC in BMT patients. Most cases of hemorrhagic cystitis after BMT are usually self-limited, but may persist for several weeks. Supportive therapy includes hydration, and bladder irrigation as needed to avoid clot obstruction. There have been few case reports suggesting the beneficial effects of two antiviral agents, vidarabine and cidofovir, in patients with BKV-associated HC after BMT. In these case reports, HC resolved after anti-viral therapy was given and was associated with disappearance of virus from blood.[20-24] Others have observed no response to cidofovir.[25] Despite case reports of remission of HC after anti-viral therapy,[26] the natural history of HC is one of spontaneous remission with supportive therapy so little can be concluded from these cases regarding the role of anti-viral therapy in the treatment of BKV associated HC.

In conclusion, it is clear that reactivation of latent BKV is common in recipients of both allogeneic and autologous bone marrow transplants. Hemorrhagic cystitis occurs in up to 50-64% of these patients with viral reactivation, and in those with HC, BK viruria can be demonstrated in as many as 56-80% of the cases. Although the majority of the evidence shows a strong, likely causal, association between BKV viruria and HC in recipients of BMT, the data is very suggestive of a multi-factorial relationship including viral reactivation bladder injury and the occurrence of HC.

BKV-Non-Renal Solid Organ Transplant

Non-renal solid organ transplant recipients are at risk of BKV reactivation in the native kidney and urinary tract. There is very limited data in heart transplant recipients regarding BK viruia. No association with either renal dysfunction or hematuria has been identified in this group.[27,28]

Like renal transplant patients, recipients of a pancreas transplant alone (PTA) can experience BK nephropathy. The first case of BK nephropathy in a PTA patient was confirmed by renal biopsy that showed typical cytopathic changes in the renal tubular cells (Fig. 1) along with decoy cells in the urine.[29] This report clearly showed that in the absence of allogeneic microenvironment of a renal graft, native kidneys in recipients of pancreas transplant alone are at risk of BK reactivation and associated parenchymal damage. This same group screened 38 PTA recipients for evidence of BK viruria by urine cytology.[30] After an average of 16 months following transplantation, viruria was detected in four patients. To date, there have been no published reports of BKV detection after liver, small bowel or lung transplantation.

It is clear that BK infection is associated with significant morbidity among BMT patients. The role of BK infection in non-renal solid organ transplantation is not as clearly understood and may be minimal due to the lack of concomitant renal or uroepithelial injury. Prospective studies are needed to answer outstanding questions such as the method and frequency of monitoring for active infection and its role in affecting recipients of other solid organ transplants. Further investigation is needed to clarify the role of BKV in hemorrhagic cystitis after BMT, and to develop effective antiviral agents with efficacy in suppressing viral reactivation. The limited finding that BKV causes disease in the native kidneys of the recipients of non-renal solid organ grafts points to the need for the transplantation and infectious disease communities to better characterize the extent of the effects of BKV in non-renal solid organ transplantation and to optimize our diagnostic and therapeutic options.

References

1. Reploeg M., Storch GA, Clifford DB. BK virus: a clinical review. Clin Inf Dis 2001; 33:91-202.
2. Myelonakis E, Goes N, Rubin RH et al. BK virus in solid organ transplant recipients: an emerging syndrome. Transplantation 2001; 72:1587-92.
3. Demeter L. JC, BK, and other polyomaviruses; progressive leukoencephalopathy. In: Mandell GL, ed. Principles and Practice of Infectious Diseases. New York: Churchill Livingston, 200:1645-1651.
4. Dorries K, Molecular biology and pathogenesis of human polyomavirus infections. Dev Biol Stand 1998; 94:71-9.
5. Shah K, Human polyomavirus BKV and renal disease. Nephrol Dial Transplant 2000; 15:754-55.
6. O'Reilly R., Lee FK, Grossbard E et al. Papovavirus excretion following marrow transplantation: incidence and association with hepatic dysfunction. Transplant Proc 1981; 13:262-6.
7. Efros M., Ahmed T, Coombe N et al. Urologic complications of high-dose chemotherapy and bone marrow transplantation. Urology 1994; 43(3):355-60
8. Ilhan O, Koc H, Akan H et al. Hemorrhagic cystitis as a complication of bone marrow transplantation. J Chemother 1997; 9(1):56-61.
9. Arthur R, Shah KV, Baust SJ et al. Association of BK viruria with hemorrhagic cystitis in recipients of bone marrow transplants. N Engl J Med 1986; 315:230-4.
10. Priftakis P, Bogdanovic G, Kokhaei P et al. BK virus (BKV) quantification in urine samples of bone marrow transplanted patients is helpful for diagnosis of hemorrhagic cystitis, although wide individual variations exist. J Clin Virol 2003; 26(1):71-7.
11. Apperley J, Rice SJ, Bishop JA et al. Late-onset hemorrhagic cystitis associated with urinary excretion of polyomaviruses after bone marrow transplantation. Transplantation 1987. 43:108-12.
12. Chan P, Ip KW, Shiu SY et al. Association between polyomaviruria and microscopic hematuria in bone marrow transplant recipients. J Infect 1994; 29: 139-46.
13. Bedi A, Miller CB, Hanson JL et al. Association of BK virus with failure of prophylaxis against hemorrhagic cystitis following bone marrow transplantation. J Clin Oncol 1995; 12:1103-9.
14. Azzi A, Fanci R, Bosi A et al. Monitoring of polyomavirus BK viruria in bone marrow transplantation patients by DNA hybridization assay and by polymerase chain reaction: an approach to assess the relationship between BK viruria and hemorrhagic cystitis. Bone Marrow Transplant 1994; 14:235-40.

15. Azzi A, Cesar S, Laszlo D et al. Human polyomavirus BK (BKV) load and haemorrhagic cystitis in bone marrow transplantation patients. J Clin Virol 1999; 14:79-86.
16. Bogdanovic G, Ljungman P, Wang F et al. Presence of human polyomavirus DNA in the peripheral circulation of bone marrow transplant patients with and without hemorrhagic cystitis. Bone Marrow Transplant 1996; 17:573-76.
17. Priftakis P, Bogdanovic G, Kalantari M et al. Overrepresentation of point mutations in the Sp1 site of the non-coding control region of BK virus in bone marrow transplanted patients with haemorrhagic cystitis. J Clin Virol 2001; 21:1-7.
17a. Azzi A, Fanci R, Bosi A et al. Monitoring of polyomavirns BK viruria in bone marrow transplantation patients by DNA hybridization assay and by polymerase chain reation: an approach to assess the relationnship between BK viruria and hemarrhagic cystitis. Bone Marrow Transplant 1994; 14(2):235-40
18. Leung A, Suen CK, LieA et al. Quantification of polyoma BK viruria in hemorrhagic cystitis complicating bone marrow transplantation. Blood 2001; 98: 1971-78.
19. Akiyama H, Kurosu T, Sakashita C et al. Adenovirus is a key pathogen in hemorrhagic cystitis associated with bone marrow transplantation. CID 2001; 32: 1325-30.
20. Chapman C, Flower AJE, Durrant STS. The use of vidarabine in the treatment of human polyomavirus associated acute haemorrhagic cystitis. Bone Marrow Transplant 1991; 7:481-83.
21. Held T, Biel SS, Nitsche A et al. Treatment of BK virus-associated hemorrhagic cystitis and simultaneous CMV reactivation with cidofovir. Bone Marrow Transplant 2000; 26:47-50.
22. Kawakami M, Ueda S, Maeda T et al. Vidarabine therapy for virus-associated cystitis after allogeneic bone marrow transplantation. Bone Marrow Transplant 1997; 20:485-90.
23. Vianelli N, Renga M, Azzi A et al. Bone Marrow Transplant 2000; 25:319-20.
24. Hatakeyama N, Suzuki N, Kudoh T et al. Successful cidofovir treatment of adenovirus -associated hemorrhagic cystitis and renal dysfunction after allogenic bone marrow transplant. Pediatr Infect Dis J 2003; 22(10):928-9.
25. Barouch DH, Faquin WC, Chen Y et al. BK virus-associated hemorrhagic cystitis in a Human Immunodeficiency Virus-infected patient. Clin Infect Dis 2002; 35(3):326-9.
26. Gonzalez-Fraile M, Canizo C, Caballer D et al. Cidofovir treatment of human polyomavirus-associated acute haemorrhagic cystitis. Transpl Infect Dis 2001; 3: 44-6.
27. Etienne I, Francois A, Redonnet M et al. Does polyomavirus infection induce renal failure in cardiac transplant recipients? Transplant Proc 2000; 32:2794-5.
28. Masuda K, Akutagawa K, Yutani C et al. Persistent infection with human polyomavirus revealed by urinary cytology in a patient with heart transplantation: a case report. Acta Cytol 1998; 42:803.
29. Haririan A, Ramos ER, Drachenberg CB et al. Polyomavirus nephropathy in native kidneys of a solitary pancreas transplant recipient. Transplantation 2002; 73:1350-53.
30. Haririan A, Hamze O, Drachenberg CB et al. Polyomavirus reactivation in native kidneys of pancreas alone allograft recipients. Transplantation 2003; 75(8):1186-90.

Latent and Productive Polyomavirus Infections of Renal Allografts:
Morphological, Clinical, and Pathophysiological Aspects

Volker Nickeleit, Harsharan K. Singh and Michael J. Mihatsch

Abstract

Polyomavirus allograft nephropathy, also termed BK virus nephropathy (BKN) after the main causative agent, the polyoma-BK-virus strain, is a major complication following kidney transplantation. BKN is the most common viral infection affecting the renal allograft with a reported prevalence of 1% up to 10%. It often leads to chronic allograft dysfunction and graft loss. BKN is most likely caused by the reactivation of latent BK viruses which, under sustained and intensive immunosuppression, enter a replicative/productive cycle. Viral disease, i.e., BKN, is typically limited to the kidney transplant. It is histologically defined by the presence of intranuclear viral inclusion bodies in epithelial cells and severe tubular injury. Virally induced tubular damage is the morphological correlate for allograft dysfunction. In this chapter, different variants of polyomavirus intranuclear inclusion bodies [types 1 through 4] and adjunct techniques [immunohistochemistry, in-situ hybridization, electron microscopy and polymerase chain reaction (PCR)] that are used for proper characterization of disease are described. Special emphasis is placed on the clinical and pathophysiological significance of different histological stages of BKN.

Introduction

General aspects of polyomaviruses and polyomavirus infections are discussed in detail elsewhere in this book. Here, we will focus primarily on the morphology and clinicopathological aspects of polyomavirus associated allograft nephropathy which we will refer to as "BK virus nephropathy" (BKN) since kidney disease is nearly always caused by a productive infection with the polyomavirus-BK-strain. A minority of cases (approximately one third) show coactivation of BK- and JC-viruses simultaneously with, as yet, undetermined biological significance.[1,2] Polyomavirus nephropathies that are only caused by a productive JC virus infection or by the coactivation of BK and SV40 viruses are exceptionally rare and do not seem to be clinically significant.[3,4] In severely immunocompromised nontransplant patients, BK viruses can also enter into a productive/replicative cycle in native kidneys and demonstrate histological changes identical to those found in renal allografts.[5,6]

BKN affecting a kidney transplant was first described as a single case report by the pathologist Mackenzie in 1978.[7] In subsequent years however, during the era of cyclosporine and azathioprine based immunosuppression, BKN was largely 'forgotten'.[8,9] The clinical scenario changed dramatically in the mid 1990s when new third generation immunosuppressive drugs, specifically, high dose tacrolimus and mycophenolate-mofetil were introduced into the routine management of kidney transplant recipients in many centers worldwide.[8-12] Interestingly, one

Polyomaviruses and Human Diseases, edited by Nasimul Ahsan. ©2006 Eurekah.com and Springer Science+Business Media.

of the largest initial series of patients suffering from BKN was reported from the University of Pittsburgh which was one of the first transplant centers that had largely replaced cyclosporine with tacrolimus.[13] Risk factors for BKN, however, are still not fully understood, and "high dose immunosuppression" with new drugs is likely only one component in a multi-factorial risk profile promoting viral disease.[14-16] Currently BKN is reported with a prevalence of 1% up to 10% with rising incidence rates.[14,17-22] BKN is by far the most important infectious complication affecting kidney transplants. It exceeds productive CMV infections of renal allografts by approximately 20 - 30 times. Since effective anti-viral treatment strategies are poorly defined, BKN often leads to severe allograft dysfunction and graft loss.[8,9,14,17,19,22-24] Graft failure rates, especially when BKN is diagnosed late or treatment strategies fail, can reach 50% to 100% within 24 months following the initial diagnosis.[18,25,26] Improved graft survival has recently been reported from centers with vigorous patient screening programs which facilitate an early diagnosis of BKN and better outcome.[14,15,27-29]

BKN in renal allograft recipients is typically limited to the transplanted kidney. Depending on the extent of virally induced tubular injury, patients clinically present with varying degrees of allograft dysfunction. Serum creatinine levels vary from normal (BKN stage A) to markedly increased (BKN stages B and C).[14,15,21] The native kidneys are free of disease and systemic signs of an infection (fatigue, fever) are generally absent. BK-virus associated hemorrhagic cystitis, often seen after bone marrow transplantation, is not found in the setting of BKN in renal allograft recipients. Early observations linking productive infections of BK viruses with ureteral stenosis could not be confirmed in recent reports.[9,14,19,30] A definitive diagnosis of BKN requires a kidney biopsy and the detection of characteristic histologic changes.

Morphologic Characterization of BK Virus Allograft Nephropathy (BKN)

Histology

Two morphologic features define BKN: (i) intranuclear viral inclusion bodies in epithelial cells, and (ii) virally induced tubular epithelial cell injury and necrosis (Fig. 1).[9,10,13-15,23] BK viruses use the proliferative "machinery" of the host cells for replication. The formation of intranuclear viral inclusion bodies in tubular epithelial cells and glomerular parietal epithelial cells is a characteristic histologic sign of a productive polyomavirus infection, i.e., BKN. Four distinct variants of viral intranuclear inclusion bodies as well as "hybrid forms" exist which can often be seen side by side (Fig. 2 A-D): *type 1* (the most frequent form; Fig. 2A)—an amorphous basophilic ground-glass inclusion body; *type 2* (Fig. 2B)—a central, eosinophilic, granular type surrounded by a (mostly incomplete) clear halo; *type 3* (Fig. 2C)—an eosinophilic finely granular form without a halo; and *type 4* (Fig. 2D)—a vesicular variant with clumped, irregular chromatin and occasional nucleoli (also see Chapter 13: "Urine cytology findings of polyomavirus infections"). It is currently undetermined whether the different phenotypes of inclusion bodies represent various stages of intranuclear viral replication and maturation and/ or potential fixation artifacts. A productive infection with polyomaviruses does not induce cytoplasmic inclusion bodies. Ultimately, the intranuclear viral replication and assembly result in lysis of the host cell and the release of mature daughter virions.

Most important are changes in the tubules since virally induced tubular epithelial cell injury and necrosis with denudation of basement membranes are the morphologic correlates for graft dysfunction (Fig. 3).[9,14,15,23] Of special note: despite marked virally induced epithelial cell damage, the tubular basement membranes remain intact (Fig. 3). They can serve as the structural skeleton for tubular regeneration and healing once the viral replication ceases. Therefore, BKN, especially stages A and B, can heal with morphologic and functional restitution.

BKN typically involves renal tubules and collecting ducts in a focal fashion. Often, severely injured tubules containing many inclusion bearing epithelial cells are located adjacent to normal tubules. This observation likely reflects the ascending route of viral spread within "infected" nephrons.

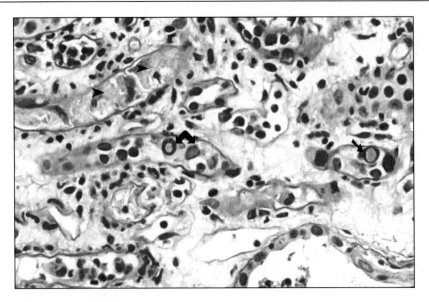

Figure 1. This is the characteristic picture of florid BKN (pattern B). Intranuclear viral inclusion bodies are seen within some of the tubular epithelial cells (arrows). One tubule demonstrates severe epithelial cell necrosis (arrowheads) and denudation of the tubular basement membrane. The interstitial compartment shows edema and scattered inflammatory cell infiltrates. Periodic Acid Schiff (PAS) stained section, x125 original magnification.

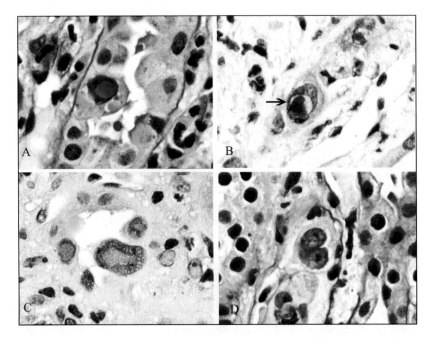

Figure 2. Different types of intranuclear polyomavirus inclusion bodies: A) Type 1. An amorphous basophilic ground glass variant (the most common form). B) Type 2. An eosinophilic variant surrounded by an incomplete halo (arrow). C) Type 3. A finely granular variant. D) Type 4. A vesicular variant with clumped chromatin and discernible nucleoli. PAS stained sections, x 400 original magnification.

Occasionally, inclusion bodies are observed in the parietal epithelial cell layer lining Bowman's capsule and in small "pseudo-crescents".[9] Signs of polyomavirus replication are characteristically absent in stromal, mesangial, endothelial, and inflammatory cells as well as in podocytes. Viral inclusion bodies can sometimes be detected in the transitional cell layer lining the renal pelvis, the ureters and/or the urinary bladder.[9] They are, however, not part of the strict histological features defining BKN (see Chapter 15: "Urine cytology findings of polyomavirus infections").

Ultrastructural Features

BK viruses are likely initially (re)activated within intrarenal or urothelial foci of latent infections. Dormant viruses can enter into a replicative and lytic cycle and subsequently spread by receptor mediated mechanisms from cell to cell via an ascending route. Virions attach to the apical surface of tubular epithelial cells in large numbers, but only relatively few seem to ultimately invade permissive target cells. Viruses enter tubular cells in small noncoated vesicles/caveolae which fuse with a network of membrane bound tubules and cisternae including the endoplasmic reticulum and the Golgi apparatus (Figs. 4 and 5). BK viruses travel through these intracytoplasmic tubules and presumably reach the nucleus through perinuclear cisternae and nuclear pores. Viral replication and assembly as well as the expression of the polyomavirus large T antigen take place in the host cell nucleus. During the final phase of intranuclear viral replication, mature daughter virions are densely packed and often arranged in crystalloid arrays surrounded by a rim of chromatin. This is the ultrastructural correlate for the histologically observed intranuclear viral inclusion bodies. Ultimately, host cells are lysed and large numbers of mature viral particles are released (Fig. 6).[31]

Ancillary Diagnostic Techniques

Although the histologic changes are characteristic for BKN, they are not pathognomonic since other viral infections caused by Herpes Simplex Virus, Adenovirus or Cytomegalovirus must be considered in the differential diagnosis.[23,32,33] Diagnostic confirmation of BKN is generally achieved by immunohistochemistry, in-situ hybridization and/or electron microscopy. These techniques are well suited to identify viral families if a productive viral infection is already suspected by light microscopy. However, their routine diagnostic use as generalized screening tools to "hunt" for a productive polyomavirus infection is neither helpful nor cost effective.[9,18]

The majority of intranuclear viral inclusion bodies in cases of BKN render a positive staining reaction with an antibody that detects the simian virus "SV-40 T antigen" which is common to all known polyomavirus strains pathogenic in humans (i.e., BK-, JC- and SV-40 strains) (Fig. 7).[14,15,23] Because the large T antigen is only expressed in abundancy during the early stages of intranuclear viral replication, some inclusion bearing cells representing late phases of virus assembly can be "SV-40 T antigen" negative. On the other hand, the expression of the SV-40 T antigen can precede the formation of intranuclear viral inclusion bodies and, consequently, a positive staining reaction may be detected in histologically normal nuclei.

In order to render the diagnosis of BKN it is clinically sufficient to document "SV-40 T positivity" since BK viruses are the causative agents in practically all cases.[9,21,34-36] Additionally, BK virus specific antibodies are also available.[14] (See refs. 14 and 23 for details on antibodies and staining protocols.)

Ultrastructurally, all polyomaviruses present as viral particles measuring between 30 and 50 nanometers in diameter, occasionally forming crystalloid structures (Figs. 4-6). Electron microscopy is not suited to distinguish between different strains of polyomaviruses. PCR techniques may be utilized to demonstrate viral DNA in tissue samples and to confirm the diagnosis of BKN.[36] However, PCR results must be interpreted with great caution. Only strong amplification signals of BK virus DNA in the setting of histologically demonstrable intranuclear viral inclusion bodies can be used to confirm the diagnosis of BKN and to distinguish clinically significant productive from clinically insignificant latent BK virus infections.[16]

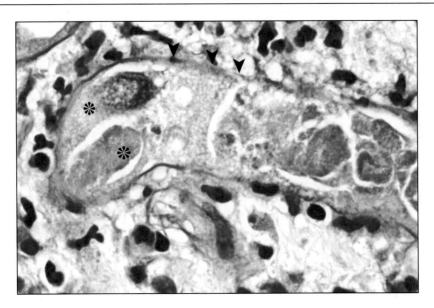

Figure 3. Florid BKN (pattern B) with severe virally induced tubular injury. Tubular epithelial cells are necrotic (asterisks) and the tubular lumen is filled with debris. The tubular basement membrane is completely denuded of the epithelial cell layer, however, it remains structurally intact (arrowheads). The interstitium shows edema and inflammatory cells. PAS stained section, x 250 original magnification.

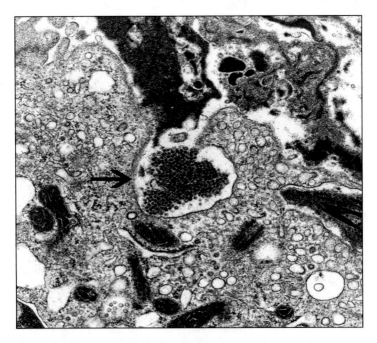

Figure 4. Electron microscopy. A cluster of polyomaviruses is seen in an infolding of the apical plasma membrane of a tubular epithelial cell (arrow). This finding represents the earliest step of viral entry into a cell. BK viruses enter permissive host cells via endocytosis in noncoated vesicles/caveolae, x 8000 original magnification.

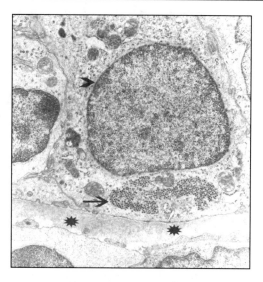

Figure 5. Electron microscopy. Virions are seen within the tubular epithelial cell cytoplasm (arrow) but not in the nucleus (arrowhead). The overall architecture of the cell is unaltered. This finding represents the passage of virions through the cytoplasm to the nucleus where viral replication takes place. Asterisk: tubular basement membrane, x 5000 original magnification.

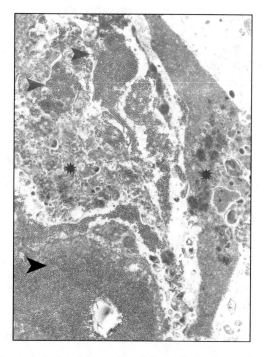

Figure 6. Electron microscopy. Lysis and destruction of a host cell after the completion of viral replication. Mature daughter virions (arranged in crystalloid arrays, arrowheads) are released into a tubular lumen. Asterisk: cellular debris. Figure 6 represents the ultrastructural correlate of the light microscopic findings illustrated in Figure 3, x 3000 original magnification.

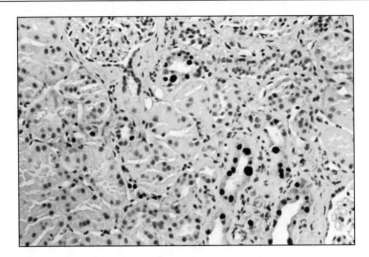

Figure 7. Immunohistochemistry. BKN (pattern A) with focal nuclear staining of tubular epithelial cells (brown staining reaction). Only scattered nephrons are involved. The tubular and interstitial architecture is normal. Formalin fixed and paraffin embedded tissue section, antibody directed against the SV-40 T antigen, x 60 original magnification.

Histologic Stages/Patterns of BKN

BKN can present with different histologic patterns and progress through various stages.[9,14,15,23,37,38] Three patterns have recently been defined at the "Polyomavirus Allograft Nephropathy Consensus Conference" (Basel, Switzerland, October 2003, in press*). They are listed here with slight modifications: (1) Pattern A (limited/early stage) (Figs. 7 and 8): Signs of viral replication in less than 25% of cortical and medullary tubular cross sections with only minimal evidence of epithelial cell necrosis and no denudation of tubular basement membranes. Interstitial inflammation, fibrosis and tubular atrophy are inconspicuous. Changes

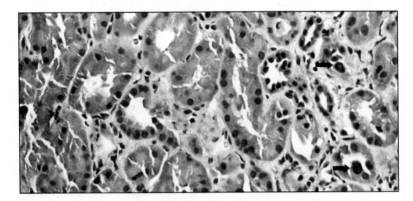

Figure 8. BKN (pattern A; early stage). Only few tubular epithelial cells show intranuclear viral inclusion bodies (arrows). The tubular and interstitial architecture is unaltered. Hematoxylin and Eosin (H&E) stained section, x 80 original magnification.

---

* The manuscript has been accepted for publication: Hirsch HH, Brennan DC, Drachenberg CB et al. Polyomavirus-associated nephropathy in renal transplantation: Interdisciplinary analyses and recommendations. Transplantation 2005, in press.

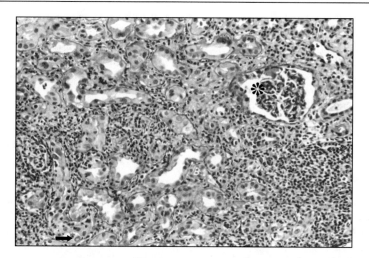

Figure 9. BKN (pattern B; florid stage). Signs of viral replication with intranuclear inclusion bodies (arrow) are associated with tubular injury. The interstitial compartment shows a diffuse predominately lymphocytic infiltrate. Asterisk: normal glomerulus. PAS stained section, x 60 original magnification.

classified as pattern A are frequently most pronounced in the renal medulla. (2) Pattern B (florid, fully developed stage) (Figs. 1, 3 and 9): Signs of viral replication in more than 10% of cortical and medullary tubular cross sections with conspicuous epithelial cell necrosis, denudation of tubular basement membranes, and interstitial edema. Inflammation, often rich in plasma cells and polymorphonuclear leukocytes, is common, whereas interstitial fibrosis and tubular atrophy are minimal. Changes classified as pattern B can be found in the renal cortex and medulla. (3) Pattern C (late, sclerosing phase) (Fig. 10): Signs of viral replication in generally less than 25% of cortical and medullary tubular cross sections associated with tubular epithelial cell injury. Interstitial inflammation can vary from minimal to marked. Interstitial fibrosis and

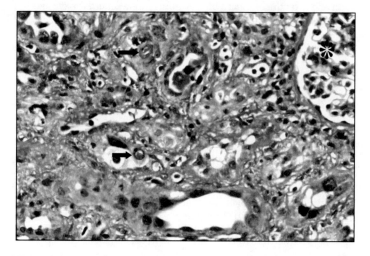

Figure 10. BKN (pattern C; late, sclerosing stage). The late, sclerosing phase of BKN is characterized by tubular atrophy and diffuse interstitial fibrosis (blue staining reaction). Viral inclusion bodies are noted in some tubular cells (arrows). Interstitial inflammation is inconspicuous. Asterisk: normal glomerulus. Trichrome stained section, x 80 original magnification.

tubular atrophy are typically seen in greater than 25% of the tissue sample. Changes classified as pattern C are frequently most pronounced in the renal cortex.

Pattern A represents the earliest stage of BKN with only scattered intranuclear viral inclusion bodies likely located in reactivated foci of latent BK virus infections. BKN-stage A, in contrast to stages B and C, responds to therapy more frequently with favorable graft survival and cessation of viral replication in up to 50% of patients.[14,21,23,27-29] Since tubular injury in pattern A is very limited (often confined to the renal medulla), graft function typically remains stable, and the optimal timing of a diagnostic graft biopsy, which is generally triggered by allograft dysfunction, becomes a clinical challenge (see Chapter 15: "Urine cytology findings of polyomavirus infections"). BKN- stage A can progress to stages B and C if productive viral replication spreads and persists over weeks to months. In one series, progression was observed in 70% of follow-up graft biopsies.[38] The therapeutic goal of BKN in stages A and B is to limit viral replication and tubular injury, to promote tubular epithelial cell regeneration, and to prevent disease progression to pattern C with irreversible interstitial fibrosis and tubular atrophy. BKN-stage C is typically associated with severe allograft dysfunction or graft loss.[9,15,38]

BKN patterns A-C are associated with varying degrees of interstitial inflammation. The inflammatory cell infiltrate, especially in pattern B, can represent "virally induced" interstitial nephritis with polymorphonuclear leukocytes located adjacent to severely injured tubules, plasma cells, and plasma cell tubulitis.[9,14,23,37] In some cases, mononuclear cell infiltrates rich in lymphocytes and a lymphocytic tubulitis can be found representing BKN and concurrent acute allograft rejection. The diagnosis of acute rejection and BKN is challenging. It can be facilitated by the detection of transplant endarteritis, transplant glomerulitis, as well as the tubular expression of MHC-class II (HLA-DR) and/or the deposition of the complement degradation product C4d along peritubular capillaries.[14,15,23,27,29,39,40] The immunohistochemical phenotyping of the inflammatory cells in BKN has shown plasma cell (CD138) as well as B (CD20) or T cell (CD3) dominant infiltrates with currently undetermined pathophysiological significance.[40-42]

Latent BK Virus Infections

Surprisingly little is known about latent infections with polyomaviruses in normal organ systems including the kidneys, ureters, and the bladder. Chesters' and colleagues studied latent BK and JC infections by the Southern blot technique more than 20 years ago.[43] They found dormant BK viruses in a focal distribution pattern in 33% of kidneys and dormant JC viruses in 10% with viral load levels of up to 5 BK virus copies and up to 40 JC virus copies per cell. These early studies are very informative since they clearly indicate that only a subgroup of kidneys harbor latent BK virus.

In order to study latent BK-virus infections in a systematic fashion we analyzed kidneys, ureters, bladders and plasma samples from 40 nontransplant patients at time of autopsy with quantitative PCR techniques. Plasma BK virus antibody titers were assessed with the hemagglutination inhibition assay. Dormant BK virus infections were found in 58% of patients and 14% of kidneys. Typically, especially in the bladder and ureters, latent viral load levels were low (less than 100 BK copies per 25,000 cell equivalents). High viral loads (more than 100 BK virus copies per 25,000 cell equivalents) were only sporadically detected in 5% of the kidneys in a focal distribution pattern in the cortex and medulla. Latent BK virus infections were not associated with morphological changes, i.e., intranuclear viral inclusion bodies were absent, and immunohistochemical incubations to detect the SV-40 T antigen were unrevealing. No BK virus DNA was found in plasma samples. 97% of patients had positive BK virus antibody titers greater than 1:128. The antibody titers did not mirror latent intrarenal BK virus load levels.

Presumably, a productive infection with BK viruses starts within intra-parenchymal foci of "high" latent BK virus loads when the right window of opportunity is provided. Thus, donor kidney organs carrying a high load of dormant BK virus may be at increased risk for the development of BKN post transplantation.[15,16] Morphologic changes of a productive infection become apparent once viral replication exceeds certain—currently undetermined—intranuclear viral load levels. When viral replication enters into the lytic cycle with necrosis of tubular epithelial cells, viral particles gain access to the blood stream via peritubular capillaries, and BK virus DNA becomes detectable in the plasma – the typical presentation of BKN.

References

1. Baksh FK, Finkelstein SD, Swalsky PA et al. Molecular genotyping of BK and JC viruses in human polyomavirus-associated interstitial nephritis after renal transplantation. Am J Kidney Dis 2001; 38(2):354-365.
2. Trofe J, Cavallo T, First MR et al. Polyomavirus in kidney and kidney-pancreas transplantation: A defined protocol for immunosuppression reduction and histologic monitoring. Transplant Proc 2002; 34(5):1788-1789.
3. Kazory A, Ducloux D, Chalopin JM et al. The first case of JC virus allograft nephropathy. Transplantation 2003; 76(11):1653-1655.
4. Li RM, Mannon RB, Kleiner D et al. BK virus and SV40 coinfection in polyomavirus nephropathy. Transplantation 2002; 74(11):1497-1504.
5. Rosen S, Harmon W, Krensky AM et al. Tubulo-interstitial nephritis associated with polyomavirus (BK type) infection. N Engl J Med 1983; 308(20):1192-1196.
6. de Silva LM, Bale P, de Courcy J et al. Renal failure due to BK virus infection in an immunodeficient child. J Med Virol 1995; 45(2):192-196.
7. Mackenzie EF, Poulding JM, Harrison PR et al. Human polyoma virus (HPV)-a significant pathogen in renal transplantation. Proc Eur Dial Transplant Assoc 1978; 15:352-360.
8. Binet I, Nickeleit V, Hirsch HH et al. Polyomavirus disease under new immunosuppressive drugs: A cause of renal graft dysfunction and graft loss. Transplantation 1999; 67(6):918-922.
9. Nickeleit V, Hirsch HH, Binet I et al. Polyomavirus infection of renal allograft recipients: From latent infection to manifest disease. J Am Soc Nephrol 1999; 10(5):1080-1089.
10. Drachenberg CB, Beskow CO, Cangro CB et al. Human polyoma virus in renal allograft biopsies: Morphological findings and correlation with urine cytology. Hum Pathol 1999; 30(8):970-977.
11. Howell DN, Smith SR, Butterly DW et al. Diagnosis and management of BK polyomavirus interstitial nephritis in renal transplant recipients. Transplantation 1999; 68(9):1279-1288.
12. Pappo O, Demetris AJ, Raikow RB et al. Human polyoma virus infection of renal allografts: Histopathologic diagnosis, clinical significance, and literature review. Mod Pathol 1996; 9(2):105-109.
13. Randhawa PS, Finkelstein S, Scantlebury V et al. Human polyoma virus-associated interstitial nephritis in the allograft kidney. Transplantation 1999; 67(1):103-109.
14. Nickeleit V, Steiger J, Mihatsch MJ. BK Virus infection after kidney transplantation. Graft 2002; 5(Dec Suppl):S46-S57.
15. Nickeleit V, Singh HK, Mihatsch MJ. Polyomavirus nephropathy: Morphology, pathophysiology, and clinical management. Curr Opin Nephrol Hypertens 2003; 12:599-605.
16. Nickeleit V, Singh HK, Gilliland MGF et al. Latent polyomavirus type BK loads in native kidneys analyzed by TaqMan PCR: What can be learned to better understand BK virus nephropathy? J Am Soc Nephrol (abstract) 2003; 14:424A.
17. Binet I, Nickeleit V, Hirsch HH. Polyomavirus infections in transplant recipients. Curr Opin Org Transplant 2000; 5:210-216.
18. Mengel M, Marwedel M, Radermacher J et al. Incidence of polyomavirus-nephropathy in renal allografts: Influence of modern immunosuppressive drugs. Nephrol Dial Transplant 2003; 18(6):1190-1196.
19. Ramos E, Drachenberg CB, Papadimitriou JC et al. Clinical course of polyoma virus nephropathy in 67 renal transplant patients. J Am Soc Nephrol 2002; 13(8):2145-2151.
20. Sachdeva MS, Nada R, Jha V et al. The high incidence of BK polyoma virus infection among renal transplant recipients in India. Transplantation 2004; 77(3):429-431.
21. Buehrig CK, Lager DJ, Stegall MD et al. Influence of surveillance renal allograft biopsy on diagnosis and prognosis of polyomavirus-associated nephropathy. Kidney Int 2003; 64(2):665-673.
22. Ramos E, Drachenberg CB, Portocarrero M et al. BK virus nephropathy diagnosis and treatment. In: Cecka, Terasaki, eds. Clinical Transplants. Los Angeles: Immunogenetics Center, 2002:143-152.
23. Nickeleit V, Hirsch HH, Zeiler M et al. BK-virus nephropathy in renal transplants-tubular necrosis, MHC-class II expression and rejection in a puzzling game. Nephrol Dial Transplant 2000; 15(3):324-332.
24. Afzal O, Hussain SA, Bresnahan BA et al. Graft loss associated with polyoma virus nephritis. Am J Transplant (abstract) 2003; 3(Suppl 5):A372.

25. Trofe J, Gaber LW, Stratta RJ et al. Polyomavirus in kidney and kidney-pancreas transplant recipients. Transpl Infect Dis 2003; 5(1):21-28.
26. Kang YN, Han SM, Park KK et al. BK virus infection in renal allograft recipients. Transplant Proc 2003; 35(1):275-277.
27. Mayr M, Nickeleit V, Hirsch HH et al. Polyomavirus BK nephropathy in a kidney transplant recipient: Critical issues of diagnosis and management. Am J Kidney Dis 2001; 38(3):E13.
28. Drachenberg CB, Papadimitriou JC, Wali R et al. Improved outcome of polyoma virus allograft nephropathy with early biopsy. Transplant Proc 2004; 36(3):758-759.
29. Hirsch HH, Knowles W, Dickenmann M et al. Prospective study of polyomavirus type BK replication and nephropathy in renal-transplant recipients. N Engl J Med 2002; 347(7):488-496.
30. Coleman DV, Mackenzie EF, Gardner SD et al. Human polyomavirus (BK) infection and ureteric stenosis in renal allograft recipients. J Clin Pathol 1978; 31(4):338-347.
31. Drachenberg CB, Papadimitriou JC, Wali R et al. BK polyoma virus allograft nephropathy: Ultrastructural features from viral cell entry to lysis. Am J Transplant 2003; 3(11):1383-1392.
32. Singh HK, Nickeleit V. Kidney Disease caused by Viral Infections. Curr Diag Pathol 2004; 10:11-21.
33. Asim M, Chong-Lopez A, Nickeleit V. Adenovirus infection of a renal allograft. Am J Kidney Dis 2003; 41(3):696-701.
34. Randhawa P, Baksh F, Aoki N et al. JC virus infection in allograft kidneys: Analysis by polymerase chain reaction and immunohistochemistry. Transplantation 2001; 71(9):1300-1303.
35. Randhawa P, Ho A, Shapiro R et al. Correlates of quantitative measurement of BK polyomavirus (BKV) DNA with clinical course of BKV infection in renal transplant patients. J Clin Microbiol 2004; 42(3):1176-1180.
36. Randhawa PS, Vats A, Zygmunt D et al. Quantitation of viral DNA in renal allograft tissue from patients with BK virus nephropathy. Transplantation 2002; 74(4):485-488.
37. van Gorder MA, Della Pelle P, Henson JW et al. Cynomolgus polyoma virus infection: A new member of the polyoma virus family causes interstitial nephritis, ureteritis, and enteritis in immunosuppressed cynomolgus monkeys. Am J Pathol 1999; 154(4):1273-1284.
38. Drachenberg RC, Drachenberg CB, Papadimitriou JC et al. Morphological spectrum of polyoma virus disease in renal allografts: Diagnostic accuracy of urine cytology. Am J Transplant 2001; 1(4):373-381.
39. Nickeleit V, Zeiler M, Gudat F et al. Detection of the complement degradation product C4d in renal allografts: Diagnostic and therapeutic implications. J Am Soc Nephrol 2002; 13(1):242-251.
40. Nickeleit V, Mihatsch MJ. Polyomavirus allograft nephropathy and concurrent acute rejection: A diagnostic and therapeutic challenge. Am J Transplant (letter) 2004; 4(5):838-839.
41. Jeong HJ, Hong SW, Sung SH et al. Polyomavirus nephropathy in renal transplantation: A clinicopathological study. Transpl Int 2003; 16(9):671-675.
42. Ahuja M, Cohen EP, Dayer AM et al. Polyoma virus infection after renal transplantation. Use of immunostaining as a guide to diagnosis. Transplantation 2001; 71(7):896-899.
43. Chesters PM, Heritage J, McCance DJ. Persistence of DNA sequences of BK virus and JC virus in normal human tissues and in diseased tissues. J Infect Dis 1983; 147(4):676-684.

Urine Cytology Findings of Polyomavirus Infections

Harsharan K. Singh, Lukas Bubendorf, Michael J. Mihatsch,
Cinthia B. Drachenberg and Volker Nickeleit

Abstract

Polyomaviruses of the BK- and JC-strains often remain latent within the transitional cell layer of the bladder, ureters and the renal pelvis as well as in tubular epithelial cells of the kidney. Slight changes in the immune status and/or an immunocompromised condition can lead to the (re)activation of latent polyomaviruses, especially along the transitional cell layer, resulting in the shedding of viral particles and infected cells into the urine. A morphologic sign of the (re)activation of polyomaviruses is the detection of typical intranuclear viral inclusion bearing epithelial cells, so-called "decoy cells", in the urine. Decoy cells often contain polyoma-BK-viruses. The inclusion bearing cells are easily identified and quantifiable in routine Papanicolaou stained urine cytology specimens. With some experience, decoy cells can also be detected in the unstained urinary sediment by phase contrast microscopy. Different morphologic variants of decoy cells (types 1 through 4) are described and ancillary techniques (immunohistochemistry, electron microscopy (EM), and fluorescence-in-situ-hybridization (FISH)) for proper identification and characterization are discussed. Special emphasis is placed on the clinical significance of the detection of decoy cells as a parameter to assess the risk for disease, i.e., polyoma-BK-virus nephropathy (BKN) in kidney transplant recipients. The sensitivity and specificity of decoy cells for diagnosing BKN is 99% and 95%, respectively, the positive predictive value varies between 27% and more than 90%, and the negative predictive value is 99%. The detection of decoy cells is compared to other techniques applicable to assess the activation of polyomaviruses in the urine (polymerase chain reaction (PCR) and EM).

Introduction

General aspects of polyomaviruses are discussed in detail elsewhere in this handbook. Here, it is important to emphasize that polyomaviruses are often not cleared from the body after the primary infection. Rather, it is assumed that primary viral entry into the host, often via an upper respiratory infection, results in transient viremia and viral spread to permissive tissues, in particular, to transitional cells and renal tubular epithelial cells. Polyomaviruses can establish life-long latency under normal cellular and humoral immuno-surveillance.[1-3] Latent polyomavirus infections cannot be identified histologically or immunohistochemically but rather require the use of molecular techniques for detection (Southern blot or PCR analyses).[1,2] Disease caused by (latent) polyomaviruses is typically not seen in the immunocompetent host. However, even slight changes in the immune surveillance can result in transient, asymptomatic and self-limiting activation of latent polyomaviruses in healthy individuals. Since the urothelium is a common site of viral latency, reactivation of polyomaviruses often occurs in the transitional

Polyomaviruses and Human Diseases, edited by Nasimul Ahsan. ©2006 Eurekah.com
and Springer Science+Business Media.

cell layer. Such viral (re)activation is characterized by the shedding of viral particles and viral inclusion bearing epithelial cells (so-called "decoy cells") into the urine. Indeed, the first strain of human polyomaviruses was isolated from the urine in 1971 and named "BK-polyomavirus" strain after the initials of the patient.[4] Based on the detection of decoy cells in the urine, transient and asymptomatic reactivation of polyomaviruses can be seen in 0.5-0.6% of all urine cytology specimens.[5,6] A high prevalence of decoy cell shedding is found in pregnant women (3%), patients suffering from cancer (13%), and diabetes mellitus (3%), as well as in healthy renal allograft (23%) and pancreas transplant (11%) recipients.[6-13] Decoy cell shedding has also been reported after heart transplantation.[14] Polyomavirus (re)activation and the shedding of decoy cells are generally not associated with kidney dysfunction, i.e., a rise in serum creatinine levels, or other renal abnormalities.[8,13]

In contrast, in severely immunocompromised patients, polyomaviruses can cause manifest disease. With the advent of new, highly potent immunosuppressive drug regimens introduced into the management of renal transplant recipients, the activation and replication of polyomaviruses of the BK-strain in renal tubules of the allograft, i.e., polyoma-BK-virus allograft nephropathy (BKN), has gained great clinical significance. BKN is characteristically associated with signs of viral activation, i.e., the shedding of decoy cells. Decoy cells contain mostly BK-virus antigens. Thus, in renal allograft recipients, the examination of urine cytology specimens and the search for polyomavirus inclusion bearing cells can be used as a clinical tool to assess the (re)activation of latent polyomaviruses and the risk for BKN (*vide intra*). In bone marrow transplant recipients, massive replication of BK-virus in the bladder mucosa and the shedding of decoy cells are associated with a hemorrhagic cystitis several weeks post grafting. However, BKN is not seen after bone marrow transplantation. A productive infection with the polyoma-JC-virus strain in the brain (i.e., in oligodendrocytes) of Acquired Immune Deficiency syndrome (AIDS) patients can cause "progressive multifocal leukoencephalopathy" which is generally not associated with renal or urinary abnormalities.

. In the following paragraphs, we will characterize polyomavirus inclusion bearing "decoy-cells". We will emphasize the clinical significance of decoy cells for assessing the risk of BKN in kidney transplant recipients. The morphological detection of decoy cells will be compared with other ancillary techniques, such as PCR analyses, electron microscopy, and FISH analyses.

Polyomavirus Inclusion Bearing "Decoy" Cells

Beginning in 1945, George Papanicolaou stressed the usefulness of urine cytology examination and the "Papanicolaou stain" for the diagnostic evaluation of cellular elements in voided urine specimens. This technique rapidly gained worldwide acceptance since it provided an easy, reliable, and inexpensive clinical tool. Approximately forty years ago, Koss and colleagues described polyomavirus inclusion bearing cells for the first time in urine cytology specimens.[15] They coined the term "decoy cells" to alert pathologists not to misdiagnose viral inclusion bearing cells as malignant cancer cells.

Decoy-Cells, Morphology and Characterization

The name "decoy cell" is a descriptive term for epithelial cells with intranuclear viral inclusion bodies that can have different phenotypes (types 1-4) depending upon the state of viral replication and maturation as well as the state of cellular preservation. The order in which the various phenotypes may occur during intranuclear viral assembly is unclear. Hybrid forms representing transitions between the different phenotypes are frequently found in the same specimen. Most common are classic decoy cells characterized by large, homogenous, amorphous ground-glass like intranuclear inclusion bodies and a condensed rim of chromatin (type 1) (Fig. 1). Sometimes, decoy cells reveal granular intranuclear inclusions surrounded by a clear halo, i.e., cytomegalovirus (CMV)-like (type 2) (Fig. 2). Occasionally, multinucleated decoy cells with granular chromatin are detected (type 3) (Fig. 3). Type 4 decoy cells show vesicular nuclei, often with clumped chromatin and nucleoli (Fig. 4). Koss called these latter inclusions the "empty post-inclusion stage".[15] Types 3 and 4 decoy cells are especially prone to misinterpretation as

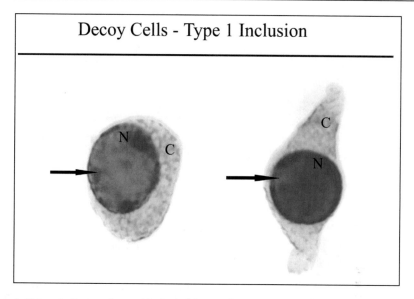

Figure 1. Urine cytology specimen with classical decoy cells (type 1) showing homogenous, amorphous, ground-glass like intranuclear inclusion bodies (arrows) in the central portion of the nuclei (N). A small condensed rim of chromatin is still visible under the nuclear membranes. Note: The cell on the right shows an eccentric "comet-like" cytoplasm (C). Papanicolaou stained preparations, 400 x original magnification.

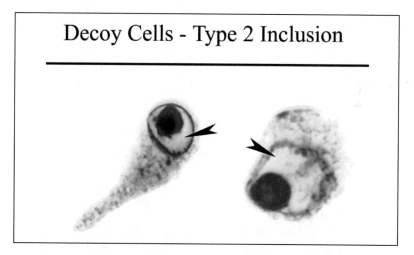

Figure 2. Type 2, "CMV-like" decoy cells showing central, intranuclear viral inclusion bodies surrounded by irregular and incomplete (intranuclear) halos (arrows). The nuclear membranes are easily discernible. The cell on the left reveals a "comet-like" cytoplasm. Papanicolaou stained preparations, 400 x original magnification.

"cancer cells". Although the nuclear features are most characteristic, many decoy cells additionally show a typical eccentric cytoplasm resembling the tail of a comet (termed "comet cells" by some, Figs. 1 and 2).[16]

Decoy cells mostly contain polyomaviruses of the BK strain or less commonly of the JC strain. Rarely, also adenoviruses may be found (Table 1).[5,17,18] Immunohistochemical and

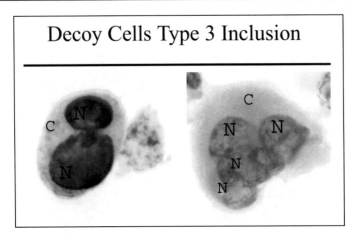

Figure 3. Type 3 decoy cells showing a granular chromatin pattern and multinucleation (N), cytoplasm (C). Papanicolaou stained preparations, 400 x original magnification.

electron microscopical analyses can easily be used to verify the presence of viruses and to identify the virus families. In general, most types 1 through 4 intranuclear inclusion bodies in decoy cells give a positive staining reaction with a commercially available antibody detecting the simian virus "SV-40 T antigen" which is common to all known polyomavirus strains pathogenic in humans (i.e., BK-, JC-, SV-40 strains, (Fig. 5); see appendix for staining protocols).[7,19] Of note: since the large T antigen is only expressed in abundancy during the early phases of viral replication, decoy cells with late stages of polyomavirus assembly may be "T antigen" negative. Using BK-virus specific antibodies or PCR techniques, most decoy cells contain polyoma-BK-virus particles.[5] Immunohistochemistry can also help to identify adenovirus containing decoy cells. Electron microscopy is well suited to detect polyomaviruses and adenoviruses based on their characteristic size of 40–50 nm and 80 nm, respectively (Fig. 6). Ultra structural analysis, however, is not suited to distinguish between different polyoma- or adenovirus strains.

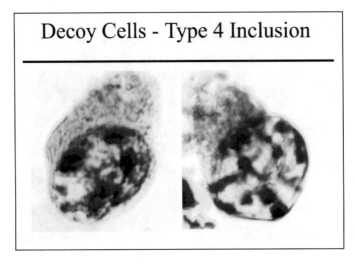

Figure 4. Type 4 decoy cells with vesicular nuclei and a distinct network of coarsely granular and clumped chromatin. Papanicolaou stained preparations, 400 x original magnification.

Table 1. Cytological changes induced by the most common viral infections observed in urine cytology specimens

Virus	Cytological Features
Polyomaviruses	**Decoy Cells** **Type 1**: Classic decoy cells show large, amorphous ground-glass like intranuclear viral inclusion bodies and a condensed rim of chromatin **Type 2**: Granular intranuclear inclusion bodies surrounded by a clear halo, i.e., CMV-like **Type 3**: Decoy cells with granular chromatin and no halo; sometimes multinucleated **Type 4**: Vesicular nuclei with a distinct network of often coarsely clumped chromatin; nucleoli can be found
Adenoviruses	**Decoy Cells** Nuclear features are identical to those seen with polyomaviruses; type 1 decoy cells are most common
Herpes simplex virus	Large multi-nucleated cells with nuclear molding, well defined nuclear inclusions of the ground-glass type (Cowdry A).
Cytomegalovirus	Large cells containing prominent intranuclear viral inclusion bodies surrounded by clear halos ("owl's eye" appearance). Additionally: eosinophilic cytoplasmic viral inclusion bodies can be found. Ground glass appearance of nuclear inclusion bodies is uncommon.

Although productive infections with cytomegalovirus, herpes simplex virus or human papillomavirus can show nuclear abnormalities including viral inclusion bodies, typical "decoy cells" as described above are generally not found in the urine in these infections (Table 1).

Decoy-Cells, Origin

The origin of decoy cells cannot be easily discerned based on morphologic grounds. It seems likely to us that they would commonly originate from the urothelium, in particular, in healthy and asymptomatic patients (Fig. 7a).[5,7] This assumption is based on the observation that the urothelium often harbors latent BK-virus infections (approximately 50% of individuals, personal observation). The replication of polyomaviruses is most pronounced in the superficial transitional cell layer, i.e., in umbrella cells, which can easily be shed.[9] As mentioned above, decoy cell shedding is often asymptomatic and renal function remains unaltered. Polyomavirus inclusion bearing cells are never seen in native kidneys of immune competent patients further arguing for an extra (renal) parenchymal origin of decoy cells found in the urine of healthy individuals.

In contrast, in immunocompromised patients BKN is characterized by intra-renal replication of BK viruses and kidney dysfunction. The morphological signs of viral replication in renal tubular epithelial cells in cases of BKN are very similar to those seen in transitional cells and decoy cells (see Chapter 14: "Latent and Productive Polyomavirus Infections of Renal Allografts: Morphological, Clinical and Pathophysiological Aspects"). Thus, in cases of BKN, decoy cells likely also originate from the renal parenchyma.[7,9,19] It is tempting to speculate that BKN may be caused by an ascending route of infection with spreading of polyomavirus replication from transitional cells to collecting ducts and proximal tubular epithelial cells in some patients in whom risk factors provide the right window of opportunity (Fig. 7b,c).[7] However, this hypopthesis has not yet been proven.

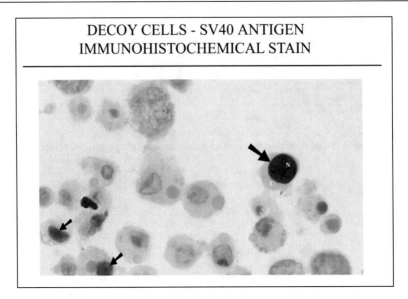

Figure 5. Immunohistochemical incubation to detect the SV-40T antigen (which is common to the SV40-, BK- and JC-polyomavirus strains). Typically, decoy cells show a distinct nuclear staining pattern (arrows). Urine cytology specimen, 200 x original magnification. N = nucleus, C = cytoplasm.

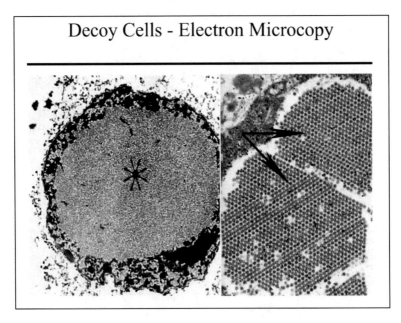

Figure 6. Electron microscopical image of decoy cells. The intranuclear viral inclusion bodies observed by light microscopy are ultrstructurally composed of densely packed viral particles (asterisk, arrows) with a diameter of approximately 40 nanometers. This is the typical size of viruses belonging to the "polyomavirus family". Occasionally, polyomaviruses are arranged in crystalloid arrays (image on the right, arrows). Note: In rare cases decoy cells can contain adenovirus particles which can easily be identified by electron micros-copy based on their large size of approximately 80 nanometers in diameter.

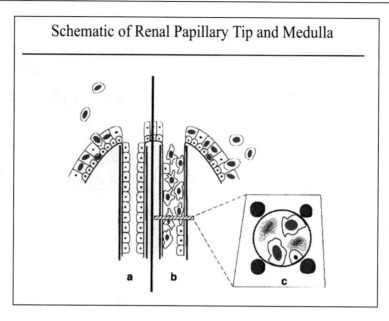

Figure 7. Intranuclear viral inclusion bodies are illustrated as large blue "dots". a) Transient and asymptomatic (re)activation of polyomaviruses with shedding of decoy cells in healthy individuals without BKN. The replication of polyomaviruses is likely limited to the urothelium/transitional cell layer from where decoy cells presumably originate; renal tubules as well as collecting ducts are normal and renal function remains unaltered. b,c) In patients with BKN—potentially due to an ascending route of infection—signs of viral replication are found in transitional cells and characteristically in renal tubular epithelial cells often resulting in kidney dysfunction. In BKN, decoy cells originate from the renal tubular compartment as well as from the urothelium. c) Cross section through a renal tubule in BKN. Lysis of tubular cells secondary to the replication of polyomaviruses releases viral particles into tubules with denuded basement membranes. Due to urine back-flow into the interstitial compartment polyomavirus particles gain access to the blood stream via the peritubular capillaries. Consequently, PCR analyses to detect viral DNA in the plasma are useful adjunct tools for diagnosing and managing BKN. (The figure is reproduced with permission from reference 7: Nephrol Dial Transplant 2000; 15:324-332; copyright release by Oxford University Press).

Decoy-Cells versus Malignant Tumor Cells

One of the most important challenges, already stressed by Koss and his colleagues, is to properly identify decoy cells and to avoid their misinterpretation as "malignant tumor cells".[15] Sound knowledge of the various phenotypes of viral inclusion bodies and the utilization of immunohistochemical and electron microscopic analyses should generally lead to their proper identification. In cases of polyomavirus activation and replication, the evaluation of "atypical cells" with proliferation markers or by DNA image cytometry can be misleading. Polyomaviruses require the "machinery" of the host cells for viral amplification. Thus, immunohistochemical stains to detect "proliferation associated antigens", such as antibodies directed against proliferating cell nuclear antigen (PCNA), KI-67 or MIB-1, give strong signals in decoy cells and inclusion bearing transitional cells. Such staining profiles should not be misinterpreted as a sign of marked "cell " proliferation, but rather indicate the replication of viral DNA. Accordingly, DNA cytometry/histograms of decoy cells invariably show aneuploidy due to the viral DNA content (Fig. 8). In contrast, FISH with chromosome enumeration probes and single locus specific identifiers (9p21) (UroVision,™ Vysis Inc., Downers Grove IL), can reliably demonstrate normal chromosome and gene copy numbers (Fig. 8).[20] The FISH profile clearly identifies decoy cells as "benign" and distinguishes them from cancer cells.[21]

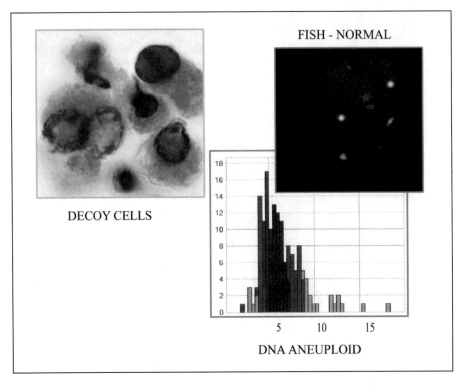

FISH - NORMAL

DECOY CELLS

DNA ANEUPLOID

Figure 8. Representative examples of DNA image cytometry and fluorescence-in-situ hybridization (FISH) analyses on decoy cells. Due to the viral DNA content, image cytometry invariably shows highly aneuploid patterns, which should not be mistaken as evidence for malignancy. FISH analyses, here with UroVysion[TM] probes to detect chromosomes 3, 7, 17 (chromosome enumeration probes—CEP), and 9p21 (single locus specific identifier—LSI) demonstrate regular copy numbers (n = 2) and confirm the benign nature of decoy cells. The DNA probes are directly labeled with the four dyes SpectrumRed (CEP 3), SpectrumGreen (CEP 7), SpectrumAqua (CEP 17), and SpectrumGold (LSI 9p21).

Decoy-Cells, Detection

Decoy cells can best be identified and quantified in standard alcohol fixed and Papanicolaou stained urine cytology specimens from either smeared or cytocentrifuged (i.e., cytospin) urine samples. In addition, the recently introduced monolayer technique is also feasible since it provides excellent preservation of nuclear details (Cytyc Inc., Boxborough, MA, and Tripath Imaging Inc., Burlington, NC). The second morning midstream voided urine specimen is best suited as the high level of cellular degeneration severely limits the first morning specimen. A few important considerations in the handling of urine specimens are the following: (1) Fresh urine specimens should be promptly transported to the cytology laboratory for immediate processing. (2) An alternative and more frequently used method is the fixation of the urine with an equal volume of 50-70% ethyl alcohol, preferably with added 2% Carbowax (polyethylene glycol). This procedure can be performed beside or in the laboratory when delayed specimen handling is anticipated. (3) Conventional cytospin or smear preparations should be obtained immediately after the specimen is received in the cytology laboratory. (4) The use of coated glass slides is recommended for adequate adherence of the cellular and noncellular elements to the slide surface.[22] It should be noted that specific guidelines for adequacy of voided urine specimens at the time of cytologic interpretation have not been firmly established and much is still dependent on the experience level of the pathologist.[22] Decoy cells can also be detected in the unstained urine sediment using phase contrast microscopy.[8,23] This technique, however, requires great experience and the quantification of decoy cells is tricky. We, therefore, recommend the analysis of standard Papanicolaou stained cytology specimens as described above.

Urine Analysis for Risk Assessment and Management of BK-Virus Nephropathy (BKN)

BKN is the most important infectious complication affecting renal allografts with a reported prevalence of 1% to 10%. It is typically caused by the replication of BK-virus in tubular epithelial cells, hence the name. The polyoma-JC and SV40 virus strains are only rarely (co)activated. BKN often results in chronic allograft dysfunction or even loss. The definitive diagnosis of BKN can only be made histologically in a renal allograft biopsy specimen showing characteristic tubular changes (see Chapter 14 "Latent and Productive Polyomavirus Infections of Renal Allografts: Morphological, Clinical and Pathophysiological Aspects").[7,9-11,19,24,25] Depending on the histologic stage in which BKN is first diagnosed, the outcome may vary. Best clinical results are seen if BKN is detected early (histological stage/pattern A), at a time when graft function is largely unaltered and irreversible graft fibrosis and tubular atrophy are absent.[7,10,19,24,26-28] Such an early diagnosis requires: (a) proper risk assessment of renal allograft recipients, and (b) optimal timing of a renal allograft biopsy. The search for decoy cells in the urine can assist in achieving these goals.[7,9-11,19,24,30] Clinical risk assessment strategies, including the search for decoy cells, were extensively discussed at the first "Polyomavirus Allograft Nephropathy Consensus Conference" held in Basel, Switzerland in October 2003 (in press).

Urine Cytology

As outlined above, the shedding of decoy cells generally indicates the (re)activation of (BK) polyomaviruses in the urothelium. Such (re)activation is a prerequisite for the potential development of BKN if the right "window of opportunity" for unrestricted viral replication in tubular epithelial cells is provided.[7,10,19] We retrospectively analyzed urine samples from more than 300 renal allograft recipients and found decoy cell shedding in 23% of patients; in 7% in high numbers, i.e., more than 5 decoy cells per 10 high power microscopic fields in cytology smears or alternatively more than 10 decoy cells per cytospin preparation.[7,11] BKN was diagnosed in 2% of patients, all of whom demonstrated abundant decoy cell shedding which often preceded the histological diagnosis of BKN by weeks to months.[7,9,10,19] These observations were confirmed in a prospective analysis.[31] In our hands, the detection of high numbers of decoy cells had a positive predictive value to indicate BKN of 27% and a negative predictive value of 99%, i.e., "no decoy cells, no BKN".[7,10] The positive predictive value can be further increased to over 90% by taking additional parameters into consideration: (a) a "dirty" cytological background, (b) decoy cell shedding in the setting of allograft dysfunction, (c) extended and persistent decoy cell shedding over more than 6 weeks, and (d) the detection of decoy cell casts.[11,19,24] The latter finding is considered to be pathognomonic for BKN since "cast material" always originates from the kidney parenchyma, i.e., the renal tubular compartment. In histologically confirmed cases of BKN, the number of decoy cells correlates with the number of inclusion bearing renal tubular epithelial cells.[24] Thus, the detection of decoy cells can also be used during therapeutic attempts to monitor for decreased viral loads and ultimately for viral "clearance" from the transplanted kidney.[7,10,19,24,31] Clinically, the search for decoy cells in the urine is frequently supplemented by (quantitative) PCR studies of BK virus DNA loads in plasma samples which can provide very valuable additional clinical information (Fig. 7c).[10,29,31-33]

Ancillary Techniques

Besides the search for decoy cells, PCR and EM analyses of urine samples have also been used to evaluate the activation of polyomaviruses and to assist with patient management.[32,34-36] All tests can provide important information, however, they vary greatly in sensitivity, specificity, feasibility, time requirement, and cost. So far, exhaustive comparative analyses have not been performed. A test should be carefully chosen in order to address specific questions.

Electron microscopy (EM) of negatively stained urine samples can be easily used to rapidly identify polyomaviruses in large numbers.[34,36] Howell and colleagues studied six patients with BKN, all of whom showed icosahedral, nonenveloped polyomavirus particles in the urine.[34] In three patients in whom BK virus replication in the kidney ceased during follow-up, i.e., BKN "cleared from the graft", viral particles also disappeared from the urine. The investigators did not find polyomaviruses in control patients (potentially due to low copy numbers below the level of detection, which varies between 10^3 and 10^9 viral particles per ml urine).[36] Thus, EM of negatively stained urine specimens provides an additional rapid, noninvasive, and relatively inexpensive diagnostic tool for the detection of large numbers of polyomaviruses. Such "crude" analyses appear to be suitable for patient management/risk assessment.

In contrast, highly sensitive PCR studies of urine samples do not seem to be of great clinical benefit in the setting of kidney or bone marrow transplantation since PCR tests often detect clinically irrelevant (low) levels of BK virus activation, i.e., low positive predictive value to indicate disease. In addition, urine PCR analyses can be technically challenging, due to non-specific endogenous inhibition of the PCR reactions or cross-contamination problems. Whether quantitative PCR tests measuring BK virus DNA or RNA loads in urine samples may be better suited for patient management has to be determined in future multicenter studies.[32,35] Not surprisingly, one report suggests that viral load levels in the urine have to be very high and exceed 10^7 BK virus DNA copies per ml in order to be predictive of BKN.[32]

From a clinical point of view, we propose a step-wise approach to assess the risk of renal allograft recipients for BKN. Initially (step one), patients should be screened for the activation of BK-virus. As outlined above, this goal can most easily be achieved by searching in the urine for decoy cells or alternatively for viral particles by EM. Positive test results should further be amended by quantitative PCR analyses measuring BK virus DNA loads in serum samples (step two). Serum BK-virus load levels exceeding 10,000 copies/ml indicate a very high risk for BKN.[31] This algorithmic approach will help to properly identify kidney transplant recipients in whom a diagnostic graft biopsy should be performed[7,10,19,29,31,33] This concept has largely been adopted by the "Polyomavirus Allograft Nephropathy Consensus Conference" (Basel, Switzerland, October 2003, in press).

Appendix Immunohistochemical Staining Protocols to Detect Polyomavirus Antigens in Urine Cytology Specimens (Decoy Cells)

In order to detect polyomavirus antigens in decoy cells, we generally use a monoclonal antibody directed against the large T antigen of the SV-40 polyomavirus strain (Oncogene Research Products, San Diego, CA, USA, Cat #DP02, DP02A, clone PAB 416). This antibody typically detects the T antigen of the BK-, JC-, and SV-40 strains (i.e., "pan" anti-polyomavirus antibody). Thus, the immunohistochemical detection of the SV40-T antigen can only prove the presence of polyomavirus antigens; different polyomavirus strains cannot be differentiated. The antibody typically gives a crisp nuclear staining reaction in some, but not all decoy cells (likely due to different stages of viral assembly and maturation since the large T antigen is expressed during early viral replication).

BK-viruses can be detected with a monoclonal antibody specifically directed against the T region of the polyoma-BK-virus strain (Chemicon, Mab8505, clone BK-T1). This antibody does not cross-react with JC-viruses. The antibody often shows increased background staining.

For all cytology specimens, we use antigen retrieval by microwaving for 5 minutes at 80 degrees Celsius followed by overnight incubation with the primary antibody at a dilution of 1:20.000 at 4 degrees Celsius. Subsequent to the incubation with a secondary antibody AEC is used as a chromogen. Histological sections of known cases of BKN can serve as positive staining controls.

References

1. Nickeleit V, Singh HK, Gilliland MGF et al. Latent polyomavirus type BK loads in native kidneys analyzed by Taqman PCR: What can be learned to better understand BK virus nephropathy? J Am Soc Nephrol 2003; 14:42-4A.
2. Chesters PM, Heritage J, McCance DJ. Persistence of DNA sequences of BK virus and JC virus in normal human tissues and in diseased tissues. J Infect Dis 1983; 147(4):676-684.
3. Heritage J, Chesters PM, McCance DJ. The persistence papovavirus BK DNA sequences in normal human renal tissue. J Med Virol 1981; 8:143-150.
4. Gardner SD, Field AM, Coleman DV et al. New human papovavirus (B.K.) isolated from urine after renal transplantation. Lancet 1971; 1:1253-1257.
5. Itoh S, Irie K, Nakamura Y et al. Cytologic and genetic study of polyomavirus-infected or polyomavirus-activated cells in human urine. Arch Pathol Lab Med 1998; 122(4):333-337.
6. Kahan AV, Coleman DV, Koss LG. Activation of human polyomavirus infection-detection by cytologic technics. Am J Clin Pathol 1980; 74(3):326-332.
7. Nickeleit V, Hirsch HH, Zeiler M et al. BK-virus nephropathy in renal transplants-tubular necrosis, MHC-class II expression and rejection in a puzzling game. Nephrol Dial Transplant 2000; 15(3):324-332.
8. Binet I, Nickeleit V, Hirsch HH et al. Polyomavirus disease under new immunosuppressive drugs: A cause of renal graft dysfunction and graft loss. Transplantation 1999; 67(6):918-922.
9. Nickeleit V, Hirsch HH, Binet IF et al. Polyomavirus infection of renal allograft recipients: From latent infection to manifest disease. J Am Soc Nephrol 1999; 10(5):1080-1089.
10. Nickeleit V, Singh HK, Mihatsch MJ. Polyomavirus nephropathy: Morphology, pathophysiology, and clinical management. Curr Opin Nephrol Hypertens 2003; 12:599-605.
11. Drachenberg CB, Beskow CO, Cangro CB et al. Human polyoma virus in renal allograft biopsies: Morphological findings and correlation with urine cytology. Hum Pathol 1999; 30(8):970-977.
12. Hogan TF, Padgett BL, Walker DL et al. Survey of human polyomavirus (JCV, BKV) infections in 139 patients with lung cancer, breast cancer, melanoma, or lymphoma. Prog Clin Biol Res 1983; 105:311-324.
13. Haririan A, Hamze O, Drachenberg CB et al. Polyomavirus reactivation in native kidneys of pancreas alone allograft recipients. Transplantation 2003; 75(8):1186-1190.
14. Masuda K, Akutagawa K, Yutani C et al. Persistent infection with human polyomavirus revealed by urinary cytology in a patient with heart transplantation, a case report. Acta Cytol 1998; 42(3):803-806.
15. Koss LG. The urinary tract in the absence of cancer. In: Koss LG, ed. Diagnostic Cytology and Its Histopathologic Basis. 4th ed. Philadelphia: J.B. Lippincott 1992; 2:890-933.
16. Crabbe JG. "Comet" or "decoy" cells found in urinary sediment smears. Acta Cytol 1971; 15(3):303-305.
17. De Las Casas LE, Hoerl HD, Bardales RH et al. Utility of urinary cytology for diagnosing human polyoma virus infection in transplant recipients: A study of 37 cases with electron microscopic analysis. Diagn Cytopathol 2001; 25(6):376-381.
18. Asim M, Chong-Lopez A, Nickeleit V. Adenovirus infection of a renal allograft. Am J Kidney Dis 2003; 41(3):696-701.
19. Nickeleit V, Steiger J, Mihatsch MJ. BK virus infection after kidney transplantation. Graft 2002; 5(DecemberSuppl):S46-S57.
20. Nickeleit V, Bubendorf L, Zeiler M et al. Polyomavirus-infected decoy cells in urine cytology specimens of renal allograft recipients: Clinicopathological considerations. Lab Invest 2002; 82(1):82A.
21. Dalquen P, Kleiber B, Grilli B et al. DNA image cytometry and fluorescence in situ hybridization for noninvasive detection of urothelial tumors in voided urine. Cancer 2002; 96(6):374-379.
22. Bardales RH. Constituents of urinary tract specimens in the absence of disease. In: Bardales RH, ed. Practical Urologic Cytopathology. New York: Oxford University Press, 2002:38-52.
23. Fogazzi GB, Cantu M, Saglimbeni L. 'Decoy cells' in the urine due to polyomavirus BK infection: Easily seen by phase-contrast microscopy. Nephrol Dial Transplant 2001; 16(7):1496-1498.
24. Drachenberg RC, Drachenberg CB, Papadimitriou JC et al. Morphological spectrum of polyoma virus disease in renal allografts: Diagnostic accuracy of urine cytology. Am J Transplant 2001; 1(4):373-381.
25. Randhawa PS, Finkelstein S, Scantlebury V et al. Human polyoma virus-associated interstitial nephritis in the allograft kidney. Transplantation 1999; 67(1):103-109.
26. Drachenberg CB, Papadimitriou JC, Wali R et al. Improved outcome of polyoma virus allograft nephropathy with early biopsy. Transplant Proc 2004; 36(3):758-759.

27. Buehrig CK, Lager DJ, Stegall MD et al. Influence of surveillance renal allograft biopsy on diagnosis and prognosis of polyomavirus-associated nephropathy. Kidney Int 2003; 64(2):665-673.
28. Mayr M, Nickeleit V, Hirsch HH et al. Polyomavirus BK nephropathy in a kidney transplant recipient: Critical issues of diagnosis and management. Am J Kidney Dis 2001; 38(3):E13.
29. Nickeleit V, Klimkait T, Binet IF et al. Testing for polyomavirus type BK DNA in plasma to identify renal-allograft recipients with viral nephropathy. N Engl J Med 2000; 342(18):1309-1315.
30. Nickeleit V, Steiger J, Mihatsch MJ. Re: Noninvasive diagnosis of BK virus nephritis by measurement of messenger RNA for BK virus VP1. Transplantation 2003; 75(12):2160-2161.
31. Hirsch HH, Knowles W, Dickenmann M et al. Prospective study of polyomavirus type BK replication and nephropathy in renal-transplant recipients. N Engl J Med 2002; 347(7):488-496.
32. Randhawa P, Ho A, Shapiro R et al. Correlates of quantitative measurement of BK polyomavirus (BKV) DNA with clinical course of BKV infection in renal transplant patients. J Clin Microbiol 2004; 42(3):1176-1180.
33. Limaye AP, Jerome KR, Kuhr CS et al. Quantitation of BK virus load in serum for the diagnosis of BK virus-associated nephropathy in renal transplant recipients. J Infect Dis 2001; 183(11):1669-1672.
34. Howell DN, Smith SR, Butterly DW et al. Diagnosis and management of BK polyomavirus interstitial nephritis in renal transplant recipients. Transplantation 1999; 68(9):1279-1288.
35. Ding R, Medeiros M, Dadhania D et al. Noninvasive diagnosis of BK virus nephritis by measurement of messenger RNA for BK virus VP1 in urine. Transplantation 2002; 74(7):987-994.
36. Biel SS, Nitsche A, Kurth A et al. Detection of human polyomaviruses in urine from bone marrow transplant patients: Comparison of electron microscopy with PCR. Clin Chem 2004; 50(2):306-312.

CHAPTER 16

Diagnosis and Treatment of BK Virus-Associated Transplant Nephropathy

Abhay Vats, Parmjeet S. Randhawa and Ron Shapiro

Abstract

The incidence of polyoma virus infection, particularly that of BK virus (BKV) in kidney transplant recipients has been increasing steadily since early 1990s. The diagnosis is generally made by a renal allograft biopsy. However the diagnosis can sometimes be difficult because of the pathological similarities between BKV associated nephropathy (BKVAN) and acute cellular rejection. In addition to the difficulties in making a diagnosis, the treatment of BKVAN can also be very complex. Reduction in immunosuppression is generally advocated as the initial therapeutic option for the management of BKVAN. Despite reduced immunosuppression, BKV can persist in the renal allograft and lead to gradual loss of kidney function. Hence, new therapeutic options are being evaluated for treatment of BKVAN. Cidofovir, an anti-viral agent with known nephrotoxic effects, has been successfully used in very low doses to treat patients with BKVAN, with serial measurement of the blood and urine BKV load with PCR assays. More recently several other agents have also been utilized to treat BKVAN, with variable success. This chapter summarizes the current diagnostic modalities and therapeutic options for BKVAN.

Introduction

BK, JC, and SV40 viruses are three closely related members of the polyomavirus family. Serological studies have shown that BK and JC virus infections occur worldwide and in childhood.[1,2] However, very little is known about the epidemiology of these viruses, including routes of infection, the modes of spread, or clinical spectrum of disease. Both JC and BK viruses appear to be strictly human viruses, but the prevalence of SV40 infections in humans is unclear. Of the three viruses, BK virus associated nephropathy (BKVAN) of renal allograft has emerged as a major cause of renal allograft dysfunction worldwide since early 1990s.[3-5] This emergence seems to have coincided with the widespread availability and administration of potent immunosuppressive drugs.[6,7] However, the diagnosis of BKVAN can be a challenge in the initial stages of the disease and treatment can be even more complex and demanding. BKVAN can be a difficult clinical problem and has been associated with a graft loss rate of more than 50% in some series.[3,4,6,8] Since the recognition of BKV as a major cause of both acute and chronic allograft dysfunction, different treatment modalities have been proposed in an attempt to prolong graft survival in patients who develop BKVAN. This chapter focuses on the current state of diagnostic testing and therapeutic options for this difficult and poorly understood condition.

Polyomaviruses and Human Diseases, edited by Nasimul Ahsan. ©2006 Eurekah.com and Springer Science+Business Media.

Clinical Presentation of BKVAN

BKVAN can present in many different ways and can affect both children and adult renal transplant recipients. In early studies, the prevalence of BKVAN in renal transplant recipients was reported to be 2-3%.[1,9] More recent data, however, indicate that the incidence is progressively increasing and may affect 5- 7% of kidney transplant recipients.[3,8,10,11] The rise in BKVAN over the last few years has been attributed to a number of factors, including increased awareness, more frequent use of biopsies, improved methods for diagnosis and the introduction of new and more potent immunosuppressive drugs such as tacrolimus, microemulsion cyclosporine, mycophenolate mofetil, and sirolimus.[12]

Generally BKVAN is diagnosed on a kidney biopsy in asymptomatic patients presenting with a rise in serum creatinine during routine follow-up and with no obvious preceding or concurrent symptoms.[6,13,14] BK-virus is known to be tropic for tubular epithelial cells and in most cases BKVAN is presumed to result from reactivation of virus latent in the renal tubules. However, affected children may have a primary infection with BKV especially if recipient is very young (less than 5-7 years of age).[14] Glomerular capillary tufts remain uninvolved by viral replication and significant proteinuria or hematuria are generally not clinically observed in BKVAN.[6,7] It is not uncommon to find that many patients are diagnosed with and treated for acute rejection in the months preceding the diagnosis of BKVAN.[14] Many such rejection episodes are generally only partially responsive to therapy. Thus, a high index of suspicion is needed for diagnosis of BKVAN especially in patients presenting with episodes of acute rejection that are refractory to steroid therapy or those presenting with late acute rejection (more than 6 months - 1 year after transplantation). In addition to asymptomatic patients, BKVAN has been diagnosed in patients who have presented with features that were variably diagnosed as acute rejection, interstitial nephritis, and ureteral stenosis.[14-17] A viral prodrome can sometimes be seen in a small fraction of patients prior to onset of allograft dysfunction.[14] The prodrome may consist of low-grade fever, myalgias or mild flu-like or gastro-enteritis type symptoms. These systemic symptoms may resolve spontaneously or after specific anti-viral therapy with cidofovir. Although BKV infection is primarily limited to kidney transplants, including the allograft and ureters, native kidney involvement can also be seen in recipients of nonrenal solid organ and bone marrow transplants.[18,19] The nonrenal transplant polyoma infections are discussed elsewhere in this book.

Diagnosis of BKVAN

Since the first report of BKV in the urine of a renal transplant recipient in 1971, BKVAN has been emerging as an important cause of renal allograft dysfunction over the last decade.[1,6,7] It was virtually nonexistent in many centers till mid 1990s, even when all allograft biopsies since 1985 from patients with documented shedding of "decoy cells" (a hallmark of BKVAN and discussed further below) were systematically reexamined.[7] The first case of PVAN diagnosed by a renal allograft needle biopsy was seen in 1993 and published in 1996 from University of Pittsburgh.[20] The previous literature on histologic diagnosis was restricted to occasional observations made at the time of graft nephrectomy or autopsy, while other studies focused on the diagnosis of polyomavirus infection by serology or urine cytology. Most such studies had concluded that polyomavirus infection usually does not affect graft outcome.[1,6] However, BKVAN is now increasingly being recognized as an important contributor to graft dysfunction and failure. The diagnosis of BKVAN currently must be established by renal biopsy, which shows typically shows viral inclusions and is often associated with interstitial infiltrates that may resemble acute rejection.[6,7] The details of viral pathogenesis are discussed elsewhere (Chapter 2, Discovery and Epidemiology of the Human Polyomaviruses) while some of the various modalities that are useful in the diagnoses of BKVAN are discussed below.

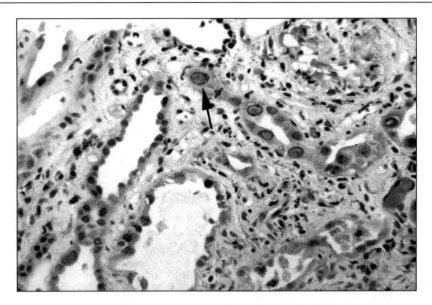

Figure 1. Renal allograft biopsy showing BKVAN. Several tubular epithelial cells contain an intranuclear viral inclusion typical of polyomavirus. The interstitium contains an active infiltrate comprised of neutrophils and mononuclear cells, which is presumably a response to viral antigens (H&E X 400).

Histopathology

The key to establishing the diagnosis of BKVAN remains the recognition of BKV inclusions in tubular and glomerular epithelial cells in renal allograft biopsy specimens[6,21,22] (Fig. 1). The renal medulla is preferentially affected during the early stages of the disease, and viral inclusions may be observed with little associated inflammation. Later phases of the disease are characterized by mononuclear infiltrates with focal invasion of the renal tubules and urothelium and involvement of cortex. Infected epithelial cells show enlarged nuclei, hyperchromatic chromatin, and intranuclear inclusions.[20-22] Cytoplasmic inclusion bodies are not seen, which helps distinguish polyomavirus infections from cytomegalovirus (CMV) infections. BKVAN can show varying degrees of tubular epithelial cell injury ranging from occasional intranuclear viral inclusion bodies, to widespread acute tubular necrosis with denudation of basement membranes. In approximately 30% of the biopsies with PVAN, a significant inflammatory infiltrate of polymorphonuclear cells is also present.[7,20] Prominence of plasma cells and changes resembling acute tubular necrosis are other features described in this clinical setting.

The initial histological changes of BKVAN can be fully reversible, and renal function may remain clinically unaltered. When viral replication spreads to the cortex and shows extensive involvement of proximal tubules with epithelial cell necrosis, allograft dysfunction almost always ensues.[16,23] Persistent and long lasting necrosis is associated with irreversible changes of interstitial fibrosis, tubular atrophy and will ultimately lead to chronic renal failure.[16,21,22] at times there can be a poor correlation between viral load, tubulitis grade, and serum creatinine. Clinical management practices can also affect renal viral load and pathology. In a recent study, we systematically examined the evolution of histologic viral load, grade of tubulitis, and graft function in BKVAN.[24] Over an 8 week period, reduced viral load in biopsies was seen in a significantly lower proportion (20% or 4/20) of patients treated initially by increased immunosuppression, compared to 83.3% (15/ 19) of patients treated with reduced immunosuppression (p =0.001). However, improvement in serum creatinine occurred in only a smaller fraction of these patients (15.8% and 5.3% respectively). Improved tubulitis was seen in a similar

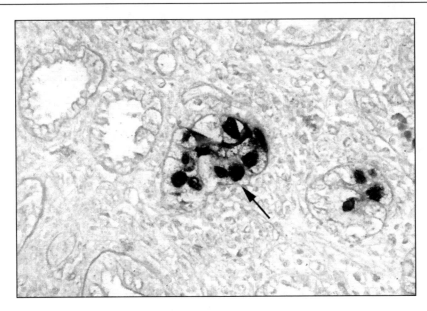

Figure 2. In-situ hybridization confirming the presence of BKV infected cells in the biopsy illustrated in Figure 1. Intranuclear hybridization signals are seen in the tubular epithelium (X 400).

proportion in the two groups. These data demonstrated that reduced immunosuppression is more effective in lowering viral load than steroid therapy but also suggested that there is a complex interplay of viral and alloimmune factors leading to graft injury.

The presence of polyomavirus protein or DNA expression in the infected cells can be confirmed by immunohistochemistry using commercially available antibodies (Fig. 2) or by in-situ hybridization.[7,20] Electron microscopy (EM) can also be used to confirm the diagnosis of BKVAN. EM typically shows intranuclear, intracytoplasmic, and extracellular virus particles (size, 40-50 nm) arranged in small clusters or crystalline arrays.[7] This size distinguishes polyomaviruses from other viruses such as adenovirus or CMV. Immunohistochemical or EM techniques are, however, not sensitive enough to detect latent virus in biopsies lacking viral inclusions by standard light microscopy. These modalities can only serve as confirmatory or adjunct diagnostic tools for the light microscopic examination, usually is performed by well trained and experienced personnel.[7,20]

BKVAN and Renal Allograft Rejection

Viral inclusions in BKVAN are often associated with a variable mononuclear interstitial infiltrate and focal tubulitis that closely resemble acute rejection. It is not clear if this resemblance reflects common mechanisms of T-cell influx or the concurrent presence of viral infection or true acute rejection. Conceivably, polyomavirus infection could precipitate acute rejection via upregulation of MHC class I or class II antigen expression, or the release of other pro-inflammatory cytokines.[7,21] Conversely, experimental evidence suggests that tubular injury associated with acute cellular rejection could secondarily increase polyomavirus replication.[25] Hence, at times it can be very difficult to separate BKVAN from its one major differential diagnosis, i.e., acute rejection. It has been proposed that the diagnosis of rejection can be suggested by the detection of strong tubular human leukocyte antigen-D related (HLA-DR) upregulation or the detection of C4d along peritubular capillaries. Both markers reportedly remain unchanged in pure BKVAN.[21,22,26,27] In another study, immunophenotyping found that there were more B cells (CD20) and fewer cytotoxic T cells in the lymphocyte infiltrates of BKVAN than in those with acute rejection.[28] The relationship between polyomavirus infection and acute, as well as chronic graft rejection thus remains to be evaluated in a systematic fashion, as it has been done for CMV.

Molecular Aids to Diagnoses

Although identification of nuclear viral inclusions by light microscopy is currently mandatory for the diagnosis, in certain circumstances (i.e., patchy renal involvement or early in the course of the disease) these findings may not be clearly evident.[20] Lately both qualitative and quantitative polymerase chain reaction (PCR) techniques have been utilized to show BK-virus DNA in biopsy tissue samples and to confirm the diagnosis.[5,10,29,30] By its inherent nature, PCR can detect BKV DNA in much smaller amounts than is possible by in-situ hybridization or by antigen detection using immunohistochemistry. In studies at our institution, quantitative PCR assay for BKV DNA was performed on biopsy tissue to see if it can aid in early diagnosis of BKVAN.[29] These studies showed that BKV DNA was present at a lower viral load (mean 216 copies/cell) in 38% of the 50 biopsies performed 1 to 164 weeks before diagnosis of BKVAN compared to a significantly higher viral load (mean 6063 viral copies/cell) in 28 biopsies of patients with active BKVAN. A BKV load exceeding 59 copies per cell identified all cases of BKVAN. Interestingly 8% of control biopsies (mostly with chronic allograft nephropathy or acute rejection) also showed a low level of BKV load (mean 3.8 copies/cell). The diagnostic sensitivity, positive predictive value, and negative predictive value of tissue quantitative PCR were 100%, 73.6%, and 100%, respectively. Thus, determination of renal BKV load by PCR may identify patients at risk for disease before histologic nephropathy develops. However, PCR-based BKVAN diagnostics is still an evolving field and only additional studies can determine if earlier recognition of at-risk patients allows application of antiviral strategies to improve graft outcome.

Another advantage of PCR based diagnostics is identification of coinfection of BKV with other polyoma and non polyoma viruses.[5,10,29-31] Lately, coinfection with both BKV and JCV was described, based on PCR amplification profiles of renal allograft biopsies, and approximately 35% of cases with BKVAN may have coexistent JCV.[31,32] Although JCV DNA has been detected in the kidneys of a significant subset of renal transplant recipients, a role for JCV as an independent etiologic agent of kidney disease has not been proven. Incidentally, coinfection with JCV and BKV has also been reported in pregnant women with viruria and in the urine and brain tissue of HIV-infected patients with progressive multifocal leukoencephalopathy (PML) and patients with HIV-related nephropathy.[33-35] Similar to JCV, detection of SV40 sequences has also been described in some patients with renal transplants but its role in allograft nephropathy needs further confirmation.[10,30]

Non-Invasive Viral Load Monitoring

Since primary isolation of human polyomaviruses is too difficult to be attempted outside of research laboratories and, at present, a definitive diagnosis of BKVAN requires a biopsy. There has been considerable interest in developing less invasive diagnostic methods that are also rapid and reproducible. Similar to other viral infections, such as CMV or Epstein-Barr virus (EBV), both qualitative and quantitative assessments of BK-virus activation can provide important clinical information that is crucial for patient management. Some of the practical noninvasive approaches have been: (a) Urine cytology and (b) PCR of blood and urine.

Urine Cytology

The hallmark of BKVAN is the presence of so-called "decoy cells", which are BKV infected cells, shed into the urine from renal tubules.[7,36,37] Different studies have shown that the detection of decoy cells in urine has a very high negative predictive value of about 100%, but a relatively low positive predictive value of 25-30% for BKVAN.[16,22] It has been found that most cases with detectable decoy cells on urine cytology are asymptomatic and transient shedding can be seen in

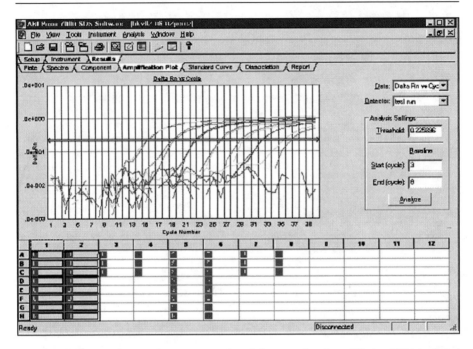

Figure 3. Real Time PCR technology is now increasingly being used to detect BK virus DNA in clinical specimens. The results of a typical real time PCR run (TaqMan™) on an Applied Biosystems, Inc. machine are shown.

up to a fourth of healthy renal allograft recipients.[3] However, the presence of inclusion-bearing decoy cells in high numbers may have a greater significance and association with active BKVAN.[36,37] A cut-off level of greater than five decoy cells per 10 high power microscopic fields has been proposed for such an association. The presence of decoy cells generally precedes the histologic diagnosis of BKVAN by 5-6 months and disappear shortly after transplant nephrectomy or clearance of the infection.[3,22] The risk for BKVAN increases significantly, with positive predictive value reaching up to 100%, if a combination of factors is taken into account; i.e.: high numbers of decoy cells that are detected persistently over months, or presence of decoy cell casts, and presence of pronounced allograft dysfunction.[36,37] Thus urine cytology is a good screening tool in renal allograft recipients, but is not diagnostic of BKVAN.[3]

Polymerase Chain Reaction (PCR)

Viral DNA can be detected in urine and blood and suspect tissues, such as kidney biopsy, by PCR. Such tests have been found to be useful for diagnosis of many other viral infections (i.e., CMV, HIV or EBV) and are increasingly being applied for the diagnosis and monitoring of BK and JC virus infections.[3,36] Unfortunately, qualitative PCR techniques reported in earlier studies varied greatly in their sensitivity and performance in different laboratories. More recently, reproducible quantitative PCR tests utilizing the newly available real time PCR technology (TaqMan™) have been developed and utilized in management of BKVAN[14,16,38-40] (Fig. 3). Many studies are currently in progress to evaluate further the role of blood and urine quantitative PCR in the diagnosis of and management BKVAN.

PCR Viral Load Measurements in the Blood

PCR analysis of blood samples (serum or plasma) to detect and quantify BK-virus DNA is rapidly becoming the test of choice for confirming the diagnosis and monitoring the progress of BKVAN.[14,36,38,39] Its sensitivity is considered to be 100%, and the specificity is about 85%.[3,16] In a single study, a serum BK-virus DNA load of more than 7700 copies / ml was predictive of BKVAN whereas several groups, including ours, now consider a titer above 10,000 copies / ml to be a significant correlate of BKVAN.[14,25,41] Also, the presence of BK DNA in blood may reflect the dynamics of the disease: the conversion of plasma from negative to positive for BKV DNA after transplantation, the presence of DNA in plasma in conjunction with the persistence of nephropathy, and its disappearance from plasma after the reduction of immunosuppression or anti-viral therapy can be various stages in the evolution of BKVAN.[14,36] In addition to confirming the diagnosis, these assays could also help monitor the response to therapy and guide the duration of therapy.[14,38,40] The ultimate goal of any BKVAN treatment should be at least a persistently negative serum PCR for BK-virus DNA.

PCR Viral Load Measurements in Urine

Urine PCR analysis can detect a very small number of viral copies. It thus has a higher sensitivity but a lower specificity than urine cytology.[3,14] Viral load measurement by PCR in the urine is not routinely performed at many centers, but has been monitored at the University of Pittsburgh since 2001 and has been reported by others.[14,34,38,42] All BKVAN patients with active disease in our studies were found to have a variable urinary viral load but it was generally more than 10 million (10^7 or 10E7) copies / ml [ranging from several thousand to more than 10 billion (10^{10} or 10E10) copies / ml]. No patient with BKVAN had a negative urinary PCR and we now consider a urine load of more than 10 million (10^7 or 10E7) copies / ml to be a significant risk factor of BKVAN. During acute BKV infection, the urinary viral load is several log orders higher (>4-6 log orders) than the plasma load. Several patients can maintain high urinary viral loads despite clearance of virus from blood. However PCR analyses for quantification of BKV loads in the urine can assume clinical significance especially if a rising titer of several log orders is noted. In our experience, several patients have been identified with a rising urinary viral load prior to their presentation with full blown BKVAN on renal biopsy and positive blood PCR.[38] Such a scenario can predict and predate the onset of overt BKVAN by several months. These assays can provide additional clinical information that may alert a physician to presence of early BKV infection, especially in clinical scenarios where the patient shows renal allograft dysfunction and the blood PCR or biopsy are negative still for BKVAN or biopsy shows mild rejection that appears to be refractory to conventional therapy with increased immunosuppression.[38,42] Besides urinary DNA PCR, there has been a recent report of using BKV messenger RNA as the substrate for amplification by real time reverse transcription-PCR (RT-PCR).[43] In this study, quantitation of urinary BKV VP1 messenger RNA was reported to be better predictor of disease activity or onset with a specificity and sensitivity of 93.8% and 93.9%, respectively.[43] However the role of BKV messenger RNA amplification in BKVAN diagnostics needs further confirmation.

Risk Factors for BKVAN

It is still not clear why only a small number of immunosuppressed patients with BKV infection develop full blown renal disease. BKV reactivation, as marked by viruria, does not necessarily indicate BKVAN, as it can be seen in 15-50% of renal allograft recipients, while the incidence of BKVAN is only 1-10 %.[4,6,8] Thus, several efforts have been made to identify risk factors for development of BKVAN. Specific immunosuppressive agents, i.e., tacrolimus and mycophenolate mofetil, are generally believed to be associated with a higher incidence of BKVAN.[6,8,44,45] In fact, most cases of BKVAN have occurred in patients treated with one or both of these drugs since 1995, after their use became widespread suggesting their role as risk factors for BKVAN.[6,8,45] However, a single prospective trial that compared the incidence of BK viremia and viruria in patients randomly assigned to receive tacrolimus or cyclosporine demonstrated no significant difference between the two agents as well as no significant association between mycophenolate mofetil and BKV infection.[46] Also several studies have reported BKVAN in association with cyclosporine and even sirolimus.[47-49] Therefore, it is more plausible that patients whose overall immunosuppression is maintained at a higher total level, rather than with a specific agent, have an increased incidence of BKVAN.[25,50] Other factors that have been associated with an increased risk of BKVAN include: a higher number of HLA mismatches between donor and recipient, the use of corticosteroid pulses to treat graft rejection, cell injury due to acute rejection or cold ischemia, male gender, older recipient age and BKV seropositivity.[16,17,25,41,51] However, many studies have also contradicted these associations too.[16,52,53] BKVAN thus seems to be promoted by the concurrent presence of several risk factors, among which potent immunosuppression appears to be a prerequisite.[3,54]

Molecular Techniques in Identification of Risk Factors for BKVAN

In addition to the factors defined above, efforts have also been made to identify variable host susceptibilities or pathogenecity of the virus that may further identify the risk factors for the development of BKVAN. Besides aiding in the diagnoses of BKVAN, molecular techniques have thus also been used to characterize possible mutations in BKV that may affect its pathogenecity. The polyomavirus genome contains a noncoding control region (NCCR), which is believed to contain the enhancer elements that are important activators of viral transcription.[25,55] DNA sequence variations, in the form of nucleotide substitutions, deletions, complex rearrangements or duplications, have been identified in several putative transcription factor binding sites in the NCCR region and these viral genomic changes have been proposed to play a role in the pathogenesis of BKVAN. Changes were most commonly found in binding sites for the granulocyte/macrophage stimulating factor promoter and the nuclear factor-1 transcription factor in our studies.[55] The regulatory region of BKV thus shows sequence heterogeneity in biopsy tissue, a situation that is reminiscent of genomic changes in JCV that are pathogenic and cause PML.

Besides viral genotype, it is possible that the host (renal transplant recipient) genotype may also contribute to the risk of BKVAN. There is now increasing evidence that cytokine gene polymorphisms can influence both rejection and infection outcomes after solid organ transplantation. We recently assessed whether various cytokine gene polymorphisms can be associated with the risk of development of BKVAN after renal transplantation in 86 renal allograft recipients, of whom 25 developed BKVAN and 61 did not (controls). A statistically significant correlation with BKVAN was detected between the presence of specific alleles of three genes i.e., the low expression allele of interferon (IFN)-γ (+874 A/A); and high-expression alleles of transforming growth factor (TGF-γ1) (+25 G/G); and interleukin (IL)- 6 (-174 G/G).[56] Thus, it is possible that presence of these cytokine gene polymorphisms may contribute to an imbalance between TGF β, IFN-γ and IL-6 expression and thereby increase the risk of BKVAN. Further studies are obviously needed to clarify the role of host and viral genotype in the development of BKVAN.

Clinical Management of BKVAN

BKVAN is associated with markedly compromised renal allograft survival with a variable rate of graft loss ranging from 10% to over 70 % in some series.[4,22,53] This is related to the fact that the clinical management of BKVAN has been a significant challenge. Although various therapeutic strategies have been tried, the results have often been variable and dismal. The fact that even when biopsies show tubulitis, suggesting rejection, there is little response to corticosteroids in many cases. Reduction of immunosuppression decreases the viral load, but also increases the risk of rejection. This therapeutic dilemma can result in an unfavorable clinical outcome although it has been associated with better outcomes than those seen with increasing immunosuppression. For instance, in 1993, the clinical diagnosis of BKV was first made in one of our renal transplant recipients who was treated aggressively for presumed cellular rejection. This patient subsequently lost her graft. Our initial experience in other similar patients who were treated with steroids and increased maintenance immunosuppression, instituted as treatment of the variable tubulitis seen in these patients, also resulted in graft loss in nearly 50% of such cases.[53] In view of the dismal experience associated with the ongoing treatment of tubulitis, we have attempted to treat BKVAN with reduced immunosuppression alone for the past 5-6 years. Others have also reported prolongation of graft function following an approach that involves a careful reduction of the immunosuppressive therapy with the aim of eliminating the viral load before significant scarring develops in the kidney.[3,7] This approach, although relatively successful, can still be associated with graft loss, either to chronic rejection, or to ongoing viral nephropathy, confirmed either by repeated kidney biopsies, or by plasma and urine PCR assays. This scenario has also been reported by other centers. In a study from University of Maryland, one-third of the patients diagnosed with BKVAN over a six year period lost their grafts, and a third of the remaining patients had a serum creatinine over 3 mg/dl.[41] No specific immunosuppressive agents were found to increase the incidence of BKVAN. Patients on a single immunosuppressive agent in addition to prednisone had less graft loss and a higher rate of viral clearance compared to patients on two immunosuppressant drugs and steroids. After reduction of immunosuppression, clearance of the infection and disappearance of the viral cytopathic changes in biopsies were seen in 20%; while persistence of viral replication with ongoing tubular damage occurred in the majority (70%) of the patients. Thus, early diagnosis and complete cessation of viral replication with morphological and functional restitution are the ultimate clinical goals of BKVAN therapy.

Although the optimal management of BKVAN remains controversy-ridden at this stage, we describe the management approach that is currently close to consensus and is also the approach followed at University of Pittsburgh. In most centers, BKVAN is initially treated by reducing immunosuppression and sometimes additionally by discontinuing drug regimens containing tacrolimus.[7,41] At our institutions, the first step in the treatment of BKVAN is to decrease immunosuppression.[38,53] The dose of tacrolimus is decreased (to achieve level of 5 ± 2 ng/ml), and steroids are either decreased or discontinued. If patients are on mycophenolate mofetil or sirolimus, these agents are nearly always discontinued after the diagnosis of BKVAN is established. These therapeutic attempts can sometimes result in good clinical success particularly if BKVAN is diagnosed at an early stage, viral loads and renal function tests are carefully monitored and if acute rejection is adequately controlled.[6,23,40] However, if the patient's BK viral DNA load increases (in blood and / or urine) along with worsening of renal function during the follow up of such patients, a consideration for institution of additional therapy should be made quickly. Currently, specific anti-viral strategies to treat patients with BKVAN are poorly defined, although very low dose cidofovir has been increasingly used by us and other centers with generally beneficial results.[8,14,38,40] Cidofovir is a very nephrotoxic drug and its use in BKVAN has to be carefully monitored. The role of cidofovir and additional therapeutic options for BKVAN is further discussed in another section and Figure 4 shows the flow diagram currently being practiced at University of Pittsburgh in the management and viral load monitoring of BKVAN.

Specific Anti-Viral Therapy for BKVAN: Pittsburgh Experience

Several therapies have been tried or shown to be effective in vitro for BKV infections, and these include vidarabine, cidofovir, retinoic acid derivatives, and DNA gyrase inhibitors.[57-63] We first used one such therapy, anecdotally in 1999, when low dose cidofovir was tried in a child with BKVAN with an encouraging outcome.[14,64] Since then, low dose cidofovir has been used in a number of our patients to treat BKVAN.[38,65,66] Details of cidofovir therapy in BKVAN are presented below.

Cidofovir (HPMPC, Vistide™, (S)-1-(3-hydroxy-2-phosphonylmethoxypropyl) cytosine) is an anti-viral agent that is a synthetic purine nucleotide (phosphorylated nucleoside) analog of cytosine.[67,68] It is converted via cellular enzymes to the pharmacologically active diphosphate metabolite (cidofovir diphosphate). This metabolite has in-vitro and in-vivo inhibitory activity against a large number of herpes viruses, as well as activity against adenovirus, human

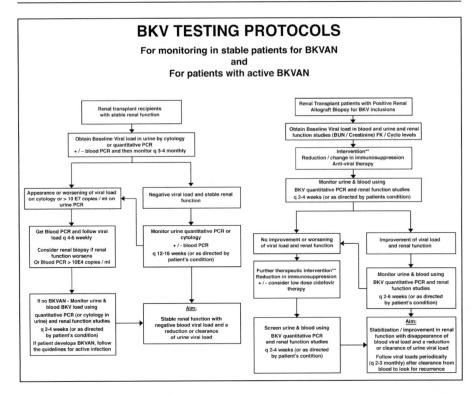

Figure 4. Flow charts showing the approach for screening patients for BKVAN and for management of a patient with active BKVAN. The antiviral treatment for BKVAN is still in evolutionary stages. Please see the text for details.

papilloma and polyoma viruses. Cidofovir diphosphate exerts its antiviral effect by interfering with DNA synthesis and inhibiting viral replication. Since this drug has an extended half-life, there is a prolonged anti-viral effect as well as an extended protection against subsequent viral infections in uninfected cells. Initial indications for the use of cidofovir were for the treatment of human CMV infection, particularly CMV retinitis in patients with acquired immunodeficiency syndrome.[68] It had also been shown to be effective in the therapy of bone marrow transplant patients with hemorrhagic cystitis due to BKV and CMV infections.[69,70] In order to prevent or reduce the nephrotoxicity of cidofovir, the dosages used in our studies were reduced to 5-20% of the recommended dose levels given to patients without renal disease. These patients were also adequately hydrated. Although probenecid (an uricosuric agent) is recommended for concomitant use with cidofovir to reduce renal excretion and possibly nephrotoxicity, withholding probenecid possibly allows for concentration of cidofovir within the proximal tubules, with an increased amount of drug excreted from the kidney. Thus the patients at our center have been treated with low dose cidofovir in the range of 0.25-1.0 mg/kg/dose given once every 2-3 weeks intravenously, without probenecid. The initial dose has tended to be 0.25-0.33 mg / Kg with incremental doses as needed.

Patient and Graft Outcome

In our report of 16 cidofovir treated BKVAN patients, the drug was effective in rendering the plasma PCR negative in a significant majority (98%) of the patients.[38] However, a few patients continued to demonstrate BKV interstitial nephritis despite negative plasma PCR

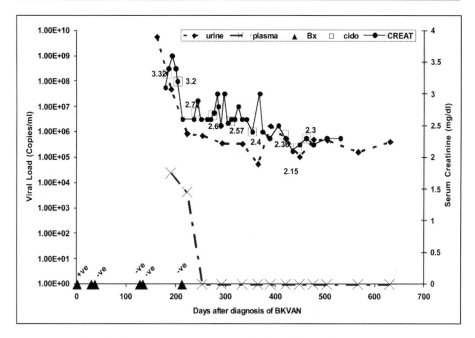

Figure 5. Typical time course events in a patient treated with cidofovir with improvement in serum creatinine, clearance of blood viral load and reduction of urinary viral load as determined by real time PCR for BKV. The cidofovir doses are represented by open squares (□), urine viral load by diamonds (♦) and blood viral load by crosses (X).

levels. This might be explained by the ongoing presence of virus in the kidney and urine without spillover into the blood stream. The continued presence of the virus is the kidney can lead to progressive destruction of the graft. This can be monitored by serial urinary titers or, if necessary, renal allograft biopsy for BKV. Cidofovir therapy was associated with significant reduction in the urine viral load (4-6 log orders) in over half of the patients and with a transient clearance of urinary viral load in a smaller fraction (about 15 %) of patients. However, most patients remained with positive urine PCR levels despite multiple courses of low dose cidofovir, and clearance of virus from the plasma. One possible reason could be that, because of concern about cidofovir's nephrotoxicity, the dosages used were too low.

Four patients (25%) lost their allografts, one of which was related to a single inadvertent high dose (3 mg/Kg) of cidofovir. Another patient with graft loss in our series did not respond at all to cidofovir therapy and this scenario could represent infection with a drug-resistant virus. Both plasma and urine PCR levels remained elevated throughout the course of therapy and allograft nephrectomy showed ongoing severe BKV infection. Twelve (75%) patients retained prolonged graft function. Serum creatinine improved from pretreatment levels and remained less than 2 mg/dl in three patients. Figure 5 shows typical time course events in a patient treated with cidofovir with improvement in serum creatinine. Five of twelve patients had serum creatinine levels between 2.3 and 3.8 mg/dl, which were unchanged or improved when compared to the serum creatinine levels prior to the diagnosis and treatment of BKVAN.

To date we have treated over thirty patients with BKVAN with reduction of immunosuppression and low dose cidofovir and three overall patterns of response have been identified by us: (1) significant improvement, based on assessment of renal function by serum creatinine, seen in approximately 25% of patients; (2) slight improvement or maintenance and preservation of renal function in approximately 50%; and (3) ongoing worsening of renal function in another 25%.[66] Future studies are needed to identify factors or markers that contribute to the poor response to therapy and ultimate poor graft outcome seen in some of these patients. Identification of various biomarkers including viral drug sensitivity, and viral and host genotypes along with their correlation with clinical outcomes may shed more light on these observations.

Thus our experience demonstrates the ability to use cidofovir safely, and efficaciously and shows low dose therapy administered every 1-3 weeks at a dose of 0.25-1 mg/kg without probenecid can be useful in the management of BKVAN. A gradual increase in the dosage of cidofovir with each treatment for BKVAN would perhaps allow for an earlier clearance of the virus and a shorter course of infection and treatment. Most importantly, this potentially nephrotoxic therapy should be carefully monitored by serial assessment of renal function and viral load. The quantitation of the viral load in blood and urine can allow a close monitoring of the patient's response to cidofovir. Systematic assessment of the kidney by biopsy can be useful in determining the progression and/or deterioration of renal function and may need to be undertaken if viral load determination is not helpful. The role of cidofovir in BKVAN needs to be further investigated in a larger cohort of patients in a multi-center setting to arrive at a consensus regarding the optimum dose and duration of therapy.

Additional Approaches for BKVAN Management

The timing of the initial diagnosis of BKVAN is very critical for therapeutic success and a good outcome, since graft failure rates can be very high. In addition to cidofovir, anecdotal evidence suggests that leflunomide, a new anti-arthitic and immunosuppressive agent with antiviral properties, may also be effective in BKVAN.[71,72] Additional agents that have been recently reported to have a potential therapeutic benefit include intravenous immunoglobulin and even steroid therapy given along with reduction in other immunosuppression.[73,74] It is quite possible that BKVAN therapy in future may evolve to include simultaneous or sequential use of one or more of these or other yet-to-be-identified agents.

Retransplantation and BKVAN

Once a graft has been lost due to BKVAN, consideration has to be given regarding retransplantation and its timing. There is now growing evidence that retransplantation is a safe therapeutic option, either with or without graft nephrectomy.[8,75,76] Recently, the characteristics and outcome in the largest series so far of 10 patients from five transplant centers who underwent retransplantation after losing their renal grafts to BKVAN was reported.[8] These patients underwent retransplantation a mean of 13.3 months after failure of the first graft. Nephroureterectomy of the first graft was performed in seven patients, while maintenance immunosuppression regimens after the first and second grafts were similar. BKVAN recurred in only one patient, but subsequent stabilization of graft function was achieved with a decrease in immunosuppression and treatment with low-dose cidofovir in this patient. After a mean follow-up of 34.6 months, all patients were found to have good graft function with a mean creatinine of 1.5 mg/dL. Thus the risk of recurrence does not seem to be increased in comparison with the first graft, and retransplantation should be offered to such patients after the active disease has subsided and the BKV PCR in the blood has turned negative.

Conclusion

There have been several recent advances, specifically viral load monitoring by quantitative PCR and cidofovir therapy that have both facilitated a better understanding of the natural course of BKVAN and also improved its management. However, anti-viral treatment strategies, that will enable complete cessation of BK-virus replication and functional graft recovery with minimal side effects, still need to be optimized. There are still a large number of unanswered questions. For example, why do only some of the patients develop the full blown BKVAN syndrome even though seroprevalance is over 85%, or why do some patients with BKVAN respond better to therapy (either reduced immunosuppression or cidofovir) while others have a much poorer outcome. Thus, risk factors associated with BKVAN should be carefully studied and it will be of great clinical interest if biomarkers other than PCR or serum creatinine could be identified that would correlate with disease activity or progression. Finally, there is also an urgent need for high throughput assays capable of screening currently available libraries of chemical compounds for anti-polyomavirus activity that are safer to use and not as nephrotoxic as cidofovir.

References

1. Shah K. Polyomaviruses. In: Fields B, Knipe D, Howley P, eds. Fields Virology. Philadelphia: Lippincott-Raven, 1996:2:2027-2043.
2. Shah KV, Daniel RW, Warszawski RM. High prevalence of antibodies to BK virus, an SV40-related papovavirus, in residents of Maryland. J Infect Dis 1973; 128:784-787.
3. Kazory A, Ducloux D. Renal transplantation and polyomavirus infection: Recent clinical facts and controversies. Transpl Infect Dis 2003: 5:65-71.
4. Hirsch HH, Steiger J. Polyomavirus BK. Lancet Infect Dis 2003; 3:611-623.
5. Baksh FK, Finkelstein SD, Swalsky PA et al. Molecular genotyping of BK and JC viruses in human polyomavirus-associated interstitial nephritis after renal transplantation. Am J Kidney Dis 2001; 38:354-365.
6. Randhawa PS, Demetris AJ. Nephropathy due to polyomavirus type BK. N Engl J Med 2000; 342:1361-1363.
7. Nickeleit V, Singh HK, Mihatsch MJ. Polyomavirus nephropathy: Morphology, pathophysiology, and clinical management. Curr Opin Nephrol Hypertens 2003; 12:599-605.
8. Ramos E, Vincenti F, Lu WX, et al. Retransplantation in patients with graft loss caused by polyoma virus nephropathy. Transplantation 2004; 77:131-133.
9. Gardner SD, MacKenzie EF, Smith C, et al. Prospective study of the human polyomaviruses BK and JC and cytomegalovirus in renal transplant recipients. J Clin Pathol 1984; 37:578-586.
10. Li RM, Mannon RB, Kleiner D et al. BK virus and SV40 coinfection in polyomavirus nephropathy. Transplantation 2002; 74:1497-1504.
11. Trofe J, Gaber LW, Stratta RJ et al. Polyomavirus in kidney and kidney-pancreas transplant recipients. Transpl Infect Dis 2003; 5:21-28.
12. Binet I, Nickeleit V, Hirsch HH et al. Polyomavirus disease under new immunosuppressive drugs: A cause of renal graft dysfunction and graft loss. Transplantation 1999; 67:918-922.
13. Nickeleit V, Hirsch HH, Binet IF et al. Polyomavirus infection of renal allograft recipients: From latent infection to manifest disease. J Am Soc Nephrol 1999; 10:1080-1089.
14. Vats A, Shapiro R, Singh Randhawa P et al. Quantitative viral load monitoring and cidofovir therapy for the management of BK virus-associated nephropathy in children and adults. Transplantation 2003; 75:105-112.
15. Gardner SD, Field AM, Coleman DV et al. New human papovavirus (B.K.) isolated from urine after renal transplantation. Lancet 1971; 1:1253-1257.
16. Hirsch HH, Knowles W, Dickenmann M et al. Prospective study of polyomavirus type BK replication and nephropathy in renal-transplant recipients. N Engl J Med 2002; 347:488-496.
17. Ramos E, Drachenberg CB, Papadimitriou JC et al. Clinical course of polyoma virus nephropathy in 67 renal transplant patients. J Am Soc Nephrol 2002; 13:2145-2151.
18. Haririan A, Ramos ER, Drachenberg CB et al. Polyomavirus nephropathy in native kidneys of a solitary pancreas transplant recipient. Transplantation 2002; 73:1350-1353.
19. Etienne I, Francois A, Redonnet M et al. Does polyomavirus infection induce renal failure in cardiac transplant recipients? Transplant Proc 2000; 32:2794-2795.
20. Pappo O, Demetris AJ, Raikow RB et al. Human polyoma virus infection of renal allografts: Histopathologic diagnosis, clinical significance, and literature review. Mod Pathol 1996; 9:105-109.
21. Nickeleit V, Hirsch HH, Zeiler M et al. BK-virus nephropathy in renal transplants-tubular necrosis, MHC-class II expression and rejection in a puzzling game. Nephrol Dial Transplant 1996; 15:324-332.
22. Nickeleit V, Steiger J, Mihatsch MJ. BK virus infection after kidney transplantation. Graft 2002; 5(Supplement December):S46-S57.
23. Buehrig CK, Lager DJ, Stegall MD et al. Influence of surveillance renal allograft biopsy on diagnosis and prognosis of polyomavirus-associated nephropathy. Kidney Int 2003; 64:665-673.

24. Celik B, Shapiro R, Vats A et al. Polyomavirus allograft nephropathy: Sequential assessment of histologic viral load, tubulitis, and graft function following changes in immunosuppression. Am J Transplant 2003; 3:1378-1382.

25. Randhawa PS, Vats A, Weck K et al. BK virus: Discovery, epidemiology, and biology. Graft 2002; 5(Supplement December):S19-S27.

26. Mayr M, Nickeleit V, Hirsch HH et al. Polyomavirus BK nephropathy in a kidney transplant recipient: Critical issues of diagnosis and management. Am J Kidney Dis 2001; 38:E13.

27. Nickeleit V, Zeiler M, Gudat F et al. Detection of the complement degradation product C4d in renal allografts: Diagnostic and therapeutic implications. J Am Soc Nephrol 2002; 13:242-251.

28. Ahuja M, Cohen EP, Dayer AM et al. Polyoma virus infection after renal transplantation. Use of immunostaining as a guide to diagnosis. Transplantation 2001; 71:896-899.

29. Randhawa PS, Vats A, Zygmunt D et al. Quantitation of viral DNA in renal allograft tissue from patients with BK virus nephropathy. Transplantation2002; 74:485-488.

30. Li RM, Branton MH, Tanawattanacharoen S et al. Molecular identification of SV40 infection in human subjects and possible association with kidney disease. J Am Soc Nephrol 2002; 13:2320-2330.

31. Randhawa P, Baksh F, Aoki N et al. JC virus infection in allograft kidneys: Analysis by polymerase chain reaction and immunohistochemistry. Transplantation 2001; 71:1300-1303.

32. Boldorini R, Omodeo-Zorini E, Suno A et al. Molecular characterization and sequence analysis of polyomavirus strains isolated from needle biopsy specimens of kidney allograft recipients. Am J Clin Pathol 2001; 116:489-494.

33. Chang D, Wang M, Ou WC et al. Genotypes of human polyomaviruses in urine samples of pregnant women in Taiwan. J Med Virol 1996; 48:95-101.

34. Boldorini R, Zorini EO, Vigano P et al. Cytologic and biomolecular diagnosis of polyomavirus infection in urine specimens of HIV-positive patients. Acta Cytol 2000; 44:205-210.

35. Giri JA, Gregoresky J, Silguero P et al. Polyoma virus JC DNA detection by polymerase chain reaction in CSF of HIV infected patients with suspected progressive multifocal leukoencephalopathy. Am Clin Lab 2001; 20:33-35.

36. Nickeleit V, Klimkait T, Binet IF et al. Testing for polyomavirus type BK DNA in plasma to identify renal-allograft recipients with viral nephropathy. N Engl J Med 2000; 342:1309-1315.

37. Drachenberg RC, Drachenberg CB, Papadimitriou JC et al. Morphological spectrum of polyoma virus disease in renal allografts: Diagnostic accuracy of urine cytology. Am J Transplant 2001; 1:373-381.

38. Scantlebury V, Randhawa P, Shapiro R et al. Cidofovir: A Method of Treatment for BK Virus-Associated Transplant Nephropathy. Graft 2002; 5(Supplement December):S82-S87.

39. Limaye AP, Jerome KR, Kuhr CS et al. Quantitation of BK virus load in serum for the diagnosis of BK virus-associated nephropathy in renal transplant recipients. J Infect Dis 2001; 183:1669-1672.

40. Kadambi PV, Josephson MA, Williams J et al. Treatment of refractory BK virus-associated nephropathy with cidofovir. Am J Transplant 2003; 3:186-191.

41. Ramos E, Drachenberg CB, Portocarrero M et al. BK virus nephropathy diagnosis and treatment: Experience at the university of Maryland renal transplant program. Clin Transpl 2002:143-153.

42. Ginevri F, De Santis R, Comoli P et al. Polyomavirus BK infection in pediatric kidney-allograft recipients: A single-center analysis of incidence, risk factors, and novel therapeutic approaches. Transplantation 2003; 75:1266-1270

43. Ding R, Medeiros M, Dadhania D et al. Noninvasive diagnosis of BK virus nephritis by measurement of messenger RNA for BK virus VP1 in urine. Transplantation 2002; 74:987-994.

44. Kitamura T, Yogo Y, Kunitake T et al. Effect of immunosuppression on the urinary excretion of BK and JC polyomaviruses in renal allograft recipients. Int J Urol 1994; 1:28-32.

45. Hirsch HH. Polyomavirus BK nephropathy: A (re)emerging complication in renal transplantation. Am J Transplant 2002; 2:25-30.

46. Lopez-Rocafort L, Wang C, Miller B et al. A prospective evaluation of BK virus infection in renal transplant patients. (abstract) Am J Transplant 2002; 2:S260.

47. Barri YM, Ahmad I, Ketel BL et al. Polyoma viral infection in renal transplantation: The role of immunosuppressive therapy. Clin Transplant 2001; 15:240-246.

48. Howell DN, Smith SR, Butterly DW et al. Diagnosis and management of BK polyomavirus interstitial nephritis in renal transplant recipients. Transplantation 1999; 68:1279-1288.

49. Hirsch HH, Mohaupt M, Klimkait T. Prospective monitoring of BK virus load after discontinuing sirolimus treatment in a renal transplant patient with BK virus nephropathy. J Infect Dis 2001; 184:1494-1495, author reply 1495-1496.

50. Hodur DM, Mandelbrot D. Immunosuppression and BKV Nephropathy. N Engl J Med 2002; 347:2079-2080, author reply 2079-2080.
51. Andrews CA, Shah KV, Daniel RW et al. A serological investigation of BK virus and JC virus infections in recipients of renal allografts. J Infect Dis 1988; 158:176-181
52. Priftakis P, Bogdanovic G, Tyden G et al. Polyomaviruria in renal transplant patients is not correlated to the cold ischemia period or to rejection episodes. J Clin Microbiol 2000; 38:406-407.
53. Randhawa PS, Finkelstein S, Scantlebury V et al. Human polyoma virus-associated interstitial nephritis in the allograft kidney. Transplantation 1999; 67:103-109.
54. Mengel M, Marwedel M, Radermacher J et al. Incidence of polyomavirus-nephropathy in renal allografts: Influence of modern immunosuppressive drugs. Nephrol Dial Transplant 2003; 18:1190-1196.
55. Randhawa P, Zygmunt D, Shapiro R et al. Viral regulatory region sequence variations in kidney tissue obtained from patients with BK virus nephropathy. Kidney Int 2003; 64:743-747.
56. Swarup S, Randhawa P, Singla I et al. Cytokine gene polymorphism is associated with BK virus nephropathy in renal transplantation. J Am Soc Nephrol 2003; 12, [abstract].
57. Seabra C, Perez-Simon JA, Sierra M et al. Intra-muscular vidarabine therapy for polyomavirus-associated hemorrhagic cystitis following allogeneic hemopoietic stem cell transplantation. Bone Marrow Transplant 2000; 26:1229-1230.
58. De Clercq E, Andrei G, Balzarini J et al. Antitumor potential of acyclic nucleoside phosphonates. Nucleosides Nucleotides 1999; 18:759-771.
59. Russell JK, Blalock JE. Vitamin A inhibition of polyoma virus replication. Biochem Biophys Res Commun 1984; 122:851-858.
60. Chen Y, Freund R, Listerud M et al. Retinoic acid inhibits transformation by preventing phosphatidylinositol 3-kinase dependent activation of the c-fos promoter. Oncogene 1999; 18:139-148.
61. Talmage DA, Listerud M. Retinoic acid suppresses polyoma virus transformation by inhibiting transcription of the c-fos proto-oncogene. Oncogene 1994; 9:3557-3563.
62. Portolani M, Pietrosemoli P, Cermelli C et al. Suppression of BK virus replication and cytopathic effect by inhibitors of prokaryotic DNA gyrase. Antiviral Res 1988; 9:205-218.
63. Kerr DA, Chang CF, Gordon J et al. Inhibition of human neurotropic virus (JCV) DNA replication in glial cells by camptothecin. Virology 1993; 196:612-618.
64. Vats A. Viral load monitoring in BK virus-associated nephropathy. Nephrol News Issues 2002; (Suppl):S17-19.
65. Lin PL, Vats AN, Green M. BK virus infection in renal transplant recipients. Pediatr Transplant 2001; 5:398-405.
66. Vats A, Shapiro R, Scantlebury V et al. BK Virus associated nephropathy and cidofovir: Long term experience. Am J Transplant 2003; 3 (Suppl 5):A190,[abstract].
67. De Clercq E. Acyclic nucleoside phosphonates in the chemotherapy of DNA virus and retrovirus infections. Intervirology 1997; 40:295-303.
68. De Clercq E. New inhibitors of human cytomegalovirus (HCMV) on the horizon. J Antimicrob Chemother 2003; 51:1079-1083.
69. Held TK, Biel SS, Nitsche A et al. Treatment of BK virus-associated hemorrhagic cystitis and simultaneous CMV reactivation with cidofovir. Bone Marrow Transplant 2000; 26:347-350.
70. Gonzalez-Fraile MI, Canizo C, Caballero D et al. Cidofovir treatment of human polyomavirus-associated acute haemorrhagic cystitis. Transpl Infect Dis 2001; 3:44-46.
71. Poduval R, Kadambi P, Javaid B et al. Leflunomide: A potential new therapeutic agent for BK nephropathy [abstract]. Am J Transplant 2003; 3(Suppl 5):A189.
72. Foster P, Wright F, McLean D et al. Leflunomide administration as an adjunct in treatment of BK-polyoma viral disease in kidney allografts [abstract]. Am J Transplant 2003; 3(Suppl 5):A421.
73. Cibrik D, O'Toole J, Norman S et al. IVIG for the treatment of transplant BK nephropathy. Am J Transplant 2003; 3(Suppl 5):A370, [abstract].
74. Tata S, Milgrom M, Govani M et al. Novel strategy for the management of polyoma virus nephropathy [abstract]. Am J Transplant 2003; 3(Suppl 5).
75. Poduval RD, Meehan SM, Woodle ES et al. Successful retransplantation after renal allograft loss to polyoma virus interstitial nephritis. Transplantation 2002; 73:1166-1169.
76. Ginevri F, Pastorino N, de Santis R et al. Retransplantation after kidney graft loss due to polyoma BK virus nephropathy: Successful outcome without original allograft nephrectomy. Am J Kidney Dis 2003; 42:821-825.

Chapter 17

Pharmacotherapeutic Options for the Management of Human Polyomaviruses

Julie Roskopf, Jennifer Trofe, Robert J. Stratta and Nasimul Ahsan

Abstract

Polyomaviruses [BK virus (BKV), JC virus (JCV) and simian virus 40 (SV40)] have been known to be associated with diseases in humans for over thirty years. BKV-associated nephropathy and JCV-induced progressive multifocal leukoencephalopathy (PML) were for many years rare diseases occurring only in patients with underlying severe impaired immunity. Over the past decade, the use of more potent immunosuppression (IS) in transplantation, and the Acquired Immune Deficiency Syndrome (AIDS) epidemic, have coincided with a significant increase in the prevalence of these viral complications. Prophylactic and therapeutic interventions for human polyomavirus diseases are limited by our current understanding of polyomaviral pathogenesis. Clinical trials are limited by small numbers of patients affected with clinically significant diseases, lack of defined risk factors and disease definitions, no proven effective treatment and the overall significant morbidity and mortality associated with these diseases. This chapter will focus on a review of the current and future research related to therapeutic targets and interventions for polyomavirus-associated diseases.

Introduction

Polyomaviruses (PV) are nonenveloped, double-stranded deoxyribonucleic acid (DNA) viruses that are ubiquitous in nature. Although 13 types of PV exist, only three species [simian virus 40 (SV40), JC virus (JCV), and BK virus (BKV)] have been reported to be associated with diseases affecting humans.[1] This chapter will focus on pharmacotherapeutic options for the management of BKV and JCV.

Both BKV and JCV were first isolated in immunocompromised patients in 1971.[2,3] Infection with either BKV or JCV is widespread, with seroprevalence rates of up to 90% worldwide.[4] Primary infection typically occurs during childhood, and is largely asymptomatic.[1] After being infected with BK or JC virus, antibodies remain throughout life, but the titer may fluctuate.[5] In immunocompetent hosts, both viruses are known to remain latent in the kidneys and in B-lymphocytes.[5,6] Unlike BKV, JCV may also persist in brain tissue.[1] It is not uncommon for patients to have asymptomatic viruria with BKV or JCV. Viruria is known to occur in 0.3% of nonimmunosuppressed patients,[7] 3.2% of pregnant women,[8] and in 25-44% of patients after kidney transplantation.[1,5,9,10] Clinically significant disease due to PV is primarily found in patients with severely impaired cellular immunity. This would include immunosuppressed recipients of organ, stem cell and bone marrow transplants, patients with primary immunodeficiency diseases, human immunodeficiency virus (HIV) infection, or patients undergoing immunosuppressive chemotherapy.[1,11]

Polyomaviruses and Human Diseases, edited by Nasimul Ahsan. ©2006 Eurekah.com and Springer Science+Business Media.

JC Virus

Upon prolonged suppression of the immune system, JCV replication may result in a fatal demyelinating disease of the central nervous system known as progressive multifocal leukoencephalopathy (PML).[3] JCV has shown oncogenic potential in laboratory animals and has recently been reported to be associated with human medulloblastomas, brain tumors[12-15] and colorectal cancers.[16] There are currently no prophylactic therapies directed at JCV replication to prevent oncogenic related disorders or PML.

Progressive Multifocal Leukoencephalopathy

PML is a neurodegenerative disease of the human central nervous system causing demyelinization of the white matter of the brain, resulting from a lytic infection of oligodendrocytes by JCV.[17] The pathogenesis of JCV in PML is not well understood, and consequently the development of therapeutic targets for the prevention and treatment of JCV-induced PML has been limited. For example, it is unknown if PML is a consequence of initial JCV entry into the central nervous system via infected lymphocytes in the blood,[6] or whether it is a result of reactivation of latent infection.[18,19] Further defining the cellular mechanisms of JCV leading to PML occurrence, could aid in the development of specific therapeutic interventions. Potential targets may be aimed at inhibiting viral entry into the central nervous system, preventing viral activity by blocking JCV cell receptor attachment, or interfering with subsequent processes necessary for viral replication.[20,21]

Although several cases of PML have been reported in patients without an underlying disorder,[22] the majority of patients presenting with PML have a significant degree of immune system suppression due to predisposing conditions such as malignancy, organ transplantation or, more recently, HIV infection.[23] Therefore, in the absence of specific antiviral treatments, a potential target for therapeutic intervention in PML patients is to partially or completely reverse the underlying condition responsible for causing the immune system suppression.[24-28] In patients with HIV infection, as immune reconstitution occurs [usually as a result of administration of highly active antiretroviral therapy (HAART)], an inflammatory response may develop. This inflammatory response is thought in most cases to be beneficial and may eventually prevent PML disease progression.[29] In contrast, rapid immune reconstitution due to HAART may paradoxically worsen the course of PML and, therefore, gradual reversal of immune deficiency might be associated with better outcomes.[30] A report based on 43 HIV-infected patients with PML has proposed that HAART associated immune reconstitution may play a role in the development of PML. Eight (19%) patients presented with PML symptoms 21-55 days after the initiation of HAART, concomitant with a decrease in HIV load and an increase in CD4 cell count. Four (50%) subsequently died of PML. Apart from baseline viral load, no other variable could distinguish these cases of PML occurring during immune reconstitution from those occurring in patients either untreated or failing to respond to therapy. A subset of 23 patients untreated with HAART at the time of onset of PML was compared for viroimmunological response to patients who initiated HAART and developed PML, but no different pattern of response to HAART was observed between patients who either died or survived. Therefore, the authors concluded that although no direct deleterious effect of HAART on PML could be identified, prompt initiation of HAART after PML diagnosis and subsequent successful response to HAART were often associated with poor PML outcomes.[31] Certainly, the benefits, and detrimental effects of the inflammatory response in HIV-infected patients with PML requires further investigation.

HIV infection is currently the most common underlying disorder associated with PML, with up to 5% of all HIV-infected patients eventually developing this infectious complication.[32] The reason why PML has seemed to increase disproportionately in HIV infection compared to other predisposing immune system altering conditions (such as organ transplantation or malignancy), is uncertain.[33] One proposed explanation is that the presence of HIV infection may contribute to a state of more profound immunosuppression (IS) than that seen with other

PML predisposing conditions, or HIV may directly play a role in JCV pathogenesis.[33-35] Although HAART targets HIV infection, the multifactorial pathogenic role of HIV infection in JCV-induced PML requires more study.

Historically, the prognosis of PML in patients with HIV infection was poor, with death occurring within three to four months from the time of initial disease manifestations.[27] To date, none of the antiviral treatments, including cytarabine (Ara-C), alpha-interferon, cidofovir and topotecan, have shown a clearly defined beneficial effect on disease progression.[36-40] Conversely, the introduction of HAART has had a significant impact on opportunistic infections and has improved the survival of patients with PML.[26,30,41] Median survival from PML in the HAART era has increased from 4 months to 10.5 months.[26] The increase in survival may be attributed to disease stabilization in approximately half of the patients, whereas the remainder do not show any longer survival than before the introduction of HAART.[42] Recently, definitions for consensus PML terminology[43] and clinical trial guidelines[44] to test the efficacy of therapeutic agents in PML with patient survival as the primary endpoint have been proposed.

BK Virus

BKV is most frequently associated with nephropathy and ureteral stenosis in renal transplant recipients, and nonhemorrhagic and hemorrhagic cystitis (HC) in bone marrow and stem cell transplant recipients.[45,46] Clinical disease with BKV manifests principally in the genitourinary tract, because the virus is known to remain latent in transitional epithelium.[45,46] There is currently no standardized treatment available for patients diagnosed with BKV-associated disease. The most common treatment strategy is to reduce or discontinue immunosuppressive drugs and treatments, if possible. This approach is designed to reduce viral replication, but may be associated with risks such as acute rejection and graft loss in renal transplant recipients, so patients must be monitored closely.[11,47]

BKV-Associated Hemorrhagic Cystitis

Hemorrhagic cystitis (HC) is a well-defined complication following treatment with high-dose cyclophosphamide, which is often used in bone marrow or stem cell transplant patients. HC typically occurs within 48 hours of cyclophosphamide infusion. HC associated with viruses, including adenovirus, JCV and BKV, differ in that it most commonly occurs late and is long lasting. Review of the literature suggests that reactivation of latent BKV is common in both autologous and allogeneic bone marrow transplant recipients, occurring in 60% to 100% of patients. In patients with viruria, 50% to 64% develop HC. In patients with HC, BK viruria has been detected in 56% to 80% of patients.[48,49] Late onset HC is strongly associated with BKV viruria, however, a causal link has never been fully established. Renal dysfunction associated with HC is the result of clot retention and urinary tract obstruction, without direct involvement of the renal parenchyma.[48,50]

The treatment of HC is largely supportive and usually includes hydration, alkalinization of the urine, bladder irrigation, pain management, antibiotics, and maintaining an adequate platelet count.[45,51-53] The intravesical instillation of drugs such as formalin, alum, silver nitrate and prostaglandin E2 (PGE2) may also be used for severe cases of HC, but side effects such as bladder spasms limit their clinical utility.[54,55] Several case reports have described the use of two antiviral agents, vidarabine and cidofovir, to successfully treat BKV-associated HC. This is described in detail later in this chapter.

Polyomavirus-Associated Nephropathy in Transplant Recipients

Historically, the majority of PVN was due to BKV. Although some studies have found the presence of JCV and SV40 in conjunction with BKV on renal biopsies of patients with PVN, the pathogenic role of SV40 or JCV remains unknown.[56-58] Recent studies have demonstrated that BKV causes nephropathy in up to 8% of kidney transplant patients, and leads to kidney allograft failure in as many as 70% of PVN cases.[10,47,59-71] Certain risk factors, such as multiple acute rejection episodes and the availability of more potent immunosuppressive medications [including tacrolimus and mycophenolate mofetil (MMF)], have been associated with PVN.[69,72] However, prospective studies to date have been unable to identify either antibody induction therapy, or any specific maintenance immunosuppressive agent or combination, as the cause of PVN.[9,10] In a prospective, 2:1 randomized evaluation of kidney transplant recipients receiving rabbit anti-thymocyte globulin and either tacrolimus (n = 32) or cyclosporine (n = 18) in combination with MMF/azathioprine and corticosteroids, an interim analysis at 43 weeks showed no difference in the incidence of viruria or viremia between the tacrolimus and cyclosporine groups, and PVN was not observed.[9] This is the only study to date that has examined whether a reduction in IS when BKV is detected early, may prevent the development of clinically significant PVN.

Even though IS seems to be a prerequisite for PVN, the interaction between several factors such as IS, preexisting recipient factors, and tubular injury (due to a variety of causes such as drug toxicity, ischemic injury, and rejection episodes), may be responsible for the development of PVN.[73-77] Patients have been diagnosed with PVN between 2-60 months after transplant, but are most commonly diagnosed within the first 12 months post-transplant.[59,77,78] Patients often present with an asymptomatic rise in serum creatinine (SCr), necessitating further investigation. Unfortunately, in most cases, renal dysfunction is representative of a late stage of PVN, occurring as a result of BKV-associated renal allograft injury.[70,79] Confirmation of the diagnosis requires biopsy of the allograft and the use of either immunohistochemical analysis, in situ hybridization, or BKV PCR on the renal transplant biopsy specimen.[80] These advanced techniques are needed to distinguish if the tubular injury is due to the virus or the presence of concurrent acute rejection.[47,68,77,81]

A better understanding of how to manage PVN is slowly evolving. Historically, it was difficult to exclude concurrent acute rejection on biopsy. Therefore, many patients were given intensified immunosuppressive regimens to treat acute rejection. Based on the following data, most authors have concluded that it is best to avoid anti-T-cell agents such as muromonab-CD3 (Orthoclone® OKT3) and anti-thymocyte preparations after a diagnosis of PVN has been made. However, if acute rejection is found concomitantly on tissue biopsy, patients may benefit from pulsed steroid therapy followed by a reduction in baseline IS.[74,77]

Hussain et al[82] described their experience in patients diagnosed with PVN (Table 1). They compared seven patients who received OKT3 or equine antithymocyte globulin (Atgam®) at the time of diagnosis, to seven patients who did not. In the OKT3/Atgam group, all 7 (100%) grafts were lost, whereas only 2 (29%) grafts were lost in the other group. Randhawa and colleagues[47] reported their initial experience with 12 patients diagnosed with PVN. All patients were given empiric steroids. Only 1/12 (8%) patients cleared the virus, and 3/12 (25%) had a partial response. The other eight patients that did not respond were managed with a reduction in baseline IS, with graft failure occurring in 8/12 (67%) patients. Ahuja et al[68] also treated ten patients with PVN; 9/10 (90%) were given steroids at diagnosis and one patient also received Atgam followed by OKT3. This approach resulted in a 70% rate of graft loss. Mengel et al[72] prospectively evaluated all biopsies performed at the Hannover Medical School in Germany. Seven patients were diagnosed with PVN. Acute rejection was found in 6/7 biopsies. In the first three patients, no change or an intensification in IS was made. In the next four patients, IS was initially reduced. Overall, 5/7 (71%) of grafts were lost to PVN, and another graft was lost in a patient who died from heart failure. In another study by Nickeleit and colleagues,[63-66] 11 patients diagnosed with PVN were given antirejection therapy if concurrent acute rejection was detected on biopsy. As their awareness of PVN evolved, patients were managed with an initial decrease in IS. The overall rate of graft loss was 5/11 (45%).

Other authors have reported better outcomes associated with the initial use of antirejection therapy in the setting of PVN. Howell et al[62] diagnosed PVN at nephrectomy in one patient who was given antirejection therapy and an increase in maintenance IS. In three patients initially given antirejection therapy followed later by a decrease in IS, and in three other patients

Table 1. *Management and outcomes in polyomavirus-associated nephropathy*

| Source | PVN Cases | Anti-Rejection Therapy | Baseline Immunosuppression | | | Graft Loss Due to PVN |
			Decrease	Increase	No Change	
Hussain et al[82]	14	11	14	—	—	9/14 (64%)
Randhawa et al[47]	22	12	16	—	6	10/22 (45%)
Ahuja et al[68]	10	9	10	—	—	7/10 (70%)
Mengel et al[72]	7	—	4	1	2	5/7 (71%)
Nickeleit et al[63-66]	11	n/a	n/a	n/a	n/a	5/11 (45%)
Howell et al[62]	7	4	6	1	—	1/7 (14%)
Huralt de Ligny et al[83]	10	9	8	2	—	2/10 (20%)
Rahamimov et al[84]	7	7	6	—	1	1/7 (14%)
Li et al[57]	6	3	6	—	—	1/6 (17%)
Ramos et al[78]	67	—	52	—	15	11/67 (16%)
Buehrig et al[70]	18	3	18	—	—	7/18 (39%)
Trofe et al[60]	13	—	10	—	3	7/13 (54%)
Trofe et al[58]	10	—	10	—	—	1/10 (10%)
Barri et al[69]	8	3	7	—	1	2/8 (25%)
Ginevri et al[61]	5	—	5	—	—	1/5 (20%)
Hirsch et al[9]	5	4	5	—	—	0/5 (0%)
Totals	220	63 (29%)	177 (80%)	4 (2%)	28 (13%)	69/220 (31%)

PVN—polyomavirus-associated nephropathy; n/a—data not available.

managed with an initial decrease in IS, no patient experienced graft loss. Hurault de Ligny and colleagues[83] diagnosed ten patients with PVN. Nine patients were given treatment for acute rejection at the time of PVN diagnosis. Two patients managed with an increase in basal IS experienced graft loss, while the other eight patients managed by a reduction in IS stabilized their renal function. Rahamimov et al[84] diagnosed seven patients with PVN; one patient was given anti-thymocyte globulin to treat rejection, and the other six were given increased oral steroids along with a reduction in basal IS. The overall rate of graft loss was 1/7 (14%). Li et al[57] identified six patients with PVN; all were managed with a decrease in IS, but three received pulsed steroids to treat acute rejection. Five patients have maintained graft function while the remaining patient (1/6 = 17%) experienced graft loss.

Several authors have reported their clinical experience with decreasing IS when PVN is initially diagnosed. The largest experience to date is by Ramos et al,[78] who diagnosed PVN in 67 patients between June 1997 and March 2001. An initial decrease in IS was performed in 52 patients, while no specific IS intervention was made in 15 patients. The overall rate of graft loss was 11/67 (16.4%). Buehrig and colleagues[70] reported their experience with 18 patients diagnosed with PVN; all patients were ultimately managed with a decrease in maintenance IS, but three were given a steroid bolus or a modest temporary increase in baseline IS to initially treat acute rejection. Satisfactory results occurred in 11 patients (61%), while the remaining seven (39%) had poor outcomes (graft loss, increased severity of PVN on repeat biopsy, or SCr > 3 mg/dl at 6 months after diagnosis). Trofe et al[60] reported their experience at the University of Tennessee-Memphis with 13 patients diagnosed with PVN; ten patients were managed with a decrease in maintenance IS, while three patients (who received a kidney-pancreas transplant) were not. Graft loss occurred in 7/13 (54%) of patients. Trofe et al[58] also reported the results of ten patients at the University of Cincinnati diagnosed with PVN. All patients were managed with an initial decrease in baseline IS. Graft loss occurred in only one patient (10%). Barri et al[69] reported their experience with eight patients diagnosed with PVN; three patients were given antirejection therapy followed by a decrease in maintenance IS, baseline IS was reduced in four patients, and one patient had no intervention. Graft loss occurred in 2/8 (25%) of patients, but one patient was lost to follow-up and stopped taking their IS. Ginevri and colleagues[61] managed five pediatric kidney transplant recipients with PVN; a decrease in baseline IS was performed in all patients, and one patient was treated with cidofovir. Only one patient (20%) experienced graft loss.

Although the majority of data describing PVN in kidney transplantation is based on retrospective analyses, one prospective study has been published to date. Hirsch et al[10] followed 78 renal transplant patients at University Hospitals in Basel, Switzerland. The primary outcomes were the detection of decoy cells in the urine using the Papanicolaou method, the detection of BKV DNA in the plasma, and the development of PVN in allograft biopsy specimens. Routine screening for viruria was performed every month for the first six months, during any hospitalization, if allograft function declined, or if a biopsy was performed. BKV DNA was measured in the plasma using a nested PCR assay at three, six and twelve months, and when viruria was present. A biopsy was performed if the SCr increased by ≥ 25%, and all biopsies were stained for polyomavirus specific antigen. The median follow-up was 85 weeks (range 43-130). Viruria developed in 23 patients, viremia developed in ten patients, and PVN was detected on biopsy in five patients. Using a Kaplan-Meier analysis, the probability of developing viruria was 30% (95% CI 20-40%), the probability of developing viremia was 13% (95% CI 5-21%), and the probability of developing PVN was 8 % (95% CI 1-15%). Concurrent acute rejection was detected in 4/5 (80%) patients. Three patients were treated with steroids and one patient was given anti-T-cell therapy. Baseline IS was modified in all patients at the time PVN was diagnosed. The overall graft survival rate in the group was 96%, with no graft loss due to PVN. Factors found to contribute to BKV reactivation/disease included the use of steroids to treat acute rejection, but BKV did not correlate with the induction IS therapy used. The authors concluded that screening for decoy cells in the urine is simple and always precedes PVN, and that the use of quantitative BKV viremia can be useful since the mean viral load was significantly higher in patients with PVN (28,000 vs. 2,000 copies/ml, P < 0.001 by the Mann-Whitney U test).

Better diagnostic testing and more experience suggest that in the case of PVN, early detection is imperative. It is also important to distinguish PVN from acute rejection so that anti-rejection therapy is not given inappropriately. The mainstay of therapy is to lower the amount of maintenance IS in an attempt to allow the patient's immune defenses to overcome the viral infection.[47,62,68,69] Several approaches have been advocated, including reducing or stopping azathioprine, MMF, or sirolimus; using lower target concentrations of the calcineurin inhibitors (cyclosporine or tacrolimus); switching from one calcineurin inhibitor to another; or stopping the calcineurin inhibitor completely. These approaches have resulted in a variety of different outcomes (Table 1). A better prognosis is likely if PVN is suspected and diagnosed early, followed by an immediate reduction in IS. Many patients, however, may still have persistent allograft dysfunction that may progress to chronic allograft nephropathy with eventual graft loss. This has led to the search for novel therapeutic agents that may be used as an adjunct to treat PVN.

Targets for Pharmacotherapeutic Intervention (Table 2)

The receptors for viral entry differ for polyomaviruses. BKV, JCV, and murine polyomavirus use sialoglycoproteins as primary receptors for viral entry.[21,85-87] In contrast, SV40 has receptors related to the MHC system.[85,88] Many viruses enter host cells using the endocytic pathway that utilizes clathrin-coated vesicles.[89] JC virions have recently been shown to use this endocytic pathway for cell entry.[87] SV40 and murine polyomavirus, however, are internalized in nonclathrin-coated vesicles called caveolae.[21] Recently, BK virions have also been shown to enter renal tubular cells in smooth monopinocytotic vesicles consistent with caveolae.[88] Chlorpromazine has been shown to inhibit clathrin dependent endoctyosis of JCV, but has no significant activity against BKV.[90] Since chlorpromazine is associated with the development of extrapyramidal symptoms that may be heightened in HIV-infected patients (due to basal ganglia deficits in AIDS patients), clozapine, an atypical anti-pyschotic agent that is associated with less severe side effects, has also been evaluated for antiviral activity against JCV.[91] Clozapine was found to be as effective as chlorpromazine at inhibiting infection. Furthermore, the combination of low dose chlorpromazine and clozapine was shown to synergistically inhibit infection in vitro in glial cells. It is unknown, however, if these drugs can inhibit already active infection.[91] Therefore, further in vitro studies followed by initiation of clinical trials are necessary to determine the efficacy and safety of these drug combinations in the treatment of PML.

In vitro, nystatin inhibits caveolae activity associated with SV40 and BKV entry, but to date, has not been evaluated in vivo for BKV.[92-94] Further research into the efficacy and dosing of nystatin necessary to inhibit PVN in vivo are required prior to recommending it for therapeutic use.

Caveolae containing either SV40 or BK virions appear to use an extensive network of tubules and vesicles to transport the virions to the nucleus. The mechanism of nuclear entry, however, remains unclear for all of the polyomaviruses. The virus multiplies in the nucleus and involves the structural proteins VP1, VP2, and VP3. Polyomaviruses do not encode viral DNA polymerases, but they rely extensively on host-cell enzymes, thereby providing potential targets for therapeutic intervention.[74] The majority of virions in infected cells appear to remain within the nucleus until released by cell lysis.[88]

Retinoic acids, 5-bromo-2'-deoxyuridine and prokaryotic DNA gyrase inhibitors have been shown to inhibit PV in vitro but have not been tested in clinical trials.[95-99] Several other compounds have been evaluated in vitro for their inhibitory activity against murine polyomavirus and SV40 strains. Many compounds, including acyclovir, ganciclovir, penciclovir, brivudine, ribavirin, vidarabine [Ara-A], and foscarnet, were found to have minimal or no activity against polyomavirus replication, whereas cidofovir [HPMPC: (S)-1-(3-hydroxy-2-phosphonylmethoxypropyl)cytosine] and cyclic HPMPC were found to be the most selective inhibitors.[100-102] Leflunomide [N-(4-trifluoromethylphenyl)-5-methylisoxazole-4-carboxamide] is a known immunosuppressive agent that is reported to have antiviral properties, and may have a role in the management of PVN.[71,103] The malononitrilamide (MNA) compound FK-778 {2-cyano-3-hydroxy-N-[4-(trifluoromethyl)phenyl]-2-hepten-6-yonic acid amide} is currently being evaluated in a phase II clinical trial in kidney transplant recipients. It is a derivative of leflunomide's active metabolite A77-1726 and has been shown in vitro to possess activity against polyomavirus.[104] Cytarabine (Ara-C) and topotecan have shown in vitro activity against JCV, and clinical data exists in humans. Another potential therapeutic target that is currently being studied are the antisense oligonucleotides.[35] These agents

Table 2. Potential targets for therapeutic intervention

	JC Virus	BK Virus
Modulation of overall immune status	yes	yes
Chlorpromazine/clozapine	yes	no
Nystatin	no	yes
Retinoic acids	yes	yes
DNA gyrase inhibitors	yes	yes
Vidarabine/cytarabine	yes	yes
Cidofovir	no	yes
Leflunomide	?	yes
Topotecan	yes	?
Antisense oligonucleotides	?	?
Interferon-alpha	no	yes
Interferon-beta	?	?
Intravenous immune globulin	?	yes

Yes—in vivo/in vitro data shows activity; no—in vivo/in vitro data shows no activity; ?—no data available.

have been shown to inhibit viral DNA replication and transcription[105] and techniques for drug delivery to the brain are currently being studied.[106]

The remainder of this chapter will focus on a review of therapeutic agents that have been used to treat polyomavirus related diseases (PML, HC and PVN) in humans.

Specific Pharmacotherapeutic Intervention

Cidofovir

Cidofovir (Vistide®) is currently approved for use in the treatment of CMV retinitis in patients with acquired immunodeficiency syndrome (AIDS).[107] It is often reserved for patients who are intolerant, unresponsive or relapse on drugs such as ganciclovir or foscarnet.[102,108] Cidofovir is being evaluated for its activity against other viruses, including BKV and JCV, however, it is not approved for use in these settings.

Mechanism of Action

Cidofovir is an acyclic nucleoside phosphonate that is active against virtually all herpesviruses, as well as polyomaviruses, papillomaviruses, adenoviruses, iridoviruses, and poxviruses (Fig. 1). The spectrum of activity for cidofovir is very different from classic acyclic nucleoside analogues such as acyclovir, penciclovir and ganciclovir. To exert antiviral activity, these agents require phosphorylation by viral nucleoside kinases. In contrast, this initial phosphorylation step is not needed for cidofovir.[109] In murine models, cidofovir is more effective than acyclovir against herpes simplex virus (HSV) infection, and more effective than ganciclovir against cytomegalovirus (CMV) infection.[101,102] The active intracellular metabolite, cidofovir diphosphate, suppresses viral replication by interfering with DNA transcription following incorporation into the growing DNA chain.[109]

Pharmacokinetics

Cidofovir is extensively metabolized intracellularly. It is phosphorylated by cellular enzymes to its active diphosphate form. Cidofovir has minimal protein binding (0.5%), and is not thought to undergo systemic metabolism. When 5 mg/kg doses of cidofovir are used with probenecid and hydration, the volume of distribution is 300 ml/kg, and the renal clearance is 80 ml/kg/hr. The half life of the parent compound is 2.5 hours, however, the antiviral activity is related to the intracellular concentrations of the active phosphorylated metabolite (half-life 65 hours).[102,110] The accumulation of this metabolite allows for a prolonged antiviral effect with infrequent dosing. The majority of each cidofovir dose (70-85%) is excreted renally within 24 hours as unchanged drug in patients who have received probenecid, and approximately 80-100% of the drug is excreted unchanged without probenecid.

Dosing and Adverse Events

The dosing of cidofovir recommended for AIDS patients is 5 mg/kg once each week for two doses (induction phase) followed by the same dose every other week (maintenance phase). Each dose is diluted in 100 ml normal saline and infused intravenously (IV) at a constant rate over 1 hour. Cidofovir is contraindicated in patients with a SCr >1.5 mg/dl, a calculated creatinine clearance ≤ 55 ml/min, or a urine protein ≥ 100 mg/dl. The dose must also be reduced or discontinued if the patient's renal function deteriorates during therapy. To minimize the risk of nephrotoxicity when treating CMV retinitis, cidofovir is routinely given with high-dose oral probenecid (used to block the uptake of cidofovir by the proximal tubular cells), and saline hydration (at least one liter of sodium chloride 0.9%) prior to each dose. When cidofovir is used to treat CMV retinitis, the most common clinical adverse events reported include nephrotoxicity (specifically proteinuria), nausea, vomiting, and fever.[111] Cidofovir has also been associated with neutropenia and intraocular inflammation (uveitis).

Clinical Experience

Progressive Multifocal Leukoencephalopathy

Although an initial in vitro study showed the efficacy of cidofovir against SV40 and murine polyomaviruses,[100] a second in vitro study found it to be ineffective at inhibiting JCV replication.[112] Anecdotal PML experiences have shown some benefit with cidofovir treatment in both HIV and nonHIV-infected patients,[113-118] while others have advocated a role for combined HAART and cidofovir for HIV-infected patients with PML.[108,119,120] In contrast, other studies have found no benefit of cidofovir for the treatment of PML.[113,121,122] These results, however, are difficult to interpret due to small sample sizes and the coadministration of HAART in HIV-infected patients.

A multicenter, observational study evaluated consecutive HIV-infected patients with virologically or histologically proven PML treated with either HAART alone (n = 26) or HAART plus cidofovir 5 mg/kg IV per week for 12 weeks and alternate weeks thereafter (n = 14).[123] After two months of therapy, 5/12 (42%) patients receiving HAART alone and 7/8 (87%) patients receiving HAART and cidofovir, reached undetectable JCV DNA in the cerebrospinal fluid (CSF) (Chi-square, P = 0.04). Furthermore, 24% of HAART alone patients and 57% of HAART plus cidofovir patients showed neurological improvement or stability (P = 0.038). One-year cumulative probability of survival was 0.67 with cidofovir and 0.31 without (log-rank test, P = 0.01). Variables found to be independently associated with longer survival were the use of cidofovir, HAART prior to the onset of PML, a baseline JCV DNA load in CSF < 4.7 log10 copies/ml, and a baseline Karnofsky performance status ≥ 60. The authors concluded that in HIV-infected patients with PML, cidofovir added to HAART was associated with more effective control of JCV replication, with improved neurological outcome and survival compared with HAART alone. An extended follow-up for this study at a median of 132 weeks post diagnosis found that the one-year cumulative probability of survival was 0.61 with cidofovir and 0.29 without (log rank test, P = 0.02).[124] After adjusting for baseline CD4 counts, JCV load in the CSF, Karnofsky performance status, and use of HAART prior to the onset of PML, the use of cidofovir was still found to be independently associated with a reduced risk of death (hazard ratio, 0.21; 95% confidence interval, 0.07-0.65; P = 0.005).

In contrast, a single center observational study compared 22 patients treated with HAART alone to 24 patients treated with cidofovir and HAART for PML in HIV-infected patients. At six months, JCV load in the CSF was below the detection level in 8/24 (33%) patients in the cidofovir plus HAART group and 7/18 (39%) patients in the HAART alone group (P = 0.71). One-year cumulative probability of survival was 62% in the cidofovir plus HAART group and 53% in the HAART alone group (P = 0.72). The authors concluded that the addition of cidofovir to HAART had no significant benefit.[40]

Because of these conflicting results, a prospective, multicenter, open-label, pilot study was recently conducted. Twenty-four HIV-infected patients with symptoms of PML for 90 days or less, received cidofovir 5 mg/kg IV at baseline and one week, followed by infusions every two weeks with dose adjustments for renal function. Probenecid was administered based on weight and saline infusions were administered before and after each cidofovir dose. Eligibility criteria did not include the use of antiretroviral agents, and no specific regimen or duration of therapy was required. Seventeen (71%) patients also received potent antiretroviral therapy defined as at least three antiretroviral agents at study entry. For 15 (88%) patients, the regimen included a protease inhibitor. Follow-up continued to 24 weeks. Results showed that a higher CD4-cell count at study entry was significantly associated with survival (P = 0.02). Two (8%) patients underwent cidofovir dose reduction for neutropenia and elevated serum creatinine, respectively. Five (21%) patients discontinued cidofovir treatment because of toxicity; a 50% or greater decrease in intraocular pressure in either eye (n = 4), and proteinuria (n = 1). Twelve (50%) deaths occurred, with 11 (46%) patients dying from PML during the 24 weeks of follow-up. As a result of toxicity or patient death, 14 (58%) patients discontinued study treatment by week 12, and only seven of the ten remaining patients completed 24 weeks of treatment. The median duration of treatment was seven weeks (range 1-23) and the median number of cidofovir doses was five (range 1-13). Only two (8%) patients experienced a 25% or greater improvement in neurological examination scores at week eight. The authors concluded that cidofovir did not improve neurological examination scores at week eight. In a secondary analysis, patients who entered the study with suppressed plasma HIV RNA levels (500 copies/ml or less), had significantly better scores at eight weeks compared to patients who entered the study with plasma HIV RNA levels of greater than 500 copies/mL. The authors proposed that cidofovir may confer some benefit in patients who have already had a virological response to potent antiretroviral therapy, or who are controlling HIV infection by their own immune mechanisms.[37] The authors also propose that their results may simply mean that individuals with control of HIV infection may have a less aggressive clinical course of PML. Since a control group was not evaluated in this study, the authors cannot differentiate between these two theories, and a prospective controlled study would be required to determine whether cidofovir confers a benefit beyond that of potent antiretroviral therapy for PML. Nevertheless, this prospective trial failed to show significant benefit of cidofovir for PML in HIV-infected patients above that seen with antiretroviral therapy alone.

In summary, although some positive experiences with cidofovir have been reported, cidofovir was not found to be effective for PML in HIV-infected patients in a prospective multi-center trial.[37] Moreover, HIV-infected patients with high JCV load and/or low CD4-cell counts do not respond to potent antiretroviral or antiretroviral plus cidofovir combinations.[124,125] The current belief is that immune reconstitution is a requisite for clinical improvement.[35]

BKV-Associated Hemorrhagic Cystitis

There are several case reports describing the use of cidofovir for BKV-associated HC in bone marrow and stem cell transplant recipients.[51,52,126,127] In one patient, after palliative treatment of HC failed, cidofovir was initiated at 5 mg/kg/week IV for two weeks, followed by 5 mg/kg IV every two weeks for a month (total of four doses over six weeks) with concurrent probenecid to minimize the risk for nephrotoxicity. Symptoms improved after two weeks, and BK viruria cleared. The patient experienced nausea and vomiting, thought to be secondary to probenecid, and also a slight increase in SCr that resolved in one week with IV hydration.[51] Another patient, who had CMV reactivation in addition to BKV-associated HC, was treated with cidofovir. Cidofovir was given as an initial 5 mg/kg infusion, and was repeated at one week and three weeks. Probenecid and IV hydration were also given simultaneously. As the BK viruria improved, the patients symptoms of HC improved, and the CMV antigenemia became negative. During treatment, the SCr fluctuated, but it never exceeded 1.8 mg/dl and always returned to baseline.[126] In a third patient, cidofovir was used for BKV-associated HC, but treatment failed and the patient underwent cystectomy.[52] In another case report, a 15 year old male developed HC and renal dysfunction after allogeneic BMT. Both BKV and adenovirus type 11 were detected in the urine. Initially, a course of IV vidarabine was given (10 mg/kg/day for 5 days) without improvement. He was later given cidofovir (1 mg/kg IV three times a week) along with probenecid. He complained of mild nausea (likely due to probenecid) but otherwise tolerated the regimen well. After seven doses of cidofovir his renal function normalized and the HC resolved.[127] Based on these and other anecdotal reports, cidofovir may be safe and effective for treating HC in the setting of BKV, and should be considered for patients who fail conventional methods for controlling HC.

Polyomavirus-Associated Nephropathy

Based on in vitro findings, attention has focused on the therapeutic use of cidofovir as an adjunct to managing patients with PVN. The successful use of cidofovir has been described in several case reports,[128-132] (Table 3) but the largest experience to date has been reported from the University of Pittsburgh. Cidofovir was used in 16 renal transplant patients diagnosed with PVN.[131,132] In addition to a kidney transplant, two had also received a simultaneous pancreas transplant, and one patient had previously received a liver transplant. In 12 patients, the diagnosis of PVN was made using renal biopsy specimens, and in four patients the diagnosis was made by plasma DNA-PCR assay (two patients diagnosed using both methods simultaneously). Patients had a median age of 48.5 years (range 6-70), the time to diagnosis was 3-73 months, and the male-to-female ratio was 13:3. IS was decreased in all patients at the time of diagnosis. Tacrolimus was decreased and steroids were decreased or discontinued. If patients were on MMF or sirolimus, it was almost always stopped. Cidofovir was administered as 0.2-1 mg/kg/dose every 1-4 weeks IV for a total of 1-7 doses (mean 2.7 doses per patient). Low doses (5-20% of the dose recommended for the treatment of CMV retinitis, given less often) were used, since the majority of cidofovir (80-100%) is excreted unchanged in the kidney, and the goal was to treat virus localized in the kidney. Overall, the SCr improved in five (31%) patients and stabilized in five (31%). In two (13%) patients the SCr increased but then stabilized, and the remaining four (25%) patients developed graft failure. Using a quantitative polymerase chain reaction (PCR) assay for BKV, the majority of patients [14/16 (88%)] showed clearance of viremia. Most patients [15/16 (94%)] also had either a transient clearance or reduction in viruria. No lasting nephrotoxicity was attributed to the use of low dose cidofovir. Only one patient appeared to be completely unresponsive to intervention with cidofovir and it is possible that this patient was infected with a drug-resistant virus. Several patients have had recurrence of the viruria, and therefore, after treatment, patients still need to be monitored closely. The authors suggest that quantitative PCR testing can be used to diagnose and manage the course of PVN, and that cidofovir therapy may be beneficial in select patients, especially those who have not responded to a reduction in IS. The authors also state that patients may benefit from a gradual increase in the cidofovir dose with each treatment in an attempt to clear the virus earlier.

When cidofovir is used to treat PVN, lower doses must be used. This helps to minimize the risk for developing adverse events such as dose-dependent nephrotoxicity. Probenecid has not been advocated for use in patients being treated for PVN, to allow for maximal excretion of the drug by the kidney, but prehydration with normal saline is still recommended. In addition, a second liter of fluid may be given over 1-3 hours during or after the cidofovir infusion if the patient will tolerate it.

Table 3. Use of cidofovir in polyomavirus-associated nephropathy

Source	Patient #	Pharmacologic Management	Outcome/Comments
Bjorang et al[128]	1	Decrease IS	SCr improved and stabilized
		• 8 months later required antirejection therapy and after 4 months polyoma detected again Decrease IS further and given cidofovir	
Keller et al[129]	1	Decrease IS and given cidofovir	SCr improved and plasma viral load became negative *Overall graft failure: 0/1 (0%)*
			SCr improved, plasma viral load became negative and repeat biopsy negative for polyomavirus *Overall graft ailure: 0/1 (0%)*
Kadambi et al[130]	2	2 patients: Decrease IS and given cidofovir	2/2 SCr improved, plasma viral load became negative and repeat biopsies negative for polyomavirus *Overall graft failure: 0/2 (0%)*
Vats et al[131]	4	3 patients: Decrease IS 1 patient: No decrease IS All patients given cidofovir	4/4 SCr improved and in 3 patients initially with positive viremia, viremia cleared before viruria *Overall graft failure: 0/4 (0%)*
Scantlebury et al[132]	16 13 KTX 2 KPTX 1 KALTX	16 patients: Decrease IS All patients given cidofovir	5/16 (31%) SCr improved 5/16 (31%) SCr stabilized 2/16 (13%) SCr increased but then stabilized 4/16 (25%) graft loss *Overall graft failure: 4/16 (25%)*
Total	24	—	Overall Graft Failure: 4/24 (16.7%)

IS—immunosuppression; KTX—kidney transplant; KPTX—kidney-pancreas transplant; KALTX—kidney after liver transplant; SCr—serum creatinine.

Leflunomide

Leflunomide (Arava®) is a novel disease modifying anti-rheumatic drug (DMARD) with anti-inflammatory, anti-proliferative and immunomodulative properties that was approved for the treatment of active rheumatoid arthritis in 1998.[133] Leflunomide is chemically unrelated to other immunosuppressants including cyclosporine and tacrolimus, and it is currently being evaluated in many different disease states including transplantation.

Mechanism of Action

Leflunomide is an isoxazole derivative. Its immunosuppressive properties are due to the inhibition of the enzyme dihydroorotate dehydrogenase (DHODH), as well as its ability to interfere with protein tyrosine kinases. DHODH interferes with the de novo synthesis of pyrimidine nucleotides, and ultimately induces cell-cycle arrest and inhibits lymphocyte clonal expansion.[134-136] Leflunomide has also demonstrated antiviral activity against cytomegalovirus (CMV) and herpes simplex virus-1 (HSV-1).[134,137,138] In vitro studies have shown that in contrast to other anti-CMV and anti-HSV agents used today, leflunomide acts at a late stage in virion assembly, rather than interfering with viral DNA synthesis.

Pharmacokinetics

Leflunomide is a prodrug that is rapidly metabolized to the active major metabolite, A77-1726. This metabolite is a MNA compound and is responsible for the large majority of its pharmacologic activity. Pharmacokinetic studies have primarily evaluated the plasma concentrations of the active metabolite A77-1726, since leflunomide concentrations are usually undetectable after oral administration. Peak plasma levels of the active metabolite occur between 6-12 hours after an oral dose. A loading dose of leflunomide is recommended due to the long half-life of A77-1726 of approximately 15 days. Using a loading dose will help to achieve steady state concentrations of the active metabolite after approximately 2-3 weeks. In contrast, without a loading dose, it would likely take about two months to reach steady state.[111,135] The active metabolite has a low volume of distribution (0.13 L/kg) and is highly protein bound to albumin (>99.3%). It is eliminated by further metabolism and subsequent renal and biliary excretion.

Leflunomide pharmacokinetics are known to vary with renal function. In a study by Williams et al,[139] renal transplant patients with diminished renal function were more likely to have lower serum levels of active metabolite, despite comparable doses. This is likely due to the fact that protein binding of the active metabolite is reduced in uremia, and results in a higher fraction of unbound drug. This may lead to increased elimination, thus necessitating higher doses in patients with renal dysfunction.

Dosing and Adverse Events

The dosing of leflunomide recommended for patients with rheumatoid arthritis is 100 mg each day for three days followed by 20 mg each day. This dosing regimen is designed to produce a steady state serum concentration of the active metabolite of approximately 25-45 mcg/ml. Higher maintenance doses are not recommended, and if a patient experiences adverse events, the dose may be decreased to 10 mg per day.

Adverse reactions associated with leflunomide in rheumatoid arthritis patients include nausea, diarrhea, alopecia, rash, anemia and elevated liver enzymes.[111] It appears that the side effect profile may differ slightly in different patient populations. In kidney transplant patients, the main side effect reported has been anemia, while in liver transplant patients, an elevation in liver enzymes was found.[139]

It was noted that side effects were more common in patients with lower total serum concentrations and diminished renal function, and this may be attributed to a higher unbound fraction. The assay that the authors utilized to measure A77-1726 detected total (both bound and unbound) concentrations, and in patients with renal dysfunction, this assay is not likely to accurately reflect the amount of pharmacologically active drug.[139]

Clinical Experience

Progressive Multifocal Leukoencephalopathy and BKV-Associated Hemorrhagic Cystitis

Currently, there are no data describing the use of leflunomide to treat PML or BKV-associated HC. Moreover, the time period that would be necessary to achieve therapeutic concentrations with leflunomide may prohibit its use in PML or HC.

Polyomavirus-Associated Nephropathy

Several investigators are starting to use leflunomide to manage PVN, but clinical experience is limited. Foster and colleagues described the use of leflunomide in place of MMF in two patients with PVN who showed no clinical improvement after they were switched from tacrolimus to cyclosporine. Immunosuppressive doses were used with a target blood concentration of 60-90 mcg/ml. Renal function improved in both patients, and BK virus was no longer detected in the blood.[103] Poduval and colleagues described the use of leflunomide in six patients diagnosed with PVN. All patients were on tacrolimus, MMF and prednisone. After diagnosis, MMF was stopped and replaced with leflunomide. A loading dose of 100 mg per day for 3-5 days was used and then a 40-60 mg maintenance dose was given every day. Patients were followed with BK viral load by PCR in blood, SCr measurements, and follow-up biopsy as indicated. Within 60 days of leflunomide therapy, the SCr decreased from 2.8 ± 1.6 mg/dl to 2.4 ± 0.7 mg/dl. After 90 days, the SCr was 2.1 ± 0.6 mg/dl. At diagnosis, blood PCR was positive in 4/6 patients and became negative in all patients. The urine PCR was positive in five patients tested initially, but with treatment, there was a significant reduction in viruria. No rejection or graft loss was reported with a follow-up of 147 ± 67 days. The authors concluded that this unique drug, with both antiviral and antirejection properties, may be useful in the setting of PVN.[71] The optimal dosing strategy to maximize clinical outcome and minimize adverse effects in patients with PVN remains unclear.

Topotecan

Data from in vitro studies have shown that the topoisomerase I inhibitors, camptothecin and topotecan, can block parts of JCV replication in glioblastoma cells at drug levels that were not toxic to the host cells.[140] Topotecan is a semi-synthetic derivative of the drug camptothecin, and is approved for the treatment of ovarian and small lung cancer.[141] Recently, topotecan, has been evaluated in a phase II trial to treat HIV patients with JCV-induced PML.[36]

Mechanism of Action

The mechanism of action of topotecan involves inhibition of topoisomerase I. Topoisomerase I is an enzyme that produces single strand breaks in DNA and promotes unwinding of supercoiled DNA to allow for DNA replication to proceed and subsequently repairs the strands. Inhibiting topoisomerase I prevents S-phase DNA replication and translocation, resulting in cell death.

Pharmacokinetics

Topotecan exhibits multiexponential pharmacokinetics with a terminal half-life of two to three hours. Total exposure is approximately dose proportional. Topotecan is about 35% protein bound and achieves significant concentrations in the CSF. Mean half-life, estimated in three renally impaired patients was approximately five hours. Hepatic function impairment may also slightly increase the terminal half-life of topotecan. Approximately 30% of topotecan is eliminated by renal excretion. Some topotecan is also eliminated via the biliary route.

Dosing and Adverse Events

Topotecan treatment of cancer is usually continued for a minimum of four cycles. In clinical studies, the median time to response was 9-12 weeks, and responses may be missed if therapy is discontinued prematurely. The usual dose of topotecan for ovarian cancer and small cell lung cancer is 1.5 mg/m^2 of body surface area given IV over 30 minutes for five consecutive days, repeated every 21 days.

Due to its myelosuppressive and hematologic effects, the manufacturer recommends that topotecan should only be administered to patients with adequate bone marrow reserves (baseline neutrophil count of at least 1,500 cells/mm^3. In order to monitor the occurrence of bone marrow suppression, primarily neutropenia, which may be severe and result in infection and death, frequent peripheral blood cell counts should be performed. Neutropenia is not cumulative over time. If severe topotecan-induced anemia, neutropenia or thrombocytopenia occur during treatment, subsequent courses of topotecan should be delayed until the hemoglobin recovers to at least 9 gm/dl (with transfusion if necessary), neutrophil counts recover to greater than 1000 cells/mm^3, and platelet counts recover to greater than 100,000 cells/mm^3.

In patients with mild renal impairment (creatinine clearance 40-60 ml/minute), topotecan clearance was decreased to 67% of the value seen in patients with normal renal function. In patients with moderate renal impairment (creatinine clearance 20-39 ml/minute), topotecan clearance was reduced to approximately 34% of the value in control patients, with an increase in half-life. The manufacturer does not recommend dose adjustment for patients with mild renal impairment, but does recommend dose adjustment to 0.75 mg/m^2 for patients with moderate renal impairment. There are insufficient data to provide dosage recommendations for patients with severe renal impairment (creatinine clearance less than 19 ml/minute). There is no dose adjustment recommended for patients with impaired hepatic function (plasma bilirubin >1.5 to < 10 mg/dl).[141]

Clinical Experience

Progressive Multifocal Leukoencephalopathy

Based on the in vitro effects of camptothecins inhibiting JCV,[140] topotecan has recently been evaluated in a phase II clinical trial for PML treatment in HIV-infected patients.[36] Data was evaluated in 11 of 12 HIV-infected patients with PML, all of whom were on a HAART combination, at the time of initiation of topotecan therapy. A total of 38 treatment courses were administered to 11 patients, the majority at a dose of 0.3 gm/m^2/day or higher, over the 2.5 year study period. The maximum dose administered was 0.6 mg/m^2/day. Overall, responders had higher pretreatment Karnofsky performance scores and lower Kurtzke expanded disability status scale scores than nonresponders. Only three patients responded to therapy, with two alive at the time of publication. The time to radiographic response was approximately two months for all three patients, and the time to clinical response was less than one month in one patient, and more prolonged in the other two patients. Additionally, one patient was treated off protocol and showed a response to therapy. In this patient, progression of disease occurred after the first dose, however, a partial radiographic response was noted after five doses. Seven patients did not respond to treatment and died of PML within 30 days of treatment initiation with topotecan. Furthermore, one study patient died of hematologic toxicity from an accidental topotecan overdose (2.42 mg/m^2/day). Despite using lower doses of topotecan than those used in oncology, moderate to severe neutropenia, anemia and thrombocytopenia developed in 10 (90%), 6 (54%) and 5 (45%) patients, respectively. The authors speculated that one reason the incidence of hematologic adverse events was still high despite using lower doses of topotecan may be that HIV infection itself could have contributed to the observed hematologic toxicities. However, by adjusting treatment doses according to the protocol, and administering granulocyte colony stimulating factors (G-CSF) and blood transfusions, the hematologic effects eventually resolved. The most frequently reported nonhematologic effects were nausea in 4 (36%) patients, vomiting in 3 (27%) patients, fever in 3 (27%) patients, and diarrhea, fatigue, rash, and alopecia developing in two patients (18%) each, respectively. The authors concluded that due to the small number of patients, and the late stage of PML at time of entry into the protocol, further studies are needed to assess the efficacy of topotecan for PML. The study was closed due to poor recruitment and the fact that the early data did not suggest a beneficial effect.[36]

Topotecan is also limited by its parenteral formulation. However, development of an oral formulation of topotecan is underway. Future studies of topotecan with larger patient enrollment, stratification by treatment group, interim analyses, use of a toxicity grading system that incorporates multiple etiologic factors,[44] and defined earlier PML at study entry[43] may allow for better assessment of topotecan efficacy and safety in the treatment of PML in HIV-infected patients.[36]

BKV-Associated Hemorrhagic Cystitis and Polyomavirus-Associated Nephropathy

Topotecan has not been evaluated for use in BKV-associated HC or PVN mainly due to its significant hematologic toxicities, which could result in fatal opportunistic infections in the immunosuppressed transplant recipient. Moreover, since the drug is renally eliminated, many patients presenting with PVN may have significant renal dysfunction which may require dose adjustment. The manufacturer does not have guidelines for dosing in severe renal dysfunction, and accumulation of doses could theoretically lead to further hematologic toxicity.

Vidarabine and Cytarabine

Clinical Experience

Progressive Multifocal Leukoencephalopathy

Vidarabine (Ara-A) was administered to two patients with advanced cases of PML in the 1970s, but the therapy was unsuccessful.[142] Cytarabine (Ara-C) has been shown to inhibit JCV replication in vitro.[112] Cytarabine is a synthetic pyrimidine nucleoside that is thought to inhibit DNA polymerase activity. Cytarabine is associated with significant bone marrow toxicity, which is reported to occur within the first seven days of treatment and manifests as neutropenia, anemia and thrombocytopenia in greater than 10% of patients.[143] In anecdotal reports, cytarabine has induced remission of PML in patients with and without HIV infection.[144-146] However, in a randomized, multicenter, prospective trial of cytarabine for the treatment of PML in HIV patients, cytarabine was not effective for PML in this patient population.[38] Fifty-seven patients with HIV infection and a diagnosis of PML established within two months of study entry were randomly assigned to receive one of three treatments: antiretroviral therapy alone, antiretroviral therapy plus IV cytarabine, or antiretroviral therapy plus intrathecal cytarabine. For most patients, antiretroviral therapy consisted of zidovudine plus either didanosine or stavudine. This study was undertaken prior to the advent of HAART. After a lead-in period of 1 to 2 weeks, active treatment was given for 24 weeks. An external performance and safety monitoring board reviewed the results at a second interim (when 50% of the expected results had occurred) and concluded that no treatment was likely to show a survival benefit, even if the study was continued to completion. The study was terminated at 24 months. Median follow-up was 8.7 weeks and outcomes did not differ significantly among the three treatment groups. Only seven (12%) patients completed the 24 week treatment. Forty-two (74%) patients (14 in each treatment group) had died, and there were no significant differences in survival among the three groups (log-rank test, P = 0.85). Thirty seven (88%) patients died from PML. The median survival times (11, 8, and 15 weeks, respectively) were similar to those in previous studies. Anemia and thrombocytopenia were more frequent in patients who received antiretroviral therapy in combination with intravenous cytarabine. The authors concluded that cytarabine administered either IV or intrathecally did not improve the prognosis of HIV-infected patients with PML who were treated with antiretroviral therapy.[38]

In contrast to the cytarabine experience in PML patients with HIV infection, an open-label, retrospective study of 19 nonHIV-infected patients with PML treated with IV cytarabine at 2 mg/kg/day for five days found that 7/19 (36%) patients treated with cytarabine and followed for 2-4.5 years had neurologic improvement.[147] All patients who experienced neurologic improvement also exhibited radiologic improvement on magnetic resonance imaging (MRI) scans. Cytarabine treatment was associated with significant bone marrow toxicity. Eleven patients experienced pancytopenia, with five requiring transfusion of blood products. Interestingly, all who survived their neurologic disease also recovered from their pancytopenia. However, 12 patients showed no evidence of response and died rapidly of PML after treatment (range 8 days-6 months). The authors concluded that cytarabine, when used to treat PML in nonHIV-infected patients, is associated with a 36% chance of disease stabilization at one year. Although treatment was associated with significant bone marrow toxicity, the 36% one year survival was higher than expected for PML patients.

In summary, in vitro data has shown cytarabine to be effective at inhibiting JCV replication.[112] However, cytarabine failed to show efficacy in a multi-center, randomized trial for PML in HIV-infected patients.[38] Some investigators have proposed that the failure of cytarabine in this trial was due to insufficient drug delivery through traditional IV and intrathecal routes. An alternative convection–enhanced intraparenchymal delivery of cytarabine is currently being studied.[148] Although cytarabine has not been shown to be beneficial in patients with HIV infection and PML,[38] it has shown a small benefit in the treatment of nonHIV-infected patients with PML.[147] Bone marrow toxicity is the main limiting factor in cytarabine administration, and treatment is not recommended in patients without adequate bone marrow reserve, or in those presenting with severe pancytopenia. Currently, cytarabine may be an effective choice for some nonHIV-infected patients with PML. Due to the lack of in vitro data, and the lack of availability in parenteral form in the United States, vidarabine (Ara-A), has not been used routinely to treat PML in nonHIV or HIV-infected patients.

BKV-Associated Hemorrhagic Cystitis

Several different drugs have been used to treat BKV-associated HC found in patients after either allogeneic bone marrow or stem cell transplant. The nucleoside analogue vidarabine (adenine arabinoside or Ara-A), is known to be active against several double-stranded DNA viruses.[142] It appears to exert its antiviral effects by interfering with the early steps in viral DNA synthesis.[149] Ara-A use has been described in several case reports. Chapman et al[150] successfully treated a 23-year-old man with BKV-associated HC with Ara-A 10 mg/kg/day for five days, given IV over 12 hours. Within two days, his symptoms improved, and after seven days, he was symptom free. On day 16 of therapy, the virus was cleared from the urine. In another case series, Ara-A (10 mg/kg/day for five days, given IV over 2-3 hours) was used in one patient with polyomavirus associated cystitis, and in two patients with asymptomatic polyoma viruria.[53] With Ara-A therapy, the viral inclusion bodies in urinary sediments disappeared in all three patients. In one patient, the viruria recurred, and was successfully cleared with another course of Ara-A. In another case report, severe polyomavirus associated HC was treated with Ara-A (10 mg/kg/day for five days, given intramuscular), resulting in resolution of HC within 24 hours of starting therapy, and clearance of the virus from the urine after four days of treatment.[151] Intramuscular Ara-A may be an alternative when patients have an adequate platelet count and do not have IV access. In another case, a 48 year-old male with CMV antigenemia 60 days after allogeneic bone marrow transplant, developed HC.[152] Acute obstructive renal failure developed with bilateral hydronephroses. Initially, tests for polyomavirus were negative, and ureteric stents were placed with improvement. Symptoms of HC resolved and then relapsed. Further laboratory testing later in the course revealed the presence of BKV by PCR. On day 174 after transplant, treatment with vidarabine was started (10 mg/kg/day IV for five days given as 12 hour infusions). Symptoms resolved within one week, but because of recurrence, vidarabine was repeated twice.

The most common side effects of Ara-A include nausea, vomiting, diarrhea, increased liver function tests, headache, confusion and tremor.[33] In the case reports above, Ara-A was associated with fatigue, nausea, vomiting, diarrhea, claustrophobia and a transient increase in liver function tests.[53,150,151] Ara-A appears to be a safe and effective therapeutic alternative for BKV-associated HC, however, parenteral Ara-A is no longer available in the United States. Historically, Ara-A was used to treat varicella-zoster and herpes simplex virus infections, but drugs such as acyclovir are now used to treat these types of viruses.[149]

Polyomavirus-Associated Nephropathy

Cytarabine and vidarabine have not been evaluated for use in the management of PVN due to the lack of in vitro activity.[100] The potential hematologic toxicity would also limit these agents' clinical utility.

Intravenous Immune Globulin

Clinical Experience

Progressive Multifocal Leukoencephalopathy and BKV-Associated Hemorrhagic Cystitis

Intravenous immune globulin (IVIG) has not been evaluated for use in PML or HC.

Polyomavirus-Associated Nephropathy

IVIG has been administered empirically for PVN, but there are limited data to support its efficacy.[59] Recently, an in vitro study has shown that IVIG contains antibodies to BKV,[153] suggesting that IVIG may provide a therapeutic option for patients with PVN. IVIG has also been used to treat steroid resistant acute rejection, and may offer an advantage for a patient with PVN who has concurrent acute rejection.[154] Based on this recent finding, IVIG has been used at a dose of 500 mg/kg/day for seven days in conjunction with IS reduction in four renal transplant patients to treat PVN.[155] When comparing these four patients to two patients who received IS reduction alone, patients in the latter group failed to clear viremia by 45 weeks post-treatment. In contrast, 2/4 (50%) patients treated with IVIG cleared BK viremia at 12 and 19 weeks after initiation of treatment and their SCr concentrations stabilized. The other two patients have had much shorter follow-up and were still viremic at four weeks post-treatment. To date, no patient has experienced graft loss.

Interferons

Progressive Multifocal Leukoencephalopathy

Interferons have also been considered for use in treating PML in an effort to reconstitute the immune system.[156] A retrospective, open label, study of 77 HIV-infected patients with PML, prior to the availability of HAART, was conducted.[157] Patients received a minimum treatment of 3 weeks of 3 million units of alpha-IFN daily (n = 21) and were compared to untreated historical controls (n = 32). In patients who died, median survival of treated patients was 128 days longer than in untreated patients (Chi-square = 4.21, P = 0.04). When living and deceased treated patients were combined, the median survival was 325 days (range 35 - 1634) versus 121 days (range 46 - 176) in untreated patients (Chi-square = 13.47, P < 0.001). When survival times in untreated patients were censored to account for possible survivorship bias in treated patients, survival in treated patients remained significantly prolonged (325 days versus 176 days, Chi-square = 4.65, P = 0.03). In addition, use of alpha-IFN was associated with a significant delay in the onset of memory loss (Chi-square = 8.59, P < 0.01). Seven alpha-IFN treated patients showed sustained remissions of several months to over a year, with documented improvements in mental status, aphasia, dysarthria, dysphagia, paresis, and dyscoordination. Moreover, four IFN-treated patients had evidence of regression of MRI lesions, although this was not always correlated with clinical remission. Four of 32 untreated patients also reported transient symptomatic improvements. The authors concluded that alpha-IFN may delay progression, palliate symptoms, and significantly prolong survival in HIV-associated PML, and therefore, recommended that a controlled clinical trial is warranted.

The long term follow-up of the study described above has recently been reported.[39] The retrospective analysis compared the survival of 97 HIV-infected patients with PML prior to the HAART era, during the HAART era, ± alpha-interferon. No benefit was found for alpha-interferon therapy. Likewise, a multivariate analysis showed no difference in survival among patients on none, one, or two forms of antiretrovirals. However, survival was significantly greater for those on HAART. Whereas alpha-interferon use was shown to be associated with longer survival (P < 0.057), this effect was not independent of the effects of HAART. The authors concluded that HAART significantly increases survival for patients with PML and AIDS; however, alpha-interferon does not appear to provide additional benefit.

In summary, although interferon appeared to possibly have benefit in PML prior to the HAART era,[157] it does not appear to have any benefit above that seen with HAART in treating PML in HIV-infected patients.[39] However, due to the lack of other effective therapy against JCV induced PML in HIV-infected patients, and the prevalence of PML in the HAART era, researchers now propose that agents such as interferon-beta should be explored in clinical trials.[20] Interferon-beta has been reported to inhibit HIV transcription in macrophages, and may potentially have an antiviral effect on JCV in PML. Moreover, researchers have proposed that its efficacy in treating multiple sclerosis, another central nervous system demyelinating condition, and its known toxicity profile in humans, make it a therapeutic alternative worth considering in a clinical trial setting.[158]

BKV-Associated Hemorrhagic Cystitis
Interferon therapy has not been evaluated for use in BKV-associated HC.

Polyomavirus-Associated Nephropathy
The effects of human leukocyte interferon on BKV infection were studied in 41 renal transplant recipients as part of a randomized, double-blind, placebo-controlled trial.[159] Eight transplant recipients demonstrated a fourfold or greater rise in antibody to BKV, and three excreted BKV in urine. Neither seroconversion nor excretion was reduced by interferon administration. No clinical syndromes could be clearly linked to BKV infection. BKV was also relatively resistant to the in vitro effects of interferon. Pretreatment of interferon-sensitive human fibroblasts with up to 620 units of interferon/ml resulted in a loss of viral infectivity of one log or less. Continuous exposure of infected cultures to these interferon levels reduced BKV titers by 1.5-2.9 logs, whereas continuous exposure to lower concentrations of interferon had less effects. The levels shown to be marginally effective in vitro were considerably higher than those achieved in patient sera. Based on the lack of activity of interferon and the fear of promoting rejection in transplant recipients, interferon therapy has not been used for PVN.

Algorithms for Clinical Interventions (Fig. 1)
Several authors have devised algorithms for the screening, diagnosis and monitoring of patients with PVN.[65,77,160,161] These include the use of urine cytology to screen for decoy cells in renal transplant patients. Ramos et al[160] recommends monitoring for viruria at 3, 6, 9 and 12 months post-transplant, and every 12 months thereafter. Screening may also be intensified in patients who receive treatment for acute rejection.[77] Mayr and colleagues[161] suggest that if >5 decoy cells per 10 high power fields are found repeatedly, then a plasma PCR to check for BKV is indicated. Likewise, Ramos et al[160] also recommend that a quantitative viral load in the plasma should be checked in the presence of viruria. If > 10,000 copies of BK virus/ml are present, then an allograft biopsy should be performed. If the diagnosis of PVN is made, overall IS is decreased. If acute rejection is also present on the biopsy, the authors recommend the use of pulsed steroids to treat the acute rejection, followed either by repeat urine cytology and quantitative viral load in the plasma or by a reduction in IS. Based on the current data available, an algorithm for the pharmacologic management of PVN has been developed (Fig. 1). Many authors support the reduction or discontinuation of the antimetabolite agent in addition to reducing the target concentrations of the calcineurin inhibitor.[58,62,68,69,160,162,163] If the antimetabolite is discontinued, leflunomide may be added to take advantage of both its antiviral and antirejection properties. A loading dose of 100 mg per day for 3-5 days is suggested followed by a maintenance dose of 40-60 mg every day.[71] Preliminary data suggest that a target range of 60-90 mcg/ml should be achieved, however, this warrants further investigation, since

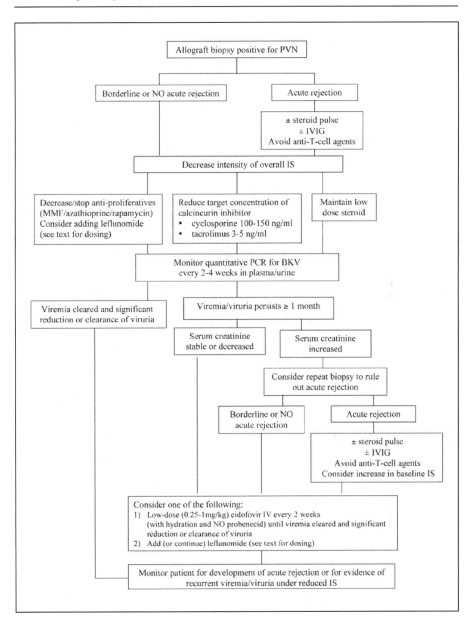

Figure 1. Proposed algorithm for the pharmacological management of patients with polyomavirus-associated nephropathy.

leflunomide pharmacokinetics are known to vary with renal function.[103] Leflunomide or cidofovir should be considered for patients who have persistent viremia/viruria despite a reduction in IS, especially if renal function continues to worsen. Further studies are needed to determine if utilizing this approach to treat PVN will stabilize or improve renal function and ultimately prevent graft loss.

Conclusion

In conclusion, the pathogenesis and treatment of the complications associated with polyomavirus disease (PML, HC, and PVN) in humans remains to be defined. It is clear that the development of clinically significant disease with polyomavirus is related to the degree of overall IS. Immune reconstitution through influencing the underlying immune defect such as reducing IS in transplant recipients with PVN, or HAART administration in HIV-infected patients with PML theoretically should impact disease prevention and progression. However, these interventions alone are apparently not sufficient, as these diseases are still associated with significant morbidity and mortality such as renal allograft loss in PVN and death in PML. Our current understanding of polyomavirus disease pathogenesis is limited. Consequently, the availability and development of effective prophylactic and therapeutic agents are lacking.

Efforts are focused on improving clinical outcomes through early diagnosis and monitoring for polyomavirus diseases. Current therapies for PML including cidofovir, cytarabine, topotecan and alpha-interferon have not been shown to be effective in prospectively conducted trials for PML treatment in HIV-infected patients. However, cytarabine may be of some benefit in nonHIV-infected patients with PML. Likewise, cidofovir, IVIG and leflunomide may have some benefit in PVN, but have not been studied in large prospective trials. Furthermore, no agent has been studied in a prospective trial for HC. Chlorpromazine and clozapine have been shown to inhibit the growth of JCV in vitro, but not active infection in vivo. With further in vitro study, consideration may be given to using chlorpromazine and clozapine in clinical trials. Similarly, due to its known efficacy in multiple sclerosis and its reported inhibitory effects on HIV transcription in macrophages, interferon-beta is also being considered for use in clinical trials to treat PML. FK-778, a nonnephrotoxic immunosuppressive and antiviral agent, has shown in vitro activity against polyomaviruses and may be beneficial in the treatment of PVN. Nystatin has also been shown to inhibit BKV cell entry in vitro and further in vitro research is underway.

In the future, these compounds may be added to the current armamentarium of agents used to treat polyomavirus-induced diseases. Future research efforts focused on further delineating the pathogenesis of polyomaviral disease may allow for the development of more specific therapeutic targets. Clinical trials designed to enroll large numbers of patients, with broad inclusion criteria and stratification based on treatment groups and utilizing consensus definitions for disease states are necessary to determine the safety and efficacy of current and future management techniques (screening, diagnostic and monitoring) and therapeutic interventions for polyomavirus diseases.

References

1. Shah KV. Polyomaviruses. In: Fields BN, Knipe DM, eds. Fields Virology. 3rd ed. Philadelphia: Lippincott-Raven, 1996:2027-43.
2. Gardner SD, Field AM, Coleman DV et al. New human papovavirus (B.K.) isolated from urine after renal transplantation. Lancet 1971; 1(7712):1253-7.
3. Padgett BL, Walker DL, ZuRhein GM et al. Cultivation of papova-like virus from human brain with progressive multifocal leucoencephalopathy. Lancet 1971; 1(7712):1257-60.
4. Knowles W. The epidemiology of BK virus and the occurence of antigenic and genomic subtypes. In: Khalili K, Stoner GL, eds. Human Polyomaviruses: Molecular and Clinical Perspectives. New York: Wiley-Liss, 2001:527-60.
5. Major EO. Human polyomavirus. In: Knipe DM, Howley PM, eds. Fields Virology. 4th ed. Philadelphia: Lippincott Williams and Wilkins, 2001:2:2175-96.
6. Houff SA, Major EO, Katz DA et al. Involvement of JC virus-infected mononuclear cells from the bone marrow and spleen in the pathogenesis of progressive multifocal leukoencephalopathy. N Engl J Med 1988; 318(5):301-5.
7. Kahan AV, Coleman DV, Koss LG. Activation of human polyomavirus infection - detection by cytologic techniques. Am J Clin Pathol 1980; 74:326-32.
8. Coleman DV, Wolfendale MR, Daniel RA et al. A prospective study of human polyomavirus infection in pregnancy. J Infect Dis 1980; 142(1):1-8.

9. Agha IA, Brennan DC. BK virus and current immunosuppressive therapy. Graft 2002; 5(Suppl):S65-72.
10. Hirsch HH, Knowles W, Dickenmann M et al. Prospective study of polyomavirus type BK replication and nephropathy in renal-transplant recipients. N Engl J Med 2002; 347(7):488-96.
11. Mylonakis E, Goes N, Rubin RH et al. BK virus in solid organ transplant recipients: An emerging syndrome. Transplantation 2001; 72(10):1587-92.
12. Dorries K, Loeber G, Meixensberger J. Association of polyomaviruses JC, SV40, and BK with human brain tumors. Virology 1987; 160(1):268-70.
13. Del Valle L, Gordon J, Enam S et al. Expression of human neurotropic polyomavirus JCV late gene product agnoprotein in human medulloblastoma. J Natl Cancer Inst 2002; 94(4):267-73.
14. Khalili K. Human neurotropic JC virus and its association with brain tumors. Dis Markers 2001; 17(3):143-7.
15. Boldorini R, Pagani E, Car PG et al. Molecular characterisation of JC virus strains detected in human brain tumours. Pathology 2003; 35(3):248-53.
16. Laghi L, Randolph AE, Chauhan DP et al. JC virus DNA is present in the mucosa of the human colon and in colorectal cancers. Proc Natl Acad Sci USA 1999; 96(13):7484-9.
17. Safak M, Khalili K. An overview: Human polyomavirus JC virus and its associated disorders. J Neurovirol 2003; 9(Suppl 1):3-9.
18. Corral I, Quereda C, Hellin T et al. Relapsing and remitting leukoencephalopathy associated with chronic HIV infection. Eur Neurol 2002; 48(1):39-41.
19. White FA, Ishaq M, Stoner GL et al. JC virus DNA is present in many human brain samples from patients without progressive multifocal leukoencephalopathy. J Virol 1992; 66(10):5726-34.
20. Joseph J, Major EO. Basic, clinical, and epidemiological studies of progressive multifocal leukoencephalopathy: Implications for therapy. J Neurovirol 2003; 9(Suppl 1):1-2.
21. Atwood WJ. Cellular receptors for the polyomaviruses. In: Khalili K, Stoner G, eds. Human Polyomaviruses: Molecular and Clinical Perspectives. New York: Wiley-Liss, 2001:53-72.
22. Mahmut S, Khalili K. An overview: Human polyomavirus JC virus and its associated disorders. J Neurovirol 2003; 9(Suppl 1):3-9.
23. Berger JR, Nath A. Clinical progressive multifocal leukoencephalopathy: Diagnosis and treatment. In: Khalili K, Stoner G, eds. Human Polyomaviruses: Molecular and Clinical Perspectives. New York: Wiley-Liss, 2001:237-56.
24. Koralnik IJ, Du Pasquier RA, Kuroda MJ et al. Association of prolonged survival in HLA-A2+ progressive multifocal leukoencephalopathy patients with a CTL response specific for a commonly recognized JC virus epitope. J Immunol 2002; 168(1):499-504.
25. Du Pasquier RA, Kuroda MJ, Schmitz JE et al. Low frequency of cytotoxic T lymphocytes against the novel HLA-A*0201-restricted JC virus epitope VP1(p36) in patients with proven or possible progressive multifocal leukoencephalopathy. J Virol 2003; 77(22):11918-26.
26. Clifford DB, Yiannoutsos C, Glicksman M et al. HAART improves prognosis in HIV-associated progressive multifocal leukoencephalopathy. Neurology 1999; 52(3):623-5.
27. Berger JR, Levy RM, Flomenhoft D et al. Predictive factors for prolonged survival in acquired immunodeficiency syndrome-associated progressive multifocal leukoencephalopathy. Ann Neurol 1998; 44(3):341-9.
28. Weber F, Goldmann C, Kramer M et al. Cellular and humoral immune response in progressive multifocal leukoencephalopathy. Ann Neurol 2001; 49(5):636-42.
29. Du Pasquier RA, Koralnik IJ. Inflammatory reaction in progressive multifocal leukoencephalopathy: Harmful or beneficial? J Neurovirol 2003; 9(Suppl 1):25-31.
30. Cinque P, Pierotti C, Vigano MG et al. The good and evil of HAART in HIV-related progressive multifocal leukoencephalopathy. J Neurovirol 2001; 7(4):358-63.
31. Cinque P, Bossolasco S, Brambilla AM et al. The effect of highly active antiretroviral theapy-induced immune reconstitution on development and outcome of progressive multifocal leukoencephalopathy: Study of 43 cases with reveiw of the literature. J Neurovirol 2003; 9(Suppl 1):73-80.
32. Berger JR, Concha M. Progressive multifocal leukoencephalopathy: The evolution of a disease once considered rare. J Neurovirol 1995; 1(1):5-18.
33. Berger JR. Progressive multifocal leukoencephalopathy in acquired immunodeficiency syndrome: Explaining the high incidence and disproportionate frequency of the illness relative to other immunosuppressive conditions. J Neurovirol 2003; 9(Suppl 1):38-41.
34. Berger JR, Chauhan A, Galey D et al. Epidemiological evidence and molecular basis of interactions between HIV and JC virus. J Neurovirol 2001; 7(4):329-38.
35. Seth P, Diaz F, Major EO. Advances in the biology of JC virus and induction of progressive multifocal leukoencephalopathy. J Neurovirol 2003; 9(2):236-46.

36. Royal W, Dupont B, McGuire D et al. Topotecan in the treatment of acquired immunodeficiency syndrome-related progressive multifocal leukoencephalopathy. J Neurovirol 2003; 9(3):411-9.
37. Marra CM, Rajicic N, Barker DE et al. A pilot study of cidofovir for progressive multifocal leukoencephalopathy in AIDS. Aids 2002; 16(13):1791-7.
38. Hall CD, Dafni U, Simpson D et al. Failure of cytarabine in progressive multifocal leukoencephalopathy associated with human immunodeficiency virus infection. AIDS Clinical Trials Group 243 Team. N Engl J Med 1998; 338(19):1345-51.
39. Geschwind MD, Skolasky RI, Royal WS et al. The relative contributions of HAART and alpha-interferon for therapy of progressive multifocal leukoencephalopathy in AIDS. J Neurovirol 2001; 7(4):353-7.
40. Gasnault J, Kousignian P, Kahraman M et al. Cidofovir in AIDS-associated progressive multifocal leukoencephalopathy: A monocenter observational study with clinical and JC virus load monitoring. J Neurovirol 2001; 7(4):375-81.
41. De Luca A, Giancola ML, Ammassari A et al. The effect of potent antiretroviral therapy and JC virus load in cerebrospinal fluid on clinical outcome of patients with AIDS-associated progressive multifocal leukoencephalopathy. J Infect Dis 2000; 182(4):1077-83.
42. De Luca A, Ammassari A, Cingolani A et al. Disease progression and poor survival of AIDS-associated progressive multifocal leukoencephalopathy despite highly active antiretroviral therapy. Aids 1998; 12(14):1937-8.
43. Cinque P, Koralnik IJ, Clifford DB. The evolving face of human immunodeficiency virus-related progressive multifocal leukoencephalopathy: Defining a consensus terminology. J Neurovirol 2003; 9(Suppl 1):88-92.
44. Yiannoutsos C, De Luca A. Designs for clinical trials to test the efficacy of therapeutics in progressive multifocal leukoencephalopathy. J Neurovirol 2001; 7:369-74.
45. Reploeg MD, Storch GA, Clifford DB. BK virus: A clinical review. Clin Infect Dis 2001; 33(2):191-202.
46. Hirsch HH, Mohaupt M, Klimkait T. Prospective monitoring of BK virus load after discontinuing sirolimus treatment in a renal transplant patient with BK virus nephropathy. J Infect Dis 2001; 184(11):1494-5, author reply 5-6.
47. Randhawa PS, Finkelstein S, Scantlebury V et al. Human polyoma virus-associated interstitial nephritis in the allograft kidney. Transplantation 1999; 67(1):103-9.
48. Haririan A, Klassen D. BK virus infection after nonrenal transplantation. Graft 2002; 5(Suppl):S58-S64.
49. Arthur RR, Shah KV, Baust SJ et al. Association of BK viruria with hemorrhagic cystitis in recipients of bone marrow transplants. N Engl J Med 1986; 315(4):230-4.
50. Leung AY, Mak R, Lie AK, et al. Clinicopathological features and risk factors of clinically overt haemorrhagic cystitis complicating bone marrow transplantation. Bone Marrow Transplant 2002; 29(6):509-13.
51. Gonzalez-Fraile MI, Canizo C, Caballero D, et al. Cidofovir treatment of human polyomavirus-associated acute haemorrhagic cystitis. Transpl Infect Dis 2001; 3(1):44-6.
52. Garderet L, Bittencourt H, Sebe P et al. Cystectomy for severe hemorrhagic cystitis in allogeneic stem cell transplant recipients. Transplantation 2000; 70(12):1807-11.
53. Kawakami M, Ueda S, Maeda T et al. Vidarabine therapy for virus-associated cystitis after allogeneic bone marrow transplantation. Bone Marrow Transplant 1997; 20(6):485-90.
54. Goddard AG, Saha V. Late-onset hemorrhagic cystitis following bone marrow transplantation: A case report. Pediatr Hematol Oncol 1997; 14(3):273-5.
55. Laszlo D, Bosi A, Guidi S et al. Prostaglandin E2 bladder instillation for the treatment of hemorrhagic cystitis after allogeneic bone marrow transplantation. Haematologica 1995; 80(5):421-5.
56. Randhawa P, Baksh F, Aoki N et al. JC virus infection in allograft kidneys: Analysis by polymerase chain reaction and immunohistochemistry. Transplantation 2001; 71(9):1300-3.
57. Li RM, Mannon RB, Kleiner D et al. BK virus and SV40 coinfection in polyomavirus nephropathy. Transplantation 2002; 74(11):1497-504.
58. Trofe J, Cavallo T, First MR et al. Polyomavirus in kidney and kidney-pancreas transplantation: A defined protocol for immunosuppression reduction and histologic monitoring. Transplant Proc 2002; 34(5):1788-9.
59. Randhawa PS, Demetris AJ. Nephropathy due to polyomavirus type BK. N Engl J Med 2000; 342(18):1361-3.
60. Trofe J, Gaber LW, Stratta RJ et al. Polyomavirus in kidney and kidney-pancreas transplant recipients. Transpl Infect Dis 2003; 5(1):21-8.

61. Ginevri F, De Santis R, Comoli P et al. Polyomavirus BK infection in pediatric kidney-allograft recipients: A single-center analysis of incidence, risk factors, and novel therapeutic approaches. Transplantation 2003; 75(8):1266-70.
62. Howell DN, Smith SR, Butterly DW et al. Diagnosis and management of BK polyomavirus interstitial nephritis in renal transplant recipients. Transplantation 1999; 68(9):1279-88.
63. Binet I, Nickeleit V, Hirsch HH et al. Polyomavirus disease under new immunosuppressive drugs: A cause of renal graft dysfunction and graft loss. Transplantation 1999; 67(6):918-22.
64. Nickeleit V, Hirsch HH, Binet IF et al. Polyomavirus infection of renal allograft recipients: From latent infection to manifest disease. J Am Soc Nephrol 1999; 10(5):1080-9.
65. Nickeleit V, Hirsch HH, Zeiler M et al. BK-virus nephropathy in renal transplants-tubular necrosis, MHC-class II expression and rejection in a puzzling game. Nephrol Dial Transplant 2000; 15(3):324-32.
66. Nickeleit V, Klimkait T, Binet IF et al. Testing for polyomavirus type BK DNA in plasma to identify renal-allograft recipients with viral nephropathy. N Engl J Med 2000; 342(18):1309-15.
67. Binet I, Nickeleit V, Hirsch HH. Polyomavirus infections in transplant recipients. Current Opinions in Organ Transplantation 2000; 5:210-16.
68. Ahuja M, Cohen EP, Dayer AM et al. Polyoma virus infection after renal transplantation. Use of immunostaining as a guide to diagnosis. Transplantation 2001; 71(7):896-9.
69. Barri YM, Ahmad I, Ketel BL et al. Polyoma viral infection in renal transplantation: The role of immunosuppressive therapy. Clin Transplant 2001; 15(4):240-6.
70. Buehrig CK, Lager DJ, Stegall MD et al. Influence of surveillance renal allograft biopsy on diagnosis and prognosis of polyomavirus-associated nephropathy. Kidney Int 2003; 64(2):665-73.
71. Poduval RD, Kadambi P, Javaid B et al. Leflunomide-a potential new therapeutic agent for BK nephropathy. Am J Transplant 2003; 3(Suppl 5):189, (Abstract 44).
72. Mengel M, Marwedel M, Radermacher J et al. Incidence of polyomavirus-nephropathy in renal allografts: Influence of modern immunosuppressive drugs. Nephrol Dial Transplant 2003; 18(6):1190-6.
73. Fishman JA. BK virus nephropathy—polyomavirus adding insult to injury. N Engl J Med 2002; 347(7):527-30.
74. Hirsch HH, Steiger J. Polyomavirus BK. The Lancet Infectious Diseases 2003; 3(10):611-23.
75. Kazory A, Ducloux D. Renal transplantation and polyomavirus infection: Recent clinical facts and controversies. Transpl Infect Dis 2003; 5(2):65-71.
76. Nickeleit V, Steiger J, Mihatsch MJ. BK virus infection after kidney transplantation. Graft 2002; 5(Suppl):S46-57.
77. Nickeleit V, Singh H, Mihatsch M. Polyomavirus nephropathy: Morphology, pathophysiology, and clinical management. Curr Opin Nephrol Hypertens 2003; 12(6):599-605.
78. Ramos E, Drachenberg CB, Papadimitriou JC et al. Clinical course of polyoma virus nephropathy in 67 renal transplant patients. J Am Soc Nephrol 2002; 13(8):2145-51.
79. Drachenberg RC, Drachenberg CB, Papadimitriou JC et al. Morphological spectrum of polyoma virus disease in renal allografts: Diagnostic accuracy of urine cytology. Am J Transplant 2001; 1(4):373-81.
80. Celik B, Shapiro R, Vats A et al. Polyomavirus allograft nephropathy: Sequential assessment of histologic viral load, tubulitis, and graft function following changes in immunosuppression. Am J Transplant 2003; 3(11):1378-82.
81. Drachenberg CB, Beskow CO, Cangro CB et al. Human polyoma virus in renal allograft biopsies: Morphological findings and correlation with urine cytology. Hum Pathol 1999; 30(8):970-7.
82. Hussain S, Bresnahan BA, Cohen EP et al. Rapid kidney allograft failure in patients with polyoma virus nephritis with prior treatment with antilymphocyte agents. Clin Transplant 2002; 16(1):43-7.
83. Hurault de Ligny B, Etienne I, Francois A et al. Polyomavirus-induced acute tubulo-interstitial nephritis in renal allograft recipients. Transplant Proc 2000; 32(8):2760-1.
84. Rahamimov R, Lustiga S, Tovar A et al. BK polyoma virus nephropathy in kidney transplant recipient: The role of new immunosuppressive agents. Transplant Proc 2003; 35(2):604-5.
85. Atwood WJ, Norkin LC. Class I major histocompatibility proteins as cell surface receptors for simian virus 40. J Virol 1989; 63(10):4474-7.
86. Liu CK, Wei G, Atwood WJ. Infection of glial cells by the human polyomavirus JC is mediated by an N-linked glycoprotein containing terminal alpha(2-6)-linked sialic acids. J Virol 1998; 72(6):4643-9.
87. Liu CK, Hope AP, Atwood WJ. The human polyomavirus, JCV, does not share receptor specificity with SV40 on human glial cells. J Neurovirol 1998; 4(1):49-58.
88. Drachenberg CB, Papadimitriou JC, Wali R et al. BK polyoma virus allograft nephropathy: Ultrastructural features from viral cell entry to lysis. Am J Transplant 2003; 3(11):1383-92.

89. Schweighardt B, Atwood WJ. Virus receptors in the human central nervous system. J Neurovirol 2001; 7(3):187-95.
90. Atwood WJ. A combination of low-dose chlorpromazine and neutralizing antibodies inhibits the spread of JC virus (JCV) in a tissue culture model: Implications for prophylactic and therapeutic treatment of progressive multifocal leukencephalopathy. J Neurovirol 2001; 7(4):307-10.
91. Baum S, Ashok A, Gee G et al. Early events in the life cycle of JC virus as potential therapeutic targets for the treatment of progressive multifocal leukoencephalopathy. J Neurovirol 2003; 9(Suppl 1):32-7.
92. Anderson HA, Chen Y, Norkin LC. Bound simian virus 40 translocates to caveolin-enriched membrane domains, and its entry is inhibited by drugs that selectively disrupt caveolae. Mol Biol Cell 1996; 7(11):1825-34.
93. Chen Y, Norkin LC. Extracellular simian virus 40 transmits a signal that promotes virus enclosure within caveolae. Exp Cell Res 1999; 246(1):83-90.
94. Gilbert JM, Goldberg IG, Benjamin TL. Cell penetration and trafficking of polyomavirus. J Virol 2003; 77(4):2615-22.
95. Portolani M, Pietrosemoli P, Cermelli C et al. Suppression of BK virus replication and cytopathic effect by inhibitors of prokaryotic DNA gyrase. Antiviral Res 1988; 9(3):205-18.
96. Chen Y, Freund R, Listerud M et al. Retinoic acid inhibits transformation by preventing phosphatidylinositol 3-kinase dependent activation of the c-fos promoter. Oncogene 1999; 18(1):139-48.
97. Talmage DA, Listerud M. Retinoic acid suppresses polyoma virus transformation by inhibiting transcription of the c-fos proto-oncogene. Oncogene 1994; 9(12):3557-63.
98. Ferrazzi E, Peracchi M, Biasolo MA et al. Antiviral activity of gyrase inhibitors norfloxacin, coumermycin A1 and nalidixic acid. Biochem Pharmacol 1988; 37(9):1885-6.
99. Tarabek J, Zemla J, Bacik I. Northern blot hybridization analysis of polyoma virus-specific RNA synthesized under the block of virus replication by 5-bromo-2'-deoxyuridine. Acta Virol 1991; 35(4):305-12.
100. Andrei G, Snoeck R, Vandeputte M et al. Activities of various compounds against murine and primate polyomaviruses. Antimicrob Agents Chemother 1997; 41(3):587-93.
101. De Clercq E. Acyclic nucleoside phosphonates in the chemotherapy of DNA virus and retrovirus infections. Intervirology 1997; 40(5-6):295-303.
102. De Clercq E. In search of a selective antiviral chemotherapy. Clin Microbiol Rev 1997; 10(4):674-93.
103. Foster PF, Wright F, McLean D et al. Leflunomide administration as an adjunct in treatment of BK-polyoma viral disease in kidney allografts [abstract]. Am J Transplant 2003; 3(Suppl 5):421.
104. Snoeck R, Andrei G, Lilja H et al. Activity of malononitrilamide compounds against murine and simian polyomavirus. Geneva, Switzerland: Paper presented at: 5th International Conference on New Trends in Clinical and Experimental Immunosuppression 2002, [abstract].
105. Ma DD, Doan TL. Antisense oligonucleotide therapies: Are they the "magic bullets"? Ann Intern Med 1994; 120(2):161-3.
106. Levy RM, Ward S, Schalgeter K et al. Alternative delivery systems for antiviral nucleosides and antisense oligonucleotides to the brain. J Neurovirol 1997; 3(Suppl 1):S74-5.
107. Package insert. Vistide® (cidofovir injection). Foster City, CA: Gilead Sciences Inc., 2000.
108. Portilla J, Boix V, Roman F et al. Progressive multifocal leukoencephalopathy treated with cidofovir in HIV-infected patients receiving highly active anti-retroviral therapy. J Infect 2000; 41(2):182-4.
109. Cundy KC. Clinical pharmacokinetics of the antiviral nucleotide analogues cidofovir and adefovir. Clin Pharmacokinet 1999; 36(2):127-43.
110. Cassady KA, Whitley RJ. New therapeutic approaches to the alphaherpesvirus infections. J Antimicrob Chemother 1997; 39(2):119-28.
111. Package insert. Arava® Tablets (leflunomide). Kansas City, MO: Aventis Pharmaceuticals Inc., 2003.
112. Hou J, Major EO. The efficacy of nucleoside analogs against JC virus multiplication in a persistently infected human fetal brain cell line. J Neurovirol 1998; 4(4):451-6.
113. Houston S, Roberts N, Mashinter L. Failure of cidofovir therapy in progressive multifocal leukoencephalopathy unrelated to human immunodeficiency virus. Clin Infect Dis 2001; 32(1):150-2.
114. Dodge RT. A case study: The use of cidofovir for the management of progressive multifocal leukoencephalopathy. J Assoc Nurses AIDS Care 1999; 10(4):70-4.
115. Cardenas RL, Cheng KH, Sack K. The effects of cidofovir on progressive multifocal leukoencephalopathy: An MRI case study. Neuroradiology 2001; 43(5):379-82.
116. Salmaggi A, Maccagnano E, Castagna A et al. Reversal of CSF positivity for JC virus genome by cidofovir in a patient with systemic lupus erythematosus and progressive multifocal leukoencephalopathy. Neurol Sci 2001; 22(1):17-20.

117. Razonable RR, Aksamit AJ, Wright AJ et al. Cidofovir treatment of progressive multifocal leukoencephalopathy in a patient receiving highly active antiretroviral therapy. Mayo Clin Proc 2001; 76(11):1171-5.
118. Haider S, Nafziger D, Gutierrez JA et al. Progressive multifocal leukoencephalopathy and idiopathic CD4+lymphocytopenia: A case report and review of reported cases. Clin Infect Dis 2000; 31(4):E20-2.
119. Zimmermann T, Stingele K, Hartmann M et al. Successful treatment of aids related PML with HAART and cidofovir. Eur J Med Res 2001; 6(5):190-62.
120. Roberts MT, Carmichael A, Lever AM. Prolonged survival in AIDS-related progressive multifocal leucoencephalopathy following anti-retroviral therapy and cidofovir. Int J Antimicrob Agents 2003; 21(4):347-9.
121. Antinori A, Cingolani A, Lorenzini P et al. Clinical epidemiology and survival of progressive multifocal leukoencephalopathy in the era of highly active antiretroviral therapy: Data from the Italian Registry Investigative Neuro AIDS (IRINA). J Neurovirol 2003; 9(Suppl 1):47-53.
122. Kiewe P, Seyfert S, Korper S et al. Progressive multifocal leukoencephalopathy with detection of JC virus in a patient with chronic lymphocytic leukemia parallel to onset of fludarabine therapy. Leuk Lymphoma 2003; 44(10):1815-8.
123. De Luca A, Giancola ML, Ammassari A et al. Cidofovir added to HAART improves virological and clinical outcome in AIDS-associated progressive multifocal leukoencephalopathy. Aids 2000; 14(14):F117-21.
124. De Luca A, Giancola ML, Ammassari A et al. Potent anti-retroviral therapy with or without cidofovir for AIDS-associated progressive multifocal leukoencephalopathy: Extended follow-up of an observational study. J Neurovirol 2001; 7(4):364-8.
125. Taoufik Y, Delfraissy JF, Gasnault J. Highly active antiretroviral therapy does not improve survival of patients with high JC virus load in the cerebrospinal fluid at progressive multifocal leukoencephalopathy diagnosis. Aids 2000; 14(6):758-9.
126. Held TK, Biel SS, Nitsche A et al. Treatment of BK virus-associated hemorrhagic cystitis and simultaneous CMV reactivation with cidofovir. Bone Marrow Transplant 2000; 26(3):347-50.
127. Hatakeyama N, Suzuki N, Kudoh T et al. Successful cidofovir treatment of adenovirus-associated hemorrhagic cystitis and renal dysfunction after allogenic bone marrow transplant. Pediatr Infect Dis J 2003; 22(10):928-9.
128. Bjorang O, Tveitan H, Midtvedt K et al. Treatment of polyomavirus infection with cidofovir in a renal-transplant recipient. Nephrol Dial Transplant 2002; 17(11):2023-5.
129. Keller LS, Peh CA, Nolan J et al. BK transplant nephropathy successfully treated with cidofovir. Nephrol Dial Transplant 2003; 18(5):1013-4.
130. Kadambi PV, Josephson MA, Williams J et al. Treatment of refractory BK virus-associated nephropathy with cidofovir. Am J Transplant 2003; 3(2):186-91.
131. Vats A, Shapiro R, Singh Randhawa P et al. Quantitative viral load monitoring and cidofovir therapy for the management of BK virus-associated nephropathy in children and adults. Transplantation 2003; 75(1):105-12.
132. Scantlebury V, Shapiro R, Randhawa P et al. Cidofovir: A method of treatment for BK virus-associated transplant nephropathy. Graft 2002; 5(Suppl):S82-7.
133. Mayer DF, Kushwaha SS. Transplant immunosuppressant agents and their role in autoimmune rheumatic diseases. Curr Opin Rheumatol 2003; 15(3):219-25.
134. Sanders S, Harisdangkul V. Leflunomide for the treatment of rheumatoid arthritis and autoimmunity. Am J Med Sci 2002; 323(4):190-3.
135. Goldenberg MM. Leflunomide, a novel immunomodulator for the treatment of active rheumatoid arthritis. Clin Ther 1999; 21(11):1837-52; discussion 21.
136. Lednicky JA, Stewart AR, Jenkins III JJ et al. SV40 DNA in human osteosarcomas shows sequence variation among T-antigen genes. Int J Cancer 1997; 72(5):791-800.
137. Waldman WJ, Knight DA, Blinder L et al. Inhibition of cytomegalovirus in vitro and in vivo by the experimental immunosuppressive agent leflunomide. Intervirology 1999; 42(5-6):412-8.
138. Waldman WJ, Knight DA, Lurain NS et al. Novel mechanism of inhibition of cytomegalovirus by the experimental immunosuppressive agent leflunomide. Transplantation 1999; 68(6):814-25.
139. Williams JW, Mital D, Chong A et al. Experiences with leflunomide in solid organ transplantation. Transplantation 2002; 73(3):358-66.
140. Kerr DA, Chang CF, Gordon J et al. Inhibition of human neurotropic virus (JCV) DNA replication in glial cells by camptothecin. Virology 1993; 196(2):612-8.
141. Package insert. Hycamtin® (topotecan hydrochloride). Research Triangle Park, North Carolina: GlaxoSmithKline Pharmaceuticals, 2003.

142. Rand KH, Johnson KP, Rubinstein LJ et al. Adenine arabinoside in the treatment of progressive multifocal leukoencephalopathy: Use of virus-containing cells in the urine to assess response to therapy. Ann Neurol 1977; 1(5):458-62.
143. Package Insert. Cytarabine. Irvine, California: GensiaSicor Pharmaceuticals, 1999.
144. Nicoli F, Chave B, Peragut JC et al. Efficacy of cytarabine in progressive multifocal leucoencephalopathy in AIDS. Lancet 1992; 339(8788):306.
145. O'Riordan T, Daly PA, Hutchinson M et al. Progressive multifocal leukoencephalopathy-remission with cytarabine. J Infect 1990; 20(1):51-4.
146. Steiger MJ, Tarnesby G, Gabe S et al. Successful outcome of progressive multifocal leukoencephalopathy with cytarabine and interferon. Ann Neurol 1993; 33(4):407-11.
147. Aksamit AJ. Treatment of nonAIDS progressive multifocal leukoencephalopathy with cytosine arabinoside. J Neurovirol 2001; 7(4):386-90.
148. Levy RM, Major E, Ali MJ et al. Convection-enhanced intraparenchymal delivery (CEID) of cytosine arabinoside (AraC) for the treatment of HIV-related progressive multifocal leukoencephalopathy (PML). J Neurovirol 2001; 7(4):382-5.
149. Hoffmann RP, Lewis IK. Vidarabine (Drug Evaluation). In: Hutchinson TA, Shahan DR, eds. DRUGDEX® System. MICROMEDEX, Greenwood Village, Colorado (Edition expires 9/2002).
150. Chapman C, Flower AJ, Durrant ST. The use of vidarabine in the treatment of human polyomavirus associated acute haemorrhagic cystitis. Bone Marrow Transplant 1991; 7(6):481-3.
151. Seabra C, Perez-Simon JA, Sierra M et al. Intra-muscular vidarabine therapy for polyomavirus-associated hemorrhagic cystitis following allogeneic hemopoietic stem cell transplantation. Bone Marrow Transplant 2000; 26(11):1229-30.
152. Vianelli N, Renga M, Azzi A et al. Sequential vidarabine infusion in the treatment of polyoma virus-associated acute haemorrhagic cystitis late after allogeneic bone marrow transplantation. Bone Marrow Transplant 2000; 25(3):319-20.
153. Puliyanda D, Amet N, Archana D et al. IVIG contains antibodies reactive with polyomaviruses BK and may represent a therapeutic option for BK virus and may represent a therapeutic option for BK nephropathy. Am J Transplant 2003; 3(Suppl 5):393 (Abstract 941).
154. Casadei DH, Rial MDC, Opelz G et al. A randomized and prospective study comparing treatment with high-dose intravenous immunoglobulin with monoclonal antibodies for rescue of kidney grafts with steroid-resistant rejection. Transplantation 2001; 71(1):53-8.
155. Cibrik DM, O Toole JF, Norman SP et al. IVIG for the treatment of BK nephropathy. Am J Transplant 2003; 3(Suppl 5):370 (Abstract 850).
156. Berger JR. Progressive Multifocal Leukoencephalopathy. Curr Treat Options Neurol 2000; 2(4):361-8.
157. Huang SS, Skolasky RL, Dal Pan GJ et al. Survival prolongation in HIV-associated progressive multifocal leukoencephalopathy treated with alpha-interferon: An observational study. J Neurovirol 1998; 4(3):324-32.
158. Clifford DB. Challenges for clinical trials to treat progressive multifocal leukoencephalopathy. J Neurovirol 2003; 9(Suppl 1):68-72.
159. Cheeseman SH, Black PH, Rubin RH et al. Interferon and BK Papovavirus—clinical and laboratory studies. J Infect Dis 1980; 141(2):157-61.
160. Ramos E, Drachenberg CB, Portocarrero M et al. BK virus nephropathy diagnosis and treatment: Experience at the University of Maryland Renal Transplant Program. In: Cecka J, Terasaki P, eds. Clinical Transplants 2002. Los Angeles: UCLA Immunogenetics Center; 2003:143-53.
161. Mayr M, Nickeleit V, Hirsch HH et al. Polyomavirus BK nephropathy in a kidney transplant recipient: Critical issues of diagnosis and management. Am J Kidney Dis 2001; 38(3):E13.
162. Scantlebury V, Shapiro R, Justin G et al. Graft function after diagnosis of BK virus in adult kidney transplant recipients under tacrolimus-based immunosuppression [abstract]. Am J Transpl 2001; 1(Suppl 1):404.
163. Loertscher R, Suri R, Lipman M et al. Deliberate reduction of immunosuppression benefits patients with polyoma BK virus infection in kidney allografts [abstract]. Am J Transpl 2002; 2(Suppl 3):262.

CHAPTER 18

Leflunomide in Solid Organ Transplantation and Polyoma Virus Infection

Michelle A. Josephson, Basit Javaid, Pradeep V. Kadambi,
Shane M. Meehan and James W. Williams

Introduction

Leflunomide, trade name Arava® (Aventis Pharmaceuticals Incorporation, Bridgewater, New Jersey, U.S.A.), belongs to a family of drugs called the malonitrilamides. Some, like leflunomide, have substantial immune suppressive activity in experimental allograft models. In addition to experimental data suggesting leflunomide's value in preventing[1-5] and reversing acute[1,5] and chronic rejection,[6,7] it has been shown to inhibit human cytomegalovirus (CMV) and herpes simplex virus (HSV) in vitro.[8-10] Because it is a drug with a variety of biologic activities, it has been investigated for diseases as disparate as cancer and autoimmunity. Leflunomide was approved for the treatment of rheumatoid arthritis and has been used in more than 300,000 patients worldwide with efficacy and a favorable side effect profile. In this chapter, we will discuss the immunemodulatory effects of leflunomide and its metabolite A77 1726 that prevent organ rejection. We will also share our experience in the treatment of polyomavirus infections.

Clinical Pharmacology

Leflunomide, a pro-drug, is rapidly metabolized to A77 1726. A77 1726, a malononitrileamide, accounts for the in vivo and in vitro activity of leflunomide as well as its toxicity. The pharmacokinetic behavior of this drug is very different in humans from all other species tested. The half life of the drug in dogs, rats, mice, cats, and non human primates is 9 to 24 hours while in normal human volunteers and patients with rheumatoid arthritis, the half life is 15 to 30 days.[11] The half life in patients with reduced renal function is much shorter, approximately 10 days.[12] The reason for this phenomenon is not well understood but may be linked to a reduction in protein binding as kidney function worsens.[11]

Leflunomide and similar analogues (malononitrile amides) inhibit both immune and nonimmune cell responses to various cytokines and signaling molecules.[1,13-21] Experimental features of this drug include the following: (1) inhibition of T Cell activation and control of acute rejection in rodents[1,13-15,17-21] and dogs;[22] (2) inhibition of B cell activity[5,6,18,20] and control of xeno-rejection;[3,4,7] (3) ability, in rodents to reverse an on-going acute rejection refractory to cyclosporine;[5] (4) synergistic interaction with the calcineurin inhibitors in vitro and in vivo;[5,6,23] (5) the ability to reverse established pathological features of chronic rejection in rodents;[6,7] (6) inhibition of CMV replication in vitro and in vivo at concentrations readily attained in humans;[8-10] (7) inhibition of polyoma BK virus replication in vitro. The two areas of leflunomide activity that are relevant to transplantation immunosuppression are cytokine

Polyomaviruses and Human Diseases, edited by Nasimul Ahsan. ©2006 Eurekah.com
and Springer Science+Business Media.

driven immune suppressive activity and nonimmune anti-proliferative activity involving cells of mesenchymal origin.

A77 1726's mechanism of action involves at least two properties: the inhibition of a mitochondrial enzyme, dihydroorotic acid dehydrogenase (DHODH), in the de novo synthesis of uridine,[13,24-27] and the inhibition of selected tyrosine kinases involved in T cell, B cell, vascular smooth muscle cell and fibroblast signaling cascades.[13,17-20] It also has been reported to block NFkB and AP-1 activation in peripheral blood lymphocytes in vitro.[28]

Immunosuppressive Properties: Mechanisms of Immunosuppression

Consensus on the basic mechanism of action of this drug has been slow to evolve. In 1996 it was established and subsequently confirmed, that the active metabolite, A77,1726, at low molar concentrations reversibly inhibits a mitochondrial enzyme (DHODH) in de novo pyrimidine synthesis.[13,25-27,29] Because rapidly proliferating lymphocytes tend to rely on de novo pyrimidine synthesis rather than the salvage pathways, the inhibition of this enzyme can impede lymphocyte proliferation [peripheral blood lymphocytes (PBL) and cell lines]. However, while high concentration mitogen stimulated lymphocyte proliferation is controlled, lower mitogen concentrations and other proliferative stimuli are not controlled by pyrimidine (DHODH) inhibition.[26] We[1,20] and others[30] have shown that if adequate supply of pyrimidine is provided the salvage pathway is adequate to restore intracellular stores of uridine/pyrimidines in the lymphoid, splenic, hepatic and myeloid compartments. Restoring pyrimidine levels in vitro reverses the anti proliferative effects at the lower concentration of A77 1726, but not at concentrations of drug above 50 uM where other mechanisms of activity are encountered.[13,15,18,19]

This observation has been replicated in experimental animals, with intra peritoneal (IP) pyrimidine supplementation reversing the toxicity of high dose leflunomide, but not reversing the control of acute allograft rejection.[1] In a xenograft model (Hamster to Lewis rat), a potent stimulus to both T and B Cell proliferation, 15 mg/kg leflunomide alone effectively delays rejection to more than 45 days, and exogenous pyrimidine replacement (uridine IP) reduces graft survival to ~ 15 days. In the presence of exogenous uridine a leflunomide dose of 30 mg/kg, restores the control of xeno-rejection, extending graft survival to 40 + days.[7] A number of other drug effects, including the anti-polyoma and anti-CMV activities, are similarly not explained by the DHODH mechanism (Table 1).

In 1993 Mattar et al[16] reported that A77 1726 blocks phosphorylation by protein tyrosine kinases (PTKs) and these observations have been confirmed by other investigators. The protein tyrosine kinases shown to be blocked by A77 1726 are listed in Table 1. The molecule has no effect against serine/threonine kinases or phosphatases. Evidence has been reported that the molecule inhibits activation of NFκB[28] but this has not been confirmed by other laboratories. Because A77 1726 blocks phosphorylation of several tyrosine kinase cellular signaling molecules important for immune responses at inhibitory concentrations (IC50) attained in animals and humans, (Table 1) and because the toxicity, but not the efficacy, is reversed by pyrimidine repletion in rats, we have proposed that the mechanism of action is primarily related to the ability to interrupt these signaling molecules.

Relationship of in Vitro Kinase Activity to Mechanism of Action in Vivo

Assigning a relevant protein kinase inhibitory mechanism to the in vivo action to leflunomide has been resisted[30-32] for three principal reasons: (1) in rats the concentration of drug needed to inhibit the PTKs is 100 to 1000 times the concentration needed for inhibition of rat DHODH (and the affinity of A77 1726 for the rat isoform is approximately 3 logs greater than the human DHODH), (2) the drug levels attained in leflunomide treated rats were not well defined, and (3) until recently there were essentially no data on the blood levels attained in human subjects with organ transplantation.

Table 1. In vitro activity not dependent on DHODH inhibition

Inhibition of by A771726		References
PDGF-B	IC_{50} 30 uM	*17,21
PDGF-B	IC_{50} 75 uM	
EGF	IC_{50} 30-40 uM	16,21
	IC_{50} 150-200 uM	
JAK/STAT	IC_{50} 75-100 uM	13,18
LCK, FYN	IC_{50} 50-100 uM	19
ζ chain TCR	IC_{50} 35uM	19
PLC-γ1	IC_{50} 44uM	19
Adhesion		50
Chemotaxis, Neutrophil		51
Inhibition of Cytokine Production		
TNF, IL-1, IL652		
Antibody phenomena		
Isotype Switch		18
No uridine reversal of Ab inhibition at A77 1726		53
conc of 100uM		
Blocks Allo IgG		6
Class Switch, IgG and IgE		54
PGE and IL6		55
Sepsis Protection		Unpublished data, Ma Y et al
B cell and T cell, differential reversal by uridine		56
Endothelial cell proliferation		57
Viral Replication		9

* Leflunomide rather than A77,1726 used for in vitro studies in reference 18.

It now appears that the difference in IC 50 for DHODH and PTK inhibition in humans is approximately 50 fold (IC 50 for human DHODH is ~1-3 µM and PTK's is 50 to 150 µM). More importantly, it is now clear that transplant patients tolerate A77,1726 blood levels of 150 µM to 250 µM with minimal side effects.[12] *

Leflunomide and PDGF (Platelet Derived Growth Factor)

PDGF (A and B isoforms) are potent mitogens for smooth muscle cell (SMC) and mesangial cell proliferation and chemotaxis.[33] This cytokine is thought to mediate vascular remodeling in models of immune and non immune arterial injury as well as mesangial proliferation and, in concert with other signaling molecules, influence arterial and mesangial matrix deposition. While other cytokines are invoked in the repair process (TGFβ, epidermal growth factor [EGF] for example), blockade of this receptor signaling, binding of the ligand by antibody or genetic deletion, eliminates or substantially reduces the observed fibrosis and mesangial injury endpoints in several models of experimental renal injury and vascular responses.[34-49]

We and others have shown that leflunomide (A77 1726) prevents PDGF receptor phosphorylation at an IC 50 of approximately 50 µM.[17,21] This corresponds to approximately 16 µg/ml, well within the blood levels clinically attained in transplant patients. Because there appears to be limited requirement for PDGF functioning in adult life, blockade of this receptor is not likely to be associated with significant morbidity.

*Blood levels of A77 1726 are reported as ug/ml, and 150 mM corresponds to a blood level of 50 mg/ml.

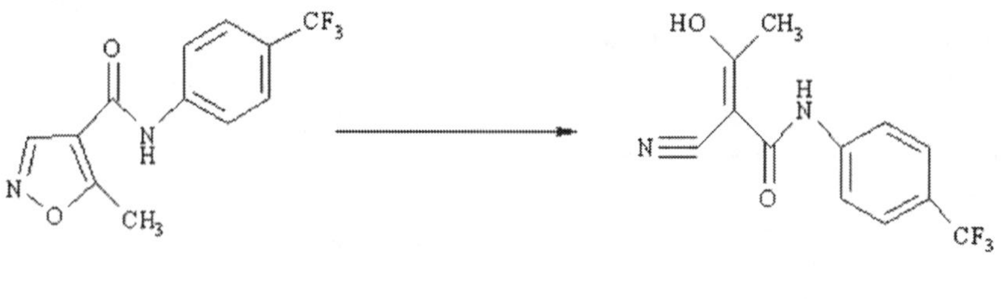

Figure 1. The isonazde ring is immediately opened after oral dosing and only A77 1726 is found in blood.

Leflunomide Control of Acute Rejection: Data and Possible Mechanisms

Once leflunomide was shown to control acute rejection in rodents at a wide range of doses[1,5-7,22] a number of laboratories, in addition to ours, began to study the effects of A77,1726 on lymphocyte function in vitro (Table 1). The molecular activities ascribed to leflunomide, aside from pyrimidine synthesis inhibition, that may explain its control of acute T and B cell activation in an allograft include the following:

Inhibition PTK(phosphorylation)
1. Inhibition of theta chain of TCR
2. Inhibition of src family kinases P56 lck and P59 fyn
3. JAK STATs
4. Activation of PLCγ

A77,1726 blocks the phosphorylation of these proteins at IC50 concentrations of 50 to 150 μM, levels now known to be attained in the blood of animals and patients receiving leflunomide following organ transplantation. While it is intuitive to conclude that the effective blockade of these molecules (either alone or as a group) would prevent T and B cell activation and thus control acute rejection, little in the way of direct proof of this concept in vivo exists. While Xu et al[20] have demonstrated that leflunomide treatment reduced phosphorylation of various substrates in the *lpr/lpr* mouse that coincided with reduced lupus-like manifestations, these studies have not been done in transplant models.

Leflunomide Control of Chronic Rejection: Data and Possible Non Immune Mechanisms

In addition to its effects in acute rejection, a considerable amount of work in rodents has shown leflunomide to be effective in both the prevention[58] and reversal[7,31] of chronic allograft rejection and in controlling acute and chronic xeno rejection.[3,4,7] Using the Lewis to Fisher chronic cardiac rejection model, the combination of leflunomide and cyclosporine starting 30-45 days after surgery, reversed the arterial vasculopathy almost to baseline with 60 days of therapy[59] (Table 2). In this model cyclosporine is not significantly better at controlling vasculopathy or interstitial fibrosis than no treatment. The potency of this drug combination in this and other models has been reproduced by others.[4,30,60]

Because an immune suppressive drug alone cannot (or at least has not been able to) control chronic rejection, it is likely that nonimmune suppressing activities of leflunomide account for its experimental control of chronic rejection and vascular remodeling. The ability of leflunomide (unpublished data from our laboratory), as well as other malononitrile amide analogues,[61] to control the exuberant intimal expansion in rat carotid artery catheter injury support this position.

Despite the descriptive data in chronic vascular remodeling, there are no data directly addressing the molecular mechanisms of action behind this feature. However, the ability of leflunomide to inhibit PDGFR signaling at low drug concentrations is an attractive hypothesis.

Table 2. Score of chronic arterial lesions with various treatments

| | N | Arteries Scored | Arterial Score | | | % of Art Injured |
			Day 30	Day 60	Day 90	
Control	17	508	2.3 ± 0.9	2.7 ± 1.3	3.4 ± 0.9	92% ± 10
CyA	12	404		1.6 ± 0.8	2.8 ± 1.0	83% ± 20*
Lef	12	442		1.6 ± 0.5	1.4 ± 0.9*	48% ± 18*
CyA and Lef	12	480		0.8 ± 0.3	0.7 ± 0.4*	37% ± 12

*p< 0.05. Modified from Xiao et al. Transplantation 1995; 60:1065.[59]

Clinical Immunosuppression Efficacy in Transplantation

The evaluation of leflunomide in clinical transplantation is not extensive. Its use in 53 transplant patient with a variety of clinical issues has been published.[5] A study of 22 patients with clinical evidence of chronic allograft nephropathy (CAN) by Hardinger et al[62] supports leflunomide's safety and potential efficacy in renal allograft recipients. Active metabolite blood level monitoring of a targeted blood level between 50 and 100 µg/ml (150 to 300 µM) requires doses higher than those more commonly used for rheumatoid arthritis.

Anti-Viral Properties: In Vitro Activity of A77 1726

CMV

The first evidence that leflunomide had anti viral activity was developed in collaboration with Waldman et al[9,10] who showed that human and rat CMV are inhibited by A77 1726 in vitro in a dose dependent manner with an IC 50 of 50 µM and that the effect is independent of pyrimidine deficiency. In collaboration with Waldman, we have shown that A77 1726, significantly inhibits replication of rat CMV in vivo.[10] Herpes virus Type I is similarly inhibited in vitro and all of these anti viral effects are unrelated to inhibition of pyrimidine production. Waldman suggests that while neither CMV viral DNA nor viral protein synthesis are affected, tegumentation and viral assembly are impaired. This defective viral assembly prevents production of infectious virions.

Clinical evaluation of leflunomide in the treatment of CMV is limited to a small number of patients with CMV who have been treated with leflunomide when all else had failed. Five of these cases have been reported.[63,64] In four other patients treated by the authors, (one liver, one heart, and two kidney allograft recipients) CMV became undetectable in the blood with leflunomide therapy.[65]

Polyoma

Atwood and colleagues have tested polyoma BK and polyoma JC viral strains in vitro for sensitivity to the active metabolite of leflunomide, A77 1726 (manuscript in preparation). SVG-A and Vero cells were grown in Eagles minimal essential media with 10% fetal bovine serum. Sub-confluent 6-well culture plates were pretreated for 45 minutes with 100 uM uridine alone or in combination with 18 µM, 39 µM and 390 µM A77 1726 (leflunomide active metabolite). The cells were then infected with JCV (SVG-A cells) or BKV (Vero cells). Following incubation with virus the cells were washed three times with PBS and then maintained in media with or without drug and uridine. At 72 hours post-infection the cells were washed three times with phosphate buffer solution (PBS), acetone-fixed, and stained with an anti-V antigen monoclonal antibody followed by goat anti-rabbit fluorescein isothiocyanate (FITC) conjugated secondary antibody. Infected cells were visualized and counted on a Nikon E800 epi-fluorescent microscope.

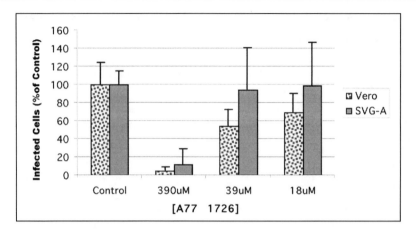

Figure 2. Effects of A77 1726 (leflunomide) on infection of cells by the human polyomaviruses, JCV and BKV. Vero cells and SVG-A cells were infected with either BKV or JCV in the absence and presence of increasing concentrations of A77,1726. At three days post-infection cells were fixed and scored for expression of the late viral protein V antigen by indirect immunofluorescent analysis. The percentage of infected cells in drug treated samples was compared to the percentage of infected cells in untreated cells which was set at 100%. The presence of uridine at 100 μM had no effect on viral inhibition. Data used with permission from Walter J. Atwood.

Figure 2 shows the effect of increasing concentrations of active metabolite A77,1726 on replication of JC and BK virus in vitro. Data are presented as the estimated proportion of infected cells, relative to an untreated control, plus the corresponding estimate of standard error for each concentration. These data suggest that the IC 50 for polyoma BK virus is approximately 40uM. However, unlike CMV, polyoma viruses lack a tegument, and so a different mechanism of viral inhibition from that seen with CMV must be involved.

Reconciliation of Immune Suppression and Anti-Viral Activity

Anti-viral activity from a potent immune suppressive molecule seems to defy the conventional principles in immune suppressive therapy. Some of the previously described features of the drug allow us to speculate about what might account for this paradox. Experimental data from in vitro and in vivo studies clearly show that the anti viral activity[8-10] and substantial immune suppression occur independently of the pyrimidine inhibition.[1] The active metabolite, A77 1726, and structural analogues of this molecule have also been shown to block signaling mediated by several tyrosine kinases including PDGF,[17,19] EGF,[14,16,21] JAK 3,[13,18] Bruton's Tyrosine Kinase[15] ξ chain of T cell receptor (TCR), PLCγ1,[19] and the Src family kinases p56 lck and fyn,[19] molecules which are involved in signaling within T and B cell and other populations. Thus, drug induced interference with the phosphorylation of molecules causing the virally infected cell to proliferate, such as the Src family of kinases or others known to be inhibited by leflunomide, could be the link between the drug's ability to inhibit viral replication and at least part of its ability to prevent rejection.

The relevance of leflunomide's PTK inhibition demonstrated in vitro to its clinical immune suppression efficacy has been disputed[30,31] because levels required in vitro for PTK inhibition are higher than those observed for DHODH inhibition. However, the blood levels of A77 1726 found clinically to be efficacious in reducing polyoma BK viral loads, above 40 μg/ml (120 μM), exceed the IC 50 concentrations demonstrated in vitro for inhibition of BK virus. These blood levels also exceed the in vitro IC 50 concentrations required for inhibition of PDGF B signaling,[17,21] EGF signaling,[16,21] JAK/STAT, PLCγ, LCK, FYN, and ξ chain TCR signaling.[13,18,19]

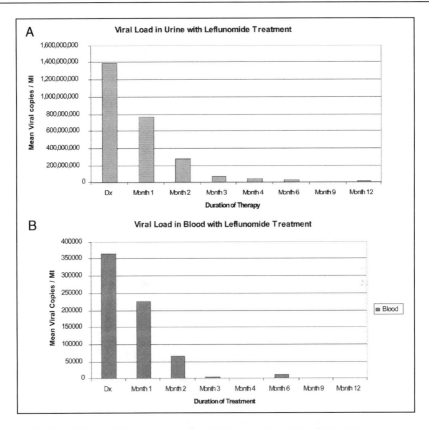

Figure 3. Copies of Polyoma BK virus measured by PCR in urine (A) and blood (B) in 15 patients sustaining blood levels of A771726 above 40 µg/ml. Modified from Williams JW, Javid B, Kadambi PV et al, N Engl J Med (letter) 2005; 352:1157-8.

Leflunomide in BKN

From July 2001 to April 2004 we used leflunomide as the initial anti viral therapy for 16 patients with biopsy proven BKN. All but one of these patients was receiving tacrolimus, prednisone and mycophenolate mofetil at the time of diagnosis. Mycophenolate mofetil was stopped, tacrolimus was targeted at trough levels of 4-6 ng/ml, and the prednisone dose generally was not altered. Leflunomide was dosed to a targeted blood level of 50 to 100 µg/ml using a loading dose of 100 mg daily for five days and maintenance doses of 20 mg to 60 mg/day. Treatment was monitored by serial determinations of viral load in blood and urine (PCR), serum creatinine, hematologic and liver functions, A77 1726 blood levels and allograft rebiopsy when clinically needed.

All patients maintaining blood levels of A77 1726 above 40 µg/ml either cleared the virus or have had progressive reduction in viral load in blood and urine (p<.001) (Fig. 3). Seven patients cleared the viremia and five of these have cleared the viruria. Although viruria persists (at significantly reduced levels) in 11 patients, viremia has not recurred in any of them.

Two of these 16 patients did not sustain blood levels of A77 1726 above 40 µg/ml using a 60 mg daily dose and both graft histology and viral load failed to improve. With continued leflunomide dosing, a short course of cidofovir was given to these two patients. The viremia then cleared in one and the viral load continues to fall in the other.

Serum creatinine levels stabilized in those with therapeutic A771726 levels, and have not changed significantly from base line. There were no significant dose limiting changes in

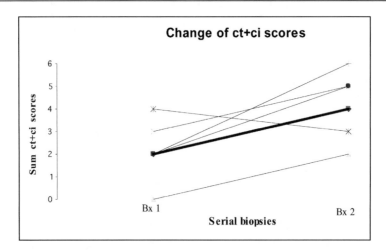

Figure 4. Change in ct +ci score in index (B x 1) and follow up biopsies (B x 2). The ct +ci score is the sum of the Banff 97 chronic score indices for tubular atrophy and intersitial fibrosis.[66] The median sum score was 2 (range 0-4) for the index biopsies (B x 1), and 4 (range 2-6) for the follow-up biopsies (B x 2), p = 0.01. The dark bolded line represents the median trend-line.

hematocrit or white blood cell counts. One patient had an elevation of serum alkaline phosphatase to 5 times that of the baseline value requiring dose reduction.

It is important to note that the protocol described above, using leflunomide for anti viral therapy, employs doses higher than those recommended in the drug "package insert." The insert states that the maximum dose for Arava® (leflunomide) is 20 mg/day. The increased dosing protocol used for anti-viral therapy was only used when drug levels were monitored closely and doses adjusted as needed. Doses higher than 20 mg/day should not be prescribed if drug levels cannot be monitored closely.

The Consequences of Late Diagnosis and Intervention

The experience described above is consistent with in vitro data demonstrating leflumomide's anti-polyoma virus activity. Though these observations are encouraging, we are left with the question: did leflunomide use improve the dismal graft survival that might otherwise be expected in BK nephropathy? In the absence of a controlled clinical trial, it is difficult to answer that question. However, examining the kidney biopsies of treated patients gave us some insight into the potential for BK nephropathy to cause irreversible and progressive damage, despite viral resolution. Eight patients with a history of leflunomide only treated BK nephropathy underwent repeat biopsy. These biopsies revealed either complete resolution of or significant reduction in the extent of tubular T antigen expression. Despite the decreased extent of T antigen expression, interstitial fibrosis and tubular atrophy had developed in the graft parenchyma. The chronic changes were more apparent in the follow-up biopsy compared to the index diagnostic biopsy (Fig. 4). This patient cohort had likely been diagnosed late in their disease course and the virus and inflammation had been present for a considerable but indeterminate duration. Early diagnosis and intervention before the onset of fibrosis may allow resolution of the virus without long term fibrosis and impaired graft survival. This hypothesis implying early viral screening deserves further study.

Conclusion

Leflunomide was approved in 1998 in the United States for the treatment of rheumatoid arthritis. The drug appears to be efficacious in the treatment of rheumatoid arthritis in patients refractory to methotrexate. Though generally well tolerated, the most common side effects include gastrointestinal complaints, hair loss and skin rash. In the first 100,000 patients receiving the drug serious liver complications were seen in approximately 15 patients with liver failure and death in 10, most of whom had known preexisting liver disease or were taking other hepatotoxic drugs. When these conditions were avoided and liver enzymes were monitored during the first few months of therapy, this complication has fallen substantially. In addition to its use as a disease modifying agent in rheumatoid arthritis there are multiple reports of successful outcomes with the use of this drug in various clinical conditions including autoimmune diseases, solid organ transplantation, and viral infections specifically in immune compromised individuals. The unique immunomodulatory and antiproliferative properties of this drug, and its evolving role as an antiviral agent, has generated a great deal of interest for this compound in the field of transplantation. The mechanism of leflunomide antiviral activity is a topic of active research. Preliminary observations with the successful use of leflunomide in patients with BKN warrant additional clinical studies to further define the role of this drug in the field of solid organ transplantation.

References

1. Chong AS, Huang W, Liu W et al. In vivo activity of leflunomide: Pharmacokinetic analyses and mechanism of immunosuppression. Transplantation 1999; 68:100-109.
2. Kuchle CC, Thoenes GH, Langer KH et al. Prevention of kidney and skin graft rejection in rats by leflunomide, a new immunomodulating agent. Transplant Proc 1991; 23:1083-1086.
3. Lin Y, Waer M. In vivo mechanism of action of leflunomide: Selective inhibition of the capacity of B lymphocytes to make T-independent xenoantibodies. Transplant Proc 1996; 28:3085.
4. Lin Y, Goebels J, Xia G et al. Induction of specific transplantation tolerance across xenogeneic barriers in the T-independent immune compartment. Nat Med 1998; 4:173-180.
5. Williams JW, Xiao F, Foster P et al. Leflunomide in experimental transplantation. Control of rejection and alloantibody production, Reversal of acute rejection, and interaction with cyclosporine. Transplantation 1994; 57:1223-1231.
6. Xiao F, Chong A, Shen J et al. Pharmacologically induced regression of chronic transplant rejection. Transplantation 1995; 60:1065-1072.
7. Xiao F, Shen J, Chong A et al. Control and reversal of chronic xenograft rejection in hamster-to-rat cardiac transplantation. Transplant Proc 1996; 28:691-692.
8. Knight DA, Hejmanowski AQ, Dierksheide JE et al. Inhibition of herpes simplex virus type 1 by the experimental immunosuppressive agent leflunomide. Transplantation 2001; 71:170-174.
9. Waldman WJ, Knight DA, Lurain NS et al. Novel mechanism of inhibition of cytomegalovirus by the experimental immunosuppressive agent leflunomide. Transplantation 1999; 68:814-825.
10. Waldman WJ, Knight DA, Blinder L et al. Inhibition of cytomegalovirus in vitro and in vivo by the experimental immunosuppressive agent leflunomide. Intervirology 1999; 42:412-418.
11. Sponsor: Hoechst Marion Roussel. Summary of Nda 20-905. Clinical Pharmacology/Biopharmaceutics Review 1998; 31-33.
12. Williams JW, Mital D, Chong A et al. Experiences with leflunomide in solid organ transplantation. Transplantation 2002; 73:358-366.
13. Elder RT, Xu X, Williams JW et al. The immunosuppressive metabolite of leflunomide, A77 1726, affects murine T cells through two biochemical mechanisms. J Immunol 1997; 159:22-27.
14. Ghosh S, Zheng Y, Jun X et al. Alpha-cyano-beta-hydroxy-beta-methyl-N-[4-(Trifluoromethoxy)phenyl] propenamide: An inhibitor of the epidermal growth factor receptor tyrosine kinase with potent cytotoxic activity against breast cancer cells. Clin Cancer Res 1998; 4:2657-2668.
15. Mahajan S, Ghosh S, Sudbeck EA et al. Rational design and synthesis of a novel anti-leukemic agent targeting bruton's tyrosine kinase (Btk), Lfm-A13 [Alpha-Cyano-Beta-Hydroxy-Beta-Methyl-N-(2, 5-Dibromophenyl)propenamide]. J Biol Chem 1999; 274:9587-9599.
16. Mattar T, Kochhar K, Bartlett R et al. Inhibition of the epidermal growth factor receptor tyrosine kinase activity by leflunomide. Febs Lett 1993; 334:161-164.
17. Shawver LK, Schwartz DP, Mann E et al. Inhibition of platelet-derived growth factor-mediated signal transduction and tumor growth by N-[4-(Trifluoromethyl)-Phenyl]5-Methylisoxazole-4-Carboxamide. Clin Cancer Res 1997; 3:1167-1177.
18. Siemasko K, Chong AS, Jack HM et al. Inhibition of Jak3 and Stat6 tyrosine phosphorylation by the immunosuppressive drug leflunomide leads to a block in Igg1 production. J Immunol 1998; 160:1581-1588.

19. Xu X, Williams JW, Bremer EG et al. Inhibition of protein tyrosine phosphorylation in T cells by a novel immunosuppressive agent, leflunomide. J Biol Chem 1995; 270:12398-12403.

20. Xu X, Blinder L, Shen J et al. In vivo mechanism by which leflunomide controls lymphoproliferative and autoimmune disease in Mrl/Mpj-Lpr/Lpr mice. J Immunol 1997; 159:167-174.

21. Xu X, Shen J, Mall JW et al. In vitro and in vivo antitumor activity of a novel immunomodulatory drug, leflunomide: Mechanisms of action. Biochem Pharmacol 1999; 58:1405-1413.

22. Mcchesney LP, Xiao F, Sankary HN et al. An evaluation of leflunomide in the canine renal transplantation model transplantation 1994; 57:1717-1722.

23. Sankary HN, Yin DP, Chong AS et al. Fk506 treatment in combination with leflunomide in hamster-to-rat heart and liver Xenograft transplantation. Transplantation 1998; 66:832-837.

24. Cherwinski HM, Cohn RG, Cheung P et al. The immunosuppressant leflunomide inhibits lymphocyte proliferation by inhibiting pyrimidine biosynthesis. J Pharmacol Exp Ther 1995; 275:1043-1049.

25. Davis JP, Cain GA, Pitts WJ et al. The immunosuppressive metabolite of leflunomide is a potent inhibitor of human dihydroorotate dehydrogenase. Biochemistry 1996; 35:1270-1273.

26. Knecht W, Loffler M. Species-related inhibition of human and rat dihydroorotate dehydrogenase by immunosuppressive isoxazol and cinchoninic acid derivatives. Biochem Pharmacol 1998; 56:1259-1264.

27. Williamson RA, Yea CM, Robson PA et al. Dihydroorotate dehydrogenase is a high affinity binding protein for A77 1726 and mediator of a range of biological effects of the immunomodulatory compound. J Biol Chem 1995; 270:22467-22472.

28. Manna SK, Aggarwal BB. Immunosuppressive leflunomide metabolite (A77 1726) blocks tnf-dependent nuclear factor-kappa B activation and gene expression. J Immunol 1999; 162:2095-2102.

29. Cherwinski HM, Byars N, Ballaron SJ et al. Leflunomide interferes with pyrimidine nucleotide biosynthesis. Inflamm Res 1995; 44:317-322.

30. Silva Jr HT, Cao W, Shorthouse RA et al. In vitro and in vivo effects of leflunomide, brequinar, and cyclosporine on pyrimidine biosynthesis. Transplant Proc 1997; 29:1292-1293.

31. Allison AC. Immunosuppressive drugs: The first 50 years and a glance forward. Immunopharmacology 2000; 47:63-83.

32. Nair RV, Cao W, Morris RE. Inhibition of smooth muscle cell proliferation in vitro by leflunomide. A new immunosuppressant, is antagonized by uridine immunol. Lett 1995; 47:171-174.

33. Heldin CH, Westermark B. Mechanism of action and in vivo role of platelet-derived growth factor. Physiol Rev 1999; 79:1283-1316.

34. Border WA, Okuda S, Languino LR et al. Suppression of experimental glomerulonephritis by antiserum against transforming growth factor beta 1. Nature 1990; 346:371-374.

35. Buchdunger E, Zimmermann J, Mett H et al. Selective inhibition of the platelet-derived growth factor signal transduction pathway by a protein-tyrosine kinase inhibitor of the 2-phenylaminopyrimidine class. Proc Natl Acad Sci USA 1995; 92:2558-2562.

36. Doi T, Vlassara H, Kirstein M et al. Receptor-specific increase in extracellular matrix production in mouse mesangial cells by advanced glycosylation end products is mediated via platelet-derived growth factor. Proc Natl Acad Sci USA 1992; 89:2873-2877.

37. Floege J, Eng E, Young BA et al. Infusion of platelet-derived growth factor or basic fibroblast growth factor induces selective glomerular mesangial cell proliferation and matrix accumulation in rats. J Clin Invest 1993; 92:2952-2962.

38. Floege J, Johnson RJ. Multiple roles for platelet-derived growth factor in renal disease. Miner Electrolyte Metab 1995; 21:271-282.

39. Floege J, Ostendorf T, Janssen U et al. Novel approach to specific growth factor inhibition in vivo: Antagonism of platelet-derived growth factor in glomerulonephritis by aptamers. Am J Pathol 1999; 154:169-179.

40. Gilbert RE, Kelly DJ, Mckay T et al. Pdgf signal transduction inhibition ameliorates experimental mesangial proliferative glomerulonephritis. Kidney Int 2001; 59:1324-1332.

41. Iida H, Seifert R, Alpers CE et al. Platelet-derived growth factor (Pdgf) and Pdgf receptor are induced in mesangial proliferative nephritis in the rat. Proc Natl Acad Sci USA 1991; 88:6560-6564.

42. Isaka Y, Fujiwara Y, Ueda N et al. Glomerulosclerosis induced by in vivo transfection of transforming growth factor-beta or platelet-derived growth factor gene into the rat kidney. J Clin Invest 1993; 92:2597-2601.

43. Isaka Y, Brees DK, Ikegaya K et al. Gene therapy by skeletal muscle expression of decorin prevents fibrotic disease in rat kidney. Nat Med 1996; 2:418-423.

44. Johnson RJ, Raines EW, Floege J et al. Inhibition of mesangial cell proliferation and matrix expansion in glomerulonephritis in the rat by antibody to platelet-derived growth factor. J Exp Med 1992; 175:1413-1416.

45. Ostendorf T, Kunter U, Grone HJ et al. Specific antagonism of Pdgf prevents renal scarring in experimental glomerulonephritis. J Am Soc Nephrol 2001; 12:909-918.

46. Ostendorf T, Kunter U, Van Roeyen C et al. The effects of platelet-derived growth factor antagonism in experimental glomerulonephritis are independent of the transforming growth factor-beta system. J Am Soc Nephrol 2002; 13:658-667.

47. Tang WW, Ulich TR, Lacey DI et al. Platelet-derived growth factor-bb induces renal tubulointerstitial myofibroblast formation and tubulointerstitial fibrosis. Am J Pathol 1996; 148:1169-1180.

48. Throckmorton DC, Brogden AP, Min B et al. Pdgf and Tgf-beta mediate collagen production by mesangial cells exposed to advanced glycosylation end products. Kidney Int 1995; 48:111-117.

49. Yagi M, Kato S, Kobayashi Y et al. Beneficial effects of a novel inhibitor of platelet-derived growth factor Receptor autophosphorylation in the rat with mesangial proliferative glomerulonephritis. Gen Pharmacol 1998; 31:765-773.

50. Dimitrijevic M, Bartlett RR. Leflunomide, A novel immunomodulating drug, Inhibits homotypic adhesion of mononuclear cells in rheumatoid arthritis. Transplant Proc 1996; 28:3086-3087.

51. Kraan MC, De Koster BM, Elferink JG et al. Inhibition of neutrophil migration soon after initiation of treatment with leflunomide or methotrexate in patients with rheumatoid arthritis: Findings in a prospective, randomized, double-blind clinical trial in fifteen patients. Arthritis Rheum 2000; 43:1488-1495.

52. Miljkovic D, Samardzic T, Drakulic D et al. Immunosuppressants leflunomide and mycophenolic acid inhibit fibroblast Il-6 production by distinct mechanisms. Cytokine 2002; 19:181-186.

53. Siemasko KF, Chong AS, Williams JW et al. Regulation of B cell function by the immunosuppressive agent leflunomide. Transplantation 1996; 61:635-642.

54. Mizushima Y, Amano Y, Kitagawa H et al. Oral administration of leflunomide (Hwa486) results in prominent suppression of immunoglobulin E formation in a rat type 1 allergy model. J Pharmacol Exp Ther 1999; 288:849-857.

55. Burger D, Begue-Pastor N, Benavent S et al. The active metabolite of leflunomide, A77 1726, inhibits the production of prostaglandin E(2), matrix metalloproteinase 1 and interleukin 6 in human fibroblast-like synoviocytes. Rheumatology (Oxford) 2003; 42:89-96.

56. Pinschewer DD, Ochsenbein AF, Fehr T et al. Leflunomide-mediated suppression of antiviral antibody and T cell responses: Differential restoration by uridine. Transplantation 2001; 72:712-719.

57. Waldman WJ, Bickerstaff A, Gordillo G et al. Inhibition of angiogenesis-related endothelial activity by the experimental immunosuppressive agent leflunomide. Transplantation 2001; 72:1578-1582.

58. Swan SK, Crary GS, Guijarro C et al. Immunosuppressive effects of leflunomide in experimental chronic vascular rejection. Transplantation 1995; 60:887-890.

59. Xiao F, Chong A, Shen J et al. Pharmacologically induced regression of chronic transplant rejection. Transplantation 1995; 60:1065-72.

60. Kemp E, Dieperink H, Jensen J et al. Newer immunosuppressive drugs in concordant Xenografting-transplantation of hamster heart to rat. Xenotransplantation 1994; 1:102-108.

61. Savikko J, Von Willebrand E, Hayry P. Leflunomide analogue Fk778 is vasculoprotective independent of its immunosuppressive effect: Potential applications for restenosis and chronic rejection. Transplantation 2003; 76:455-458.

62. Hardinger KL, Wang CD, Schnitzler MA et al. Prospective, Pilot, Open-label, Short-term study of conversion to leflunomide reverses chronic renal allograft dysfunction. Am J Transplant 2002; 2:867-871.

63. Avery RK, Bolwell BJ, Yen-Lieberman B et al. Use of leflunomide in an allogeneic bone marrow transplant recipient with refractory cytomegalovirus infection. Bone Marrow Transplant 2004.

64. John GT, Manivannan J, Chandy S et al. Leflunomide therapy for cytomegalovirus disease in renal allograft recepients. Transplantation 2004; 77:1460-1461.

65. Josephson MA, Kadambi PV, Javaid B et al. The use of Leflunomide in virally infected transplant patients. J Am Soc Nephrol 2004; 15:523a.

66. Racusen LC, Solez K, Colvin RB et al. The Banff 97 working classification of renal allograft pathology. Kidney Int 1999; 55:713-723.

CHAPTER 19

JC Virus Can Infect Human Immune and Nervous System Progenitor Cells:
Implications for Pathogenesis

Jean Hou, Pankaj Seth and Eugene O. Major

Abstract

Recent advances in stem cell biology have called attention to the role these cells may play in the pathogenesis of systemic and nervous system diseases. Although not capable of indefinite self renewal and pluripotentiality as stem cells are, progenitor cells can give rise to cells of different lineages. It is infection of these differentiated cells that has tradition- ally been associated with the pathology and symptoms of viral-induced disease. However, neural progenitor cells have been shown, in vitro, to be susceptible to infection by neurotro- pic viruses such as the human polyomavirus, JCV, and the lentivirus, HIV-1. These progeni- tor cells, which exist during development as well as in the fully developed adult brain, could therefore be involved in neuropathogenesis. Morever, JCV can also infect progenitor cells of the hematopoietic system, derivatives of which have been implicated in the trafficking of virus from the periphery to the brain. Interestingly, susceptibility to and molecular regula- tion of JCV infection in hematopoietic cells closely parallels what has been observed in glial cells. The biological interaction between the immune and nervous systems that exists in the dissemination of virus from periphery to nervous system and the susceptibility of both sys- tems to JCV infection provide potential for hematopoietic and neural progenitor cell in- volvement in JCV pathogenesis.

Introduction

The human polyomavirus, JCV, is the etiologic agent responsible for the fatal demyeli- nating disease, Progressive Multifocal Leukoencephalopathy (PML).[1] Although the majority of the healthy human population has circulating antibodies against JCV,[2] it is only during periods of severe immune deficiency that the virus will reactivate and cause disease. PML was initially associated with immunosuppressive disorders such as lymphomas and leuke- mias,[3] however, it has recently become a more common concern for patients undergoing transplant or particularly, for patients with AIDS. It has been estimated that 5% of the AIDS population will eventually develop PML, which has since been added to the list of AIDS defining-illnesses.[4]

After an asymptomatic initial infection early in childhood, the virus may remain latent in several body compartments, including the tonsils, kidneys, lymphoid tissues and bone marrow.[5] However, in the immune-compromised host, reactivation of the latent infection can ultimately lead to lytic infection of oligodendrocytes, resulting in demyelination and

Polyomaviruses and Human Diseases, edited by Nasimul Ahsan. ©2006 Eurekah.com and Springer Science+Business Media.

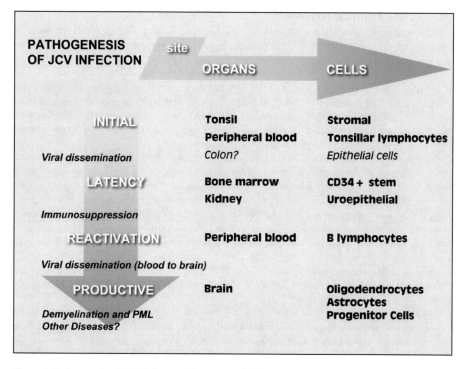

Figure 1. Pathogenesis of JCV infection. The proposed pathway from initial infection to demyelination, through different tissues and susceptible cell types.

associated clinical symptoms of PML. Figure 1 outlines the pathogenesis of JCV as we understand it to date, including susceptible cell types. It is not known precisely when the virus enters the brain; whether JCV is already present in a latent state or whether it enters only after reactivation has occurred elsewhere in the periphery. A hematogenous route of JCV dissemination had been implicated, where infected, circulating B lymphocytes function to traffic the virus across the blood brain barrier.[6] This was further supported by later studies which demonstrated the presence of JCV nucleotide sequences in B lymphocytes isolated from patients with PML and other immunosuppressive disorders.[7] The susceptibility of lymphoid cells to JCV also raised the possibility that hematopoietic precursor cells might support viral infection. Indeed, two CD34+ hematopoietic progenitor cell lines (KG-1 and KG-1a), as well as primary CD34+ hematopoietic progenitor cells isolated from human fetal liver did demonstrate evidence of infection following JC virus exposure.[8]

Similarly, primary human CNS progenitor cells have also been shown to support JCV infection in vitro, as well as astrocyte lineage cells derived from the progenitor population.[9] These results mirror data obtained from primary human brain cell cultures, where astrocytes demonstrate a high susceptibility to JCV.[10] Although lytic infection during the actual course of PML occurs in oligodendrocytes, there is also evidence of infected astrocytes in vivo,[11] raising the possibility of astrocytic involvement in the spread of infection to neighboring cells. Since JCV can infect progenitor and some progenitor derived cells of both the immune and nervous system, these undifferentiated precursor cells may play roles in JCV pathogenesis and the development of PML. Furthermore, current data suggest that the susceptibility to JCV infection in the neural and hematopoietic cells is linked by a common mechanism of molecular regulation.

JCV in the Immune System

JCV was originally believed to be a neurotropic virus with a restricted cellular tropism. However, in the last decade significant progress has been made to define the possible route of infection and widen the range of susceptible cell types to JC virus, in order to include other tissues such as kidney, heart, spleen, bone marrow, lung, liver and colon.[12] The route of primary infection is unknown, however the widespread nature of infection points towards a common route such as respiratory inhalation. The discovery of JCV in tonsillar stromal cells supports the hypothesis that if JCV enters the human body by inhalation, tonsillar tissue may then be a likely site for initial infection, with dissemination occurring via circulating B lymphocytes that come in contact with the infected stromal cells.[13]

Previous reports have shown that B-lymphocytes are susceptible to JCV infection, which strongly points to a role in the dissemination of the virus throughout the body via a circulatory route. Viral DNA sequences have been documented to be present in sites such as the bone marrow and spleen of PML patients[6] as well as in circulating peripheral lymphocytes from both PML[7] and otherwise immunocompromised patients.[14] However, not much is known about the sites and mechanisms of JCV latency and reactivation. As primary exposure to JCV occurs in childhood and is not associated with any known clinical manifestations, it has been suggested that the onset of PML originates from a reactivation of latent JCV infection rather than from an isolated primary exposure event. Serological data also support this hypothesis, as the majority of circulating antibodies are of the IgG subtype, and not IgM, which would be indicative of a primary infection.

The initial evidence of JCV infection in hematopoietic progenitor cells was provided in 1996 with the first description of the infection of primary human CD34+ cells isolated from fetal liver tissue and primary human B lymphocytes. Consistent with these results was the demonstrated susceptibility of CD34+ hematopoietic cell lines KG-1 and KG-1a. (Monaco 1996). Infection and subsequent differentiation of hematopoietic progenitor cells in peripheral lymphoid tissues could be a factor in explaining how the virus can be disseminated and repopulated in the body. A better understanding of the expanded JCV cellular tropism was made available with studies taking advantage of unique properties of the CD34+ hematopoietic cell line KG-1. These JCV susceptible CD34+ precursors could be further differentiated into either a lymphocyte lineage, or with exposure to phorbol 12-myristate 13-acetate (PMA), into a monocyte/macrophage lineage. JC viral infection was maintained only in the lymphocytic cells. Consistent with results from primary tissue, cells that were differentiated into a macrophage-like lineage were nonsusceptible to infection.[15]

Closer examination of the cellular host range of JCV was based on previous studies demonstrating the presence of several nuclear transcription binding sites in the regulatory region of the JCV genome.[16] It was hypothesized that the cell type susceptibility could be regulated at the transcriptional level, through interactions with transcription factors. One binding site in particular served as a consensus sequence for the nuclear transcription factor 1 (NF-1) family,[17,18] which is made up of four different class members.[19] It had been previously demonstrated that the expression of NF1-D message was significantly higher in JCV susceptible cell types such as primary human fetal brain cells and an immortalized human glial cell line, SVG, as compared to a completely non susceptible cell type, HeLa.[20] Based on Northern blot and PCR analysis of the three hematopoietic populations, it was later shown that the level of NF1-D expression was significantly higher in the KG-1 (precursors) and KG-1a cells (lymphocytes) which supported JCV infection, and lower in the nonsusceptible PMA treated KG-1 cells (macrophages). Furthermore, overexpression of NF1-D using an expression construct in the PMA treated cells initiated susceptibility to JCV infection, as measured by in situ DNA hybridization for viral sequences, as well as immunocytochemistry against the early viral protein Large T.[15] Collectively, the data generated from these and previous studies suggest that susceptibility to JCV infection is controlled at the level of transcription, and that the NF1-D transcription factor plays an important role in cellular tropism. Furthermore, the ability of JCV to

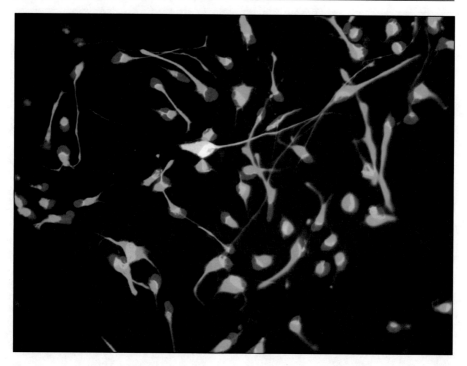

Figure 2. JCV infection of human CNS progenitor cells. Immunocytochemical staining of human CNS progenitor cells following JC Virus exposure. Cells were stained with antibodies against the human stem cell marker, nestin (green), the major JC Viral capsid protein, Vp1 (red), and nuclear dye, bisbenzimide (blue). Images were overlaid to detect the presence of JC viral proteins in nestin-postivie human CNS progenitor cells (yellow, center of field).

infect undifferentiated hematopoietic progenitor cells could play a role in the dissemination of the virus in the periphery either upon differentiation of infected precursor cells or infection of differentiated cell types.

JCV in the CNS

In the central nervous system, lytic infection of oligodendrocytes by JCV leads to demyelination and the hallmark neurological symptoms in patients with PML.[21] However, in vitro, the virus has also been shown to infect astrocytes, while neuronal cells are nonsusceptible to infection.[10,22] Indeed, there has been evidence of JCV infection in astrocytes of PML lesions, while neurons within the demyelinated plaques are largely spared from infection.[23] Added to this in vitro data is the recent surprising finding that human brain derived progenitor cells can also support JCV infection (Fig. 2),[9] raising interesting questions about the role these cells play in the pathogenesis of this disease. As yet, JCV infected progenitor cells have not been identified in PML brain tissue, but efforts are currently underway to further examine this possibility.

In order to study the regulation of JCV infection in human brain derived cells, a multipotential CNS derived progenitor cell culture model was established.[9] Primary human progenitor cells were isolated from an 8 week gestation human fetal brain and established as adherent cultures. The cell population is positive for the human stem and progenitor cell marker, nestin, but negative for markers indicative of other fully differentiated neural cell types. This undifferentiated phenotype could be maintained for long periods of time in culture, without loss of nestin expression. Once established, the progenitor cell culture model eliminated the need to

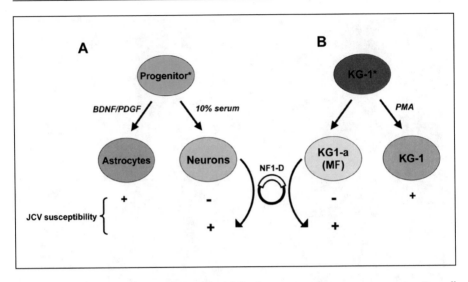

Figure 3. Schematic representation of JCV susceptibility in nervous and immune system progenitor cell systems. *Both progenitor populations are susceptible to JCV infection. However, differentiation of the neural progenitor cells into an astrocyte lineage greatly increases susceptibility while differentation into a neuronal lineage does not. Similarly, differentiation of the KG-1 cells into a macrophage lineage following phorbol ester treatment abolishes susceptibilty to infection. In both neuronal cells and PMA treated KG-1a cells, overexpression of the NF1-D plasmid confers susceptibility to JCV infection in previously nonsusceptible cell types.

work with primary tissues and mixed cultures which could not easily be separated into highly purified substituent populations. These CNS progenitor cells can be selectively differentiated into a neuronal or astrocytic lineage, dependening on growth factors supplied in the cell culture medium. The ability to shift phenotypes in this culture system provided a useful model to study JCV infection in highly purified neural cell populations, as well as at different stages of differentiation.

Much has been learned about the molecular regulation of JCV susceptibility using this human CNS progenitor cell culture system. Identical to primary cultures, JCV robustly infects primary and progenitor derived astrocytes, while primary neurons and progenitor derived neuronal cells remain nonsusceptible to infection. Following exposure to JC virion particles, only progenitor cells and progenitor derived astrocytes demonstrated evidence of active viral infection, as demonstrated by in situ DNA hybridization using a JCV specific DNA probe and by immunocytochemical detection of viral proteins Large T and Vp1. Although the numbers of infected cells were much higher in the astrocyte population, a small percentage of the progenitor cell population did show evidence of viral DNA replication and protein production. No evidence of infection was ever detected in the progenitor derived neuronal population.

Similar to the hematopoietic system, susceptibility to infection has been linked to the expression of the NF1-D transcription factor. The differential expression of the different NF1 class members was examined in progenitor cells as well as the progenitor-derived neurons and astrocytes. The results demonstrated that susceptibility to infection correlated to the level of NF1-D expression, with astrocytes showing the highest level, as compared to the nonsuceptible neurons. Progenitor cells, which were shown to support a modest infection, demonstrated median levels of NF1-D expression. Transfection of the NF1-D plasmid construct into the neuronal cells once again conferred susceptibility to JCV infection (Fig. 3), demonstrating a crucial role for this transcription factor not only in the hematopoietic system, but also in the CNS cell culture model.

The role of CNS progenitor cells in the pathogenesis of PML is currently unknown. Although the progenitors can support JCV infection in vitro, efforts are underway to identify them in tissue sections from PML patients. The susceptibility of progenitor cells to JCV raises an interesting question as to when the virus actually enters the brain. The possibility exists that infected progenitor cells could give rise to other infected cell types such as astrocytes and oligodendrocytes. Alternatively, infection of the neural progenitor cells could prevent them from performing normal functions such as repopulation of cell types within the brain. The presence and proliferation of adult neural progenitor and stem cells has been documented in the case of other brain injury models.[24] If these cells continue to exist in small numbers in the adult brain, viral infection at any point, either before or during immunosuppression, could have profound implications. Current studies are also examining JCV infected progenitor cells as they differentiate into an astrocytic lineage. Assays for viral DNA replication and virion production at different stages early in the differentiation process may yield more information on the molecular regulation of JCV infection during CNS development. Furthermore, it may also reveal some data as to the role that these cells play in vivo, from initial infection to the development of PML.

Therapeutic Purposes

Studying viral susceptibility in progenitor cell culture models would provide a new way to examine the fate of infection in target cells as they differentiate into different lineage pathways. Such studies could reveal more information on the molecular regulation of susceptibility, or viral pathogenesis in cases where it not yet completely understood. The progenitor cells provide a renewable, multipotential source of tissue that largely avoids many of the ethical concerns associated with working with primary human fetal tissue. Studies examining HIV-1 infection of immature neural cells in the past were severely impaired by the lack of true primary human stem or progenitor cells and relied mainly on cell lines with what were termed "immature phenotypes."[25] Other CNS viral infections such as Cocksackie have been studied as well, but with rodent neural stem cells rather than human, most likely due to restrictions and the lack of available human stem cell lines for research purposes.[26] Recently, due to better characterization methods and increased capacity to culture hematopoietic stem cells, HIV-1 infection is also being studied in human CD34+ cells isolated from patients with HIV, where differentiation into dendritic cells with strong T-cell stimulatory capacity could prove useful as a future immunotherapy to combat infection.[27] Evidence of HIV-1 infection has also been demonstrated in vitro in human CNS progenitor cells,[28] and efforts are currently underway to identify infected progenitor cells in the brains of patients with HIV-1 encephalopathy.

Perhaps the most apparent connection between progenitor cells and human disease is their potential role in cancer. This is of particular interest since many of the same pathways involved in self renewal are also involved in tumorigenesis.[29,30] Indeed, there have been attempts to identify and isolate cancer stem cells from tumor tissue in both humans as well as from animal models. Mutations in either the stem cells or at the level of restricted progenitors could explain the heterogeneity of tumors, despite the fact that that most of the cells are derived from a single clone. The potential association of stem cells with cancer is not only causative, however, as hematopoietic stem cells hold great potential as therapeutic agents in combating lymphoproliferative disorders. CD34+ hematopoietic stem cells are routinely isolated, enriched, and transplanted back into patients undergoing immunotherapy.[30] Although autologous transplant largely avoids the potential of graft versus host disease, potential infection of the CD34+ stem cells by either of the human polyomaviruses could have severe implications in the setting of allogeneic transplants into an immunosuppressed host.

Just as the progenitor cell culture models have proven useful for studying the pathogenesis of certain neurodegenerative diseases, the stem cells provide a powerful therapeutic potential in combination with genetic engineering and transplant.[31] Neural stem cell lines are currently being studied as therapeutic agents against brain tumors. The migratory capacity of these cells could be utilized to deliver therapeutic agents in the brain. Genetically modified stem cell lines have been transplanted at or near tumor sites in animal models, with efficient distribution throughout the tumor. Successful transplantation of progenitor cells points toward the possibility of differentiating CNS progenitor cells into specific cell types and transplanting these populations into the brain as a therapy for neurodegenerative disorders. Included in this list would be transplantation of dopaminergic neurons for Parkinson's disease, as well as transplantation of oligodendrocytes to combat demyelinating diseases such as multiple sclerosis and PML.

Conclusion

While a clear understanding of the site and mechanism of JCV reactivation in the human host continues to elude the investigators in this field, majority of evidence suggests immunosupression to be the major cause of reactivation and setting in of PML. Significant progress has been made in determining the cell types that are initially infected and recent studies have provided convincing data to help understand the mechanism of JCV infection in CNS as well as non-CNS cells. The finding that JCV and HIV-1 can infect progenitor cells of the CNS and immune system is of particular importance, since latently infected CD34+ cells or CNS progenitors could produce virus upon reactivation and differentiation, as demonstrated by the tissue culture models. Progenitor and stem cells hold great potential for studies of viral tropism and pathogenesis, as well as therapeutic potential to combat viral induced infections and other neurodegenerative and neoplastic disorders.

References

1. Padgett BL, Walker DL, ZuRhein GM et al. Cultivation of papova-like virus from human brain with progressive multifocal leucoencephalopathy. Lancet 1971; 1(7712):1257-60.
2. Walker DL, Padgett BL. The epidemiology of human polyomaviruses. Prog Clin Biol Res 1983; 105:99-106.
3. Astrom KE, Mancall EL, Richardson EP. Progressive multifocal leukoencephalopathy. Brain 1958; 81:93-127.
4. Stoner GL, Ryschkewitsch CF, Walker DL et al. JC papovavirus large tumor (T)-antigen expression in brain tissue of acquired immune deficiency syndrome (AIDS) and nonAIDS patients with progressive multifocal leukoencephalopathy. Proc Natl Acad Sci USA 1986; 83(7):2271-5.
5. Sabath BF, Major EO. Traffic of JC virus from sites of initial infection to the brain: The path to progressive multifocal leukoencephalopathy. J Infect Dis 2002; 186(Suppl 2):S180-6.
6. Houff SA, Major EO, Katz DA et al. Involvement of JC virus-infected mononuclear cells from the bone marrow and spleen in the pathogenesis of progressive multifocal leukoencephalopathy. N Engl J Med 1988; 318(5):301-5.
7. Tornatore C, Berger JR, Houff SA et al. Detection of JC virus DNA in peripheral lymphocytes from patients with and without progressive multifocal leukoencephalopathy. Ann Neurol 1992; 31(4):454-62.
8. Monaco MC, Atwood WJ, Gravell M et al. JC virus infection of hematopoietic progenitor cells, primary B lymphocytes, and tonsillar stromal cells: Implications for viral latency. J Virol 1996; 70(10):7004-12.
9. Messam CA, Hou J, Gronostajski RM et al. Lineage pathway of human brain progenitor cells identified by JC virus susceptibility. Ann Neurol 2003; 53(5):636-46.
10. Major EO, Vacante DA. Human fetal astrocytes in culture support the growth of the neurotropic human polyomavirus, JCV. J Neuropathol Exp Neurol 1989; 48(4):425-36.
11. Aksamit Jr AJ. Nonradioactive in situ hybridization in progressive multifocal leukoencephalopathy. Mayo Clin Proc 1993; 68(9):899-910.
12. Seth P, Diaz F, Major EO. Advances in the biology of JC virus and induction of progressive multifocal leukoencephalopathy. J Neurovirol 2003; 9(2):236-46.
13. Monaco MC, Jensen PN, Hou J et al. Detection of JC virus DNA in human tonsil tissue: Evidence for site of initial viral infection. J Virol 1998; 72(12):9918-23.
14. Schneider EM, Dorries K. High frequency of polyomavirus infection in lymphoid cell preparations after allogeneic bone marrow transplantation. Transplant Proc 1993; 25(1 Pt 2):1271-3.
15. Monaco MC, Sabath BF, Durham LC et al. JC virus multiplication in human hematopoietic progenitor cells requires the NF-1 class D transcription factor. J Virol 2001; 75(20):9687-95.

16. Frisque RJ. Regulatory sequences and virus-cell interactions of JC virus. Prog Clin Biol Res 1983; 105:41-59.

17. Amemiya K, Traub R, Durham L et al. Interaction of a nuclear factor-1-like protein with the regulatory region of the human polyomavirus JC virus. J Biol Chem 1989; 264(12):7025-32.

18. Amemiya K, Traub R, Durham L et al. Adjacent nuclear factor-1 and activator protein binding sites in the enhancer of the neurotropic JC virus. A common characteristic of many brain-specific genes. J Biol Chem 1992; 267(20):14204-11.

19. Gronostajski RM. Roles of the NFI/CTF gene family in transcription and development. Gene 2000; 249(1-2):31-45.

20. Sumner C, Shinohara T, Durham L et al. Expression of multiple classes of the nuclear factor-1 family in the developing human brain: Differential expression of two classes of NF-1 genes. J Neurovirol 1996; 2(2):87-100.

21. Itoyama Y, Webster HD, Sternberger NH et al. Distribution of papovavirus, myelin-associated glycoprotein, and myelin basic protein in progressive multifocal leukoencephalopathy lesions. Ann Neurol 1982; 11(4):396-407.

22. Assouline JG, Major EO. Human fetal schwann cells support JC virus multiplication. J Virol 1991; 65(2):1002-6.

23. Aksamit Jr AJ. Progressive multifocal leukoencephalopathy: A review of the pathology and pathogenesis. Microsc Res Tech 1995; 32(4):302-11.

24. Lie DC, Song H, Colamarino SA et al. Neurogenesis in the adult brain: New strategies for central nervous system diseases. Annu Rev Pharmacol Toxicol 2004; 44:399-421.

25. Ensoli F, Ensoli B, Thiele CJ. HIV-1 gene expression and replication in neuronal and glial cell lines with immature phenotype: Effects of nerve growth factor. Virology 1994; 200(2):668-76.

26. Feuer R, Mena I, Pagarigan RR et al. Coxsackievirus B3 and the neonatal CNS: The roles of stem cells, developing neurons, and apoptosis in infection, viral dissemination, and disease. Am J Pathol 2003; 163(4):1379-93.

27. Gruber A, Chen I, Kuhen KL et al. Generation of dendritic cells from lentiviral vector-transduced CD34+ cells from HIV+ donors. J Med Virol 2003; 70(2):183-6.

28. Lawrence DM, Durham LC, Schwartz L et al. HIV-1 infection of human brain-derived progenitor cells, in press.

29. Sharpless NE, DePinho RA. Telomeres, stem cells, senescence, and cancer. J Clin Invest 2004; 113(2):160-8.

30. Kawabata Y, Hirokawa M, Komatsuda A et al. Clinical applications of CD34+ cell-selected peripheral blood stem cells. Therap Apher Dial 2003; 7(3):298-304.

31. Jakel RJ, Schneider BL, Svendsen CN. Using human neural stem cells to model neurological disease. Nat Rev Genet 2004; 5(2):136-44.

CHAPTER 20

The Polyomavirus, JCV, and Its Involvement in Human Disease

Kamel Khalili, Jennifer Gordon and Martyn K. White

Abstract

The human neurotropic polyomavirus, JC virus (JCV), is the etiologic agent of progressive multifocal leukoencephalopathy (PML), a fatal demyelinating disease of the central nervous system that occurs mainly in immunosuppressed patients. JCV has also been found to be associated with human tumors of the brain and other organs. In this chapter, we describe JC virus and its role in human diseases.

An Introduction to JC Virus

JC virus (JCV) belongs to the genus of viruses known as the polyomaviruses which are nonenveloped DNA viruses with icosahedral capsids containing small, circular, double-stranded DNA genomes. Polyomaviruses have been isolated from multiple species including humans, monkeys, rodents and birds. Each polyomavirus exhibits a very limited host range and does not usually productively infect other species.[1,2] Mouse polyoma virus[3] and simian vacuolating virus 40 (SV40)[4] were the first polyomaviruses to be discovered. These two archetypal polyomaviruses have been intensively studied as model systems for the study of the basic eukaryotic molecular biology of cell processes such as DNA replication, transcription, malignant transformation and signal transduction. In 1971, two human polyomaviruses were discovered. BK virus (BKV) was isolated from the urine of a kidney allograft recipient with chronic pyelonephritis and advanced renal failure.[5] JC virus was isolated from the brain of a patient suffering from progressive mutifocal leucoencephalopathy (PML).[6] The designations BK and JC were derived from the initials of the patients involved.

JCV is very similar to its cousins, SV40 and BKV, with respect to size (~5.2 Kb), genome organization and DNA sequence. The circular genome of JCV contains two regions of approximately equal size known as the early and late transcription units. Transcription of both units is initiated from a common nontranscribed regulatory region which contains the origin of DNA replication. Starting from this region, early transcription proceeds in a counterclockwise direction while late transcription proceeds clockwise on the opposite strand of the DNA. The JCV late region encodes the capsid structural proteins VP1, VP2 and VP3 that are encoded by alternatively spliced mRNAs derived from the same primary late transcript and a small regulatory protein known as Agnoprotein. The JCV early region encodes the alternatively spliced transforming proteins large T-antigen and small t-antigen. These proteins are important in promoting transformation of cells in culture and oncogenesis in vivo.

Polyomaviruses and Human Diseases, edited by Nasimul Ahsan. ©2006 Eurekah.com and Springer Science+Business Media.

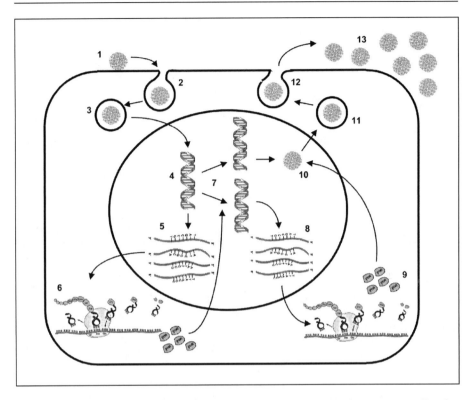

Figure 1. Life cycle of JCV. The following steps are indicated: 1—Binding of JC virions to cell surface receptor, 2—endocytosis, 3—nuclear import, 4—uncoating, 5—transcription of the early region, 6—translation of the early proteins, T-antigen and t-antigen, 7—viral DNA replication, 8—transcription of the late region, 9—translation of Agnoprotein and the capsid proteins VP1, VP2 and VP3, 10—virion assembly, 11—nuclear export, 12—virion release from the cell, 13—infectious viral particles. (Adapted from Cole, 1996).[1]

The Life Cycle of JCV (Fig. 1)

The infection of cells by JCV is initiated by the binding of the virion to a receptor on the outer cell membrane. Unlike SV40, JCV possesses hemagglutination activity reflecting the ability of the JC virion to bind to $\alpha(2\text{-}3)$- and $\alpha(2\text{-}6)$-linked sialic acid residues on the surface of cells.[7,8] Thus, oligosaccharide constitutes the cell surface receptor for JCV, unlike SV40 whose receptor has been identified as the major histocompatibility complex (MHC).[9] Since these oligosaccharides are ubiquitously present on glycoproteins and glycolipids on the surface of cells, JCV can enter a broad spectrum of mammalian cell types.[10] However, JCV replication is restricted to glial cells and lymphoid cells of the B-cell lineage due to cell-specific intra-nuclear mechanisms. This restriction dictates the tropism of JCV and is described below. Interestingly, cells that replicate JCV also express high levels of the sialic acid receptor.[11,12]

After binding to the cell surface, JCV capsids undergo endocytosis and are transported to the nucleus where the viral DNA is uncoated and transcription of the early region begins. Unlike SV40, which enters cells by caveola-mediated endocytosis,[13] JCV employs a clathrin-dependent mechanism that is blocked by tyrosine-specific protein kinase inhibition.[14,15] Recent data indicate that the nuclear localization signal of VP1 is important for nuclear entry of JCV and involves importins and the nuclear pore complex.[16] After JCV enters the nucleus of a permissive cell, the primary transcript is expressed from the early region and is alternatively spliced to give two mRNAs that encode large T-antigen and small t-antigen. JCV T-antigen is a large nuclear phosphoprotein that is an essential factor for viral DNA replication. It binds to the viral origin of DNA replication region where it promotes unwinding of the double helix and recruitment of cellular proteins that are required for DNA synthesis.[1] JCV relies on cellular enzymes and cofactors for DNA replication and these proteins are expressed in the S-phase of the cell cycle. JCV T-antigen modulates cellular signaling pathways and stimulates the cell cycle through its ability to bind to a number of cellular proteins that control cell cycle progression and apoptosis. In this manner, T-antigen can direct cells to enter S-phase thus enabling viral DNA replication. As viral replication proceeds, the late genes are then expressed. T-antigen orchestrates these events as it initiates DNA replication and then acts to stimulate transcription from the late promoter while repressing transcription from the early promoter. The gene products of the late region, the capsid proteins VP1, VP2 and VP3, assemble with the replicated viral DNA to form intranuclear virions, which are released upon cell lysis.

Tropism of JCV

JCV has a unique tropism for replication in glial cells. Earlier studies have demonstrated that the narrow tissue tropism of JCV that restricts its gene expression and replication to glial cells is largely determined at the level of viral early gene transcription which is responsible for the production of T-antigen.[17,18]

Several lines of evidence indicate that the JCV early promoter is preferentially expressed in glial cells. For example, recombinant DNA constructs, in which the JCV early promoter is linked to a reporter gene, show levels of expression that are much higher in glial cells than in nonglial cells.[19] Transgenic mice with the JCV early region selectively express T-antigen in oligodendrocytes leading to a phenotype of dysmyelination.[20] In addition, transgenic mice with constructs in which the early promoters and T-antigen regions of JCV and SV40 were exchanged showed patterns of expression that demonstrated the JCV early promoter, and not the T-antigen coding sequence, is responsible for glial-specific expression.[21] In vitro transcription assays showed that hamster glial cell extract stimulated the JCV early promoter whereas HeLa cell extract reduced production of nuclear run-off transcripts. This suggests that glial cells contain an activating factor(s) for transcription of the JCV early promoter while nonglial (HeLa) cells contain a transcriptional repressor(s).[22,23] Detailed analyses of the JCV early promoter have shown that transcription is regulated in a complex fashion. Multiple transcription factors, both general and cell-type specific, regulate the JCV early promoter including Jun, NF-1, GF-1, Sp1, Smbp-2, Purα, and YB-1.[18,24]

The Spread of JCV

The transmission of JCV is not fully understood. JCV is widespread throughout the human population with greater than 80% of adults exhibiting JCV-specific antibodies.[25] Infection occurs during early childhood and is usually subclinical. In the human body, it is thought that JCV can infect cells in the tonsils and spread from there by replication in lymphoid cells.[26] The mechanism of human-to-human transmission of JCV has not been firmly established but the presence of infectious JCV in raw sewage suggests that ingestion of contaminated water or food could represent a possible portal of entrance of JCV into the human population.[27-29] Earlier studies have revealed the presence of JCV DNA sequences in a high percentage of normal tissue samples taken from the upper and lower human gastrointestinal tract.[30,31] JCV is found in the urine and the kidney is thought to be the major organ of JCV persistence during latency.[32] Infections in humans by JCV are usually restricted by the actions of the immune system, particularly cell-mediated immunity. A general impairment of the Th1-type T-helper cell function of cell-mediated immunity has been found to be associated with the emergence of JCV from latency to cause the disease progressive multifocal leukoencephalopathy (PML).[33]

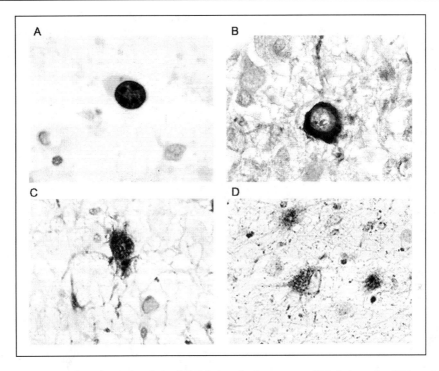

Figure 2. Immunohistochemical analysis of PML lesions for the presence of JC viral proteins. VP1 capsid protein is localized to the nucleus while Agnoprotein is observed in the perinuclear and cytoplasmic regions of inclusion bodies within infected oligodendrocytes (A and B, respectively). In bizarre astrocytes, VP1 and Agnoprotein are both detected in the nucleus and the cytoplasm (C and D, respectively).

JCV and PML

PML is a fatal demyelinating disease of the CNS which is characterized by multiple foci of demyelination caused by lytic infection of oligodendrocytes, the myelin-producing cells of the CNS.[34,35] Only individuals with severely impaired immunity, mainly Acquired Immune Deficiency Syndrome (AIDS) patients, develop PML. The occurrence of PML was very rare until the advent of the AIDS pandemic but now it is much more prevalent in that it affects ~5% of Human Immune Deficiency Virus (HIV)-infected persons.[36,37] Indeed, PML is considered as an AIDS-defining illness.[38] AIDS has been estimated to be the underlying cause of immunosuppression in 55% to more than 85% of cases of PML.[25,39] Other circumstances that incur immunosuppression are also associated with PML, e.g., autoimmune diseases, agammaglobulinemia, lymphoma, immunosuppressive drug treatment, cancer chemotherapy, etc.[36,37] Rarely, PML may occur without an underlying disease condition.

Clinically, PML patients often develop hemiplegia, visual disturbances and subcortical dementia.[37,40] Other neurological symptoms may also be found such as dipoplia, monoplegia, and akinesia. The involvement of multifocal areas of demyelination in these patients is usually detectable by magnetic resonance imaging (MRI). Although the cerebral hemispheres are usually involved, PML may develop within the white matter in any part of the CNS. The prominent histopathological finding of PML is multiple foci of myelin loss, eosinophilic, enlarged oligodendroglial nuclei, and enlarged bizarre astrocytes with lobulated hyperchromatic nuclei. Polyhedral viral particles can be observed within the inclusion bodies of oligodendrocytes by electron microscopy (Fig. 2).

The incidence of PML complicating HIV/AIDS is higher than that of any other immuno-suppressive disorder relative to their frequencies.[36] There are a number of reasons why this may be the case. First, the degree and duration of cellular immunosuppression in HIV/AIDS may be greater in AIDS compared to other immunosuppressive disorders.[36,39] JCV-specific CD4 T-cell responses are impaired in HIV-infected patients with active PML compared to PML survivors on effective and prolonged antiretroviral therapy.[41] In addition, HIV/AIDS may erode the blood brain barrier[42] and facilitate the entry of B-lymphocytes infected with JCV into the brain.[43] Finally there exist specific molecular mechanisms whereby HIV-1 may promote JCV gene expression[44,45] and participate in the pathogenesis of PML. Many studies have demonstrated cross-communication between HIV-1 and JCV through the HIV-1-encoded regulatory protein, Tat. Tat has the ability to bind to and enhance the transcription of the JCV promoter in glial cells.[44-47] In addition to transactivating JCV transcription, Tat also stimulates JC viral DNA replication.[48] Several studies, however, have reported that infection of astrocytes, and to some extent oligodendrocytes, with HIV-1 does occur suggesting the potential for coexistence of these two viruses in neural cells.[49] Of note, it is well established that Tat can be released from HIV-1-infected cells and taken up again by neighboring cells.[50,51] Thus the reactivation of JCV by HIV-1 need not require the coinfection of a glial cell with both viruses. Subsequent studies of the mechanism of Tat action demonstrated that Tat protein mediates the activation of the JCV Tat-responsive transcriptional control element by associating with the cellular nucleic acid binding protein, Purα.[47,52] The high affinity Tat/Purα complex binds to the Tat-responsive JCV element, upTAR which consists of the canonical PUR element GGAGGCGGAGGC. Tat and Purα synergistically activate JCV late gene expression resulting in >100-fold induction.[47] The interaction between Tat and Purα is mediated by RNA and involves specific regions of both Tat and Purα.[53,54]

HIV-1 transactivation of JCV can also occur by indirect mechanisms where HIV-1 causes the production of cytokines such as TNF-α,[55,56] MIP-1α,[57] and TGF-β.[58] These cytokines bind to receptors on the cell surface that signal to downstream transcription factors resulting in stimulation of the JCV promoter.

The replication and dissemination of JCV in PML causes the death of oligodendrocytes and hence the development of focal areas of progressive demyelination. The exact cause of cell death in PML is not known. It has been suggested that apoptosis of infected oligodendrocytes is involved on the basis of TUNEL assays and immunocytochemistry detecting activated caspase 3.[59] We have also detected TUNEL-positive oligodendrocytes and astrocytes in sections of PML brains (Khalili et al, unpublished observations). The TUNEL assay detects DNA breaks which may be caused directly by the effects of JCV on the cell cycle and DNA repair. In clinical samples of AIDS/PML brain, image analysis of the DNA content of inclusion-bearing oligodendrocytes and atypical astrocytes revealed DNA indices that were near tetraploid congruent with the ablation of p53 function in maintaining diploid status.[60] JCV-infected oligodendrocytes and astrocytes exhibited strong immunostaining for p53 and PCNA.[61,62] It can be envisioned that JCV early proteins T-antigen and Agnoprotein may abrogate cell cycle checkpoints (including p53 and pRb) and DNA repair in PML which would serve to drive cells into S-phase where JCV replication occurs. The cellular DNA damage accrued by oligodendrocytes and astrocytes during this process would no doubt contribute to cytotoxicity in PML and viral destruction of areas of white matter within the brain that is characteristic of PML pathogenesis. The ability of JCV to dysregulate cell growth and cause DNA damage, as discussed below, is likely also involved in JCV-mediated tumorigenesis.

JCV and Cancer: Experimental Tumorigenesis

JCV is able to transform cells in culture, particularly cells of glial origin including human fetal glial cells and primary hamster brain cells. JCV-transformed cells exhibit the phenotypic properties associated with transformation including growth in soft agar, serum-independence, changes in morphology, plasminogen activator production etc. These

Table 1. Tumors induced in transgenic mice by JCV T-antigen expression

Phenotype	Reference
Adrenal neuroblastoma	68
Neuroectodermal tumors	70
Primitive tumors originating from the cerebellum	73
Pituitary neoplasia	71
Peripheral nerve sheath tumors	72

studies have been reviewed recently.[63] The transforming ability of JCV appears to be limited to cells of neural origin and cell-type specific transcriptional regulation of the viral promoter is thought to be responsible for this property, as discussed above.

Many studies have established the highly oncogenic potential of JCV in laboratory animals, e.g., JCV induced multiple types of brain tumors when injected into the brains of newborn Golden Syrian hamsters. JCV is the only human virus that induces solid tumors in nonhuman primates. JCV caused the development of astrocytomas, glioblastomas and neuroblastomas in owl and squirrel monkeys which occurred 16-24 months after inoculation of JCV intracerebrally, subcutaneously or intravenously.[64,65] Study of monkey tissue revealed T-antigen expression but no capsid protein or infectious virions indicating monkey cells are nonpermissive for JCV replication.[25] JC viral DNA was integrated into cellular DNA in JCV-induced tumors of owl monkeys.[66] These animal studies have been reviewed recently.[63,67] As mentioned above, transgenic mice expressing JCV T-antigen can develop dysmyelinating disease. These mice can also develop adrenal neuroblastomas.[68,69] Franks et al[70] have generated a line of transgenic mice with the JCV T-antigen gene under the control of the natural JCV promoter and these mice exhibit tumors of primitive neuroectodermal origin. Transgenic mice with the JCV T-antigen gene can develop tumors that arise from the pituitary gland.[71] Recently it was reported that a small subset of these animals developed solid masses arising from the soft tissues surrounding the salivary gland, the sciatic nerve, and along the extremities that histologically resemble malignant peripheral nerve sheath tumors, rare neoplasms that occur in individuals with neurofibromatosis.[72] The phenotypes of transgenic mice expressing the JCV T-antigen are summarized in Table 1.

JCV and Cancer: Clinical Tumors

An indication that JCV may be associated with brain tumors has come from reports of brain tumors being found in patients with concomitant PML.[74] JCV has also been associated with brain tumors in patients without PML. Rencic et al[75] were able to detect JCV DNA by PCR in tumor tissue from a patient with an oligoastrocytoma. The identity of the amplified PCR product was confirmed as JCV by DNA sequencing. Moreover JCV RNA and T-antigen protein were detectable by primer extension analysis and Western blotting, respectively, in the tumor tissue indicating that JCV gene expression occurred in the tumor cells.[75] Del Valle et al[76] examined 85 samples of various tumors of glial origin for the presence of JCV DNA and T-antigen expression. It was found that, depending on the tumor type, 57-83% of tumors were positive for JCV (Fig. 3). In addition, Krynska et al[77] detected JCV T-antigen DNA sequences in 11 of 23 pediatric medulloblastomas. In another study, JCV Agnogene DNA sequences were detected in 11 of 16 medulloblastoma samples and Agnoprotein expression by immunohistochemistry was found in 11 of 20 samples. Since some of the Agnoprotein-positive medulloblastoma samples were negative for concomitant T-antigen expression, Agnoprotein may have a role in the development of JCV-associated medulloblastoma independent of T-antigen.[78] Many other studies that have employed PCR-mediated DNA amplification and/

Table 2. Detection of JC virus DNA sequences and viral protein expression in human tumors

Tumor Type	Viral DNA	Viral Protein	Reference
Oligoastrocytoma	y	y	75
	y	y	76
Xanthoastrocytoma	y	nd	79
Medulloblastoma	y	y	77
	y	y	78
Colorectal cancer	y	nd	30
	y	y	80
Astrocytoma	y	y	81
	y	y	76
Ependymoma	y	n	81
	y	y	76
Oligodendroglioma	y	y	81
	y	y	76
	y	y	82
Glioblastoma	y	y	76
	y	y	83
CNS lymphoma	y	y	84

y—positive, n—negative, nd—not done. Viral DNA was detected by PCR followed by sequencing or Southern blotting. Viral protein was detected by immunohistochemistry for T-antigen and/or Agnoprotein.

or immunohistochemistry of neural-origin tumor samples provide support for an association of JCV with a wide variety of tumors of the CNS and in other tumors such as colon cancer and CNS lymphoma. The detection of JC virus DNA sequences and viral protein expression in different types of human tumors are summarized in Table 2.

JCV DNA sequences have been found in a high percentage of normal tissue samples taken from the upper and lower human gastrointestinal tract and in colon cancer.[30,31] In a study of epithelial malignant tumors of the large intestine, 22 of 27 samples tested positive for JCV DNA sequences. Expression of JCV T-antigen and Agnoprotein was observed in >50% of the samples.[80] No expression of JCV proteins was detected in normal gastrointestinal epithelial tissue. Thus, JCV is associated with some colon cancers and evidence has been presented that dysregulation of β-catenin signaling by JCV T-antigen is involved.[80,85] The involvement of JCV in brain and nonbrain tumors has been recently reviewed.[63]

Studies of the effects of JCV on cultured cells and in animal models lend support to the findings on JCV and its association with human tumors and suggest mechanisms of JCV-mediated cellular transformation. However it remains unknown whether JCV has a causal role in human neoplasia. Problems include the following: JCV is ubiquitous in nature but JCV-associated cancer is rare. The incubation period between infection and the appearance of cancer may last many decades. The initial JCV infection is usually subclinical making it difficult to establish when exposure to the virus occurred. JCV does not productively infect animal models, thus limiting experiments which can be performed to address these questions. Environmental cofactors (e.g., cocarcinogens) or host factors (e.g., immune status) modulate pathogenesis. Zur Hausen has proposed criteria for defining a causal role for a particular infectious agent in cancer:[86] (1) epidemiological plausibility and evidence that a virus infection represents a risk factor for the development of a specific tumor; (2) regular presence and persistence of the nucleic acid of the respective agent in cells of the specific tumor; (3) stimulation of cell proliferation upon transfection of the respective genome or parts therefrom in corresponding tissue

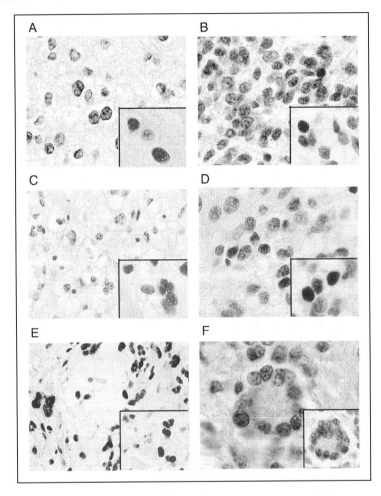

Figure 3. Immunohistochemistry of human glial tumors for JCV T-Antigen and p53. T-antigen is localized in the nuclei of tumor cells within several forms of glial-origin tumors of the central nervous system. p53 shows a similar pattern of nuclear immunolabeling in the same tumors (insets). A) oligodendroglioma; B) anaplastic oligodendroglioma; C) pilocytic astrocytoma; D) fibrillary astrocytoma; E) glioblastoma multiforme; F) ependymoma. (Reproduced with permission from Del Valle et al. Cancer Res 2001; 61:4287-4293.)[76]

culture cells; (4) demonstration that the induction of proliferation and the malignant pheno-type of specific tumor cells depend on functions exerted by the persisting nucleic acid of the respective agent. Evidence has been presented here that JCV fulfills at least the last three criteria. JCV transforms cells in culture and produces tumors in inoculated animals or transgenic mice with a pattern consistent with its putative role in human tumorigenesis. The presence of viral DNA and viral gene expression in a subset of human tumors has been established.

JCV Molecular Biology

As viruses go, JCV is tiny, weighing in with a genome size of only 5,130 base pairs and encoding only 6 viral proteins: 3 capsid structural proteins (VP1, VP2 and VP3) and 3 regula-tory proteins (T-antigen, t-antigen and Agnoprotein). Not surprisingly, the regulatory proteins of JCV have been found to be highly multifunctional. These properties have been reviewed in detail recently[87,88] and will be summarized here. As well as its role in viral DNA replication, JCV T-antigen interacts with a number of cellular proteins that are involved in regulating cell proliferation and transformation including the product of the retinoblastoma susceptibility gene,[89-91] p53,[90,92] IRS-1,[93] β-catenin,[80,85] and the neurofibromatosis type 2 gene product.[72] In addition to dysregulating cell proliferation, JCV also causes damage to cellular DNA which may be important to the pathogenesis of PML and JCV-associated tumors. Infection with JCV increases spontaneous mutation frequencies up to 100-fold in cultured lymphoid cells or human peripheral blood lymphocytes[94] and also in human colonic cells.[95] Expression of the JCV large T-antigen inhibits HR-DNA repair in cultured cells.[96] In the case of the closely related virus, SV40, large T-antigen rapidly induced numerical and structural chromosome aberrations in human fibroblasts[97,98] and disturbs the formation of the nuclear DNA-repair foci containing MRE11/Rad50/Nibrin that are involved in both HR and NHEJ DNA repair.[99] Agnoprotein also has a role in the dysregulation of DNA repair that is observed on polyomavirus infection. When expressed alone in cultured cells, JCV Agnoprotein binds p53, alters the cell cycle and inhibits NHEJ DNA repair.[100,101]

The second of the two proteins encoded by the early region of JCV is small t-antigen. Published research on small t-Ag has concentrated almost exclusively on SV40 t-antigen which has a mitogenic role in cellular transformation[102,103] by binding to and inhibiting protein phosphatase 2A[104] which is a negative regulator of many growth promoting signal transduction pathways. We are currently investigating whether or not JCV t-antigen functions in a similar manner.

Future Studies of JCV

Future studies of polyomaviruses will be aided by recent technical advances. Oligonucleotide-based microarray approaches should permit the evaluation of the expression of many thousands of genes at once to generate transcriptional profiles that can be used to examine the effects of JCV in cell culture systems and in tumors. Radhakrishnan et al[105] correlated changes in gene expression in primary human astrocytes after JCV infection with gene expression alterations that were observed in astrocytes within PML lesions of brain tissue from patients with neuro-AIDS. Proteomics-based approaches could be used to assess the status of JCV T-antigen in tumors. For example, 2-dimensional electrophoresis could be used to resolve T-antigen/p53 followed by mass spectrometry to establish the identity of the T-antigen protein (JCV as opposed to BKV or SV40) and the status of the p53 protein (wild-type or mutated).

Since JCV is associated with a significant number of human tumors, it may be possible to use the viral oncoproteins as targets for cancer therapies. The highly multifunctional transforming proteins of JCV impinge on many cellular signal transduction pathways and thus molecular strategies for the disruption of their interactions with cellular proteins may represent a fruitful avenue for the development of new types of therapeutic interventions. For example, ELISA-based assays for T-antigen/p53 interaction have been used to screen chemical libraries for agents that inhibit SV40 T-antigen binding to p53.[106] Such an approach could also be employed for JCV T-antigen. Delivery of antisense transcripts to the early region of JCV represents another possible approach. In the case of SV40, an adenoviral antisense vector achieved significant growth inhibition and apoptosis of SV40 T-antigen-expressing human mesothelioma cells in culture.[107] We have recently demonstrated the efficacy of a strategy of RNA interference using JCV T-antigen and Agnoprotein siRNA to inhibit JCV protein expression in JCV-infected human fetal astrocytes. The inhibition of T-antigen production by siRNA reduced the rate of JC viral replication.[108] Agents that target JCV proteins have the potential of providing new therapies for PML and JCV-associated cancers and of answering questions about the importance of JCV protein functions in the pathogenesis of these human diseases.

Acknowledgements

We wish to thank past and present members of the Center for Neurovirology and Cancer Biology for their insightful discussion, and sharing of ideas and reagents. We thank Dr. L. Del Valle for providing immunohistochemistry images and C. Schriver for editorial assistance and preparation of the manuscript. This work was supported by grants awarded by the NIH to KK.

References

1. Cole CN. Polyomavirinae: The viruses and their replication. In: Fields BN, Knipe DM, Howley PM, eds. Fundamental Virology. 3rd ed. Lippincott, Williams & Wilkins, Philadelphia, 917-946.
2. Imperiale MJ. The human polyoma viruses: An overview. In: Khalili K, Stoner GL, eds. Human polyomaviruses: Molecular and clinical perspective. New York: Wiley-Liss Inc., 2001:53-71.
3. Stewart SE, Eddy BE, Borgese NG. Neoplasms in mice inoculated with a tumor agent carried in tissue culture. J Natl Cancer Inst 1958; 20:1223-1243.
4. Sweet BH, Hilleman MR. The vacuolating virus, SV40. Proc Soc Exp Biol Med 1960; 105:420-427.
5. Gardner SD, Field AM, Coleman DV et al. New human papovavirus (B.K.) isolated from urine after renal transplantation. Lancet 1971; 1:1253-1257.
6. Padgett BL, Walker DL, ZuRhein GM et al. Cultivation of papova-like virus from human brain with progressive mutifocal leucoencephalopathy. Lancet 1971; 1:1257-1260.
7. Komagome R, Sawa H, Suzuki T et al. Oligosaccharides as receptors for JC virus. J Virol 2002; 76:12992-13000.
8. Liu CK, Wei G, Atwood WJ. Infection of glial cells by the human polyomavirus JC is mediated by an N-linked glycoprotein containing terminal alpha(2-6)-linked sialic acids. J Virol 1998; 72:4643-4649.
9. Norkin LC. Simian virus 40 infection via MHC class I molecules and caveolae. Immunol Rev 1999; 168:13-22.
10. Suzuki S, Sawa H, Komagome R et al. Broad distribution of the JC virus receptor contrasts with a marked cellular restriction of virus replication. Virology 2001; 286:100-112.
11. Eash S, Tavares R, Stopa EG et al. Differential distribution of the JC virus receptor-type sialic acid in normal human tissues. Am J Pathol 2004; 164:419-428.
12. Wei G, Liu CK, Atwood WJ. JC virus binds to primary human glial cells, tonsillar stromal cells and B-lymphocytes, but not to T-lymphocytes. J Neurovirol 2000; 6:127-136.
13. Anderson HA, Chen Y, Norkin LC. Bound simian virus 40 translocates to caveolin-enriched membrane domains, and its entry is inhibited by drugs that selectively disrupt caveolae. Mol Biol Cell 1996; 7:1825-1834.
14. Pho MT, Ashok A, Atwood WJ. JC virus enters human glial cells by clathrin-dependent receptor-mediated endocytosis. J Virol 2000; 74:2288-2292.
15. Querbes W, Benmerah A, Tosoni D et al. A JC virus-induced signal is required for infection of glial cells by a clathrin- and eps15-dependent pathway. J Virol 2004; 78:250-256.
16. Qu Q, Sawa H, Suzuki T et al. Nuclear entry mechanism of the human polyomavirus JC virus like particle: Role of importins and the nuclear pore complex. J Biol Chem 2004; 279:27735-27742.
17. Henson JW, Schnitker BL, Lee T-S et al. Cell-specific activation of the glial-specific JC virus early promoter by large T antigen. J Biol Chem 1995; 270:13240-13245.
18. Kim H-S, Henson JW, Frisque RJ. Transcription and replication in the human polyomaviruses. In: Khalili K, Stoner GL, eds. Human polyomaviruses: Molecular and clinical perspective. New York: Wiley-Liss Inc., 2001:73-126.
19. Kenny S, Natarajan V, Strike D et al. JC virus enhancer-promoter activity in human brain cells. Science 1984; 226:1337-1339.
20. Trapp BD, Small JA, Pulley M et al. Dysmyelination in transgenic mice containing JC virus early region. Ann Neurol 1988; 23:38-48.
21. Feigenbaum L, Hinrichs SH, Jay G. JC virus and SV40 enhancers and transforming proteins: Role in determining tissue specificity and pathogenicity in transgenic mice. J Virol 1992; 66:1176-1182.
22. Ahmed S, Chowdhury M, Khalili K. Regulation of a human neurotropic virus promoter, JCV(E): Identification of a novel activator domain located upstream from the 98 bp enhancer promoter region. Nucleic Acids Res 1990; 18:7417-7423.
23. Ahmed S, Rappaport J, Tada H et al. A nuclear protein derived from brain cells stimulates transcription of the human neurotropic virus promoter JCVE, in vitro. J Biol Chem 1990; 265:13899-13905.
24. Raj G, Khalili K. Transcriptional regulation: Lessons from the human neurotropic polyomavirus, JCV. Virology 1995; 213:283-291.

25. Major EO, Amemiya K, Tornatore CS et al. Pathogenesis and molecular biology of progressive multifocal leukoencephalopathy, the JC virus-induced demyelinating disease of the human brain. Clin Microbiol Rev 1992; 5:49-73.
26. Monaco MC, Jensen PN, Hou J et al. Detection of JC virus DNA in human tonsil tissue: Evidence for site of initial viral infection. J Virol 1998; 72:9918-9923.
27. Bofill-Mas S, Girones R. Excretion and transmission of JCV in human populations. J Neurovirol 2001; 7:345-349.
28. Bofill-Mas S, Formiga-Cruz M, Clemente-Casares P et al. Potential transmission of human polyomaviruses through the gastrointestinal tract after exposure to virions or viral DNA. J Virol 2001; 75:10290-10299.
29. Bofill-Mas S, Clemente-Casares P, Major EO et al. Analysis of the excreted JC virus strains and their potential oral transmission. J Neurovirol 2003; 9:498-507.
30. Laghi L, Randolph AE, Chauhan DP et al. JC virus DNA is present in the mucosa of the human colon and in colorectal cancers. Proc Natl Acad Sci USA 1999; 96:7484-7489.
31. Ricciardiello L, Laghi L, Ramamirtham P et al. JC virus DNA sequences are frequently present in the human upper and lower gastrointestinal tract. Gastroenterology 2000; 119:1228-1235.
32. Chesters PM, Heritage J, McCance DJ. Persistence of DNA sequences of BK virus and JC virus in normal human tissues and in diseased tissues. J Infect Dis 1983; 147:676-684.
33. Weber F, Goldmann C, Kramer M et al. Cellular and humoral immune response in progressive multifocal leukoencephalopathy. Ann Neurol 2001; 49:636-642.
34. Gordon J, Khalili K. The human polyomavirus, JCV, and neurological diseases (review). Int J Mol Med 1998; 1:647-655.
35. Safak M, Khalili K. An overview: Human polyomavirus JC virus and its associated disorders. J Neurovirol 2003; 9(Suppl 1):3-9.
36. Berger JR. Progressive multifocal leukoencephalopathy in acquired immuno-deficiency syndrome: Explaining the high incidence and disproportionate frequency of the illness relative to other immunosuppressive conditions. J Neurovirol 2003; 9(Suppl 1):38-41.
37. Berger JR, Concha M. Progressive multifocal leukoencephalopathy: The evolution of a disease once considered rare. J Neurovirol 1995; 1:5-18.
38. Berger JR, Kaszovitz B, Post MJ et al. Progressive multifocal leukoencephalopathy associated with human immunodeficiency virus infection. A review of the literature with a report of sixteen cases. Ann Intern Med 1987; 107:78-87.
39. Berger JR, Chauhan A, Galey D et al. Epidemiological evidence and molecular basis of interactions between HIV and JC virus. J Neurovirol 2001; 7:329-338.
40. Brooks BR, Walker DL. Progressive multifocal leukoencephalopathy. Neurol Clin 1984; 2:299-313.
41. Gasnault J, Kahraman M, de Goer de Herve MG et al. Critical role of JC virus-specific CD4 T-cell responses in preventing progressive multifocal leukoencephalopathy. AIDS 2003; 17:1443-1449.
42. Power C, Kong PA, Crawford TO et al. Cerebral white matter changes in acquired immunodeficiency syndrome dementia: Alterations of the blood-brain barrier. Ann Neurol 1993; 34:339-350.
43. Gallia GL, Houff SA, Major EO et al. Review: JC virus infection of lymphocytes—revisited. J Infect Dis 1997; 176:1603-1609.
44. Chowdhury M, Taylor JP, Tada H et al. Regulation of the human neurotropic virus promoter by JCV-T antigen and HIV-1 tat protein. Oncogene 1990; 5:1737-1742.
45. Tada H, Rappaport J, Lashgari M et al. Trans-activation of the JC virus late promoter by the tat protein of type 1 human immunodeficiency virus in glial cells. Proc Natl Acad Sci USA 1990; 87:3479-3483.
46. Chowdhury M, Kundu M, Khalili K. GA/GC-rich sequence confers Tat responsiveness to human neurotropic virus promoter, JCVL, in cells derived from central nervous system. Oncogene 1993; 8:887-892.
47. Krachmarov CP, Chepenik LG, Barr-Vagell S et al. Activation of the JC virus Tat-responsive transcriptional control element by association of the Tat protein of human immunodeficiency virus 1 with cellular protein Pur alpha. Proc Natl Acad Sci USA 1996; 93:14112-14117.
48. Daniel DC, Wortman MJ, Schiller RJ et al. Coordinate effects of human immunodeficiency virus type 1 protein Tat and cellular protein Puralpha on DNA replication initiated at the JC virus origin. J Gen Virol 2001; 82:1543-1553.
49. Del Valle L, Croul S, Morgello S et al. Detection of HIV-1 Tat and JCV capsid protein, VP1, in AIDS brain with progressive multifocal leukoencephalopathy. J Neurovirol 2000; 6:221-228.
50. Ensoli B, Buonaguro L, Barillari G et al. Release, uptake, and effects of extracellular human immunodeficiency virus type 1 Tat protein on cell growth and viral transactivation. J Virol 1993; 67:277-287.

51. Frankel AD, Pabo CO. Cellular uptake of the tat protein from human immunodeficiency virus. Cell 1988; 55:1189-1193.
52. Chepenik LG, Tretiakova AP, Krachmarov CP et al. The single-stranded DNA binding protein, Puralpha, binds HIV-1 TAR RNA and activates HIV-1 transcription. Gene 1998; 210:37-44.
53. Gallia GL, Darbinian N, Tretiakova A et al. Association of HIV-1 Tat with the cellular protein, Puralpha, is mediated by RNA. Proc Natl Acad Sci USA 1999; 96:11572-11577.
54. Wortman MJ, Krachmarov CP, Kim JH et al. Interaction of HIV-1 Tat with Puralpha in nuclei of human glial cells: Characterization of RNA-mediated protein-protein binding. J Cell Biochem 2000; 77:65-74.
55. Darbinian N, Sawaya BE, Khalili K et al. Functional interaction between cyclin T1/cdk9 and Puralpha determines the level of TNFalpha promoter activation by Tat in glial cells. J Neuroimmunol 2001; 121:3-11.
56. Rappaport J, Joseph J, Croul S et al. Molecular pathway involved in HIV-1-induced CNS pathology: Role of viral regulatory protein, Tat. J Leukoc Biol 1999; 65:458-465.
57. Bonwetsch R, Croul S, Richardson MW et al. Role of HIV-1 Tat and CC chemokine MIP-1alpha in the pathogenesis of HIV associated central nervous system disorders. J Neurovirol 1999; 5:685-694.
58. Enam S, Sweet TM, Amini S et al. Evidence for involvement of transforming growth factor beta1 signaling pathway in activation of JC virus in human immunodeficiency virus 1-associated progressive multifocal leukoencephalopathy. Arch Pathol Lab Med 2004; 128:282-291.
59. Richardson-Burns SM, Kleinschmidt-DeMasters BK, DeBiasi RL et al. Progressive multifocal leukoencephalopathy and apoptosis of infected oligodendrocytes in the central nervous system of patients with and without AIDS. Arch Neurol 2004; 59:1930-1936.
60. Ariza A, Mate JL, Serrano S et al. DNA amplification in glial cells of progressive multifocal leukoencephalopathy: An image analysis study. J Neuropathol Exp Neurol 1996; 55:729-733.
61. Ariza A, Mate JL, Fernandez-Vasalo A et al. p53 and proliferating cell nuclear antigen expression in JC virus-infected cells of progressive multifocal leukoencephalopathy. Hum Pathol 1994; 25:1341-1345.
62. Lammie GA, Beckett A, Courtney R et al. An immunohistochemical study of p53 and proliferating cell nuclear antigen expression in progressive multifocal leukoencephalopathy. Acta Neuropathol 1994; 88:465-471.
63. Del Valle L, Gordon J, Ferrante P et al. JC virus in experimental and clinical brain tumorigenesis. In: Khalili K, Stoner GL, eds. Human polyomaviruses: Molecular and clinical perspective. New York: Wiley-Liss Inc., 2001:409-430.
64. London WT, Houff SA, Madden DL et al. Brain tumors in owl monkeys inoculated with a human polyomavirus (JC virus). Science 1978; 201:1246-1249.
65. London WT, Houff SA, McKeever PE et al. Viral-induced astrocytomas in squirrel monkeys. In: Sever JL, Madden DL, eds. Polyomaviruses and human neurological diseases. New York: Alan R Liss Inc., 1983:227-237.
66. Miller NR, McKeever PE, London W et al. Brain tumors of owl monkeys inoculated with JC virus contain the JC virus genome. J Virol 1984; 49:848-856.
67. Khalili K, Del Valle L, Otte J et al. Human neurotropic polyomavirus, JCV, and its role in carcinogenesis. Oncogene 2003; 22:5181-5191.
68. Small JA, Khoury G, Jay G et al. Early regions of JC virus and BK virus induce distinct and tissue-specific tumors in transgenic mice. Proc Natl Acad Sci USA 1986; 83:8288-8292.
69. Small JA, Scangos GA, Cork L et al. The early region of human papovavirus JC induces dysmyelination in transgenic mice. Cell 1986; 46:13-18.
70. Franks RR, Rencic A, Gordon J et al. Formation of undifferentiated mesenteric tumors in transgenic mice expressing human neurotropic polyomavirus early protein T-antigen. Oncogene 1996; 12:2573-2578.
71. Gordon J, Del Valle L, Otte J et al. Pituitary neoplasia induced by expression of human neurotropic polyomavirus, JCV, early genome in transgenic mice. Oncogene 2000; 19:4840-4846.
72. Shollar D, Valle LD, Khalili K et al. JCV T-antigen interacts with the neurofibromatosis type 2 gene product in a transgenic mouse model of malignant peripheral nerve sheath tumors. Oncogene 2004; 23:5459-5467.
73. Krynska B, Otte J, Franks R et al. Human ubiquitous JCV•CY T-antigen gene induces brain tumors in experimental animals. Oncogene 1999; 18:39-46.
74. Gallia GL, Safak M, Khalili K. Interaction of single-stranded DNA binding protein, Puralpha, with human polyomavirus, JCV, early protein, T-antigen. J Biol Chem 1998; 273:32662-32669.

75. Rencic A, Gordon J, Otte J et al. Detection of JC virus DNA sequence and expression of the viral oncoprotein, tumor antigen, in brain of immunocompetent patient with oligoastrocytoma. Proc Natl Acad Sci USA 1996; 93:7352-7357.
76. Del Valle L, Gordon J, Assimakopolou M et al. Detection of JC virus DNA sequences and expression of the viral regulatory protein, T-antigen, in tumors of the central nervous system. Cancer Res 2001; 61:4287-4293.
77. Krynska B, Del Valle L, Croul S et al. Detection of human neurotropic JC virus DNA sequence and expression of the viral oncogenic protein in pediatric medulloblastomas. Proc Natl Acad Sci USA 1999; 96:11519-11524.
78. Del Valle L, Gordon J, Enam S et al. Expression of human neurotropic polyomavirus JCV late gene product Agnoprotein in human medulloblastoma. J Natl Cancer Inst 2002; 94:267-273.
79. Boldorini R, Caldarelli-Stefano R, Monga G et al. PCR detection of JC virus DNA in the brain tissue of a 9-year-old child with pleomorphic xanthoastrocytoma. J Neurovirol 1998; 4:242-245.
80. Enam S, Del Valle L, Lara C et al. Association of human polyomavirus JCV with colon cancer: Evidence for interaction of viral T-antigen and beta-catenin. Cancer Res 2002; 62:7093-7101.
81. Caldarelli-Stefano R, Boldorini R, Monga G et al. JC virus in human glial-derived tumors. Hum Pathol 2000; 31:394-395.
82. Del Valle L, Enam S, Lara C et al. Detection of JC polyomavirus DNA sequences and cellular localization of T-antigen and agnoprotein in oligodendrogliomas. Clin Cancer Res 200b; 8:3332-3340.
83. Del Valle L, Delbue S, Gordon J et al. Expression of JC virus T-antigen in a patient with multiple sclerosis and glioblastoma multiforme. Neurology 2002; 58:895-900.
84. Del Valle L, Enam S, Lara C et al. Primary central nervous system lymphoma expressing the human neurotropic polyomavirus, JC virus, genome. J Virol 2004; 78:3462-3469.
85. Gan DD, Khalili K. Interaction between JCV large T-antigen and beta-catenin. Oncogene 2004; 23:483-490.
86. zur Hausen H. Viruses in human cancers. Eur J Cancer 1999; 35:1878-1885.
87. White MK, Khalili K. Signaling pathways and polyomavirus oncoproteins: Importance in malignant transformation. Gene Ther Mol Biol 2004; 8:19-30.
88. White MK, Khalili K. Polyomaviruses and human cancer: Molecular mechanisms underlying patterns of tumorigenesis. Virology 2004; 324:1-16.
89. Cress WD, Nevins JR. Use of the E2F transcription factor by DNA tumor virus regulatory proteins. Curr Top Microbiol Immunol 1996; 208:63-78.
90. Krynska B, Gordon J, Otte J et al. Role of cell cycle regulators in tumor formation in transgenic mice expressing the human neurotropic virus, JCV, early protein. J Cell Biochem 1997; 67:223-230.
91. Tavis JE, Trowbridge PW, Frisque RJ. Converting the JCV T antigen Rb binding domain to that of SV40 does not alter JCV's limited transforming activity but does eliminate viral viability. Virology 1994; 199:384-392.
92. Bollag B, Chuke WF, Frisque RJ. Hybrid genomes of the polyomaviruses JC virus, BK virus, and simian virus 40: Identification of sequences important for efficient transformation. J Virol 1989; 63:863-872.
93. Lassak A, Del Valle L, Peruzzi F et al. Insulin receptor substrate 1 translocation to the nucleus by the human JC virus T-antigen. J Biol Chem 2002; 277:17231-17238.
94. Theile M, Grabowski G. Mutagenic activity of BKV and JCV in human and other mammalian cells. Arch Virol 1990; 113:221-233.
95. Ricciardiello L, Baglioni M, Giovannini C et al. Induction of chromosomal instability in colonic cells by the human polyomavirus JC virus. Cancer Res 2003; 63:7256-7262.
96. Trojanek J, Ho T, Del Valle L et al. T-antigen from human polyomavirus JC attenuates faithful DNA repair by forcing nuclear interaction between IRS-1 and Rad51. Mol Cell 2004; in press.
97. Ray FA, Peabody DS, Cooper JL et al. SV40 T antigen alone drives karyotype instability that precedes neoplastic transformation of human diploid fibroblasts. J Cell Biochem 1990; 42:13-31.
98. Ray FA, Meyne J, Kraemer PM. SV40 T antigen induced chromosomal changes reflect a process that is both clastogenic and aneuploidogenic and is ongoing throughout neoplastic progression of human fibroblasts. Mutat Res 1992; 284:265-273.
99. Digweed M, Demuth I, Rothe S et al. SV40 large T-antigen disturbs the formation of nuclear DNA-repair foci containing MRE11. Oncogene 2002; 21:4873-4878.
100. Darbinyan A, Darbinian N, Safak M et al. Evidence for dysregulation of cell cycle by human polyomavirus, JCV, late auxiliary protein. Oncogene 2002; 21:5574-5581.
101. Darbinyan A, Siddiqui K, Slonina D et al. Role of JCV agnoprotein in DNA repair. J Virol 2004; 78:8593-8600.

102. Martin RG, Setlow VP, Edwards CA et al. The roles of the simian virus 40 tumor antigens in transformation of Chinese hamster lung cells. Cell 1979; 17:635-643.
103. Sleigh MJ, Topp WC, Hanich R et al. Mutants of SV40 with an altered small t protein are reduced in their ability to transform cells. Cell 1978; 14:79-88.
104. Pallas DC, Shahrik LK, Martin BL et al. Polyoma small and middle T antigens and SV40 small t antigen form stable complexes with protein phosphatase 2A. Cell 1990; 12:167-176.
105. Radhakrishnan S, Otte J, Enam S et al. JC virus-induced changes in cellular gene expression in primary human astrocytes. J Virol 2003; 77:10638-10644.
106. Carbone M, Rudzinski J, Bocchetta M. High throughput testing of the SV40 large T antigen binding to cellular p53 identifies putative drugs for the treatment of SV40-related cancers. Virology 2003; 315:409-414.
107. Waheed I, Guo ZS, Chen GA et al. Antisense to SV40 early gene region induces growth arrest and apoptosis in T-antigen-positive human pleural mesothelioma cells. Cancer Res 1999; 59:6068-6073.
108. Radhakrishnan S, Gordon J, Del Valle L et al. Intracellular approach for blocking JCV gene expression using RNA interference during viral infection. J Virol 2004; 78:7264-7269.

CHAPTER 21

Transforming Activities of JC Virus Early Proteins

Richard J. Frisque, Catherine Hofstetter and Shiva K. Tyagarajan

Abstract

Polyomaviruses, as their name indicates, are viruses capable of inducing a variety of tumors in vivo. Members of this family, including the human JC and BK viruses (JCV, BKV), and the better characterized mouse polyomavirus and simian virus 40 (SV40), are small DNA viruses that commandeer a cell's molecular machinery to reproduce themselves. Studies of these virus-host interactions have greatly enhanced our understanding of a wide range of phenomena from cellular processes (e.g., DNA replication and transcription) to viral oncogenesis.

The current chapter will focus upon the five known JCV early proteins and the contributions each makes to the oncogenic process (transformation) when expressed in cultured cells. Where appropriate, gaps in our understanding of JCV protein function will be supplanted with information obtained from the study of SV40 and BKV.

Introduction

Human Polyomaviruses

The first isolations of JCV and BKV from humans were reported in 1971, and subsequent studies have failed to identify additional animal hosts. Serologic data indicate that asymptomatic infections often occur in young children, with 80-90% of the population eventually becoming seropositive for one or both viruses. Given stable anti-viral antibody levels and the frequent occurrence of viruria in infected individuals, it is likely that JCV and BKV persist for the lifetime of their host (reviewed in ref. 1).

The natural host of SV40 is the rhesus monkey; however, humans were exposed to this virus by contaminated lots of poliovirus and adenovirus vaccines administered during the mid-1950s to early 1960s. It is estimated that at least 30 million of the 98 million people in the United States receiving these vaccines were given preparations containing live SV40. Prior to the advent of highly sensitive polymerase chain reaction (PCR) technologies, little evidence was available to support the suggestion that SV40 circulates in the human population. However, during the last decade, numerous reports have surfaced that require the field to reconsider this possibility (reviewed in refs. 2-4).

Association of JCV with Its Human Host

JCV may establish latent, persistent or active infections in vivo depending upon the immune status of the host, the tissue infected, and the JCV variant involved. JCV has routinely been detected in kidney tissue and urine, and it has been suggested that the virus replicates at

Polyomaviruses and Human Diseases, edited by Nasimul Ahsan. ©2006 Eurekah.com and Springer Science+Business Media.

relatively low levels (persistent infection) in renal proximal tubule cells. The form of virus usually detected in urine is called archetype JCV, a variant that contains a single copy of the viral promoter-enhancer sequences within its transcriptional control region (TCR). A second variant, called rearranged JCV, has been associated with active infections in brain that lead to disease in severely immunocompromised individuals (see below). Several laboratories have reported the detection of these rearranged TCR sequences in healthy brain as well. Few amplicons are amplified from this tissue, and it is possible that a latent infection is established at this site. Relative to the archetype TCR, the promoter-enhancer sequences of a rearranged TCR have undergone deletion and duplication events that result in a virus with altered tissue tropism and pathogenic potential. In addition to the brain and kidney, one or both JCV TCR variants have been detected in tonsils, a possible primary site of infection, in peripheral blood mononuclear cells, which may seed virus to secondary sites of infection, and in colon tissue (reviewed in refs. 5,6).

JCV Infection and Human Disease

JCV actively infects oligodendrocytes, the myelin-producing cells of the central nervous system (CNS), and abortively infects astrocytes, a second glial cell type. The infected astrocytes take on a transformed appearance, whereas the oligodendrocytes are destroyed, leading to multiple foci of demyelination in the CNS (progressive multifocal leukoencephalopathy [PML]) and a variety of debilitating symptoms with the type and severity depending upon the region of the brain affected. Death usually occurs within a year of the onset of symptoms. PML patients nearly always have an underlying immune deficiency. Prior to the AIDS epidemic, PML was considered rare, and it occurred mostly in the elderly with lymphoproliferative diseases. PML is now common in younger individuals with AIDS, and it is the cause of death in ~5% of these patients (reviewed in ref. 1). It is unclear whether oligodendrocyte death results from an apoptotic or necrotic event, although two groups have recently reported evidence of apoptosis within and near PML lesions.[7,8] JCV has also been linked to polyomavirus-associated nephropathy (PAN); however, BKV is considered to be the more likely cause of this emerging disease in renal allograft recipients (reviewed in ref. 9).

Polyomaviruses go through their entire life cycle during an active infection (e.g., PML), with the outcome being the release of large numbers of infectious virions from the lysed cell. However, these viruses may enter certain cell types that do not support replication (nonpermissive cells) and the infection is aborted. A subset of the viral proteins (the early/tumor/regulatory proteins) may be expressed in these cells, thereby altering cell survival and proliferation responses and resulting in tumor induction in vivo or cellular transformation in vitro. The ability of viral proteins to induce proliferation by effecting transcriptional activation of critical cellular genes and through interactions with key cell cycle regulators and cell survival factors has become an area of intense interest.

The possibility that primate polyomaviruses might cause human cancer has been considered ever since SV40 was found as a contaminant in the early poliovirus vaccines; however, subsequent studies generally failed to identify adverse outcomes associated with this accidental exposure. It wasn't until the development of sensitive nucleic acid and protein detection methods that evide-nce was uncovered linking SV40, as well as JCV and BKV, to human oncogenesis. In the past decade, SV40 has been associated routinely with four types of cancer: brain tumors (ependymomas, medulloblastomas and glioblastomas), osteosarcoma, mesothelioma and non-Hodgkin lymphoma (reviewed in refs. 10,11). Similarly, JCV sequences have been found in tumors of the CNS (medulloblastomas, glioblastomas, oligodendrogliomas, astrocytomas, ependymomas and B cell lymphomas), colon and prostate.[12-14]

Lytic and Oncogenic Potential of JCV in Vivo

An animal model has not been developed to study productive JCV infections. Under some conditions, transgenic mice containing JCV sequences exhibit neurological problems associated with dysmyelination of their CNS. Such mice developed a shaking disorder that resembles that of myelin-deficient strains of *quaking* or *jimpy* mice.[15] However, this phenotype does not involve cytolytic destruction of oligodendrocytes, but rather a down-regulation of myelin-specific genes by the JCV large T antigen (TAg).[16,17] In addition, PML-like disease has been reported in SV40-infected rhesus monkeys immunosuppressed by simian immunodeficiency virus.[18]

SV40 was first identified as a tumor virus following the appearance of sarcomas in Syrian golden hamsters injected subcutaneously with the virus.[19] Later studies involving injection of virus or creation of transgenic animals expressing viral tumor protein(s) revealed that several rodent hosts are susceptible to tumor induction by SV40, JCV and BKV. These studies indicated that JCV displays a predilection for inducing tumors in neural tissues, including medulloblastomas, primitive neuroectodermal tumors, glioblastomas, pineocytomas, retinoblastomas, neuroblastomas and meningiomas. Particularly relevant to the question of polyomaviruses and human cancer, was the observation that JCV inoculation of primates (owl and squirrel monkeys) results in the appearance of astrocytomas. Compilation of data from several animal systems indicate that tumor type and incidence depend upon a number of parameters, including the viral variant employed, inoculum amount, route of injection, and immune status of the host (reviewed in ref. 1).

Lytic and Oncogenic Potential of JCV in Vitro

A major obstacle to the study of JCV, in contrast to that of SV40 and BKV, is its highly restricted host range. JCV replicates efficiently only in primary human fetal glial (PHFG) cells and in transformed cells derived from these heterogeneous primary cultures (e.g., POJ and SVG cells). Much effort has been expended in attempts to identify a more convenient cell system (reviewed in ref. 20). Varying success has been achieved in propagating virus in human tonsillar stromal cells, astrocytes, Schwann cells, B lymphocytes, embryonic kidney cells and brain cell lines, but none of these cells support infection as efficiently as PHFG cells. Productive JCV infections involve early and late gene expression (see below), phases of the lytic cycle that are separated temporally by the process of viral DNA replication. In contrast, transformation of cells in culture requires only early gene expression. SV40, and to a lesser extent BKV, induce oncogenic transformation in cells derived from a variety of tissues and host species. Somewhat surprisingly, given its oncogenic potential in vivo, JCV transforms only a few cultured cell types (mostly rodent fibroblasts and brain cells). The inability of JCV to efficiently convert cells to a transformed state is related to both the reduced expression and activity of the JCV tumor proteins.[21,22]

Organization of the JCV and SV40 Genomes

The organization of the primate polyomavirus genomes is highly conserved (Fig. 1). Each genome can be divided into three regions: the early and late coding regions and the regulatory region. The TCR positioned within the latter region contains viral promoters that direct transcription of the early and late genes. Alternative splicing of the precursor transcripts yields mature mRNAs that encode the early and late viral proteins. The early proteins regulate virus-cell interactions through a number of mechanisms. For example, these proteins exhibit transactivating functions that are effected through interactions with cellular transcription factors and DNA. They also bind and inactivate cellular tumor suppressor proteins, thereby influencing cell cycle progression and survival. Furthermore, the viral tumor proteins alter the activities of a number of cellular factors that regulate such diverse processes as DNA replication, intracellular signaling, protein degradation and apoptosis. It is hypothesized that these interactions prepare the cellular environment for a lytic infection; in some cells these events result in malignant transformation, a biological dead end for the virus.

The JCV early precursor mRNA is alternatively spliced to yield five transcripts encoding TAg, small t antigen (tAg), T'_{165}, T'_{136}, or T'_{135} (Fig. 1). All five proteins share their amino-terminal (N-terminal) 81 amino acids, whereas TAg and the three T' proteins also share the contiguous 51 amino acids. Furthermore, each protein has a unique carboxy-terminus

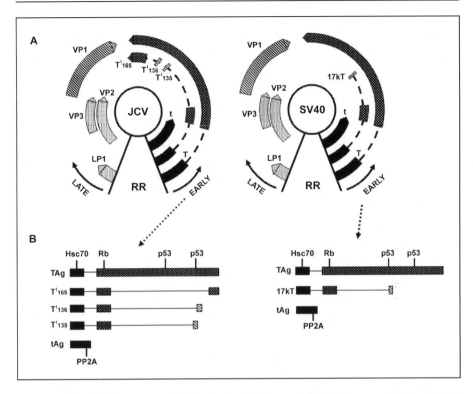

Figure 1. JCV and SV40 genomes. A) The circular, double-stranded DNA genomes of JCV and SV40 represented by the inner circles are slightly greater than 5 kilobases in length. The genomes are divided into early and late coding regions and a regulatory region (RR) containing replication and transcription signals. The single early precursor mRNA is alternatively spliced to yield mature transcripts encoding 5 (JCV) or 3 (SV40) proteins. The 3 JCV T' proteins share their N-terminal 81 amino acids with tAg and 132 amino acids with TAg; coding sequences are indicated by shaded arcs and different shading patterns indicate the exon was translated in an alternate reading frame. The T' proteins have unique C-termini of 3 (T'$_{135}$), 4 (T'$_{136}$), or 33 (T'$_{165}$) amino acids (coding sequences for all 3 T' proteins are denoted by the same arc). The late region encodes 3 capsid proteins and a fourth protein, LP1 (also called Agnoprotein). B) The early coding region is expanded below each genome, and the positions of viral sequences binding to cellular Hsc70, Rb family members, p53 and PP2A are shown.

(C-terminus), except for TAg and T'$_{165}$ that have overlapping C-termini. The presence of shared sequences among the JCV early proteins suggests that functional domains identified within the N-terminus of TAg may also be active in one or more of the smaller tumor proteins. On the other hand, it is likely that removal of TAg sequences during the processing of tAg and T' mRNAs leads to the production of proteins with distinct structures, post-translational modifications and stabilities. Such alterations might modify or abolish functions that the JCV early proteins are predicted to share.

The JCV regulatory region contains numerous, overlapping cis-acting sequences, including the early and late promoters, the enhancer and the core and auxiliary origins of DNA replication. Following early gene expression in a permissive cell, TAg binds specifically to a pentanucleotide motif within the origin sequences to initiate viral DNA replication. Once replication occurs, late gene expression ensues, leading to the production of Agnoprotein (also called LP1) and three capsid proteins, VP1, VP2, and VP3. Agnoprotein influences the assembly of the SV40 virion, whereas the related JCV protein was found recently to play roles in viral gene transcription and DNA replication and to influence cell cycle progression and DNA repair mechanisms.[23,24] Because this chapter focuses on the transforming functions of the JCV early proteins, the reader is referred to other chapters in this book for a more complete discussion of JCV replication signals and late protein functions.

JCV TAg Functions

The TAg of the primate polyomaviruses functions as the viral replication protein through (i) direct interactions with a host of cellular factors involved in regulating cell cycle progression and survival (Table 1), and (ii) its ability to transregulate viral and cellular promoters to alter gene expression. TAg is modified post-translationally in a number of ways; most work has focused upon the phosphorylation of two clusters of serine and threonine residues located in N- and C-terminal domains of the protein. Phosphorylation influences a wide range of TAg activities, including nuclear import, oligomerization and modulation of viral DNA replication (reviewed in refs. 26,27).[25,25a]

TAg-Mediated Viral DNA Replication

The multifunctional TAg is the sole JCV protein required for viral DNA replication.[28] Replication is initiated within a 68 base pair (bp) sequence, the core origin, that includes three domains, (i) TAg binding site II (BSII) composed of four copies of the pentanucleotide

Table 1. JCV early protein interactions

Protein[a]	Sequences[b]	Binding Partner	References[c]
E, T′$_{135}$	J domain	Hsc70	Bollag et al, in prep.
TAg	J domain	Tst-1	Renner et al, 1994
TAg	N.R. [d]	Pur-α	Gallia et al, 1998
TAg	AA# 266-628	YB-1	Safak et al, 1999
TAg	AA# 82-628	c-Jun	Kim et al, 2003
TAg	LXCXE domain	pRB	Dyson et al, 1989
T′	LXCXE domain	pRB	Bollag et al, 2000
TAg	LXCXE domain	p107	Dyson et al, 1990
T′	LXCXE domain	p107	Bollag et al, 2000
TAg, T′	LXCXE domain	p130	Bollag et al, 2000
TAg	N.R.	β-catenin	Enam et al, 2002
TAg	N.R.	IRS-1	Lassak et al, 2002
TAg	Bipartite p53 domain	p53	Frisque et al, 1980
TAg	N.R.	JCV Agnoprotein	Del Valle et al, 2002
TAg	N.R.	JCV TAg	Bollag et al, 1996
TAg	DNA binding domain	DNA: BSI, BSII	Tavis and Frisque, 1991
			Bollag et al, 1996
TAg	N.R.	DNA: non-specific	Bollag et al, 1996

[a] JCV early protein(s) shown to directly interact with a viral or cellular protein or with DNA (see text for details). In some experiments it was not possible to determine if more than one early protein (denoted by "E") was involved in binding. Some interactions involved all three T′ proteins (T′) or a single T′ protein (e.g., T′$_{135}$). In many instances it is expected that tAg and/or T′ proteins will contribute to the interactions already confirmed for TAg. [b] Sequences (specific amino acids [AA] or functional domain) within the JCV early protein(s) demonstrated to be involved in binding. Identification of these sequences is based upon analyses of JCV mutants and chimeras, in addition to comparisons with SV40 results. [c] The first report of a particular interaction is given in the listed reference; some papers also identify the specific viral protein sequences involved in that binding. [d] N.R.= not reported.

sequence GAGGC embedded within a 25 bp dyad symmetry, (ii) a 15 bp imperfect palindrome (IP) and (iii) a 15 bp AT-rich region.[29-31] Sequences adjacent to the core origin that enhance, but are not required for DNA replication, include TAg BSI and a pentanucleotide repeat (AGGGA AGGGA) referred to as the lytic control element (LCE). The LCE motif is bound by the transcription factors YB-1 and Pur-α and influences viral transcription as well as replication.[29,31-33]

Polyomavirus TAgs influence both the initiation and elongation steps of DNA replication, and our understanding of these processes relies primarily on studies with SV40 TAg. Upon binding to TAg BSII, the protein oligomerizes into a double hexamer structure that leads to the distortion and unwinding of origin sequences and the recruitment of the cellular replication machinery.[34-36] Upon transition from the initiation to elongation phase of DNA replication, TAg displays helicase and ATPase activities resulting in the appearance of two replication forks. Replication proceeds bidirectionally as DNA is threaded through the hexameric structures and two cellular polymerases copy the unwound template strands. The rate-limiting step in the replication process occurs at the termination stage, perhaps because steric constraints begin to interfere with replication fork movement.[37]

Several in vivo and in vitro approaches have been taken to compare the replication potential of the primate polyomaviruses. The viral replication components, TAg and the core origin, exhibit a high degree of sequence similarity. Combinations of mutant, chimeric or naturally occurring variant origins have been examined to identify the basis for observed differences in JCV, BKV and SV40 DNA replication behavior (reviewed in ref. 38). These studies reveal that JCV TAg binds to both the JCV and SV40 replication origins, but with reduced efficiency relative to its SV40 counterpart. While the BKV and SV40 TAgs interact productively with the JCV origin, the JCV TAg promotes replication only from its own origin. The inability of the JCV TAg to drive replication from the SV40 origin has been mapped to amino acids 82-411[39] and to 3 nucleotide differences between the AT-rich regions of the two viral core origins.[29] Overall, JCV TAg mediates replication, even from its own origin, less efficiently than do the BKV and SV40 proteins.[29,31]

JCV-SV40 early region chimeras have been used to investigate the well-established observation that JCV exhibits a more restricted host range than SV40 or BKV. When a series of constructs containing different portions of the JCV and SV40 TAg coding regions were introduced into human and monkey cells, JCV replication was extended to the latter cells if the C-terminal host range (HR) region of JCV TAg was replaced with that of SV40 TAg (Fig. 2).[39] It should be noted that Smith and Nasheuer[40] recently revisited the prediction that JCV's strict species specificity reflects the inability of its TAg to interact productively with a nonhuman DNA polymerase α-primase complex. Previous work with SV40 and mouse polyomavirus in fact supported this hypothesis,[41,42] but surprisingly, the JCV TAg, unlike the SV40 TAg, was found to promote DNA replication in an in vitro system employing DNA polymerase α-primase of either human or murine origin.

TAg Transformation Functions: Interactions with Rb and p53 Tumor Suppressor Proteins

Multiple TAg functional domains contribute to viral transformation by altering cellular signaling pathways regulating proliferation and survival. At least three regions of SV40 TAg are involved in these processes, the N-terminal J domain and the Rb (LXCXE) and p53 binding domains[43] (reviewed in ref. 44); these motifs have also been identified in the JCV TAg. In addition, the LXCXE and J domains are present in the T' and 17kT proteins, and the J domain is found in the small tAg of each virus (Fig. 1).

To understand the mechanisms by which polyomaviruses induce transformation, researchers have focused much of their attention on the interaction of viral tumor proteins with the cellular tumor suppressors pRB and p53. Polyomavirus infection of permissive or nonpermissive cells may induce the cell's progression into S phase, with the outcome being either a lytic infection or transformation. Sheng and coworkers[45] proposed a model to explain the ability of

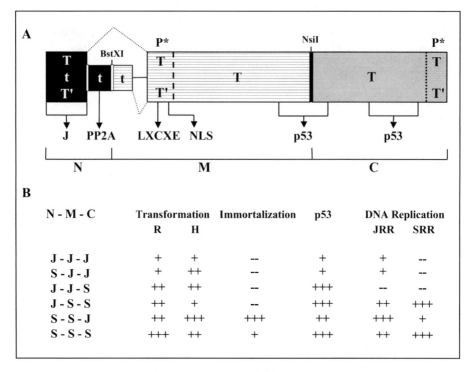

Figure 2. JCV-SV40 chimeric early regions. A) JCV-SV40 chimeras were constructed by exchanging the amino-terminal (N; dark shading), middle (M; horizontal lines) and carboxy-terminal (C; light shading) early coding sequences. The restriction enzymes *BstXI* and *NsiI*, used to swap JCV and SV40 sequences, are located at the same positions in both viral coding regions. The structure represents the JCV early region encoding the TAg (T), tAg (t) and 3 T' proteins (T'); the SV40 coding region would be similar in appearance except that 17kT would replace the T' proteins. The first introns of the TAg, T'_{135}, T'_{136}, T'_{165} and tAg mRNAs are denoted by dotted peaks. The second introns of the three T' mRNAs are not shown, however, the locations of the shared donor (dashed vertical line) and unique T'_{165} acceptor (dotted vertical line) sites are indicated. Region N includes amino acids 1-81 of JCV TAg, T'_{135}, T'_{136}, T'_{165} and 1-131 of tAg. Region M includes amino acids 82-411 of JCV TAg, 82-132 of T'_{135}, T'_{136}, T'_{165} and 132-172 of tAg. Region C includes amino acids 412-688 of JCV TAg, 133-135 of T'_{135} (unique C-terminus, not shown), 133-136 of T'_{136} (unique C-terminus, not shown), and 133-165 of T'_{165} (T'; shared C-terminus with TAg). Functional domains are indicated in the appropriate position above (P*, phosphorylation sites) and below (J, PP2A, LXCXE, NLS, p53) the early region structure. B) The JCV (J) and SV40 (S) sequences comprising the N, M and C regions of the 6 constructs are indicated to the left of the figure. These parental and hybrid early coding regions were linked to the SV40 regulatory region (SRR) and transfected into rat fibroblasts (R) and human brain cells (H). Relative transformation (rat and human cells), immortalization (rat cells) p53 binding (p53; rat cells) and DNA replication (DNA Rep; human cells) activities are denoted by pluses and minuses. DNA replication activity was also tested using the 6 early coding regions linked to the JCV regulatory region (JRR).

TAg to initiate this event. Members of the Rb family of tumor suppressor proteins (pRB, p107, p130) bind to the E2F family of transcription factors to negatively regulate cell cycle progression from G_0/G_1 to S phase.[46] Under the appropriate conditions, cyclin-dependent kinases (cdks) phosphorylate Rb proteins, leading to the release of the transcription factors and promotion of G_1 to S phase transition. The model suggests that TAg disrupts this regulation by first binding to Rb-E2F complexes through its LXCXE domain. Once bound, TAg, via its J domain, recruits the molecular chaperone, Hsc70, and activates this cellular protein's intrinsic

ATPase function. These interactions are believed to cause the release of E2F from the complex, thereby making it available to activate genes involved in S phase progression. Sullivan et al have confirmed and extended several features of this model, especially in regards to the TAg-chaperone interaction.[47,48] Relevant to the current discussion of JCV tumor proteins, these investigators have shown that a chimeric SV40-JCV TAg containing a JCV J domain supports viral replication and transformation, but with reduced efficiency relative to the intact SV40 protein.[49] Furthermore, they reported that an N-terminal truncated form of SV40 TAg (TN136), that shares features with the JCV T′ proteins, fails to form a stable complex with Hsc70, suggesting that sequences C-terminal to the J and LXCXE domains might be essential for stable interaction with Hsc70.[50] It should be noted that interactions between viral TAgs and Hsc70 appear to influence a wide range of activities in addition to cell cycle regulation and transformation, including viral DNA replication, transactivation of viral and cellular promoters, and virion assembly (reviewed in ref. 51).

By promoting unscheduled cell cycle progression through the release of active E2F, small DNA tumor viruses may provoke a counter response by a cell that leads to stabilization and elevated levels of p53. Because this transcription factor regulates a wide variety of cellular processes including cell cycle arrest, DNA repair and apoptosis, p53 is an additional key target of several viral tumor proteins. To prevent this tumor suppressor protein from interfering with critical viral functions, DNA tumor viruses have evolved mechanisms to inactivate it; polyomaviruses accomplish this feat, in part, by binding to and inactivating p53. This latter event suppresses induction of the cyclin-dependent kinase inhibitor (CKI), p21, a key downstream p53 effector that promotes arrest of cells in the G1 phase of the cell cycle. JCV TAg was first shown to bind p53 in transformed hamster brain cells using a co-immunoprecipitation approach.[52] As noted below, a smaller subpopulation of JCV TAg, compared to SV40 TAg, appears to bind p53. Through this binding, p53 is stabilized and its levels increase dramatically in primate and rodent transformed and tumor cells. Recently, SV40 small tAg was found to contribute to p53 stabilization by an unknown mechanism;[53] a similar role for the JCV tAg has not yet been demonstrated.

Several in vivo and in vitro studies have confirmed that the JCV TAg interacts with cellular pRB, p107, p130, Hsc70 and p53.[52,54-58] As with other comparisons of the JCV, BKV and SV40 TAgs, the JCV protein appears to be less robust in binding to and overriding the functions of these cellular factors. A limited number of mutations have been introduced into the J and LXCXE domains of the JCV TAg. Initial studies created two JCV TAg LXCXE mutants, one (RbS) in which the JCV sequence was converted to an SV40-like domain and the second (RbN) designed to disrupt the Rb binding region (Table 2). The first mutant exhibited increased DNA binding activity, wild type transforming activity and, surprisingly, decreased pRB binding. The latter mutant exhibited reduced DNA binding and was unable to bind pRB or transform Rat2 fibroblasts. Both mutants were defective for DNA replication and failed to produce infectious virions.[54] An additional LXCXE mutant, E109K, has been generated in the JCV sequence (Tyagarajan and Frisque, in preparation); two J domain mutants were also produced in these experiments, H42Q and H42Q/D44N (Table 2). Co-immunoprecipitation/ Western blot (IP/WB) experiments performed on extracts of cells stably expressing wild type and mutant viral proteins indicated that (i) JCV early proteins influence the phosphorylation status and stability of p107 and p130; only the faster migrating hypophosphorylated forms of p107 and p130 are detected, (ii) both hypophosphorylated and hyperphosphorylated forms p107 and p130 are present in cells expressing the LXCXE and J domain mutants, suggesting that the mutant viral proteins fail to reduce the levels of the hyperphosphorylated species and (iii) J domain, but not LXCXE domain, mutant proteins bind p107 and p130. Relevant to these findings, Howard and coworkers[58] found that induced expression of p130 resulted in elevated levels of the CKI, p27. In cells derived from tumors caused by JCV, p27 and p130 were identified as direct targets of TAg. Upon detecting a physical interaction between the two cellular proteins, these investigators suggested that p130 and p27 cooperate to negatively regulate cell

Table 2. JCV early region mutants

Mutant[a]	Protein[b]	Domain (#AA)[c]	Tfn	Rb	E2F	DB	Rep	V	S
						Mutant Phenotypes[d]			
1. H42Q (S)	E	J (42)	NT	+	+/-	NT	NT	NT	NT
2. H42Q/D44N (S)	E	J (42, 44)	NT	+	−	NT	NT	NT	NT
3. E109K (S)	TAg, T'	LXCXE (109)	NT	−	−	NT	NT	NT	NT
4. H42Q/E109K (S)	E	J, LXCXE (42, 109)	NT	+/-	−	NT	NT	−	NT
5. RbS (S, I)	TAg, T'	LXCXE (104, 108, 112, 113, 118, 120)	+	+/-	NT	++	+/-	−	NT
6. RbN (S)	TAg, T'	LXCXE (104, 105, 107, 109)	−	−	NT	+/-	+/-	−	+/-
7. T125A (S)	TAg, T'	N-terminal P* (125)	NT	NT	NT	NT	−	+	+
8. T664A (S)	TAg, T'165	C-terminal P* (664)	NT	NT	NT	+	+	+	+/-
9. T664S (S)	TAg, T'165	C-terminal P* (664)	NT	NT	NT	+	+	+	+/-
10. E666A (S)	TAg, T'165	C-terminal P* (666)	NT	NT	NT	+	+	+	+/-
11. E666S (S)	TAg, T'165	C-terminal P* (666)	NT	NT	NT	+	+	+	+/-
12. K131R (S)	TAg, T'	NLS, DNA Binding (131)	NT	NT	NT	+	+	+	NT
13. A145S (S)	TAg	DNA Binding (145)	NT	NT	NT	+	+	+	NT
14. Q149H (S)	TAg	DNA Binding (149)	NT	NT	NT	+	+/-	+	NT
15. V157L (S)	TAg	DNA Binding (157)	NT	NT	NT	+	++	+	NT
16. S159C (S)	TAg	DNA Binding (159)	NT	NT	NT	+	+/-	+	NT
17. V162I (S)	TAg	DNA Binding (162)	NT	NT	NT	+	+/-	+	NT
18. K168R (S)	TAg	DNA Binding (168)	NT	NT	NT	++	−	−	NT
19. Q149H/V157L (S)	TAg	DNA Binding (149, 157)	NT	NT	NT	+	+	+	NT
20. Q149H/V157I/ S159C (S)	TAg	DNA Binding (149, 157, 159)	NT	NT	NT	+	+	+	NT
21. A145S/Q149H/ V157I/S159C/ V162I (S)	TAg	DNA Binding (145, 149, 157, 159, 162)	NT	NT	NT	+	+/-	+	NT
22. N316K (S)	TAg	Zn finger (316)	NT	NT	NT	NT	+	+	NT

continued on next page

Table 2. Continued

Mutant[a]	Protein[b]	Domain (#AA)[c]	Mutant Phenotypes[d]						
			Tfn	Rb	E2F	DB	Rep	V	S
23. H317Y (S)	TAg	Zn finger (317)	NT	NT	NT	NT	+	+	NT
24. N316K/H317Y (S)	TAg	Zn finger (316, 317)	NT	NT	NT	NT	+	+	NT
25. ΔT' (S)	T'	5' splice site (nt# 4274)	NT	+/-	+/-	NT	+/-	+/-	—
26. ΔT'135 (S)	T'135	3' splice sites (nt# 2920, 2918, 2915, 2900, 2885, 2884, 2882)	NT	NT	NT	NT	+	+	+/-
27. ΔT'136 (S)	T'136	3' splice site (nt# 2779, 2777)	NT	NT	NT	NT	+	+	+/-
28. ΔT'165 (S)	T'165	3' splice site (nt# 2705)	NT	NT	NT	NT	+	+	+/-
29. ΔT'135/136 (S)	T'135, T'136	3' splice sites (nt# 2920, 2918, 2915, 2900, 2885, 2884, 2882, 2779, 2777)	NT	NT	NT	NT	+	+	+/-
30. ΔT'135/165 (S)	T'135, T'165	3' splice sites (nt# 2920, 2918, 2915, 2900, 2885, 2884, 2882, 2705)	NT	NT	NT	NT	+	+	+/-
31. ΔT'136/165 (S)	T'136, T'165	3' splice sites (nt# 2779, 2777, 2705)	NT	NT	NT	NT	+	+	+/-
32. ΔT'135/136/165 (S)	T'	3' splice sites (nt# 2920, 2918, 2915, 2900, 2885, 2884, 2882, 2779, 2777, 2705)	NT	NT	NT	NT	+/-	+/-	—
33. K-1 (I)	tAg	C-terminus (nt# 4502-4499)	+/-	NT	NT	NT	NT	NT	NT
34. B-B (D)	TAg, T'	Multiple (122-143)	NT	NT	NT	NT	—	—	NT

[a] Names of JCV early region substitution (S), insertion (I) and deletion (D) mutants. Mutants are described in the following references: Mutants #1 (Tyagarajan and Frisque, in preparation; Kelley and Georgopoulos, 1997), #2-4 (Tyagarajan and Frisque, in preparation), #5, 6 (Tavis et al, 1994), #7, 22-24 (Swenson et al, 1996), #8-11 (Swenson et al, 1995, 1996), #12-21, 34 (Tavis and Frisque, 1991), #25 (Trowbridge and Frisque, 1995), #26-32 (Prins and Frisque, 2001), and #33 (Mandl et al, 1987; Trowbridge and Frisque, 1993). [b] Viral proteins affected by the mutations: all five early proteins (E), all three T' proteins (T') or each individual early protein (TAg, tAg, T'135, T'136, T'165). [c] Domains within the early region affected by the mutations (see text for details). Mutants #7-11 contain alterations that are predicted to alter potential N- or C-terminal phosphorylation (N-terminal P*, C-terminal P*) sites. The deletion in mutant #34 is predicted to alter several functional domains (Multiple), including the LXCXE, N-terminal P*, NLS and DNA binding domains. The numbers in parentheses identify the amino acids (AA) altered in mutants 1-24 and 34 and refer to specific TAg residues. In the case of splice site mutants (#25-32) which retain the wild type amino acid sequence, and the tAg mutant (#33), the specific nucleotides (nt) altered are shown in parentheses. Numbering is according to Frisque et al (1984). [d] Each mutant was examined for one or more of the following phenotypes: transformation of rat fibroblasts (tfn), binding to Rb family members (Rb), release of E2F from Rb complexes (E2F), specific DNA binding (DB), DNA replication (Rep) and viability (V) in human brain cells, and altered early mRNA splicing patterns (S). Activities were listed as not tested (NT), equivalent to the negative control (—), or reduced (+/-), similar (+), enhanced (++) relative to wild type.

cycle progression, and that TAg interferes with this activity either by sequestering p27 or by altering the phosphorylation state of Rb proteins.

Earlier studies involving chimeric JCV-SV40-BKV genomes support the findings that JCV tumor proteins interact with the p53 and Rb tumor suppressor proteins, but that their ability to inactivate these key regulators is reduced relative to SV40 and BKV.[21,49,59,60] These experiments also suggest that the JCV proteins might target other cellular factors. Characterization of two sets of JCV-SV40 chimeras, generated by swapping JCV TAg sequences containing the J domain (amino acids 1-81), LXCXE domain (amino acids 82-411) or most of the p53 bipartite binding region (amino acids 412-688) (Fig. 2), led to the following observations: (i) the substitution of the J domain of JCV TAg for that in the SV40 TAg resulted in reduced dense focus formation, DNA replication and p130-E2F disruption,[47] (ii) the presence of JCV sequences in place of SV40 sequences within any of the three exchanged regions of a chimera yielded lower transformation efficiencies,[60] (iii) hybrid proteins containing most of the p53 binding domain of JCV TAg formed less stable complexes with p53 than did a TAg with an SV40 p53 binding motif[21,60] and (iv) chimeric TAgs containing the JCV C-terminal region immortalized human fibroblasts more efficiently than did the intact SV40 protein.[61] At the time many of these studies were conducted, it was not known that the exchange of sequences within the viral early coding regions would also affect the structures of JCV T′ and SV40 17kT proteins.

TAg Transformation Functions: Disruption of Wnt and IGF-IR Signaling Pathways

While most studies have examined the outcomes of interactions between polyomavirus TAgs and p53 and Rb proteins, recent work indicates that the oncogenic behavior of JCV TAg may involve the disruption of other cell signaling networks. The Wnt signal transduction pathway plays critical roles in developmental patterning events during embryogenesis; deregulation of the pathway is associated with a number of human cancers. Greater than 90% of colorectal cancers involve a genetic lesion within the Wnt pathway that leads to stabilization and nuclear import of β-catenin, a key component of this signaling cascade (reviewed in ref. 62). Nuclear β-catenin partners with the transcription factors TCF-4/LEF-1 to activate promoters of genes involved in induction of cellular proliferation. Importantly, JCV is associated with tumors of the colon and prostate and with medulloblastoma, cancers in which the Wnt pathway may be aberrantly activated (reviewed in ref. 63). Immunostaining of cells derived from these tumors shows colocalization of TAg and β-catenin in the nucleus.[64,65] Transfection of a JCV TAg-expressing vector into a colon cancer cell line indicates that TAg and wild type β-catenin form a complex and exhibit cooperativity in upregulating expression of c-myc. This latter proto-oncoprotein, a downstream target of β-catenin, is found at elevated levels in colon cancer.[66,67] These results indicate that JCV TAg may activate the Wnt pathway by altering β-catenin stability and localization, suggesting another mechanism by which TAg may exert its oncogenic potential.[64,65]

The insulin-like growth factor I receptor (IGF-IR), when activated by its major ligand, insulin receptor substrate 1 (IRS-1), elicits numerous cellular responses involving mitogenic, anti-apoptotic and transformation signals (reviewed in ref. 68). The Khalili laboratory has presented evidence that JCV TAg may mediate transforming activity through its influence upon this signaling pathway. Analyses of human medulloblastoma tissues and medulloblastoma cell lines derived from a transgenic mouse model revealed elevated levels of IGF-IR and IRS-1 in JCV TAg-positive cells. A direct interaction was observed between TAg and IRS-1, and the latter factor, which functions in the cytoplasm, was translocated to the nucleus in the presence of the viral protein.[68,69] Further, the ability of JCV TAg to induce a transformed phenotype in different murine cell lines correlated with the levels of IGF-IR present in the lines examined. Finally, cells derived from IGF-IR knockout animals, but which continue to express p53 and Rb proteins, were refractory to virally induced transformation, emphasizing the importance of a functional IGF-IR/IRS-1 pathway to JCV TAg function.[68]

TAg and Genomic Instability

The preceding discussion argues that polyomavirus tumor proteins induce transformation by directly interacting with critical cellular factors to deregulate signal transduction pathways controlling cellular proliferation, differentiation and death. Less attention has been given to the possibility that polyomavirus infections disrupt regulated cell growth by causing genomic instability. In support of this possibility, it has been shown that JCV, BKV and SV40 TAgs exhibit mutagenic activity,[70] and that JCV- and SV40-infected cells contain chromosomal abnormalities.[71,72] These and other findings support the suggestion that TAg expression sets in motion a series of mutational events that activate proto-oncogenes and/or inactivate tumor suppressor genes, thereby initiating malignant transformation. While a large body of work supports the hypothesis that continued expression of viral oncoproteins is required to maintain a transformed state, the ability of TAg to initiate a cascade of genetic defects might render the continued presence of an oncogenic virus unnecessary. Although controversial, a "hit-and-run" mechanism" has been proposed to operate in some human cancers, including medulloblastoma and colon cancer (reviewed in ref. 73).[74]

Physical and Functional Interactions between TAg and Replication and Transcription Factors

Based upon studies of SV40 TAg (reviewed in ref. 38), JCV TAg is predicted to physically interact with a number of cellular replication factors, including topoisomerase I, the single-stranded DNA binding protein RPA, and DNA polymerase α; however, such interactions have not yet been demonstrated. On the other hand, because many laboratories have focused upon the glial-specific regulation of the JCV early and late promoters, progress has been made showing TAg binding to specific components of the cell's transcriptional machinery.

The POU III domain transcription factor Tst-1 (Oct-6, SCIP) is selectively expressed in myelinating glia, the cells targeted during JCV infection. Renner and colleagues[75] discovered that the N-terminal portion of JCV TAg binds Tst-1, leading to synergistic activation of both the early and late viral promoters. Further, they proposed that if JCV TAg, like its SV40 counterpart,[76] binds TATA binding protein (TBP), then it might act as a co-activator to facilitate contact between Tst-1 and the basal transcriptional apparatus.

The cellular transcription factor, Pur-α, stimulates JCV early protein expression six fold. JCV TAg interacts with Pur-α, resulting in negative modulation of both JCV promoters.[77] Whereas TAg antagonizes the ability of Pur-α to enhance early gene transcription, Pur-α inhibits the ability of TAg to transactivate the late promoter.[78] TAg, through its C-terminal sequences, also binds YB-1, a Y-box binding protein that regulates gene expression at both the transcriptional and translational levels (see ref. 79 and references therein). TAg functionally interacts with YB-1, leading to synergistic transactivation of the JCV late promoter. In addition, YB-1 reduces TAg's negative regulation of its own promoter.[78-80] Pur-α and YB-1 modulate JCV transcription, in part, by binding to the late (A/G-rich) and early (T/C- rich) strands of the LCE motif in the viral TCR. In addition to effects on viral gene transcription, the interactions between TAg, Pur-α and YB-1 also appear to dictate the association of these factors with target DNA sequences.[77,78,81] Chen et al[82] have proposed a model to explain the mechanism by which TAg, Pur-α and YB-1 interaction leads to transition of early to late gene transcription.

Members of the Jun and Fos families of proto-oncoproteins form dimers that were initially recognized as the AP-1 family of transcription factors. These complexes activate a number of cellular and viral promoters and influence a variety of cellular events, including proliferation, apoptosis and differentiation (reviewed in ref. 83). JCV promoter function is enhanced by c-Jun and c-Fos, and c-Jun binds sequences within the JCV TCR.[84,85] Kim and coworkers[86] have reported that in the presence of JCV TAg, however, both cellular factors down-regulate TAg-mediated viral transcription and replication. A physical interaction between c-Jun and the central region of JCV TAg was demonstrated, leading to speculation that positive effects of AP-1 on JCV early transcription might be important to establishing an infection, but that once TAg was expressed, these same factors might temper TAg function through binding, thereby facilitating virus maturation.

The late coding regions of primate polyomaviruses encode a small protein called Agnoprotein or LP1. Initial studies of the SV40 protein suggested that it has several functions, including roles in VP1 localization and viral capsid assembly.[87-89] Recent experiments indicate that the JCV Agnoprotein displays additional activities. This 71 amino acid protein directly binds to TAg and to p53, and it has been hypothesized these interactions may influence cellular transformation and tumor formation.[90] In addition, JCV Agnoprotein decreases the levels of JCV late gene transcription, and inhibits viral DNA replication, both TAg-mediated activities.[91,92] Recently, Agnoprotein expression was found to enhance p21 levels in cells and to delay cell cycle progression during the G_2/M phase of the cell cycle.[24]

JCV tAg Functions

tAg Contributes to Viral Transformation

Investigations into the functions of JCV tAg are just beginning, however, several activities can be predicted based upon studies of the related SV40 protein. Early mutagenesis studies of JCV and SV40 indicated that tAg mutants are viable (Mandl et al, unpublished data),[93,94] but exhibit some defects in infectious virion production in cultured cells.[95] Transforming potential of the SV40 mutants was found to be variable and depended upon the experimental conditions.[96-98] TAg transforms many cell types in the absence of other viral proteins, but co-expression of tAg is required to initiate transformation of certain human cells.[99-102] Further, tAg enhances TAg-mediated transformation when quiescent cells are employed or under conditions in which low levels of TAg are present. Both the N-terminal portion of tAg, which is shared with TAg and the 17kT protein, and the unique C-terminal portion of tAg, influence its transformation functions. Significant effort has been expended to identify the functional domains of this 174 amino acid protein, and two key interactions with cellular factors have been reported (reviewed in ref. 103).

The J Domain of tAg

The shared N-terminal 82 amino acids of SV40 TAg and tAg represent a J domain, a conserved sequence found in the DnaJ family of molecular chaperones.[42] As discussed above, DNA tumor virus proteins, through their J domain, bind the cellular chaperone Hsc70, exhibiting a cochaperone function that contributes to viral lytic and transforming behaviors. SV40 small t protein, but not large T or truncated T (TN125 or TN136) proteins, functionally replaces the chaperone function of the *E. coli* DnaJ protein under limited growth conditions in vivo.[104] Further, tAg stimulates the ATPase activity of DnaK from *E. coli* in vitro. Differences in cochaperone activity of the individual SV40 proteins may be due to the unique tAg sequences (amino acids 83-174) that substitute for a glycine-phenylalanine-rich domain of the bacterial Type I DnaJ protein.

The SV40 tAg also exhibits transregulating activities that depend upon a functional J domain. These activities involve both the activation and repression of cell cycle regulators, including cyclins A and D1 and the CKI, p27.[100,105] In addition, tAg transregulates other cellular promoters through its binding to protein phosphatase 2A (PP2A).

tAg Interaction with PP2A

The discovery that unique C-terminal tAg sequences interact with the cellular serine/threonine phosphatase PP2A was crucial to identifying mechanisms by which tAg contributes to viral transformation.[106,107] PP2A, a modular trimeric enzyme, plays critical roles in cell signaling through the dephosphorylation of specific substrates. The large number of isoforms of the regulatory B subunit directs functional specificity when joined to the core enzyme composed of subunits A and C (reviewed in ref. 108). SV40 tAg forms a complex with the AC core, in part, through a cysteine-containing motif (amino acids 97-103). This association modifies the substrate specificity and intracellular localization of PP2A,[109] resulting in a multitude of responses that suggest mechanisms by which tAg cooperates with TAg to induce transformation.

Inhibition of PP2A by tAg results in the activation of the protein kinase C ζ isoform (PKC ζ) in quiescent cells via a mechanism requiring phosphoinositide 3-kinase (PI 3-kinase). Activated PKC ζ then upregulates the stress- and mitogen-activated protein kinase signaling cascades (SAPK and MAPK). Downstream targets of these pathways include the transcription factors, CREB, AP-1, Sp1 and NF-κB, which contribute to cellular proliferation and survival (reviewed in ref. 108).

Yuan and colleagues[110] reported that transformation and immortalization of human keratinocytes require the simultaneous expression of SV40 TAg and tAg. In parallel with these observations, the investigators detected increased phosphorylation of the protein kinase, Akt, in cells expressing both viral proteins, but not in those producing TAg only. The authors provided data supporting the hypothesis that the interaction between tAg and PP2A activates Akt, a PKC-related kinase, and telomerase, the enzyme that regulates telomere length, contributes to a cell's extended life span and displays reactivated expression in most human tumors. These experimental results fit well with earlier reports that (i) identify Akt as a target of upstream kinases of the PI 3-kinase signaling pathway and (ii) indicate activated Akt inhibits apoptosis, stimulates cell growth and enhances telomerase activity (reviewed in ref. 110).

tAg Expression and Genomic Instability

Human diploid fibroblasts expressing SV40 tAg are blocked in their progression through G_2/M, and Gaillard et al[111] observed that overexpression of the viral protein in these cells prevents formation of the mitotic spindle. This phenotype depends on the interaction between tAg and PP2A and the resulting inhibition of centrosome maturation and duplication. Such tAg effects might contribute to the TAg-mediated alterations in ploidy and genetic stability already discussed above.

tAg Expression and Effects on the Tumor Suppressor, p53

The phosphorylation state of p53 is regulated by multiple cellular kinases and phosphatases, and this post-translational modification, in turn, modulates p53 functions such as specific DNA binding, transcriptional activation, cell cycle arrest and apoptosis induction (reviewed in ref. 112). Okadaic acid and SV40 tAg, two inhibitors of PP2A, reduced p53 dephosphorylation and increased its transcriptional activity, but only okadaic acid induced p53-directed programmed cell death in these experiments.[112]

As noted above, an important step in SV40-induced transformation is the stabilization and functional inactivation of p53 following its binding to TAg. Members of the Deppert laboratory[53,113] have reported that the metabolic stabilization and high-level accumulation of p53 in SV40-infected mouse and rat cells requires co-expression of TAg and tAg. Further, they suggest that tAg influences transformation efficiency through its ability to activate an unknown cellular function that results in p53 stabilization.

JCV T' Protein Functions

The JCV early precursor mRNA is alternatively spliced to yield 5 transcripts encoding TAg, tAg, T'$_{135}$, T'$_{136}$, and T'$_{165}$.[114,115] The three T' proteins are 135, 136 and 165 amino acids in length, and share their N-terminal 132 amino acids with the multifunctional TAg, of which 81 amino acids are also shared with tAg. T'$_{165}$ shares its 33 amino acid C-terminus with TAg, while T'$_{135}$ and T'$_{136}$ have unique 3 and 4 amino acid C-termini, respectively, in a different reading frame (Fig. 1). Each T' protein retains the TAg nuclear localization signal (NLS) at the end of their second coding exon, and immunofluorescence experiments confirm that the signal is functional; tAg, which lacks this NLS, is found predominately in the cytoplasm (Bollag et al, in preparation). Unlike the 17kT protein of SV40[116] and tiny T protein of mouse polyomavirus,[117] the JCV T′ protein(s) are produced at relatively high levels in transformed and productively-infected cells (reviewed in ref. 118). Genetic and biochemical studies suggest that T′ proteins contribute both to viral replication and oncogenesis through their interaction with key cellular regulatory factors (reviewed in ref. 119).

Discovery of JCV T′ Proteins

Based upon sequence analysis of the JCV genome, the early region was initially proposed to encode two proteins, TAg and tAg.[114] Subsequent analysis of ^{35}S-methionine labeled extracts of JCV-transformed rodent cells[21,60] revealed three bands on an SDS-polyacrylamide gel representing TAg, tAg and an unidentified 17 kDa protein named T′ protein (later shown to be T′$_{136}$). Although this protein was originally thought to be a degradation product of TAg, pulse-chase experiments confirmed it to be an authentic early protein.[115] Similar studies in lytically infected PHFG cells revealed four T′ bands of 16, 17, 22 and 23 kDa. Immunoprecipitation reactions using a monoclonal antibody directed against the N-terminus of TAg recognized each T′ band, whereas an antibody directed against the C-terminus of TAg recognized only the two largest T′ bands.

RNA extracted from infected PHFG cells and subjected to reverse transcription polymerase chain reaction (RT-PCR) led to the identification of three T′ transcripts. Sequence analyses of cloned T′ cDNAs prepared from RT-PCR experiments indicated that two introns are removed during the processing of the T′ mRNAs. The first intron is removed using the TAg mRNA donor and acceptor splice sites, and the second intron, unique to T′ transcripts, is processed using a common donor site and three different acceptor sites. It will be noted that four T′ bands were observed on SDS-polyacrylamide gels, but only three T′ cDNAs were generated by RT-PCR. This discrepancy was resolved by using lambda phosphatase to identify the 23 kDa T′ band as a phosphorylated form of T′$_{165}$.[121] Subsequently, the other two T′ proteins were also found to be phosphoproteins (Bollag et al, in preparation).[120]

A single T′ protein (T′$_{136}$) was detected in JCV-transformed rat fibroblasts, whereas all three T′ proteins were observed in JCV-infected human brain cells, suggesting that T′ expression patterns either reflect differences in the species (human vs. rat), cell type (brain vs. fibroblast) or virus-cell interaction (transformed vs. infected) examined. To investigate these possibilities, Jones and Frisque (unpublished data) conducted RT-PCR on infected, transformed or tumor cells derived from different species and tissues. The results suggest that changes in T′ expression patterns are the result of differences in alternative splicing levels occurring during a lytic vs. transformation event.

Replication Function of JCV T′ Proteins

Biochemical and genetic approaches have been employed to understand the role of the T′ proteins in JCV biology. The N-terminal 132 amino acids shared by TAg and T′ proteins encompass numerous functional domains influencing both viral replication and oncogenic behavior. Early mutagenesis experiments targeted the T′ common donor splice site, thereby abrogating T′ expression. Transfection of this mutant genome (JCVΔT′) into PHFG cells resulted in a 10- to 20-fold reduction in replication, thus confirming that one or more T′ proteins contributes to TAg-mediated viral DNA replication.[115] To express these T′ proteins individually or in combination with one another, the three unique T′ acceptor sites were mutated (without changing the TAg amino acid sequence), and viral replication was measured in PHFG cells.[121] Those mutants still capable of producing one or two T′ proteins had replication activities similar to that of wild type virus, whereas the triple acceptor site mutant (no T′ proteins made) had the same defective replication phenotype as the JCVΔT′ donor site mutant.[121] It was observed that cells transfected with the initial T′$_{135}$ acceptor site mutant DNA produced new T′ mRNAs and proteins as a result of the utilization of cryptic splice sites downstream of the original T′$_{135}$ acceptor site. Therefore, these cryptic sites were altered to prevent expression of any T′$_{135}$-like transcripts.[121]

T' Proteins Influence Virus-Cell Interactions

Attempts to transform Rat2 fibroblasts with vectors expressing individual JCV early proteins have been unsuccessful (Bollag et al, in preparation). Therefore, to establish cell lines expressing each JCV tumor protein, a G418-selection protocol was employed. Constructs containing the entire JCV early coding region (JCV$_E$) or individual proteins (TAg, T'$_{135}$, T'$_{136}$ or T'$_{165}$) under the control of a cytomegalovirus (CMV) promoter were cotransfected into Rat2 cells with the pSV2-neo plasmid. Cells acquiring G418 resistance were single-cell cloned for stable and high-level protein expression. Lines expressing T'$_{135}$, T'$_{136}$ or T'$_{165}$ independently or all 5 early proteins together were readily obtained, but lines containing the TAg cDNA expressed TAg plus one or more T' proteins. Because the TAg construct retains the unique T' donor and acceptor splice sites, attempts were made to create lines expressing TAg only by using a JCVΔ T' cDNA mutant (Bollag et al, in preparation). Only 1 of the 30 lines screened produced TAg, and in this line the viral protein was produced at low levels. Sequence analysis confirmed that the integrated TAg gene was not mutated. One interpretation of these results is that TAg induces apoptosis in Rat2 cells and that one or more T' proteins block this effect. Others have shown that SV40 TAg and tAg may exhibit both proapoptotic or antiapoptotic functions depending on experimental conditions (see ref. 122 and references therein).

Analyses of cell doubling time and saturation density in media supplemented with 1% or 10% fetal bovine serum were performed on the cloned Rat2 lines expressing individual JCV proteins. Testing of 2 independent clones showed JCV$_E$ cells had accelerated growth rates and higher saturation densities, although the values were lower than those of a control transformed line isolated from a dense focus assay (Bollag et al, in preparation). Cells expressing TAg, T'$_{135}$, T'$_{136}$ or T'$_{165}$ showed growth parameters only marginally more robust than those of the parental Rat2 line. The failure of the cloned Rat2 lines to exhibit an aggressive transformed phenotype might be attributed to expression levels of the tumor proteins that are below the threshold amounts required to induce such changes.[22]

T' Proteins Interact with Key Cell Cycle Regulatory Proteins

The TAg isoforms produced by members of the Polyomavirus family, JCV T', SV40 17kT and mouse polyomavirus tiny T proteins, contain two of the three TAg transformation domains (LXCXE and J) (Fig. 1). In addition, several truncated versions of SV40 TAg constructed in vitro contain these motifs. One of these latter truncated forms, TN136, binds to Rb proteins but fails to form a stable complex with Hsc70,[50] suggesting that sequences C-terminal to the J and LXCXE domains might be essential for stable interaction with Hsc70. Riley et al[117] found that the mouse polyomavirus tiny T protein stimulates ATPase activity of Hsc70, although a direct, stable interaction between the two proteins was not reported. The SV40 17kT protein binds to and reduces the levels of p130, promotes E2F activity, and stimulates cell-cycle progression of quiescent fibroblasts.[123] Cells expressing only 17kT display a minimal transformed phenotype and the protein is underphosphorylated relative to TAg, reflecting the absence of C-terminal TAg sequences that regulate modification of the N-terminus.[124]

As discussed earlier, in vivo and in vitro studies confirm that JCV TAg interacts with cellular pRB, p107 and p130 (reviewed in ref. 119). Using an in vitro approach, Bollag et al[57] investigated the possibility that T'$_{135}$, T'$_{136}$ and T'$_{165}$ might also bind Rb family proteins. Viral proteins immunoaffinity-purified from insect cells infected with recombinant baculoviruses were mixed with extracts of human MOLT-4 cells containing pRB, p107 and p130. Each T' protein was shown to interact with the hypophosphorylated forms of the Rb proteins, and, importantly, each viral protein exhibited differential binding affinity depending on the specific interaction examined. Similar studies conducted in vivo using Rat2 cells expressing individual JCV tumor proteins revealed binding of the T' proteins to p107 and p130; the interaction between T'$_{136}$ and p107 was especially difficult to demonstrate (Bollag et al, in preparation). These experiments revealed that T' proteins not only bind to hypophosphorylated p107 and p130, but that some hyperphosphorylated species of these cellular proteins are absent in the cell lines.

Given that JCV tumor proteins interact with pRB, p107 and p130, one might predict that the five viral early proteins would also bind Hsc70 via their J domains. However, the inability to demonstrate a stable interaction between the truncated SV40 N136 peptide and this molecular chaperone raised questions about the binding potential of JCV T′ proteins. Using POJ (PHFG cells transformed with Ori defective JCV)[94] cell extracts, and a co-IP/WB assay, it was determined that at least one of the JCV early proteins bound Hsc70 (Bollag and Frisque, unpublished data). Recent experiments utilizing Rat2 cells expressing individual JCV proteins confirm that T′$_{135}$ interacts with Hsc70 (Bollag et al, in preparation).

The ability of JCV TAg and T′ proteins to bind Rb proteins and Hsc70 is expected to result in the release of E2F and the cell's progression to S phase. To address this possibility, Rat2 lines expressing individual JCV proteins were cotransfected with a β-galactosidase expression plasmid and a luciferase vector under the control of a promoter containing four E2F-1 binding sites. Luciferase data normalized to that of β-galactosidase activity indicates that the highest levels of free E2F-1 are induced in cells expressing T′$_{165}$ or all five early proteins (Tyagarajan and Frisque, in preparation). As expected, cells expressing either an LXCXE (E109K) or J (H42Q) domain mutant had relatively low levels of released E2F-1 (Table 2). Co-IP/WB experiments performed on extracts of these cells verified that the H42Q, but not the E109K, mutant proteins were capable of binding p107 and p130. Furthermore, both hypophosphorylated and hyperphosphorylated forms of p107 and p130 were detected in these cells, indicating that the mutant viral proteins fail to alter the phosphorylation states of the cellular proteins.

Summary of JCV Early Protein Function

An extensive literature details the contributions made by the SV40 multifunctional TAg and tAg to the oncogenic process. On the other hand, little is known about the17kT protein that is produced in greatly diminished amounts relative to the other SV40 early proteins. Using SV40 results as a guide, a number of studies have been conducted to examine JCV TAg functions. At the sequence level, many structural motifs (e.g., NLS, phosphorylation, zinc finger, ATP binding) and functional domains (e.g., DNA binding, transformation) have been identified that correspond to those of the SV40 TAg. Although similarities of structure and function are readily apparent, it is also clear that the JCV TAg displays less robust support of DNA replication and transformation activity in cell culture and reduced potential to interact with key cellular regulatory factors. Analyses of JCV tAg functions have only recently been initiated, and much work must be done to determine how this protein influences the transforming potential of JCV. It is expected that JCV tAg interacts with cellular proteins such as PP2A through its unique C-terminal sequences and chaperones via its J domain, thereby affecting cellular proliferation and programmed cell death. Several observations support the hypothesis that JCV T′ proteins make important contributions to the biology of the virus. Their expression is differentially regulated in permissive vs. nonpermissive cells, and they are produced at significantly elevated levels relative to their SV40 and mouse polyomavirus counterparts. In addition, T′ proteins enhance viral DNA replication and exhibit differential binding to critical cell cycle regulators. Finally, preliminary data suggest that one or more T′ proteins block apoptosis induced by JCV TAg under certain conditions. The ability to complement or antagonize activities of the multifunctional TAg may permit T′ proteins to fine-tune JCV's control over the virus-host interactions.

Acknowledgements

The authors thank Dr. Brigitte Bollag and Lisa Kilpatrick for helpful discussions. We apologize to our colleagues if we failed to cite relevant publications either because of space constraints or our own oversight. This work was supported in part by National Institutes of Health grant NS41833.

References

1. Frisque RJ, White III FA. The molecular biology of JC virus, causative agent of progressive multifocal leukoencephalopathy. In: Roos RP, ed. Molecular Neurovirology. Totowa, NJ: Humana Press; 1992:25-158.
2. Vilchez RA, Butel JS. Polyomavirus SV40 infection and lymphomas in Spain. Int J Cancer 2003; 107(3):505-506.
3. Carbone M, Bocchetta M, Cristaudo A et al. SV40 and human brain tumors. Int J Cancer 2003; 106(1):140-142.
4. Garcea RL, Imperiale MJ. Simian virus 40 infection of humans. J Virol 2003; 77(9):5039-5045.
5. Atwood WJ. Genotypes, archetypes, and tandem repeats in the molecular epidemiology and pathogenesis of JC virus induced disease. J Neurovirol 2003; 9(5):519-521.
6. Seth P, Diaz F, Major EO. Advances in the biology of JC virus and induction of progressive multifocal leukoencephalopathy. J Neurovirol 2003; 9(2):236-246.
7. Yang B, Prayson RA. Expression of Bax, Bcl-2, and p53 in progressive multifocal leukoencephalopathy. Mod Pathol 2000; 13(10):1115-1120.
8. Richardson-Burns SM, Kleinschmidt-DeMasters BK, DeBiasi RL et al. Progressive multifocal leukoencephalopathy and apoptosis of infected oligodendrocytes in the central nervous system of patients with and without AIDS. Arch Neurol 2002; 59(12):1930-1936.
9. Hirsch HH, Steiger J, Polyomavirus BK. Lancet Infect Dis 2003; 3(10):611-623.
10. Klein G, Powers A, Croce C. Association of SV40 with human tumors. Oncogene 2002; 21(8):1141-1149.
11. Vilchez RA, Madden CR, Kozinetz CA et al. Association between simian virus 40 and non-Hodgkin lymphoma. Lancet 2002; 359(9309):817-823.
12. Del Valle L, Baehring J, Lorenzana C et al. Expression of a human polyomavirus oncoprotein and tumour suppressor proteins in medulloblastomas. J Clin Pathol-Mol Pathol 2001; 54(5):331-337.
13. Laghi L, Randolph AE, Chauhan DP et al. JC virus DNA is present in the mucosa of the human colon and in colorectal cancers. Proc Natl Acad Sci USA 1999; 96:7484-7489.
14. Zambrano A, Kalantari M, Simoneau A et al. Detection of human polyomaviruses and papillomaviruses in prostatic tissue reveals the prostate as a habitat for multiple viral infections. Prostate 2002; 53(4):263-276.
15. Small JA, Scangos GA, Cork L et al. The early region of human papovavirus JC induces dysmyelination in transgenic mice. Cell 1986; 46:13-18.
16. Trapp BD, Small JA, Pulley M et al. Dysmyelination in transgenic mice containing JC virus early region. Ann Neurol 1988; 23(1):38-48.
17. Haas S, Haque NS, Beggs AH et al. Expression of the myelin basic protein gene in transgenic mice expressing human neurotropic virus, JCV, early protein. Virology 1994; 202(1):89-96.
18. Horvath CJ, Simon MA, Bergsagel DJ et al. Simian virus 40-induced disease in rhesus monkeys with simian acquired immunodeficiency syndrome. Am J Pathol 1992; 140(6):1431-1440.
19. Eddy BE, Borman GS, Berkeley WH et al. Tumors induced in hamsters by injection of rhesus monkey kidney cell extracts. Proc Soc Exp Biol Med 1961; 107:191-197.
20. Jensen PN, Major EO. Viral variant nucleotide sequences help expose leukocytic positioning in the JC virus pathway to the CNS. J Leuk Biol 1999; 65(4):428-438.
21. Bollag B, Chuke W-F, Frisque RJ. Hybrid genomes of the polyomaviruses JC virus, BK virus, and simian virus 40: Identification of sequences important for efficient transformation. J Virol 1989; 63:863-872.
22. Trowbridge PW, Frisque RJ. Analysis of G418-selected Rat2 cells containing prototype, variant, mutant, and chimeric JC-virus and SV40 genomes. Virology 1993; 196(2):458-474.
23. Safak M, Khalili K. Physical and functional interaction between viral and cellular proteins modulate JCV gene transcription. J Neurovirol 2001; 7(4):288-292.
24. Darbinyan A, Darbinian N, Safak M et al. Evidence for dysregulation of cell cycle by human polyomavirus, JCV, late auxiliary protein. Oncogene 2002; 21(36):5574-5581.
25. Barbaro BA, Sreekumar KR, Winters DR et al. Phosphorylation of simian virus 40 T antigen on Thr 124 selectively promotes double-hexamer formation on subfragments of the viral core origin. J Virol 2000; 74(18):8601-8613.
25a. Hübner S, Xiao C-Y, Jans DA. The protein kinase CK2 site (Ser111/112) enhances recognition of the simian virus 40 large T-antigen nuclear localization sequence by importin. J Biol Chem 1997; 272(27):17191-17195.
26. Prives C. The replication functions of SV40 T antigen are regulated by phosphorylation. Cell 1990; 61:735-738.

27. Fanning E. Control of SV40 DNA replication by protein phosphorylation: a model for cellular DNA replication? Trends Cell Biol 1994; 4(7):250-255.
28. Nesper J, Smith RWP, Kautz AR et al. A cell-free replication system for human polyomavirus JC DNA. J Virol 1997; 71(10):7421-7428.
29. Lynch KJ, Frisque RJ. Identification of critical elements within the JC virus DNA replication origin. J Virol 1990; 64:5812-5822.
30. Sock E, Wegner M, Grummt F. DNA replication of human polyomavirus-JC is stimulated by NF-I in vivo. Virology 1991; 182(1):298-308.
31. Sock E, Wegner M, Fortunato EA et al. Large T-antigen and sequences within the regulatory region of JC virus both contribute to the features of JC virus DNA replication. Virology 1993; 197(2):537-548.
32. Tada H, Lashgari MS, Khalili K. Regulation of JCVL promoter function: evidence that a pentanucleotide "silencer" repeat sequence AGGGAAGGGA down-regulates transcription of the JC virus late promoter. Virology 1991; 180:327-338.
33. Chang CF, Tada H, Khalili K. The role of a pentanucleotide repeat sequence, AGGGAAGGGA, in the regulation of JC virus DNA replication. Gene 1994; 148(2):309-314.
34. Chen L, Joo WS, Bullock PA et al. The N-terminal side of the origin-binding domain of simian virus 40 large T antigen is involved in A/T untwisting. J Virol 1997; 71(11):8743-8749.
35. San Martin MC, Gruss C, Carazo JM. Six molecules of SV40 large T antigen assemble in a propeller-shaped particle around a channel. J Mol Biol 1997; 268:15-20.
36. Valle M, Gruss C, Halmer L et al. Large T-antigen double hexamers imaged at the simian virus 40 origin of replication. Mol Cell Biol 2000; 20(1):34-41.
37. Ishimi Y, Sugasawa K, Hanaoka F et al. Topoisomerase-II plays an essential role as a swivelase in the late stage of SV40 chromosome replication in vitro. J Biol Chem 1992; 267(1):462-466.
38. Kim HY, Ahn BY, Cho Y. Structural basis for the inactivation of retinoblastoma tumor suppressor by SV40 large T antigen. EMBO J 2001; 20(1-2):295-304.
39. Lynch KJ, Haggerty S, Frisque RJ. DNA replication of chimeric JC virus-simian virus 40 genomes. Virology 1994; 204:819-822.
40. Smith RW, Nasheuer HP. Initiation of JC virus DNA replication in vitro by human and mouse DNA polymerase alpha-primase. Eur J Biochem 2003; 270(9):2030-2037.
41. Dornreiter I, Hoss A, Arthur AK et al. SV40 T antigen binds directly to the large subunit of purified DNA polymerase alpha. EMBO J 1990; 9:3329-3336.
42. Murakami Y, Eki T, Yamada M et al. Species-specific in vitro synthesis of DNA containing the polyoma virus origin of replication. Proc Natl Acad Sci USA 1986; 83:6347-6351.
43. Srinivasan A, McClellan AJ, Vartikar J et al. The amino-terminal transforming region of simian virus 40 large T and small t antigens functions as a J domain. Mol Cell Biol 1997; 17(8):4761-4773.
44. DeCaprio JA. The role of the J domain of SV40 large T in cellular transformation. Biologicals 1999; 27(1):23-28.
45. Sheng Q, Denis D, Ratnofsky M et al. The DnaJ domain of polyomavirus large T is required to regulate RB family tumor suppressor function. J Virol 1997; 71(12):9410-9416.
46. Zhu XY, Ohtsubo M, Bohmer RM et al. Adhesion-dependent cell cycle progression linked to the expression of cyclin D1, activation of cyclin E-cdk2, and phosphorylation of the retinoblastoma protein. J Cell Biol 1996; 133(2):391-403.
47. Sullivan CS, Cantalupo P, Pipas JM. The molecular chaperone activity of simian virus 40 large T antigen is required to disrupt Rb-E2F family complexes by an ATP-dependent mechanism. Mol Cell Biol 2000; 20(17):6233-6243.
48. Sullivan CS, Pipas JM. The virus-chaperone connection. Virology 2001; 287(1):1-8.
49. Sullivan CS, Tremblay JD, Fewell SW et al. Species-specific elements in the large T-antigen J domain are required for cellular transformation and DNA replication by simian virus 40. Mol Cell Biol 2000; 20(15):5749-5757.
50. Sullivan CS, Gilbert SP, Pipas JM. ATP-dependent simian virus 40 T-antigen-Hsc70 complex formation. J Virol 2001; 75:1601-1610.
51. Sullivan CS, Pipas JM. T antigens of simian virus 40: molecular chaperones for viral replication and tumorigenesis. Micro Mol Biol Rev 2002; 66(2):179-202.
52. Frisque RJ, Rifkin DB, Walker DL. Transformation of primary hamster brain cells with JC virus and its DNA. J Virol 1980; 35:265-269.
53. Tiemann F, Zerrahn J, Deppert W. Cooperation of simian virus 40 large and small T antigens in metabolic stabilization of tumor suppressor p53 during cellular transformation. J Virol 1995; 69(10):6115-6121.

54. Tavis JE, Trowbridge PW, Frisque RJ. Converting the JCV T antigen Rb binding domain to that of SV40 does not alter JCV's limited transforming activity but does eliminate viral viability. Virology 1994; 199:384-392.
55. Dyson N, Buchkovich K, Whyte P et al. The cellular 107K protein that binds to adenovirus E1A also associates with the large T antigens of SV40 and JC virus. Cell 1989; 58(2):249-255.
56. Dyson N, Bernards R, Friend SH et al. Large T antigens of many polyomaviruses are able to form complexes with the retinoblastoma protein. J Virol 1990; 64:1353-1356.
57. Bollag B, Prins C, Snyder EL et al. Purified JC virus T and T' proteins differentially interact with the retinoblastoma family of tumor suppressor proteins. Virology 2000; 274:165-178.
58. Howard CM, Claudio PP, De Luca A et al. Inducible pRb2/p130 expression and growth-suppressive mechanisms: evidence of a pRb2/p130, p27(Kip1), and cyclin E negative feedback regulatory loop. Cancer Res 2000; 60(10):2737-2744.
59. Chuke WF, Walker DL, Peitzman LB et al. Construction and characterization of hybrid polyomavirus genomes. J Virol 1986; 60:960-971.
60. Haggerty S, Walker DL, Frisque RJ. JC virus-simian virus 40 genomes containing heterologous regulatory signals and chimeric early regions: identification of regions restricting transformation by JC virus. J Virol 1989; 63(5):2180-2190.
61. O'Neill FJ, Frisque RJ, Xu XL et al. Immortalization of human cells by mutant and chimeric primate polyomavirus T-antigen genes. Oncogene 1995; 10(6):1131-1139.
62. Giles RH, van Es JH, Clevers H. Caught up in a Wnt storm: Wnt signaling in cancer. Biochim Biophys Acta 2003; 1653(1):1-24.
63. Kikuchi A. Tumor formation by genetic mutations in the components of the Wnt signaling pathway. Cancer Sci 2003; 94(3):225-229.
64. Gan DD, Reiss K, Carrill T et al. Involvement of Wnt signaling pathway in murine medulloblastoma induced by human neurotropic JC virus. Oncogene 2001; 20(35):4864-4870.
65. Enam S, Del Valle L, Lara C et al. Association of human polyomavirus JCV with colon cancer: Evidence for interaction of viral T-antigen and beta-catenin. Cancer Res 2002; 62(23):7093-7101.
66. Morin PJ. beta-catenin signaling and cancer. Bioessays 1999; 21(12):1021-1030.
67. Dobbie Z, Muller PY, Heinimann K et al. Expression of COX-2 and Wnt pathway genes in adenomas of familial adenomatous polyposis patients treated with meloxicam. Anticancer Res 2002; 22(4):2215-2220.
68. Del Valle L, Wang JY, Lassak A et al. Insulin-like growth factor I receptor signaling system in JC virus T antigen-induced primitive neuroectodermal tumors-medulloblastomas. J Neurovirol 2002; 8:138-147.
69. Lassak A, Del Valle L, Peruzzi F et al. Insulin receptor substrate 1 translocation to the nucleus by the human JC virus T-antigen. J Biol Chem 2002; 277(19):17231-17238.
70. Theile M, Grabowski G. Mutagenic activity of BKV and JCV in human and other mammalian cells. Arch Virol 1990; 113:221-233.
71. Ray FA, Peabody DS, Cooper JL et al. SV40 T antigen alone drives karyotype instability that precedes neoplastic transformation of human diploid fibroblasts. J Cell Biochem 1990; 42(1):13-31.
72. Neel JV, Major EO, Awa AA et al. Hypothesis: "Rogue cell"-type chromosomal damage in lymphocytes is associated with infection with the JC human polyoma virus and has implications for oncogenesis. Proc Natl Acad Sci USA 1996; 93(7):2690-2695.
73. Croul S, Otte J, Khalili K. Brain tumors and polyomaviruses. J Neurovirol 2003; 9(2):173-182.
74. Ricciardiello L, Baglioni M, Giovannini C et al. Induction of chromosomal instability in colonic cells by the human polyomavirus JC virus. Cancer Res 2003; 63(21):7256-7262.
75. Renner K, Leger H, Wegner M. The POU domain protein Tst-1 and papoviral large tumor antigen function synergistically to stimulate glia-specific gene expression of JC virus. Proc Natl Acad Sci, USA 1994; 91(14):6433-6437.
76. Gruda MC, Zabolotny JM, Xiao JH et al. Transcriptional activation by simian virus-40 large T-antigen—interactions with multiple components of the transcription complex. Mol Cell Biol 1993; 13(2):961-969.
77. Gallia GL, Safak M, Khalili K. Interaction of the single-stranded DNA-binding protein Pur alpha with the human polyomavirus JC virus early protein T-antigen. J Biol Chem 1998; 273(49):32662-32669.
78. Chen NN, Khalili K. Transcriptional regulation of human JC polyomavirus promoters by cellular proteins YB-1 and Pur α in glial cells. J Virol 1995; 69(9):5843-5848.
79. Safak M, Gallia GL, Ansari SA et al. Physical and functional interaction between the Y-box binding protein YB-1 and human polyomavirus JC virus large T antigen. J Virol 1999; 73:10146-10157.

80. Kerr D, Chang CF, Chen NC et al. Transcription of a human neurotropic virus promoter in glial cells: effect of YB-1 on expression of the JC virus late gene. J Virol 1994; 68(11):7637-7643.
81. Safak R, Gallia GL, Khalili K. Reciprocal interaction between two cellular proteins, Pur alpha and YB-1, modulates transcriptional activity of JCV(CY) in glial cells. Mol Cell Biol 1999; 19(4):2712-2723.
82. Chen NN, Chang CF, Gallia GL et al. Cooperative action of cellular proteins YB-1 and Pur alpha with the tumor antigen of the human JC polyomavirus determines their interaction with the viral lytic control element. Proc Natl Acad Sci USA 1995; 92(4):1087-1091.
83. Shaulian E, Karin M. AP-1 as a regulator of cell life and death. Nat Cell Biol 2002; 4(5):E131-136.
84. Amemiya K, Traub R, Durham L et al. Interaction of a nuclear factor-1-like protein with the regulatory region of the human polyomavirus JC virus. J Biol Chem 1989; 264(12):7025-7032.
85. Sadowska B, Barrucco R, Khalili K et al. Regulation of human polyomavirus JC virus gene transcription by AP-1 in glial cells. J Virol 2003; 77(1):665-672.
86. Kim J, Woolridge S, Biffi R et al. Members of the AP-1 family, c-Jun and c-Fos, functionally interact with JC virus early regulatory protein large T antigen. J Virol 2003; 77(9):5241-5252.
87. Carswell S, Alwine JC. Simian virus 40 agnoprotein facilitates perinuclear-nuclear localization of VP1, the major capsid protein. J Virol 1986; 60:1055-1061.
88. Ng S-C, Mertz JE, Sanden-Will S et al. Simian virus 40 maturation in cells harboring mutants deleted in the agnogene. J Biol Chem 1985; 260:1127-1132.
89. Resnick J, Shenk T. Simian virus 40 agnoprotein facilitates normal nuclear location of the major capsid polypeptide and cell to cell spread of virus. J Virol 1986; 60:1098-1106.
90. Del Valle L, Gordon J, Enam S et al. Expression of human neurotropic polyomavirus JCV late gene product agnoprotein in human medulloblastoma. J Natl Cancer Inst 2002; 94(4):267-273.
91. Safak M, Barrucco R, Darbinyan A et al. Interaction of JC virus Agno protein with T antigen modulates transcription and replication of the viral genome in glial cells. J Virol 2001; 75(3):1476-1486.
92. Safak M, Sadowska B, Barrucco R et al. Functional interaction between JC virus late regulatory agnoprotein and cellular Y-box binding transcription factor, YB-1. J Virol 2002; 76(8):3828-3838.
93. Shenk T, Carbon J, Berg P. Construction and analysis of viable deletion mutants of simian virus 40. J Virol 1976; 18:664-671.
94. Mandl C, Walker DL, Frisque RJ. Derivation and characterization of POJ cells, transformed human fetal glial cells that retain their permissivity for JC virus. J Virol 1987; 61:755-763.
95. Topp WC. Variable defectiveness for lytic growth of the dl 54/59 mutants of simian virus. J Virol 1980; 33:1208-1210.
96. Martin RG, Setlow VP, Edwards CAF et al. The roles of the simian virus 40 tumor antigens in transformation of Chinese hamster lung cells. Cell 1979; 17:635-643.
97. Frisque RJ, Rifkin DB, Topp WC. Requirement for the large T and small T proteins of SV40 in the maintenance of the transformed state. CSH Symp Quant Biol 1980; 44:325-331.
98. Sleigh MJ, Topp WC, Hanish R et al. Mutants of SV40 with an altered small t protein are reduced in their ability to transform cells. Cell 1978; 14:79-88.
99. Bikel I, Montano X, Agha ME et al. SV40 small t antigen enhances the transformation activity of limiting concentrations of SV40 large T antigen. Cell 1987; 48:321-330.
100. Porras A, Bennett J, Howe A et al. A novel simian virus 40 early-region domain mediates transactivation of the cyclin A promoter by small-t antigen and is required for transformation in small-t antigen-dependent assays. J Virol 1996; 70:6902-6908.
101. Yu J, Boyapati A, Rundell K. Critical role for SV40 small-t antigen in human cell transformation. Virology 2001; 290(2):192-198.
102. Hahn WC, Dessain SK, Brooks MW et al. Enumeration of the simian virus 40 early region elements necessary for human cell transformation. Mol Cell Biol 2002; 22(10):3562-3562.
103. Rundell K, Parakati R. The role of the SV40 ST antigen in cell growth promotion and transformation. Semin Cancer Biol 2001; 11(1):5-13.
104. Genevaux P, Lang F, Schwager F et al. Simian virus 40 T antigens and J domains: Analysis of Hsp40 cochaperone functions in Escherichia coli. J Virol 2003; 77(19):10706-10713.
105. Watanabe G, Howe A, Lee RJ et al. Induction of cyclin D1 by simian virus 40 small tumor antigen. Proc Natl Acad Sci, USA 1996; 93(23):12861-12866.
106. Rundell K. Complete interaction of cellular 56,000- and 32,000-Mr proteins with simian virus 40 small-t antigen in productively infected cells. J Virol 1987; 61:1240-1243.
107. Mungre S, Enderle K, Turk B et al. Mutations which affect the inhibition of protein phosphatase 2A by simian virus 40 small-t antigen in vitro decrease viral transformation. J Virol 1994; 68(3):1675-1681.

108. Garcia A, Cereghini S, Sontag E. Protein phosphatase 2A and phosphatidylinositol 3-kinase regulate the activity of Sp1-responsive promoters. J Biol Chem 2000; 275(13):9385-9389.
109. Yang SI, Lickteig RL, Estes R et al. Control of protein phosphatase-2A by simian virus-40 small-t antigen. Mol Cell Biol 1991; 11(4):1988-1995.
110. Yuan H, Veldman T, Rundell K et al. Simian virus 40 small tumor antigen activates AKT and telomerase and induces anchorage-independent growth of human epithelial cells. J Virol 2002; 76(21):10685-10691.
111. Gaillard S, Fahrbach KM, Parkati R et al. Overexpression of simian virus 40 small-t antigen blocks centrosome function and mitotic progression in human fibroblasts. J Virol 2001; 75(20):9799-9807.
112. Yan Y, Shay JW, Wright WE et al. Inhibition of protein phosphatase activity induces p53-dependent apoptosis in the absence of p53 transactivation. J Biol Chem 1997; 272(24):15220-15226.
113. Zerrahn J, Tiemann F, Deppert W. Simian virus 40 small t antigen activates the carboxy-terminal transforming p53-binding domain of large T antigen. J Virol 1996; 70(10):6781-6789.
114. Frisque RJ, Bream GL, Cannella MT. Human polyomavirus JC virus genome. J Virol 1984; 51:458-469.
115. Trowbridge PW, Frisque RJ. Identification of three new JC virus proteins generated by alternative splicing of the early viral mRNA. J Neurovirol 1995; 1:195-206.
116. Zerrahn J, Deppert W. Analysis of simian virus-40 small-t antigen-induced progression of rat F111 cells minimally transformed by large-T antigen. J Virol 1993; 67(3):1555-1563.
117. Riley MI, Yoo W, Mda NY et al. Tiny T antigen: an autonomous polyomavirus T antigen amino-terminal domain. J Virol 1997; 71:6068-6074.
118. Frisque RJ. Structure and function of JC virus T' proteins. J Neurovirol 2001; 7(4):293-297.
119. Frisque RJ, Bollag B, Tyagarajan SK et al. T' proteins influence JC virus biology. J Neurovirol 2003; 9 Suppl 1:15-20.
120. Swenson JJ, Frisque RJ. Biochemical characterization and localization of JC virus large T antigen phosphorylation domains. Virology 1995; 212:295-308.
121. Prins CF, Frisque RJ. JC virus T' proteins encoded by alternatively spliced early mRNAs enhance T antigen-mediated viral DNA replication in human cells. J Neurovirol 2001; 7(3):250-264.
122. Gjoerup O, Zaveri D, Roberts TM. Induction of p53-independent apoptosis by simian virus 40 small t antigen. J Virol 2001; 75(19):9142-9155.
123. Boyapati A, Wilson M, Yu J et al. SV40 17kT antigen complements dnaJ mutations in large T antigen to restore transformation of primary human fibroblasts. Virology 2003; 315(1):148-158.
124. Zerrahn J, Knippschild U, Winkler T et al. Independent expression of the transforming amino-terminal domain of SV40 large T-antigen from an alternatively spliced third SV40 early messenger RNA. EMBO J 1993; 12(12):4739-4746.

CHAPTER 22

Polyomavirus in Human Cancer Development

Winston Lee and Erik Langhoff

Abstract

In animal studies, polyoma viruses have been found to be viral agents for oncogenesis and to produce a wide range of pathological lesions in experimental animals, including a variety of neoplastic tumors. The human polyoma viruses (JCV and BKV), along with their simian cousin (SV40), are ubiquitous viruses that are primarily associated with progressive multifocal leukoencephalopathy (PML) and hemorrhagic cystitis, respectively, under specific conditions in immunocompromised individuals. Currently, polyoma viruses are now undergoing increasing scrutiny as possible causes for several human cancers. Evidence has been mounting recently that JCV, BKV as well as SV40 are potential oncogenic viruses in humans as well.

Viral Life Cycle

The molecular structure polyomavirus and its receptors have been described in great detail in several chapters and can be found elsewhere in the book. The exact mechanism in which the virus enters the host cell is not clearly defined at this time. It is known that one of the structural capsid proteins (VP1) binds to sialic acid, which is an important component of many cell receptors.[1] It is theorized that the virus uses a class of sialoglycoproteins as a conduit for cell entry. These proteins are abundantly expressed on cell surfaces. Murine polyoma virus has been shown to replicate in at least 40 different cell types in various studies.[2] Once inside the cell, it is probable that the entire particle moves into the nucleus via a nuclear pore. In the nucleus, the virus expresses "early" proteins (mainly the Large T antigen) which accumulate and recruit host DNA polymerase to the viral DNA origin. Thus the host enzymes are utilized to replicate viral DNA and produce the structural proteins. New viral particles are then formed and leave the cell by an unknown mechanism (Table 1).

Tissue tropism of polyoma viruses is determined by their enhancer regions. These regions regulate replication, and contain binding sites for multiple transcription factors which may be tissue specific. For example, Purα is a transcription factor which interacts with the enhancer region for JCV; Purα DNA-binding is only found in brain tissues.[3] Polyoma viruses are classified as archetypal or rearranged, based upon the structure of the transcriptional control region. Archetypal virus contains a single copy of the promoter and enhancer, while rearranged strains have significant variation in this region.[4,5] This may help to explain the variability of viral replication and virulence found in different strains. Rearranged virus will often have duplication of the enhancer region, which promotes viral growth. Despite this, both archetypal and rearranged strains are found in normal and diseased human tissues[6,7] and there is no known association between viral DNA structure and disease. It is probable that host factors contribute a great deal in this regard. Another possibility is that inefficient replication of archetypal virus may not elicit a strong immune response and thus create a low level persistent infection.

Polyomaviruses and Human Diseases, edited by Nasimul Ahsan. ©2006 Eurekah.com and Springer Science+Business Media.

Table 1. Components encoded by polyomavirus DNA

Structural Proteins	Function
VP1	Major structural protein thought to be a mechanism of entry into the cell.
VP2	The gene is highly conserved.
VP3	

Functional Proteins	Function
Agnoprotein	May modify Large T antigen function in JCV
Large T antigen	Share ~70% amino acid indentity between 3 viruses.
	Primary agent in cell transformation.
Small T antigen	Studied mainly in SV40
	Complementary role in cell transformation
17kT″	Found experimentally in SV40- relevance unknown
T′$_{125}$, T′$_{126}$, T′$_{165}$	Defined in JCV as products of further processing of viral transcripts-may complement or modulate Large T antigen function
T′ in BKV	Described in BKV, but relevance not fully defined

Adapted from Graft: 5, 574, 2002.

Mechanisms of Oncogenesis

The virus' T antigens, large T (LT) and small T (ST), mediate the oncogenic potential of these organisms (Table 2). The large T antigen is thought to be the primary agent in transforming cells, via three domains. Two of these regions alter the pRb (retinoblastoma susceptibility) related tumor suppressor proteins, which normally binds to transcription factor E2F. Free E2F activates transcription of genes involved in DNA synthesis, while binding of E2F by pRb represses these genes. Phosphorylation of pRb releases E2F, and leads to progression of the cell cycle and growth.[8-10] The LT of BK virus binds to the unphosphorylated form of pRb, and causes the release of E2F[11] The J domain of LT is located near the N terminal and also affects pRb by mediating degradation of pRb complexes by an independent mechanism. The N terminus contains another domain which binds to these pRb complexes.[11-13] A region of LT has the ability to bind p53,[14] whose normal function is to detect DNA damage in the cell and

Table 2. Mechanisms of cell transformation

Antigen	Function	Outcome
Large T	Binds pRb family proteins via LXCXE	Increase in cell proliferation
Large T	Binds hsc70 molecular chaperone protein affecting degradation of pRb family proteins via J domain	Increase in cell proliferation
Large T	Binds p53 tumor suppressor proteins	Blockade of apoptosis
Large T	Damages chromosomes in unknown manner	Increase in mutations
Small T	Binds PP2a affecting the cell cycle	Increase in cell proliferation under certain conditions

Adapted from Graft: 5, 574, 2002.

either pause the cell cycle or to activate an apoptotic program. Aside from these pathways, there is evidence that LT can alter the human chromosome in other unspecified ways (Table 2).[15]

There is some variability in the function of the large T antigen across different polyoma viruses. SV40 LT reaches higher concentrations compared to BKV, thus the binding of the pRb sites is more prominent in SV40, while BKV affects this system mainly via the J domain.[13] JCV LT has not been extensively studied, but it is believed to function in a similar manner.

The small T antigen (ST) has a homolgous N terminus when compared with LT, but it has a unique C-terminal end. ST is known to bind and inhibit cellular protein phosphatase 2A,[16] which regulates signal transduction pathways. ST plays a complementary role in cell transformation. Animal studies have shown that cells that are infected with SV40 strains that produce ST are more easily transformed and produce a wider range of tumors when compared to cells infected with ST deficient mutants.[17,18] It has been suggested that ST may help transform cells during times of stress, such as nutrient starvation, which would normally suppress proliferation.[19] ST has primarily been studied in SV40, but sequence homology with JCV and BKV may infer a similar mechanism of action.

There are other, smaller forms of the T antigens that arise from alternative splicing and share identity with LT. These proteins have been studied in JCV and designated T'. These T' proteins share the amino terminus with LT; the J domain and the LXCXE domain are preserved and have been shown to contribute to JCV replication.[20] There is some evidence that T' proteins may function in JCV similarly to ST in SV40. These smaller protein products have also been found in BKV infected cells,[14] but as of yet have not been further characterized (Table 3).

Evidence of Polyoma-Cancer Association

BK Virus

BKV can remain latent in a variety of tissues- the most commonly reported are kidney and brain. Evidence of BKV has also been found in leukocytes, lung, liver, bone and reproductive tissue.[21-24] The virus can be the cause of primary or reactivation disease in many sites, including brain, liver, eye, lung and kidney. There have been several strains of BK virus isolated, which may represent geographic differences as well as differences in virulence and transforming potential.

With advancements in technology, the ability to detect viral DNA in tumor specimens has become more precise over the last two decades This may in part account for discrepancies between reports of BKV in tumors from previous studies. BKV DNA has been isolated from many different types of human tumors, both integrated into the genome and episomally. Sites include bone, pancreatic islet cells, kidney, urinary tract and a wide variety of brain tissues.[23,25-31] Some of the larger studies show data as follows: BKV has been detected episomally in 4/9 tumors of pancreatic islet cells and 19/74 brain tumors via Southern blot.[28] Further work with PCR on a large group of tumor cells as well as normal tissue demonstrated BKV early DNA encoding LT in 58/68 of brain tumors, 21/27 osteosarcomas, and 5/13 Ewing's tumors. The same sequences were found in 13/13 of normal brain tissue, 2/5 normal bone tissue and 25/35 peripheral blood cells.[23] RT-PCR showed that most of these samples also expressed LT mRNA as well. A study of 18 cases of neuroblastoma showed that all 18 contained BKV DNA and 16/18 expressed LT- compared to none in the controls (adrenal medulla). These samples were further studied with immunoprecipitation to demonstrate LT binding with p53.[22] In Italy a strain of BKV designated URO1 was identified in the examination of several types of urinary tract tissues.[27] The prevalence of viral DNA was similar between neoplastic [31/52] and non-neoplastic [21/37] samples. However, BKV DNA sequences were present in sufficient amounts to be detected by Southern blot in a portion of urinary tract tumors while not in that of normals. The DNA material appeared to be integrated into the host cell genome.

The causal link between BK virus and cancer has not been established. The finding of BKV DNA in tumor specimens has not been reproduced in other studies.[32,33]

Table 3. Evidence of BKV in human tumors and tumor cell lines

Site	Evidence	Method	Reference
CNS			
Neuroblastoma	18/18 + DNA	PCR	26
	16/18 + LT	Immunohistochemistry	26
	4/5 + DNA	PCR	24
	2/6 + DNA	Southern blot	25
Astrocytoma	7/7 + DNA	PCR	24
	2/11 + DNA	Southern blot	28
Papilloma	6/6 + DNA	PCR	24
Ependymoma	10/11 + DNA	PCR	24
	1/3 + DNA	Southern blot	28
	2/3 + DNA	Southern blot	25
Glioblastoma	19/22 + DNA	PCR	24
	4/4 + LT mRNA	RT-PCR	24
	9/18 + DNA	Southern blot	28
	1/10 + DNA	Southern blot	25
	1/5 + DNA	Southern blot	31
Meningioma	5/8 + DNA	PCR	24
	1/1 + LT mRNA	RT-PCR	24
	2/20 + DNA	Southern blot	28
	2/2 + DNA	Southern blot	25
	5/6 + DNA	Southern blot	31
Oligodendroglioma	5/7 + DNA	PCR	24
	1/1 + DNA	Southern blot	28
	1/1 + DNA	Southern blot	31
Spongioblastoma	2/2 + DNA	PCR	24
	1/3 + DNA	Southern blot	28
Bone			
Giant Cell	5/5 + DNA	PCR	24
Ewing's tumor	5/13 + DNA	PCR	24
	5/5 + LT mRNA	RT-PCR	24
	1/5 + DNA	Southern blot	25
Osteosarcoma	21/27 + DNA	PCR	24
	9/14 + LT mRNA	RT-PCR	24
Kidney/Urinary tract			
Carcinomas	31/52 + DNA	PCR	27
	1/1 + DNA	Southern blot	29
Insulinoma	1/1 + DNA	Southern blot	30
	4/9 + DNA	Southern blot	28
CNS			
Medulloblastoma	22/23 + DNA	PCR	41
	4/16 + LT	Immunohistochemistry	41
	17/20 + DNA	PCR	42
	9/20 + LT	Immunohistochemistry	42
	11/20 + agnoprotein	Immunohistochemistry	42
Astrocytoma	26/25 + DNA	PCR	44
	14/30 + LT	Immunohistochemistry	44
Ependymoma/sub-ependymoma	5/6 + DNA	PCR	44
	5/6 + LT	Immunohistochemistry	44

continued on next page

Table 3. Continued

Site	Evidence	Method	Reference
CNS			
Glioblastoma/glio	13/22 + DNA	PCR	44
sarcoma	6/27 + LT	Immunohistochemistry	44
Oligodendroglioma	4/7 + DNA	PCR	44
	2/10 + LT	Immunohistochemistry	44
Meningioma	1/131 + DNA	PCR	43
Colon	12/46 + DNA (normal/cancer matched pairs)	PCR	34
	34/54 + DNA (normal/cancer matched pairs)	PCR with topoisomerase	34

Adapted from Graft: 5, 574, 2002.

JC Virus

JCV commonly resides in the kidney and may also be found in lymphoid tissue and gastrointestinal tissue.[34,35] Primary infection is generally asymptomatic. Reactivation of disease in immunosupressed hosts is thought to be the cause of progressive multifocal leukoencephalopathy, Most of the evidence for the oncogenic potential of JCV has been in experimental models: brain tumors in owl monkeys and Golden Syrian hamsters.[36,37] Several years ago, case reports began appearing of JCV DNA detected in brain tumors.[38-40] Recently, there have been more reports linking the virus with cases of human medulloblastoma as well as other brain tumors. In 1999, 23 cases of pediatric medulloblastomas were evaluated for evidence of JCV;[41] 20/23 were positive for DNA encoding the N-terminal region of LT, 13/23 contained C-terminal sequences and 20/23 had VP-1 sequences. 11/23 had all three sequences present. Further analysis showed that 4/16 available samples had detectable T antigen by immunohistochemistry. SV40 DNA was also detected in 5/23 of these samples-BKV DNA was not found. Other experiments have looked for late JCV gene products (agnoprotein) in 20 medulloblastoma specimens.[42] The function of agnoprotein is not clear at this time, but there is some evidence that it may have a complementary role in replication of the viral genome.[43] DNA sequences for LT were found in 13/20 specimens and sequences for agnoprotein in 11/16 specimens. Immunohistochemistry revealed LT in 9/20 and agnoprotein in 11/20. When different varieties of brain tumors were analyzed (including oligodendroglioma, astrocytoma, glioblastoma, gliosarcoma, ependymoma, and subependymoma-a total of 85 specimens) all types of brain tumors showed evidence of early JCV DNA sequences- ranging from 57% to 83%.[44] T antigen was also found in all the varieties of tumors except anaplastic astrocytoma, to a lesser extent. None of the samples showed immunohistochemical evidence of VP-1. JC virus has also been associated with nonneurologic disease. Studies of colorectal cancer and matched normals found 12/46 samples contained JCV DNA.[34].When another 25 pairs were analyzed after treatment with topoisomerase, 48/54 samples tested positive for JCV by PCR. Viral DNA sequences were also detected in a human colorectal cancer cell line and in colon cancer xenografts. Data from this study also suggests that JCV DNA is present at 10 times higher numbers in cancerous tissue compared to the paired normal tissue.

SV40 Virus

While similar to JCV and BKV, SV40 is not a human polyoma virus. In its natural hosts, SV40 is transmitted via urine, respiratory, oral and subcutaneous routes.[45] It has been estimated that millions of people in the US were exposed to SV40 via contaminated virus vaccines (mainly polio) from 1955 to 1963. These vaccines were prepared from infected rhesus monkey kidney cells. However, surveillance over the next 20 years failed to show any increase in the incidence of disease or cancer in this population.[46] Recently, there has been some evidence which may link SV40 with human tumors; this has led to the questioning of the initial conclusions regarding the safety of the tainted vaccines.[47] Evidence of SV40 antibodies have been found in a significant number of individuals too young to have received contaminated vaccines.[48] Considering that there are no known intermediate reservoirs or vectors, SV40 likely has a route of human to human transmission. Alternative explanations are that SV40 has been a low level human pathogen all along, or that there is some cross reactivity with other polyoma virus antibodies. There is in vitro evidence that SV40 can replicate in human cells and SV40 DNA sequences have been detected in normal human tissue.[49,50]

SV40 DNA has been reported in numerous human tumors, mainly mesotheliomas, brain and bone tumors. A large focus of study has been the association of SV40 and malignant mesothelioma. Several investigators have found evidence of the virus in this cancer; prevalence ranges from 40-50% in some areas.[51-54] Viral components have been detected with microdissection of tumor tissue[53] and with in situ hybridization.[52] There has also been some evidence that presence of SV40 may have a negative impact on prognosis in mesothelioma.[55] There is geographic variability in these findings; SV40 DNA was not found in mesothelioma samples from Finland or Turkey.[56,57] Contaminated polio vaccines were not distributed in these countries. Despite these data, the relationship between SV40 infection and mesothelioma is not defined and some investigators believe it is premature to link the two.[58] A multicenter study formed specifically to address these issues did find evidence of SV40 in 83% of samples.[54]

Studies have shown SV40 LT DNA in approximately 30% of bone tumors including osteosarcoma, giant cell tumors and various others.[59-61] One report found as high as 46% of osteosarcomas had viral sequences.[61] Various central nervous system tumors have also shown evidence of viral gene sequences, although at lower levels and with much variability.[33,41,62-65] One of these studies demonstrated LT binding with both pRb and p53.[62]

New studies have examined the correlation of this virus with nonHodgkins lymphoma. Two separate studies found that 43% of NHL patients had SV40 (compared to none in cancer and noncancer controls).[66,67] The sequences were found most commonly in B cell and follicular variants of the disease. EBV was also detected at a significantly lower level, and the association occurred in both HIV positive and negative patients.

Conclusion

In this chapter, we have reviewed the data which link the poylomaviruses with human cancer. As with most epidemiologic data, it is very difficult to establish a causal link between these organisms and human cancer. The viruses are ubiquitous and primary infection is mild; it is often impossible to determine length of infection. The incubation period after initial exposure is very long and cancers produced are very rare. There are likely to be many other environmental and host factors which play a role in the production of tumor. Studies to this point have demonstrated the presence of these viruses in human tumors, and while there is a theoretical basis for cell transformation secondary to viral infection, it is premature to state that these viruses cause cancer. Nevertheless, data is accumulating which point to an association of these viruses (especially SV40) and a role in oncogenesis.

References

1. Chen MH, Benjamin TL. Roles of N-glycans with α2,6 as well as α2,3-linked sialic acid in infection of polyoma virus. Virology 1997; 233:440-442.
2. Benjamin TL. Polyoma Virues: Old findings and new challenges. Virology 2001; 289:167-173.
3. Imperiale MJ. The human polyomaviruses, BKV and JCV: Molecular pathogenesis of acute disease and potential role in cancer. Virology 2000; 267:1-7.
4. Yogo Y, Kitamura T, Sugimoto C et al. Isolation of a possible archetypal JC virus DNA sequence from nonimmunocompromised individuals. J Virol 1990; 64:3139-3143.

5. Rubinstein R, Harley EH. BK virus DNA cloned directly from human urine confirms an archetypal structure for the transcriptional control region. Virus Genes 1989; 2:157-165.
6. Tominaga T, Yogo Y, Kitamura T et al. Persistence of archetypal JC virus DNA in normal renal tissue derived from tumor-bearing patients. Virology 1992; 186:736-741.
7. Sugimoto C, Kitamura T, Guo J et al. Typing of urinary JC virus DNA offers a novel means of tracing human migrations. Proc Natl Acad Sci USA 1997; 94:9191-9196.
8. Cole CN. Polyomavirinae: The viruses and their replication. In: Fields BN, Knipe DM, Holwey PM, Chanock RM, Melnick JL, Monath TP et al, eds. Fields Virology. 3rd ed. Philadelphia: Lippincott-Raven, 1996; 2:1997-2025.
9. Conzen SD, Cole CN. The transforming proteins of simian virus 40. Semin Virol 1994; 5:349-356.
10. Dyson N, Bernards R, Friend SH et al. Large T antigens of many polyomaviruses are able to form complexes with the retinoblastoma protein. J Virol 1990; 64:1353-1356.
11. Studbal H, Zalvide J, Campbell KS et al. Inactivation of pRB-related proteins p130 and p107 mediated by the J domain of simian virus 40 large T antigen. Mol Cell Biol 1997; 17:4979-4990.
12. Zalvide J, Stubdal H, Decaprio JA. The J domain of simian virus 40 large T antigen is required to functionally inactivate RB family proteins. Mol Cell Biol 1998; 18:1408-1415.
13. Harris KF, Christensen JB, Radany EH et al. Novel mechanisms of E2F induction by BK virus large T antigen: Requirement of both the pRb binding and J domains. Mol Cell Biol 1998; 18:1746-1756.
14. Bollag B, Chucke WF, Frisque RJ. Hybrid genomes of the polyomaviruses JC virus, BK virus and simian virus 40: Identification of sequences important for efficient transformation. J Virol 1989; 63:863-872.
15. Trabanelli C, Corallini A, Gruppioni R et al. Chromosomal aberrations induced by BK virus T antigen in human fibroblasts. Virology 1998; 243:492-496.
16. Pallas DC, Sharik LK, Martin BL et al. Polyoma small and middle T antigens and SV40 small T antigen form stable complexes with protein phosphatase 2A. Cell 1990; 60:167-176.
17. Choi YW, Lee IC, Ross SR. Requirement for the simian virus 40 small tumor antigen in tumorigenesis in transgenic mice. Mol Cell Biol 1988; 8:3382-3390.
18. Rubin H, Figge J, Bladon MT et al. Role of small t antigen in the acute transforming activity of SV40. Cell 1982; 30:469-480.
19. Hahn WC, Dessain SK, Brooks MW et al. Enumeration of the simian virus 40 early region elements necessary for human cell transformation. Mol Cell Biol 2002; 22:2111-2123.
20. Frisque RJ. Structure and function of JC virus T' proteins. J Neurovirol 2001; 7:293-297.
21. Monini P, Rotola A, De Lellis L et al. Latent BK virus infection and Kaposi's sarcoma pathogenesis. Int J Cancer 1996; 66:717-722.
22. Dorries K. Molecular biology and pathogenesis of human polyomavirus infections. Dev Biol Stand 1998; 94:71-79.
23. De Mattei M, Martini F, Corallini A et al. High incidence of BK virus large-T-antigen-coding sequences in normal human tissues and tumors of different histotypes. Int J Cancer 1995; 61:756-760.
24. Dorries K, Vogel E, Gunther S et al. Infection of human polyomaviruses JC and BK in peripheral blood leukocytes from immunocompetent individuals. Virology 1994; 198:59-70.
25. Negrini M, Rimessi P, Mantovani C et al. Characterization of BK virus variants rescued from human tumours and tumour cell lines. J Gen Virol 1990; 71:2731-2736.
26. Flaegstad T, Andresen PA, Johnsen JI et al. A possible contributory role of BK virus infection in neuroblastoma development. Cancer Res 1999; 59:1160-1163.
27. Monini P, Rotola A, Di Luca D et al. DNA rearrangements imapiring BK virus productive infection in urinary tract tumors. Virology 1995; 214:273-279.
28. Corallini A, Pagnani M, Viadana P et al. Association of BK virus with human brain tumors and tumors of pancreatic islets. Int J Cancer 1987; 39:60-67.
29. Knepper JE, diMayorca G. Cloning and characterization of BK virus-related DNA sequences from normal and neoplastic human tissues. J Med Virol 1987; 21:289-299.
30. Caputo A, Corallini A, Grossi MP et al. Episomal DNA of a BK virus variant in a human insulinoma. J Med Virol 1983; 12:37-49.
31. Dorries K, Loeber G, Meixensberger J. Association of polyomaviruses JC, SV40, and BK with human brain tumors. Virology 1987; 160:268-270.
32. Arthur RR, Grossman SA, Ronnett BM et al. Lack of association of human polyomaviruses with human brain tumors. J Neurooncol 1994; 20:55-58.
33. Weggen S, Bayer TA, von Deimling A et al. Low frequency of SV40, JC and BK polyomavirus sequences in human medulloblastomas, meningiomas and ependymomas. Brain Pathol 2000; 10:85-92.

34. Laghi L, Randolph AE, Chauhan DP et al. JC virus DNA is present in the mucosa of the human colon and in colorectal cancers. Proc Natl Acad Sci USA 1999; 96:7484-7489.

35. Monaco MC, Atwwod WJ, Gravell M et al. JC virus infection of hematopoietic progenitor cells, primary B lymphocytes, andtonsillar stromal cells: Implications for virus latency. J Virol 1996; 70:7004-7012.

36. London WT, Houff SA, Madden DL et al. Brain tumors in owl monkeys inoculated with a human polyomavirus (JCV). Science 1978; 201:1246-1249.

37. Walker DL, Padgett BL, ZuRhein GM et al. Human papovavirus (JC): Induction of brain tumors in hamsters. Science 1973; 181:674-676.

38. Gallia Gl, Gordon J, Khalili K. Tumor pathogenesis of human neurotropic JC virus in the CNS. J Neurovirol 1998; 4:175-181.

39. Rencic A, Gordon J, Otte J et al. Detection of JCV DNA sequence and expression of the viral oncogene, T-antigen, in the brain of patient with oligoastrocytoma. Proc Natl Acad Sci USA 1996; 93:7352-7357.

40. Boldorini R, Caldarelli-Stefano R, Monga G et al. PCR detection of JC virus DNA in the brain tissue of a 9-year-old child with pleomorphic xanthoastrocytoma. J Neurovirol 1998; 2:242-245.

41. Krynska B, Del Valle L, Croul S et al. Detection of human neurotropic JC virus and DNA sequence and expression of the viral oncogene protein in pediatric medulloblastomas. Proc Natl Acad Sci USA 1999; 96:11519-11524.

42. Del Valle L, Gordon J, Enam S et al. Expression of human neurotropic polyomavirus JCV late gene product agnoprotein in human medulloblastoma. J Natl Cancer Inst 2002; 94:267-273.

43. Safak M, Barrucco R, Darbinyan A et al. Interaction of JC virus agno protein with T antigen modulates transcription and replication of the viral genome in glial cells. J Virol 2001; 75:1476-1486.

44. Del Valle L, Gordon J, Assimakopoulou M et al. Detection of JC virus DNA sequences and expression of the viral regulatory protein T-antigen in tumors of the central nervous system. Cancer Res 2001; 61:4287-4293.

45. Shah K, Nathanson N. Human exposure to SV40: Review and comment. Am J Epidemiol 1976; 103:1-12.

46. Mortimer EA, Lepow ML, Gold E et al. Long-term follow-up of person inadvertently inoculated with SV40 a neonates. N Engl J Med 1981; 305:1517-1518.

47. Fisher SG, Weber L, Carbone M. Cancer risk associated with simian virus 40 contaminated polio vaccine. Anticancer Res 1999; 19:2173-2180.

48. Jafar S, Rodriguez-Barradas M, Graham DY et al. Serological evidence of SV40 infectionsin HIV-infected and HIV-negative adults. J Med Virol 1998; 54:276-284.

49. Martini F, Iaccheri L, Lazzarin L et al. SV40 early region and large T antigen in human brain tumors, peripheral blood cells, and sperm fluids from healthy individuals. Cancer Res 1996; 56:4820-4825.

50. Shein HM, Enders JF. Multiplication and cytopahtogenicity of simian vacuolating virus 40 in cultures of human tissues. Proc Soc Exp Biol Med 1962; 109:495-500.

51. Klein G, Powers A, Croce C. Association of SV40 with human tumors. Oncogene 2002; 21:1141-1149.

52. Ramael M, Nagels J, Heylen H et al. Detection of SV40 like viral DNA and viral antigens in malignant pleural mesothelioma. Eur Respir J 1999; 14:1381-1386.

53. Shivaprukar N, Wiethege T, Wistub II et al. Presence of simian virus 40 sequences in malignant mesotheliomas and mesothlial cell proliferations. J Cell Biochem 1999; 76:181-188.

54. Testa JR, Carbone M, Hirvonen A et al. A multi-institutional study confirms the presence and expression of simian virus 40 in human malignant mesotheliomas. Cancer Res 1998; 58:4505-4509.

55. Procopio A, Strizzi L, Vianale G et al. Simian virus-40 sequences are a negative prognostic cofactor in patients with malignant pleural mesothlioma. Genes Chrom Cancer 2000; 2:173-179.

56. Emri S, Kocagoz T, Olut A et al. Simian virus 40 is not a cofactor in the pathogenesis of environmentally induced malignant pleual mesothelioma in Turkey. Anticancer Res 2000; 55:110-113.

57. Hirvonen A, Mattson K, Karjalainen A et al. Simina virus 40 (SV40)-like DNA sequences not detectable in Finnish mesothelioma patients not exposed to SV40-contaminated polio vaccines. Mol Carcinog 1999; 26:93-99.

58. Shah K. Does SV40 infection contribute to the development of human cancers? Rev Med Virol 2000; 10:31-43.

59. Carbone M, Rizzo P, Procopio A et al. SV40-like sequences in human bone tumors. Oncogene 1996; 13:527-535.

60. Gamberi G, Benassi MS, Pompetti F et al. Presence and expression of the simian virus-40 genome in human giant cell tumors. Genes Chromosome Cancer 2000; 28:23-30.

61. Yamamoto H, Nakayama T, Murakami H et al. High incidence of SV40-like sequences detection in tumor and peripheral blood cells of Japanese osteosarcoma patients. Br J Cancer 2000; 82:1677-1681.

62. Zhen HN, Zhang X, Bu XY et al. Expression of the simian virus 40 large tumor antigen (Tag) and formation of Tag-p53 and Tag-pRb complexes in human brain tumors. Cancer 1999; 86:2124-2132.

63. Bergsagel DJ, Finegold MJ, Butel JS et al. DNA sequences similar to simian virus 40 in ependymomas and choroids plexus tumors of childhood. N Engl J Med 1992; 326:988-993.

64. Lednicky JA, Garcea RL, Bergsagel DJ et al. Natural simian virus 40 strains are present in human choroids plexus and ependymoma tumors. Virology 1995; 212:710-717.

65. Huang H, Reis R, Yonekawa Y et al. Identification in human brain tumors of DNA sequences specific for SV40 large T antigen. Brain Pathol 1999; 9:43-44.

66. Vilchez RA, Madden CR, Kozinetz CA et al. Association between simian virus 40 and nonHodgkin lymphoma. Lancet 2002; 359:817-823

67. Shivapurkar N, Harada K, Reddy J et al. Presence of simian virus 40 DNA sequences in human lymphomas. Lancet 2002; 359:851-852.

BK Virus, JC Virus and Simian Virus 40 Infection in Humans, and Association with Human Tumors

Giuseppe Barbanti-Brodano, Silvia Sabbioni, Fernanda Martini,
Massimo Negrini, Alfredo Corallini and Mauro Tognon

Abstract

BK virus (BKV), JC virus (JCV) and Simian Virus 40 (SV40) are polyomaviruses, highly homologous at the DNA and protein levels. While the human polyomaviruses BKV and JCV are ubiquitous in humans, SV40 is a simian virus which was introduced in the human population, between 1955 and 1963, by contaminated poliovaccines produced in SV40-infected monkey cells. Alternatively, SV40 or an SV40-like virus may have entered the human population before anti-poliovirus vaccination. Epidemiological evidence suggests that SV40 is now contagiously transmitted in the human population by horizontal infection, independently from the earlier contaminated poliovaccines. All three polyomaviruses transform rodent and human cells and are oncogenic in rodents. JCV induces tumors also in experimentally inoculated monkeys. Transformation and oncogenicity induced by BKV, JCV and SV40 are due to the two viral oncoproteins, the large T antigen (Tag) and the small t antigen (tag), encoded in the early region of the viral genome. Both proteins display several functions. The large Tag acts mainly by blocking the functions of p53 and pRB family tumor suppressor proteins and by inducing in host cells chromosomal aberrations and instability. The principal effect of small tag is to bind the catalytic and regulatory subunits of the protein phosphatase PP2A, thereby constitutively activating the β-catenin pathway which drives cells into proliferation. All three polyomaviruses are associated with specific human tumor types which correspond to the tumors induced by experimental inoculation of the three viruses in rodents and to the neoplasms arising in mice transgenic for the polyomavirus early region gene directed by the native viral early promoter-enhancer. Human tumors associated with BKV, JCV and SV40 contain viral DNA, generally episomic, express viral RNA and are positive for large Tag by immunohistochemistry. The low copy number of viral genomes in human tumors suggests that polyomaviruses may transform human cells by a "hit and run" mechanism. An autocrine-paracrine effect, involving secretion of growth factors by cells expressing polyomavirus Tag, may be responsible for recruiting to proliferation Tag-negative cells in polyomavirus-associated human tumors.

Introduction

The human polyomaviruses BK virus (BKV) and JC virus (JCV) as well as Simian Virus 40 (SV40) belong to the family *Polyomavirinae*. Both BKV and JCV have been associated with human tumors.[1-5] The recent evidence that SV40 may be a cofactor in the etiology of specific

---

Polyomaviruses and Human Diseases, edited by Nasimul Ahsan. ©2006 Eurekah.com
and Springer Science+Business Media.

human tumor types[6,7] has raised again the interest on the two human polyomaviruses as possible agents involved in human oncogenesis. In this chapter we will consider the general properties of BKV and JCV, the characteristics of the latent infection and of the ubiquitous state of these viruses in humans, their transforming capacity in vitro and oncogenicity for experimental animals, and we will critically evaluate their possible etiologic role in human tumors. We will also examine the peculiar situation of SV40 which is not a natural human virus and has been introduced recently in the human population where it seems to exert pathologic effects.

General Characteristics of BKV, JCV and SV40

The three polyomaviruses BKV, JCV and SV40 code for six viral proteins. Two early nonstructural proteins, the large tumor antigen (Tag) and the small tumor antigen (tag) are expressed before replication of the viral DNA. Four late proteins are produced after replication of the viral genome: the agnoprotein, probably involved in processing of late mRNAs and assembly of viral particles, and three capsid proteins, VP1, which is the major structural protein, VP2 and VP3.[1-11] In these viruses, the early and late genes are transcribed on different DNA strands of the circular viral genome, in a way that the transcription proceeds divergently from the transcriptional regulatory region. The three viruses show a great sequence homology. Considering the entire viral genome, the DNA sequence identity is 72% between BKV and JCV, 69% between BKV and SV40 and 68% between JCV and SV40.[1,10,11] The amino acid homology in the early region, that is in tumor antigens, is 88% between BKV and JCV, 81% between BKV and SV40 and 79% between JCV and SV40, whereas in the late region, that is in structural proteins, the homology is 86% between BKV and JCV, 85% between BKV and SV40 and 82% between JCV and SV40.[1,10,11] A low homology is detected in the regulatory region of the three polyomaviruses. This probably reflects adaptation to in vitro cell culture and most laboratory strains may have evolved from a common natural archetype.[11,12] However, the analysis of independent isolates by either direct cloning or sequencing of products obtained by polymerase chain reaction (PCR) amplification shows that different arrangements of the regulatory region are often detected in vivo.[13,14] Selection of variants with a particular cell specificity or transformation potential was proposed as a possible outcome of such variability.[12,13,15]

BKV, JCV and SV40 Infection in Humans

BKV and JCV are ubiquitous and infect a large proportion of humans all over the world, except for some segregated populations living in remote regions of Brasil, Paraguay and Malaysia.[16] Early seroepidemiological surveys showed that seroconversion to both BKV and JCV is significantly related to age.[17-21] BKV primary infection occurs in childhood. At 3 years of age BKV antibodies are detected in 50% of children, and almost all individuals are infected by the age of 10 years.[17-19] JCV primary infection occurs later. Seroconversion to JCV is observed at highest rates during adolescence and continues at lower frequency until the age of 60 years, when 50 to 75% of adults show serum antibodies against JCV.[20,21] Recent seroepidemiological data confirm that the age-specific seroprevalence is different for BKV and JCV. BKV seroprevalence reaches 91 to 98% at 5-9 years of age, remains stable at these values until the age of 30 years and then declines to 68% by age 60-69 years.[22,23] JCV seroprevalence is only 14% by age 5-9 years and raises slowly to 50-70% by age 60-69 years.[22,23] The overall rates of seropositivity for BKV and JCV, throughout all the age groups from 1 to 69 years, are 81% and 35%, respectively.[22] Thus, JCV seems to diffuse more slowly than BKV in humans, perhaps reflecting a different mechanism of transmission or a lower permissiveness of human cells to JCV infection. The age of SV40 primary infection is not known. It may be variable if different mechanisms and routes of SV40 infection exist in humans. The antigenic cross-reaction of SV40 with the two human polyomaviruses BKV and JCV has been so far the most difficult problem to study, by seroepidemiological surveys, the real diffusion of SV40 infection in humans. By virus neutralization and ELISA tests, a low number (1.3 to 16.4%) of normal human sera showed antibodies to SV40,[6,7] suggesting a limited virus circulation in the human population.

Carter et al,[24] using recombinant SV40 VP1 virus-like particles (VLPs) as antigens in an ELISA test, while detecting a percentage of SV40-positive human sera (6.6%) comparable to previous studies,[6,7] observed disappearance of SV40 antibodies after serum pre-adsorption with BKV and JCV VLPs. The authors concluded that the antibodies reacting with SV40 VLPs in human sera are not authentic SV40 antibodies but BKV and/or JCV antibodies that cross-react with SV40. According to these results, therefore, SV40 does not seem to be a prevalent human pathogen. However, due to the great homology (more than 80 %) of the VP1 structural protein in the three polyomaviruses,[1,8-11] pre-adsorption with BKV and JCV VLPs may have removed from human sera most of the SV40 antibodies, because they cross-react with the human polyomavirus capsid antigens. Conversely, recent seroepidemiological data suggest that specific SV40 antibodies can be detected in human sera. (i) In a collection of human sera from Morocco, 100% of the samples had antibodies to SV40,[25] whereas in the same study other sera from Morocco, Zaire, Sierra Leone and Poland contained SV40 antibodies in 0.4 to 5.3% of the samples,[25] a value in agreement with the results of other surveys.[6,7] All the sera in the 100% positive Moroccan collection were from cases of poliomyelitis in children under five years of age.[25] These children, therefore, had probably not been vaccinated against poliovirus. This result should not be overestimated, especially because the collection of the 100% anti-SV40-positive sera is made up of only 29 samples. Nevertheless, this observation suggests that, under particular circumstances, humans can display a great specific antibody response to SV40. Perhaps, the overt poliomyelitis syndrome has influenced the immunological reaction of affected patients to SV40. (ii) Although it is obviously difficult, due to the ubiquity of the two human polyomaviruses, to find a human serum positive for SV40 and negative for both BKV and JCV antibodies, one such serum was detected.[25] (iii) While seroconversion to BKV and JCV is age-dependent,[17-23] there is no detectable age-dependent seroconversion to SV40,[22,24,25] suggesting that most of the SV40 antibodies present in human sera are not generated by infection with BKV or JCV. (iv) In sera from two immunosuppressed renal transplant patients, that were examined sequentially for antibodies to BKV, JCV and SV40 over a period of 82 and 51 weeks, respectively, a significant rise in SV40 antibody titers was detected,[25] indicating that a latent SV40 infection, like BKV and JCV latent infection, can be reactivated in humans by immunosuppression. Moreover, during the post-transplant follow-up, the evolving profile of antibodies to SV40 was clearly different from that of antibodies to either BKV or JCV,[25] suggesting a specific immunological response to SV40 in these two patients. In our laboratory, we have set up an ELISA assay, using specific peptides of SV40 capsid proteins as antigens. These peptides do not cross-react with BKV and JCV capsid antigens. The results of this ELISA test indicate that SV40-specific antibodies could be present in a fraction of human sera larger than previously reported[7] (Corallini et al, unpublished results). These preliminary data suggest that, by using appropriate antigens, an SV40-specific antibody response can be detected in humans.

The natural history of BKV, JCV and SV40 infection in humans has been described extensively in previous reviews.[1-11,26-28] BKV and JCV primary infections are generally inapparent and rarely associated with clinical diseases. BKV, however, can cause upper respiratory or urinary tract disease,[11] while acute JCV infection has been associated with meningoencephalitis.[29] Natural infection by SV40 in humans is a rare event, restricted to people living in contact with monkeys, the natural hosts of the virus, such as inhabitants of indian villages located close to the jungle, and persons attending to monkeys in zoos and animal facilities.[30] However, massive infection of the human population by SV40 occurred between 1955 and 1963, when hundreds of millions of persons in the United States, Canada, Europe, Asia and Africa were vaccinated with both inactivated and live polio vaccines contaminated with infectious SV40.[31] Vaccines to adenoviruses, respiratory syncitial virus and hepatitis A virus also introduced SV40 in humans, although not in a massive scale.[6,7] Soon it was shown that people vaccinated with contaminated polio vaccines shed infectious SV40 in stools for at least five weeks after vaccination.[32] This observation suggested that SV40 could be transmitted by recipients of contaminated polio vaccines to contacts by the fecal-oral route, raising the possibility that SV40 would spread in humans by horizontal infection. Primary infection by BKV and JCV is followed by a persistent or latent infection which may be reactivated mainly in immunosuppressed but also in immunocompetent people. Virus isolation and Southern hybridization analysis established that the main site of BKV and JCV latency in healthy people is the kidney.[1,8-10,11] BKV and JCV viruria is detected after reactivation from latency in immunosuppressed and immuno-competent individuals.[33] The site of SV40 latent infection in humans is not known. However, detection of SV40 in human kidney and urine[34,35] points to the kidney as a site of virus latency, like in the natural monkey host.[36] The PCR technology, applied to the study of BKV and JCV latency, disclosed the presence of their DNA and RNA specific sequences in a variety of normal human tissues (Table 1).[1-5,26,37] These results indicate that BKV and JCV can establish latent infection in many more organs than previously thought. SV40 sequences were found in nor-mal brain, bone tissue and sperm fluids.[38,39] Of particular interest is detection of BKV, JCV and SV40 sequences in peripheral blood mononuclear cells (PBMC),[1-5,37-41] suggesting that infection of blood cells may represent the route of virus spread from the portal of entry to other tissues of the infected host. The modalities of inter-human virus transmission are at present not clear. Due to the high prevalence of infection and detection of BKV and JCV in tonsils,[1-5,42,43] the two human polyomaviruses were long thought to be transmitted mainly by the respiratory route. However, the recent evidence that JCV DNA is present in the gastro-intestinal tract[44-46] and that BKV, JCV and SV40 DNA sequences and virions are detected in raw urban sew-age[47,48] suggests also a fecal-oral route of transmission for the three viruses. The presence of BKV, JCV and SV40 DNA in PBMC as well as of BKV and JCV DNA in the prostate and of SV40 DNA in sperm fluids[1-5,26,38] points also to the hematic and sexual routes as possible, although perhaps less frequent, means of virus transmission in humans. Clues to the mecha-nisms and routes of SV40 transmission in humans may come from studies of SV40 natural infection in monkeys.[49] Since uninfected weaning animals do not frequently seroconvert when grouped with infected mothers and infected littermates, it seems most likely that transmission of SV40 in monkeys, under conditions of natural infection, occurs after weaning from the environment rather than directly from other animals.[49] Interestingly, these results support a rather inefficient SV40 transmission in humans from the contaminated general environment, e.g. sewage,[48] or from the home environment. This mode of restricted transmission, together with the semi-permissiveness of human cells to SV40 infection,[1,6,7] would explain, in turn, the limited SV40 circulation and the low antibody response to SV40 in humans.[6,7,22,24,25]

BKV, JCV and SV40 Cell Transformation and Experimental Oncogenicity

Transformation of rodent and human cells by polyomaviruses is induced by the two oncoproteins encoded in the early region of the viral genome, the large Tag and the small tag. Both these proteins display multiple functions. The main activity of large Tag for cell tranformation and tumorigenesis is to target key cellular proteins, such as the tumor suppressor p53 and pRB family proteins, inactivating their functions.[1-10,50-56] However, binding to p53 and pRB proteins varies for different polyomaviruses and in cells of different species. For in-stance, the amount of BKV Tag normally produced in BKV-transfected simian BSC-1 cells seems to be too low to bind a significant amount of proteins of the pRB family.[54] BKV Tag readily binds the p53 protein available in BSC-1 cells and induces serum-independence, but is unable to allow anchorage-independent growth in semisolid medium.[54] These data support the notion that BKV Tag can affect cellular growth control mechanisms, but other additional events are required for full transformation of primate cells by BKV. In addition, human p53 binds to BKV DNA in the region of the early viral promoter,[55] probably modulating the ex-pression of BKV oncoproteins. It was shown that the complex of SV40 large Tag with mouse p53 completely blocks the transactivating effect of the p53 protein, whereas the same complex in human cells allows human p53 to exert partially its transcriptional activity.[56] Owing to the great homology of SV40 large Tag with the large Tag of human polyomaviruses BKV and JCV, it is possible that the inefficiency in transformation of human cells by SV40 and human polyomaviruses may depend on the inability of their Tags to block completely the effect of the human tumor suppressor proteins pRB and p53.

The principal role of polyomavirus small tag in transformation is to bind the catalytic (36 kDa) and regulatory (63 kDa) subunits of protein phosphatase 2A (PP2A),[6,7] inactivating their function. PP2A is a serine/threonine phosphatase that regulates the phosphorylation signal activated by protein kinases[57] and has recently been shown to be a tumor suppressor gene involved in lung, colon, breast carcinoma and melanoma.[58,59] The region of small tag binding to PP2A is not part of the large Tag,[6,7] suggesting that PP2A binding is a specific function of small tag. The interaction of tag with PP2A leads to inhibition of the Wnt pathway,[60] lack of inactivation of β-catenin, its translocation to the nucleus and stimulation of cell proliferation.[61,62] The block of PP2A functions by tag induces an alteration of the actin cytoskeleton and tight junctions, resulting in loss of cell polarity and tumor invasiveness.[63] Small tag interacts with the centrosome and blocks mitosis in human cells,[64] suggesting that it may disrupt cell cycle progression. Recently, it was shown that tag activates, in human mammary epithelial cells, phosphatidylinositol 3-kinase,[65] an enzyme involved in pathways crucial for cell proliferation and transformation. In addition, SV40 small tag is able to enhance transcription from E2F-activated promoters of early growth response genes.[66,67]

Polyomavirus large Tags may lead to transformation through functions independent from inactivation of tumor suppressor proteins. In fact, BKV, JCV and SV40 large Tags induce mutations in rodent and human cells.[68,69] SV40 and BKV Tags induce chromosomal damage in human cells,[70-72] characterized by numerical and structural chromosomal alterations, such as gaps, breaks, dicentric and ring chromosomes, chromatid exchanges, deletions, duplications and translocations. Chromosome damage in human cells transfected with SV40 and BKV early region was evident before the appearance of immortalization and the morphologically transformed phenotype, suggesting that it is a cause rather than a consequence of transformation. Similar alterations were observed in cell lines from human glioblastoma multiforme, harboring the Tag coding sequences of both BKV and SV40.[73] JCV large Tag is also associated to chromosome damage and chromosomal instability in B-lymphocytes and in cells of the colorectal mucosa.[74-76] The molecular mechanism of the clastogenic effect of polyomavirus Tag may reside in its ability to bind topoisomerase I[77] and in its helicase activity[78] which could induce chromosome damage when unwinding the two strands of cellular DNA. Moreover, since polyomavirus large Tag binds the p53 protein inactivating its functions,[55,56] the direct clastogenic effect of the viral oncoprotein may be enhanced, because it inhibits p53-induced apoptosis and allows DNA-damaged cells to survive, increasing their probability to transform and acquire immortality. Recently, the X-ray diffraction structure of a hexameric SV40 large Tag with helicase activity was elucidated.[79]

BKV, JCV and SV40 transform rodent cells to the neoplastic phenotype.[1-10] In these transformation experiments, essentially all cells in the culture express Tag in their nuclei and the viral DNA is integrated into the cell genome. SV40 immortalizes and transforms human cells[80-83] which induce tumors when implanted subcutaneously in autologous and homologous hosts.[82] Transformation of human cells by BKV and JCV is inefficient and often abortive.[1-5] BKV- and JCV-infected or transfected human cells generally do not display a completely transformed phenotype, characterized by immortalization, anchorage independence and tumorigenicity in nude mice, although they show morphological alterations and an increased lifespan.[84-85] Sometimes, transformation is transient and cells revert to the original phenotype after a few passages in culture.[86] A fully transformed phenotype was observed in human embryo kidney cells transfected with a recombinant plasmid containing BKV early region and the adenovirus 12 E1A gene.[87] These cells grow as a continuous cell line suggesting that, at least in human cells, BKV Tag is competent to contribute only a partially transformed phenotype and must interact with other oncogene functions to induce a complete transformation. The recombinants pBK/*c-ras*A and pBK/*c-myc*, containing in the same plasmid BKV early region and the c-H-*ras* or c-*myc* human activated cellular oncogenes,[88-90] induced morphologic transformation of human embryo fibroblasts and kidney cells, but transformed cells were not immortalized.[91,92] Tumorigenic cell lines were established only from BKV-transformed human fetal brain cells persistently infected by BKV. Fetal brain cells had all the characteristics of transformed cells and retained viral DNA, but they were negative for Tag expression.[93] SV40 large Tag too needs cooperation for complete transformation of human cells, because a tumorigenic phenotype was obtained only after cotransfection of human cells with plasmids expressing SV40 large Tag, the catalytic subunit of telomerase and the activated c-H-*ras* oncogene.[94] Human cells transformed by BKV, JCV and SV40 harbor, in addition to integrated viral DNA, viral genomes in an episomal state, sometimes in great number.[1-10]

BKV, JCV and SV40 are highly oncogenic in rodents.[1-10] JCV induces tumors also in monkeys.[1,5,95,96] The spectrum of tumors experimentally induced in rodents is similar but distinct for each of the three viruses. All the three viruses are highly neurotropic in tumorigenesis, but induce also extraneural tumors.[1-10] Young or newborn mice, rats and hamsters developed tumors after inoculation of BKV via different routes. The frequency of tumor induction in hamsters is strictly dependent on the route of injection. In fact, BKV is weakly oncogenic when inoculated subcutaneously (s.c.), but induces tumors frequently (in the range of 73% to 88%) when inoculated intracerebrally (i.c.) or intravenously (i.v.).[1-3] Tumors induced in BKV-injected hamsters belong to a variety of histotypes, such as ependymoma, neuroblastoma, pineal gland tumors, tumors of pancreatic islets, fibrosarcoma, osteosarcoma.[1-3] However, ependymoma and choroid plexus papilloma, tumors of pancreatic islets and osteosarcomas are the most frequent histotypes, suggesting that BKV may have a marked tropism for specific organs. This tissue preference may occur because of a specific interaction between virus and cell receptors, cell type variations in the activity of the viral promoter-enhancer or the effect of viral oncoproteins on p53 and pRB in that particular tissue. The latter possibility is supported by the observation that choroid plexus cells, a tumor specific target of BKV and SV40, are unusually sensitive to p53 and RB gene mutations, leading to inactivation of the corresponding products and to rapid malignant transformation.[6,97,98] Cellular tropism is observed also in tumorigenesis by JCV. Indeed, it was shown recently that JCV tropism for glial cells is due to cell type-specific transcription and/or replication factors.[99] Tumors induced by BKV in mice and rats were fibrosarcoma, liposarcoma, ostesarcoma, nephroblastoma, glioma and choroid plexus papilloma, the latter arising only in mice.[1-3] Gardner's BKV strain seems to be more oncogenic than other isolates, such as BKV-MM, BKV-RF and BKV-IR.[1-3] Purified BKV DNA is not oncogenic when inoculated s.c. or i.v. and induces tumors at a very low frequency when inoculated i.c. in rodents.[100] It displays, however, a strong synergism with activated oncogenes. Newborn hamsters inoculated s.c. with pBK/c-*ras*A, a recombinant containing BKV early region gene and the c-H-*ras* oncogene, developed tumors within few weeks. Tumors developed at the site of injection and consisted of undifferentiated sarcomas expressing both BKV Tag and c-H-*ras* p21. Neither BKV DNA nor c-H-*ras* inoculated independently were tumorigenic.[88] The same recombinant pBK/c-*ras*A, inoculated i.c., induced brain tumors in newborn hamsters.[89] These data suggest a synergic interaction of BKV transforming functions with human oncogenes.

JCV inoculated i.c. in newborn hamsters produced brain tumors in 83% of animals.[101] Most tumors consisted of cerebellar medulloblastoma, but glioblastoma, astrocytoma, pineocytoma, thalamic gliomas and tumors of other histotypes were also observed.[5,101,102] Primitive neuroectodermal tumors were induced at a very low frequency, while neuroblastoma and retinoblastoma were consistently induced by intraocular inoculation.[103,104] Pineal gland tumors were rarely obtained with JCV strains Mad-1 or Tokyo-1, but pineocytomas were described after inoculation of JCV strain Mad-4, suggesting that, as with BKV, different JCV strains may display a different oncogenic potential or tropism.[5,101-105] Owl and squirrel monkeys inoculated with JCV either i.c., i.v. or s.c. developed, after a latency period of 14-36 months, cerebral tumors, mostly astrocytomas.[95,96] The primary monkey tumors and the derived cell lines contained integrated JCV DNA and expressed JCV Tag.[106,107] No tumors were obtained in primates inoculated with either BKV or SV40.[95,96]

SV40 inoculated s.c., i.c. or i.v. in newborn hamsters induces soft tissue sarcomas, ependymomas and choroid plexus papillomas, osteosarcomas, lymphomas, and leukemias.[1,6,7] Moreover, direct inoculation of SV40 into the pleural space induces malignant mesothelioma in 100% of the injected hamsters.[108]

The oncogenic potential of BKV, JCV and SV40 is confirmed by the generation of transgenic mice in which polyomavirus large Tag expression is regulated by the native viral early promoter-enhancer. Transgenic mice expressing BKV Tag develop hepatocellular carcinoma, renal tumors and lymphoproliferative disease.[109,110] Mice transgenic for the JCV Tag gene develop adrenal and peripheral neuroblastoma, medulloblastoma, pituitary adenoma and malignant peripheral nerve sheath tumors, according to whether the JCV early region sequence is directed by the Mad-4 or by the archetype promoter.[5,102] SV40 transgenic mice, like rodents experimentally inoculated with the virus, develop ependymomas and choroid plexus papillomas.[6,7,98,111-113] Therefore, the transgenic mice experiments confirmed that BKV, JCV and SV40 display great oncogenic potential in experimental animals.

Association of BKV, JCV and SV40 with Human Tumors

All three polyomaviruses, BKV, JCV and SV40, are associated with human tumors. However, their role as causative agents in human neoplasia is still uncertain. Fiori and Di Mayorca[114] found BKV DNA sequences by DNA–DNA reassociation kinetics in 5 of 12 human tumors and 3 of 4 human tumor cell lines. These results were confirmed by Pater et al,[115] whereas three other reports failed to support these findings.[1-3] These tumors contained full-length BKV genomes, but also rearranged and defective BKV DNA molecules. Since BKV shows a specific oncogenic tropism for the ependymal tissue, endocrine pancreas and bones in rodents,[1-3] BKV DNA sequences were searched by Southern blotting in those rare types of human tumors most frequently induced by BKV in experimental animals such as ependymomas and other brain tumors, insulinomas and osteosarcomas. BKV DNA was detected in a free, episomal state and generally at a low copy number (from 0.2 to 1 genome equivalent per cell) in 19 out of 74 (26%) human brain tumors and in four out of nine (44%) human tumors of pancreatic islets.[116] A number of tumors expressed BKV-specific RNA and Tag. Furthermore, a BKV variant DNA, BKV-IR, was detected by Southern blot hybridization in a human insulinoma.[117] Virus was rescued by transfection of human embryonic fibroblasts with tumor DNA. The genome of BKV-IR contains an IS-like structure,[118] a type of stem-loop transposable element able to integrate and excise from the host genome.[119] The IS-like sequence of BKV-IR incorporates in its loop two of the early region transcriptional enhancer repeats.[118] It may promote cell transformation by excision from viral DNA and insertion into the cell genome, thereby specifically activating the expression of cellular oncogenes or more generally as a mutagen by random integration into the cell genome. In another study, BKV DNA was detected by Southern hybridization in 46% of brain tumors of the most common histotypes.[120] In this report, BKV DNA sequences were found to be integrated into chromosomal DNA.

More recently, tumors, tumor cell lines and normal human tissues were investigated by PCR using specific primers for early region BKV DNA. In most of these studies, the amount of viral DNA detected in human tumors and normal tissues was low, generally less than one genome equivalent per cell. The results of the studies conducted by Southern blot hybridization and PCR are summarized in Table 1 which reports positive and negative data, relative to human tumors of different histotypes, obtained by various authors. Nucleotide sequence analysis of seven brain tumors, one osteosarcoma, two glioblastoma cell lines, one normal brain and one normal bone tissue specimens confirmed that the amplified sequences correspond to the expected fragment of BKV early region.[37] Expression of BKV early region was detected by Northern blot analysis or reverse transcriptase (RT)-PCR in several tumors, tumor cell lines and normal tissues[37] (Table 1). In one study, both SV40 and BKV sequences were searched in

Table 1. Presence and expression of BKV DNA in human tumors, tumor cell lines and normal tissues

Tissues and Cell Lines	BKV DNA-Positive Samples/Samples Analyzed (%)		BKV RNA-Positive Samples/Samples Analyzed	Method[a]	References
Primary Tumors					
Brain tumors	19/74	(26)		SBH	116
Brain tumors	11/24	(46)		SBH	120
Brain tumors	0/75			PCR	132
Brain tumors	50/58	(86)		PCR	37
Brain tumors	74/83	(89)		PCR	38
Brain tumors	0/10			PCR	133
Neuroblastoma	18/18	(100)		PCR	121
Bone tumors	11/25	(44)	8/11	PCR, RT-PCR	37
MED and PNET[b]	0/20			PCR	135
Insulinomas	4/9	(44)		SBH	116
Hodgkin's diseases	0/5			PCR	133
ALL[c]	0/15			PCR	134
Kaposi's sarcoma	4/20	(20)		SBH	1-3
Kaposi's sarcoma	38/38	(100)		PCR	127
Kaposi's sarcoma	0/2			PCR	133
Urinary tract tumors	31/52	(60)		PCR	26,123
Urinary tract tumors	0/15			PCR	133
Genital tumors	32/42	(76)		PCR	26,127
Cell lines from					
Brain tumors	8/10	(80)	5/5	PCR, RT-PCR	37
Brain tumors	21/26	(81)		PCR	38
MED and PNET	0/2			PCR	135
Bone tumors	20/20	(100)	6/8	PCR, RT-PCR	37
Kaposi's sarcoma	6/8	(75)		PCR	127
Kaposi's sarcoma	0/14			PCR	133
Normal tissues					
Brain	13/13	(100)		PCR	37
Bone	2/5	(40)	2/2	PCR, RT-PCR	37
Urinary tract	15/26	(58)		PCR	26,123
Adrenal gland	0/5			PCR	121
Genital tissues	28/39	(72)		PCR	26,127
PBMC[d]	25/35	(71)	8/8	PCR, RT-PCR	37
PBMC	53/79	(76)		PCR	38
Lymphnodes	4/4	(100)		PCR	127
Skin	25/33	(76)		PCR	127
Sperm	18/20	(90)		PCR	38
Sperm	18/19	(95)		PCR	127

[a]SBH: Southern blot hybridization; PCR, polymerase chain reaction; RT-PCR, reverse transcriptase PCR; [b]MED and PNET, medulloblastoma and primitive neuroectodermal tumor; [c]ALL, acute lymphoblastic leukemia; [d]PBMC, peripheral blood mononuclear cells from healthy blood donors.

human brain tumors. All the tumors harboring SV40 sequences were coinfected by BKV.[38] In three human brain tumors, we even detected the simultaneous presence of BKV, JCV and SV40 DNA sequences (Martini et al, unpublished results), suggesting a helper function of human polyomaviruses to support SV40 replication in human cells or a possible interaction of polyomaviruses in oncogenesis. It remains to be determined whether in these tumors the sequences of the different polyomaviruses are present in the same cells. In another study, Flaegstad et al[121] detected BKV DNA by PCR in 18 neuroblastomas and in none of five normal adrenal gland samples (Table 1). The presence of BKV DNA was confirmed by in situ hybridization in the tumor cells of 17 of the same neuroblastomas. The expression of BKV Tag was detected by immunohistochemistry and immunoblotting in tumor cells, but not in normal control samples. Finally, BKV Tag and p53 were coimmunoprecipitated and colocalized in tumor cells by double immunostaining, suggesting a block of p53 functions by BKV Tag.

PCR amplification of DNA sequences from BKV early and regulatory regions was carried out in urinary tract tumors. Positive samples were 31 out of 52 (60%), with a range of 50–67% in different tumor types.[26] The presence of BKV and JCV DNA in urothelial carcinomas of the renal pelvis and in renal cell carcinomas was recently confirmed.[122] In addition, BKV DNA sequences were amplified by PCR in genital papillomas and carcinomas of the uterine cervix and vulva.[26] The percentage of positive samples in the neoplastic tissues of the urinary and genital tracts was similar to that detected in the corresponding normal tissues (61 and 59%,[26] and 16 and 15%,[122] respectively). However, in tumors of the urinary bladder and prostate, two-dimensional gel electrophoresis and Southern blot hybridization analysis showed either a single integration of BKV DNA or integrated and episomal viral sequences.[123] In both the integrated and extrachromosomal viral sequences, the late region was disrupted. Viral episomes consisted of rearranged oligomers containing cellular DNA sequences, whose size was apparently incompatible with encapsidation within a viral particle. Attempts to rescue these viral sequences by transfection of tumor DNA into permissive cells failed, suggesting that in these tumors the process of integration and formation of episomal oligomers produced a rearrangement of viral sequences responsible for the elimination of viral infectivity and potentially leading to stable expression of BKV transforming functions. Recently, a metastatic bladder carcinoma, arising in an immunosuppressed transplant recipient, appeared to be causally related to BKV, because high-level expression of BKV Tag was detected immunohistochemically in the primary and metastatic tumors but not in the neighboring normal urothelium.[124] p53 was colocalized immunohistochemically with BKV Tag in the nuclei of tumor cells, suggesting stabilization and inhibition of its functions by BKV Tag binding. Zambrano et al[125] detected BKV and JCV DNA in the prostate by PCR and in situ hybridization analysis. Human papillomavirus (HPV) DNA was also frequently detected in the prostate. Interestingly, the prostatic tissue was, in same cases, coinfected by HPV and human polyomaviruses,[125] opening the question of a possible role of these mixed infections in the etiopathogenesis of prostatic cancer. The results obtained with prostate and bladder carcinoma, in connection with the evidence that the kidney is the main site of BKV and JCV latency, suggest that tumors of the urinary tract are among the best candidates for an etiological association with BKV and JCV.

Due to reactivation of BKV infection during immunosuppression, tumors typically associated with immunosuppression were also investigated and BKV DNA was detected by Southern hybridization in Kaposi's sarcoma (KS) at a frequency of 20%.[1-3] Infectious BKV DNA was rescued from two KS tissues by transfection of cellular DNA into human embryonic fibroblasts.[126] PCR analysis for BKV early and regulatory regions in 38 samples of primary KS (5 classic, 12 African and 21 AIDS-associated) revealed 100% positivity for BKV DNA sequences. Analysis by PCR of 8 KS cell lines disclosed BKV DNA sequences in 6 of them, whereas JCV and SV40 sequences were absent.[127] In addition, BKV DNA sequences were detected in 15 out of 26 (58%) prostatic tissues and in 18 out of 19 (95%) seminal fluids,[127] suggesting that BKV may be a candidate for the sexually transmitted infectious agent which was indicated by epidemiological studies to be an important cofactor in KS.[128] A specific role of the sexual route for

Table 2. JCV Tag sequences in human central nervous system tumors and colorectal carcinoma

Tumor Type	JCV Positive Samples/Samples Analyzed (%)		JCV Strain	References
Glioblastoma	12/21	(57)	ND[a]	102,142
Glioblastoma	1/1	(100)	Mad-4	143
Glioblastoma	9/22	(41)	Mad-1, Mad-4	145
Astrocytoma	4/10	(40)	Mad-4	137
Astrocytoma	18/21	(86)	ND	102,142
Oligoastrocytoma	1/1	(100)	Mad-4	136
Oligoastrocytoma	7/11	(64)	ND	102,142
Xanthoastrocytoma	1/1	(100)	Mad-4	139
Oligodendroglioma	1/5	(20)	atypical[b]	137
Oligodendroglioma	6/10	(60)	ND	102,142
Oligodendroglioma	15/20	(75)	Mad-4	144
Medulloblastoma	20/23	(87)	ND	140,141
Medulloblastoma	13/20	(65)	ND	138
Ependymoma	1/5	(20)	Mad-4	137
Ependymoma	5/6	(83)	ND	102,142
Colorectal carcinoma	24/29	(83)	Mad-1	44,46
Colorectal carcinoma	22/27	(81)	ND	148

[a]ND, not determined; [b]Rearrangement of the regulatory region not detected in known strains.

BKV transmission is suggested by the presence of JCV DNA only in 4 out of 26 (15%) prostatic tissues and in 4 out of 19 (21%) seminal fluids.[127] It is notable that polyomaviruses closely related to BKV induce angiogenic responses very similar to KS. Indeed, murine endothelial cells transformed by polyoma virus middle Tag or by SV40 large Tag induce hemangiomas or highly vascularized KS-like tumors in nude mice.[129,130] Similar lesions are induced in nude mice by mouse brain and aortic endothelial cells transformed by BKV.[131] In other reports, however, the presence of BKV DNA sequences in human brain tumors, mostly malignant glioma, medulloblastoma and primitive neuroectodermal tumors, urinary tract tumors, Kaposi's sarcoma, lymphoma and acute lymphoblastic leukemia, analysed by PCR, was not confirmed[132-135] (Table 1). The negative results obtained by Völter et al[133] may be attributed to a low sensitivity of the PCR reaction due to the use of degenerate primers, in order to detect simultaneously BKV, JCV and SV40 sequences, instead of primers specific for BKV DNA. In addition, Völter et al[133] tested human tumor tissue for the presence of BKV late sequences which code for BKV functions most likely not involved in carcinogenesis.

JCV genomic sequences and expression of Tag have been observed in a variety of human brain tumor types.[5,102,136-145] Rencic et al[136] reported the presence of JCV DNA and Tag in the oligodendroglial portion of an oligoastrocytoma by PCR and Southern blot hybridization, immunohistochemistry, and Western blotting. Subsequent analyses of oligodendrogliomas have revealed JCV DNA in 20-75% and Tag expression in up to 50% of these tumors,[5,102,137] as shown in Table 2. The two human brain tumor types most closely associated with JCV are astrocytoma and medulloblastoma.[5,95] In studies of medulloblastomas, 77% of the tumors, analysed by PCR, were shown to contain viral DNA corresponding to the N-terminal region of JCV Tag, and 36% of the tumors, analysed by immunohistochemistry, showed portions of the neoplastic tissue with nuclear positivity for JCV Tag.[5,102] An investigation of medulloblastomas showed the expression of the JCV agnoprotein, a late viral protein, in 69% of tumor

Table 3. Detection of SV40 DNA in human tumors

	Mesothelioma	Brain Tumors	Bone Tumors	Lymphoma	References
Number of articles with:					
Positive results	23	13	4	4	6,7,151-153,170-172,187
Negative results	3	3	0	4	133,157-164,167

samples.[138] The agnoprotein is a small (71 amino acids) auxiliary polyomavirus protein whose functions are at present unknown. However, it has been shown to be expressed early in viral infection and it can interact with Tag to regulate viral transcription and replication.[146] JCV agnoprotein colocalizes with tubulin[147] and may play a role in the stability of microtubules for the preservation of JCV-infected and JCV-transformed cells. JCV is also associated with non-neural tumors.[5,102] In agreement with the detection of JCV virions in raw sewage samples of urban areas [5,47] and with the possibility of JCV fecal-oral transmission, JCV DNA sequences were found in the upper and lower human gastrointestinal tract.[44-46] A series of colorectal adenocarcinomas were then surveyed for the presence of JCV by PCR and Southern blot hybridization as well as by immunohistochemistry. In one study, 83% of 29 tumor samples analysed were found to contain viral DNA sequences,[5,44] while a second study detected viral DNA in 81% of 27 samples and nuclear Tag by immunohistochemistry in 63% of the samples.[5,148] In addition, 44% of the colorectal tumors showed the presence of JCV agnoprotein.[5,148] As in JCV Tag-positive cell lines, derived from medulloblastomas arising in JCV-transgenic mice,[149] JCV Tag alters the regulation of the Wnt signaling pathway[60-61] in JCV-positive colorectal tumors.[5,148] This effect leads to constitutive expression of β-catenin and its cellular partner LEF-1 with subsequent increase in c-*myc* levels and induction of cell proliferation.[148] Recently, it was shown that JCV induces chromosomal instability in colon carcinoma cells, in an in vitro model of colorectal carcinogenesis.[76]

SV40 seems to be involved in kidney inflammatory diseases in humans,[34,35] although a recent contribution suggested that the presence of SV40 DNA in kidney and blood cells of patients with focal segmental glomerulosclerosis was an artifact due to PCR amplification of oligomers generated by the forward and reverse primers SV.For3 and SV.Rev. In fact, PCR amplification with another pair pf primers (GabE1 and GabE2) gave negative results.[150] Anyway, the main role postulated for SV40 in human pathology derives from its association with specific human tumor types: mesothelioma, lymphoma, brain and bone tumors as well as thyroid, pituitary and parotid gland tumors[1,6,7,151-153] (Table 3). These human tumors correspond in histotype to the neoplasms that are induced by SV40 experimental inoculation in rodents or by generation of transgenic mice with the SV40 early region gene directed by its own early promoter-enhancer.[1,6,7,151-153] The association of SV40 with human tumors is proved by the presence of SV40 sequences in tumor tissues and by the expression of the virus-specific RNA and proteins. The SV40 sequences were generally detected in an episomal state and rarely integrated in tumor DNA.[154,155] In addition, infectious SV40 was isolated from a choroid plexus carcinoma.[156] Negative results were also reported on the association of SV40 with human brain tumors, lymphoma and mesothelioma.[133,157-164] However, Capello et al,[157] while failing to detect SV40 sequences in lymphomas, reproducibly found them in mesotheliomas, and Völter et al,[133] as pointed out for BKV, investigated human tumor samples for the presence of SV40 late gene sequences which are unlikely to be involved in the process of SV40-induced transformation and tumorigenesis. The contribution on brain tumors by Engels et al[159] raised a controversy because the assay used in this study was estimated to be affected by low sensitivity.[165,166] A serological survey for antibodies to BKV, JCV and SV40 capsid proteins indicated no association of the three viruses with human astrocytic brain tumors.[167] It is notable that search for antibodies to polyomavirus structural proteins[158,167] may not be the best assay to evaluate polyomavirus association with human tumors. Indeed, antibodies to polyomavirus large T and small t oncoproteins should better reflect immunization against polyomavirus tumor-specific antigens. Engels et al[168] report that childhood exposure to SV40 through receipt of contaminated poliovaccines is not associated with increased risk for non-Hodgkin's B-cell lymphoma in AIDS patients. A recent commentary conveyed the skepticism of some scientists about the results linking SV40 to human tumors.[169] To settle the dispute among different results on SV40 in human neoplasia, two multi-institutional studies were performed to examine the presence of SV40 in human malignant mesotheliomas.[164,170] Unfortunately, the two investigations reached opposite conclusions leaving the question unresolved. It was therefore proposed that studies on association of SV40 with human tumors should fulfill at least three criteria: (i) analysis of primary tumor specimens and not of cell lines; (ii) inclusion of a control group; (iii) use of the same techniques for cases and controls.[171,172] The last point is very important, because different methodologies used in different studies appear to be one of the main reasons of the controversial results.

The functions of SV40 Tag must be continuously expressed in SV40-transformed rodent cells in order to establish and maintain transformation, since rodent and human cells transformed by temperature-sensitive mutants of Tag loose the transformed phenotype at the nonpermissive temperature.[173-176] This condition is in contrast with the evidence that the viral load in SV40-positive human tumors is generally low (less than one genome equivalent per cell) and Tag is expressed only in a fraction of tumor cells.[1,6,7] The situation, however, may be more complex, due to the multifunctional properties of SV40 Tag. Indeed, in human cells SV40 Tag induces chromosome aberrations[70,71] which likely affect the functions of genes involved in tumorigenesis, such as oncogenes, tumor suppressor and DNA repair genes.[177-179] Once chromosomal damage has been triggered in tumors and chromosomal aberrations have reached a threshold, genomic instability ensues,[180] due to the functional alteration of DNA repair genes, leading to more genetic lesions and tumor progression. This process does not need the maintenance of the original injury that initiated tumorigenesis. The same course of events may occur in SV40-positive human tumors, where the clastogenic activity of Tag, like a chemical or physical carcinogen, initiates the tumorigenic process by hitting the cell genome, then becomes dispensable and is lost in the progression phase of the tumor, when the accumulation of genetic alterations renders the presence of viral transforming functions unnecessary. Immunoselection may even be exerted against persistently SV40-infected cells, while genetically mutated, uninfected cells may have a proliferative advantage and become the prevalent population in the tumor. This "hit and run" mechanism was originally proposed to explain transformation of human cells by the mutagenic herpesviruses,[181,182] and has been recently demonstrated to be operative in an in vitro model of colorectal carcinogenesis associated with JCV.[76] Contrary to SV40-transformed human cells, in transformed rodent cells, where SV40 Tag is equally clastogenic, SV40 sequences are not lost during chromosomal rearrangements. This difference may depend on the fact that rodent cells are non-permissive to SV40 replication and therefore the incoming viral DNA is integrated and fixed into the cell genome.[1,6] Because human cells are semi-permissive to virus replication, most of the SV40 DNA molecules remain in an episomal state, even when cell transformation is established,[1,6,7] rendering them more prone to be lost.

Another observation explaining the low viral load in SV40-positive human tumors is that SV40 Tag induces a paracrine mechanism by which a growth factor, such as insulin-like growth factor type I (IGF-I), is secreted by SV40-positive cells[183] and may stimulate proliferation of surrounding cells that do not contain SV40. More recently, it was shown that SV40 Tag activates in human mesothelial cells an autocrine-paracrine loop, involving the hepatocyte growth factor (HGF) and its cellular receptor, the oncogene c-*met*,[184] as well as the vascular endothelial growth factor (VEGF) and its cellular receptor.[185,186] HGF and VEGF, released from SV40-positive cells, bind their receptors in neighboring and distant SV40-positive and SV40-negative cells, driving them into proliferation and tumorigenesis. Thus, it is conceivable that not every cell in the tumor needs to express SV40 Tag in order to participate in tumor growth. Mesothelioma is the human tumor most closely and convincingly related to SV40.[187] The role of SV40 Tag in the pathogenesis of human mesothelioma was shown by: (i) its ability to bind in vivo p53 and pRB family proteins in human mesothelioma samples;[188,189] (ii) activation of Notch-1, a gene promoting cell cycle progression and cell proliferation in primary human mesothelial cells;[190] (iii) induction of apoptosis in mesothelioma cells transfected with antisense DNA to the SV40 early region gene;[191] (iv) the presence of SV40 Tag specific antibodies in sera of mesothelioma patients;[192] (v) the poorer prognosis of mesotheliomas harboring SV40 early region sequences compared to SV40-negative mesotheliomas.[193] Moreover, human mesothelial cells can be infected by SV40, but they can control SV40 replication and are resistant to lysis, due to the endogenous high levels of wild-type p53[194] which maintains the cells in a resting state. As a consequence of these properties, human mesothelial cells are particularly susceptible to SV40-mediated transformation.[184,194] Instead, JCV does not infect human mesothelial cells and BKV replicates faster than SV40 in these cells, causing mesothelial cell lysis and not cellular transformation.[195] These observations may explain why mesothelioma is specifically associated with SV40 rather than with the two ubiquitous human polyomaviruses. Asbestos, which is the main cause of human mesothelioma, cooperates with SV40 in transformation of human fibroblasts, mesothelial cells and murine cells,[194,196] suggesting that SV40 and asbestos may be co-carcinogens in the pathogenesis of mesothelioma.[187,197] Fluorescent in situ hybridization analysis indicated that the RB and cyclin E/CDK2 genes undergo the same type of deregulation during the cell cycle in asbestos-treated and SV40-transformed human mesothelial cells as well as in mesothelioma cells.[198] Recently, it was shown that SV40 large T and small t antigens induce telomerase activity in human mesothelial cells, but not in human fibroblasts,[199] suggesting that both SV40 oncoproteins participate in the immortalization of mesothelial cells during mesothelioma development.

The problems of the SV40 infection in human population and of SV40 contribution to human cancer may be summarized by considering a recent evaluation by the Immunization Safety Review Committee established by the Institute of Medicine of the National Academies.[200] The Committee stated that "the evidence is inadequate to accept or reject a causal relationship between SV40-containing polio vaccines and cancer". In fact, the epidemiological studies conducted in the past are flawed by the difficulty to establish which individuals received contaminated vaccines, to determine the dosage of infectious SV40 present in different lots of vaccine (due to formalin inactivation of poliovirus which may have variably affected SV40 infectivity), and finally to follow large cohorts of subjects for several decades after virus exposure to monitor for cancer development.[201] The Committee concluded that "the biological evidence is strong that SV40 is a transforming virus, but it is of moderate strength that SV40 exposure from polio vaccine is related to SV40 infection in humans and that SV40 exposure could lead to cancer in humans under natural conditions". The Committee also recommended targeted biological research in humans as well as development of specific and sensitive serologic tests for SV40 and use of standardized techniques that should be accepted and shared by all laboratories involved in SV40 detection.

Although it may seem somehow a premature effort, the conviction that SV40 is implicated as a cofactor in the etiology of some human tumors has prompted programs to prepare a vaccine against the main viral oncoprotein, the SV40 large Tag.[202] A recombinant vaccinia vector containing a safety-modified SV40 Tag sequence was constructed.[203] Such modified Tag excludes the p53 and pRB protein binding sites as well as the amino-terminal oncogenic CRI and J domains,[203] but preserves the immunogenic regions. Tumorigenesis studies carried out in vivo indicated that this vector can efficiently prime the immune response to provide effective, antigen-specific prophylactic and therapeutic protection against SV40 Tag-expressing lethal tumors.[203] Although truncation of large Tag at the carboxyl terminus, where the p53 binding sites are located, produces unstable products,[51] these types of vaccines may represent in the future a useful immunoprophylactic and immunotherapeutic defense against human tumors associated with SV40, such as in persons exposed to asbestos at risk for mesothelioma.[187,197] Anti-SV40 vaccines to be used in human immunizatation should mainly activate CD4+ T lymphocytes of the Th2 type and induce production of IgG1 antibodies, because these immunological reactions were shown to be most effective in the anti-tumor response of mice immunized with recombinant SV40 Tag.[204]

Conclusions and Future Perspectives

This review has critically evaluated results demonstrating that polyomaviruses BKV, JCV and SV40 are latent in human tissues, disrupt normal cell growth control by expression of their large T and small t antigens, transform cells in vitro and are oncogenic in experimental animals. It appears then that polyomaviruses have the potential to be cofactors in induction and/or progression of human tumors. A "hit and run" mechanism could explain the low viral load and the low number of polyomavirus Tag-positive cells in human tumors. In fact, BKV, JCV and SV40 induce chromosomal aberrations and mutations in human cells before the appearance of the transformed phenotype. This effect may represent an important oncogenic mechanism and, once chromosomal alterations are fixed in the host cells, viral sequences may be dispensable for the maintenance of transformation and may be lost by the neoplastic tissues. It is possible therefore that, while continuous expression of polyomavirus Tag is necessary for maintenance of polyomavirus transformation in rodent cells, in human cells the transformed phenotype is maintained by mechanisms independent from stable expression of polyomavirus oncoproteins. A suggestive proof of polyomavirus causative role in human oncogenesis would be to establish whether polyomavirus-positive tumors do not carry mutations in the p53 and RB family genes. Indeed, the viral oncoproteins should functionally inactivate the gene products, substituting for mutations in these tumor suppressors genes, although mutations may subsequently appear during tumor progression toward an invasive and metastatic phenotype, as it was shown to occur in genital tumors infected by HPV.[205,206] Finally, the detection of BKV, JCV and SV40 in sewage[47,48] prompts to search for the presence of BKV and SV40 in the gastrointestinal tract and for their possible association with colorectal tumors, as already shown for JCV.[44-46]

The association of BKV, JCV and SV40 with human tumors is related to the general problem concerning the role of infectious agents in human oncogenesis.[207,208] Childhood brain tumors were recently proposed to have an infectious etiology, on the basis of epidemiological investigations.[209] There was strong evidence of space-time clustering, suggesting transmission of an infectious agent, particularly involving cases of ependymoma and astrocytoma, that are neoplastic histotypes frequently associated to all three polyomaviruses. The incidence of brain tumors has increased substantially in the last years.[210] Environmental agents have been mainly incriminated, but polyomaviruses should not be overlooked as additional risk factors for such an increased frequency of brain tumors. Massive epidemiological surveys on the incidence of brain tumors in recipients of polio vaccines were discontinued in 1980 in the United States[211] and in 1989 in the former East Germany,[212] just when a trend towards a greater incidence of certain brain tumors was observed in cohorts of vaccinated individuals.[212] In subsequent years, the latency period for SV40 oncogenicity may have elapsed and tumors may have developed in vaccinated persons. A thirty-five year follow-up of about thousand recipients of polio vaccine did not detect a significantly greater cancer mortality compared to non-vaccinated persons,[213] but the number of cases was too low to exclude SV40 as a causative agent.

While BKV and JCV natural infection in humans is essentially well known, much work remains to be done to clarify whether SV40 is now circulating in the human population, independently from the earlier contaminated poliovaccines, and whether it has become a human pathogen. To determine the real diffusion of SV40 infection in humans, it is of paramount importance to establish a specific, sensitive and easy serological assay to investigate the presence of SV40 antibodies in human sera. Our laboratory is working to set up such a test, using SV40-specific structural epitopes that do not cross-react with BKV and JCV capsid antigens.

Finally, we must recall that the classical Koch's postulates, formulated to demonstrate the etiologic role of microorganisms in infectious diseases, cannot be applied directly to prove the viral etiology of human tumors, because most tumor-associated viruses are ubiquitous in humans and produce a persistent or latent infection in many human tissues. Thus, detection of virus in a tumor does not establish causation. New rules should be considered in order to evaluate the oncogenic effect of viruses in humans:[1,214,215]

1. presence and persistence of the virus or its nucleic acid in tumor cells;
2. cell immortalization and/or neoplastic transformation after virus infection or transfection of cells with the viral genome or its subgenomic fragments;
3. demonstration that the malignant phenotype of the primary tumor and the modifications induced by infection or transfection of cultured cells depend on specific functions expressed by the viral genome;
4. epidemiologic and clinical evidence that viral infection represents a risk factor for tumor development.

BKV, JCV and SV40 fulfill at least the first three criteria. Further work will be carried out in the future to prove that BKV, JCV and SV40 infection represents a risk factor for the development and/or progression of polyomavirus-associated human tumors.

Acknowledgements

The work of the authors described in this review was supported by grants to G. Barbanti-Brodano, M. Negrini and M. Tognon from Associazione Italiana per la Ricerca sul Cancro (AIRC) and from Ministero dell'Istruzione, Università e Ricerca (MIUR), COFIN and local projects, and by grants to A. Corallini from MIUR local projects.

Note

Due to the increasing amount of literature on BKV, JCV and SV40, we could quote only part of the pertinent articles and were often forced to cite general reviews instead of primary papers. We apologize for this behavior to the authors of the omitted articles and to the readers of this chapter.

References

1. Barbanti-Brodano G, Martini F, De Mattei M et al. BK and JC human polyomaviruses and simian virus 40: natural history of infection in humans, experimental oncogenicity, and association with human tumors. Adv Virus Res 1998; 50:69-99.
2. Corallini A, Tognon M, Negrini M et al. Evidence for BK virus as a human tumor virus. In: Khalili K, Stoner GJ, eds. Human Polyomaviruses: Molecular and Clinical Perspectives. New York: Wiley-Liss, 2001:431-460.
3. Tognon M, Corallini A, Martini F et al. Oncogenic transformation by BK virus and association with human tumors. Oncogene 2003; 22:5192-5200.
4. Hurault de Ligny B, Godin M, Lobbedez T et al. Virological, epidemiological and pathogenic aspects of human polyomaviruses. Presse Med 2003; 32:656-658.
5. Khalili K, Del Valle L, Otte J et al. Human neurotropic polyomavirus, JCV, and its role in carcinogenesis. Oncogene 2002; 22:5181-5191.
6. Garcea RL, Imperiale MJ. Simian virus 40 infection of humans. J Virol 2003; 77:5039-5045.
7. Barbanti-Brodano G, Sabbioni S, Martini F et al. Simian Virus 40 infection in humans and association with human diseases: results and hypotheses. Virology 2004; 318:1-8.
8. Imperiale MJ. The human polyomaviruses, BKV and JCV: molecular pathogenesis of acute disease and potential role in cancer. Virology 2000; 267:1-7.
9. Imperiale MJ. Oncogenic transformation by the human polyomaviruses. Oncogene 2001; 20:7917-7923.

10. Imperiale MJ. The human polyomaviruses: an overview. In: Khalili K, Stoner GL, eds. Human Polyomaviruses: Molecular and Clinical Perspectives. New York: Wiley-Liss, 2001:53-71.
11. Moens U, Rekvig OP. Molecular biology of BK virus and clinical and basic aspects of BK virus renal infection. In: Khalili K, Stoner GL, eds. Human Polyomaviruses: Molecular and Clinical Perspectives. New York: Wiley-Liss, 2001:359-408.
12. Yogo Y, Sugimoto C. The archetype concept and regulatory region rearrangement. In: Khalili K, Stoner GL, eds. Human Polyomaviruses: Molecular and Clinical Perspectives. New York: Wiley-Liss, 2001:127-148.
13. Loeber G, Doerries K. DNA rearrangements in organ-specific variants of polyomavirus JC strain GS. J Virol 1988; 62:1730-1735.
14. Jorgensen GE, Hammarin AL, Bratt G et al. Identification of a unique BK virus variant in the CNS of a patient with AIDS. J Med Virol 2003; 70:14-19.
15. Negrini M, Sabbioni S, Arthur RR et al. Prevalence of the archetypal regulatory region and sequence polymorphisms in nonpassaged BK virus variants. J Virol 1991; 65:5092-5095.
16. Brown P, Tsai T, Gajdusek DC. Seroepidemiology of human papovaviruses. Discovery of virgin populations and some unusual patterns of antibody prevalence among remote peoples of the world. Am J Epidemiol 1975; 102:331-340.
17. Gardner SD. Prevalence in England of antibody to human polyomavirus (BK). BMJ 1973; 1:77-78.
18. Shah KV, Daniel RW, Warszawski RM. High prevalence of antibodies to BK virus, an SV40-related papovavirus, in residents of Maryland. J Infect Dis 1973; 128:784-787.
19. Portolani M, Marzocchi A, Barbanti-Brodano G et al. Prevalence in Italy of antibodies to a new human papovavirus (BK virus). J Med Microbiol 1974; 7:543-546.
20. Padgett BL, Walker DL. Prevalence of antibodies in human sera against JC virus, an isolate from a case of progressive multifocal leukoencephalopathy. J Infect Dis 1973; 127:467-470.
21. Taguchi F, Kajioka J, Miyamura T. Prevalence rate and age of acquisition of antibodies against JC virus and BK virus in human sera. Microbiol Immunol 1982; 26:1057-1062.
22. Knowles WA, Pipkin P, Andrews N et al. Population-based study of antibody to the human polyomaviruses BKV and JCV and the simian polyomavirus SV40. J Med Virol 2003; 71:115-123.
23. Stolt A, Sasnauskas K, Koskela P et al. Seroepidemiology of the human polyomaviruses. J Gen Virol 2003; 84:1499-1504.
24. Carter JJ, Madeleine MM, Wipf GC et al. Lack of serologic evidence for prevalent simian virus 40 infection in humans. J Natl Cancer Inst 2003; 95:1522-1530.
25. Minor P, Pipkin P, Jarzebek Z et al. Studies of neutralising antibodies to SV40 in human sera. J Med Virol 2003; 70:490-495.
26. Monini P, De Lellis L, Barbanti-Brodano G. Association of BK and JC human polyomaviruses and SV40 with human tumors. In: Barbanti-Brodano G, Bendinelli M, Friedman H, eds. DNA Tumor Viruses: Oncogenic Mechanisms. New York: Plenum Press, 1995:51-73.
27. Doerries K. Latent and persistent polyomavirus infection. In: Khalili K, Stoner GL, eds. Human polyomaviruses: molecular and clinical perspectives. New York: Wiley-Liss, 2001:197-235.
28. Hirsch HH, Steiger J. Polyomavirus BK. Lancet Infect Dis 2003; 3:611-623.
29. Blake K, Pillay D, Knowles W et al. JC virus associated meningoencephalitis in an immunocompetent girl. Arch Dis Child 1992; 67:956-957.
30. Shah KV, Nathanson N. Human exposure to SV40. Am J Epidemiol 1976; 103:1-12.
31. Carbone M, Rizzo P, Pass HI. Simian virus 40, poliovaccines and human tumors: a review of recent developments. Oncogene 1997; 15:1877-1888.
32. Melnick JL, Stinebaugh S. Excretion of vacuolating SV40 virus (papova virus group) after ingestion as a contaminant of oral poliovaccine. Proc Soc Ep Biol Med 1962; 109:965-968.
33. Ling PD, Lednicky JA, Keitel WA et al. The dynamics of herpesvirus and polyomavirus reactivation and shedding in healthy adults: A 14-month longitudinal study. J Infect Dis 2003; 187:1571-1580.
34. Li RM, Tanawattanacharoen S, Falk RA et al. Molecular identification of SV40 infection in human subjects and possible association with kidney disease. J Am Soc Nephrol 2002; 13:2320-2330.
35. Li RM, Mannon RB, Kleiner D et al. BK virus and SV40 co-infection in polyomavirus nephropathy. Transplantation 2002; 74:1497-1504.
36. Sweet BH, Hilleman MR. The vacuolating virus SV40. Proc Soc Exp Biol Med 1960; 105:420-427.
37. De Mattei M, Martini F, Corallini A et al. High incidence of BK virus large T antigen coding sequences in normal human tissues and tumors of different histotypes. Int J Cancer 1995; 61:756-760.
38. Martini F, Iaccheri L, Carinci P et al. SV40 early region and large T antigen in human brain tumors, peripheral blood cells, and sperm fluids from healthy individuals. Cancer Res 1996; 56:4820-4825.

39. Martini F, Lazzarin L, Iaccheri L et al. Different simian virus 40 genomic regions and sequences homologous with SV40 large T antigen in DNA of human brain and bone tumors and of leukocytes from blood donors. Cancer 2002; 94:1037-1048.

40. Lecatsas G, Schoub BD, Rabson AR et al. Papovavirus in human lymphocyte cultures. Lancet 1976; 2:907-908.

41. Schneider EM, Doerries K. High frequency of polyomavirus infection in lymphoid cell preparations after allogenic bone marrow transplantation. Transplant Proc 1993; 25:1271-1273.

42. Goudsmit J, Wertheim-van Dillen P, van Strien A et al. The role of BK virus in acute respiratory tract disease and the presence of BKV DNA in tonsils. J Med Virol 1982; 10:91-99.

43. Monaco MCG, Jensen PN, Hou J et al. Detection of JC virus DNA in human tonsil tissue: evidence for site of initial viral infection. J Virol 1998; 72:9918-9923.

44. Laghi L, Randolph AE, Chauhan DP et al. JC virus DNA is present in the mucosa of the human colon and in colorectal cancers. Proc Natl Acad Sci U.S.A. 1999; 96:7484-7489.

45. Ricciardiello L, Laghi L, Ramamirtham P et al. JC virus DNA sequences are frequently present in the human upper and lower gastrointestinal tract. Gastroenterology 2000; 119:1228-1235.

46. Ricciardiello L, Chang DK, Laghi L et al. Mad-1 is the exclusive JC virus strain present in the human colon, and its transcriptional control region has a deleted 98-base-pair sequence in colon cancer tissues. J Virol 2001; 75:1996-2001.

47. Bofill-Mas S, Formiga-Cruz M, Clemente-Casares P et al. Potential transmission of human polyomaviruses through the gastrointestinal tract after exposure to virions or viral DNA. J Virol 2001; 75:10290-10299.

48. Vastag B. Sewage yields clues to SV40 transmission. J Am Med Assoc 2002; 288:1337-1338.

49. Minor P, Pipkin PA, Cutler K et al. Natural infection and transmission of SV40. Virology 2003; 314:403-409.

50. Pipas JM, Levine AJ. Role of T antigen interactions with p53 in tumorigenesis. Sem Cancer Biol 2001; 11:23-30.

51. Sáenz-Robles MT, Sullivan CS, Pipas JM. Transforming functions of Simian Virus 40. Oncogene 2001; 20:7899-7907.

52. Dyson N, Buchkovich K, Whyte P et al. The cellular 107K protein that binds to adenovirus E1A also associates with the large T antigens of SV40 and JC virus. Cell 1989; 58:249-255.

53. Dyson N, Bernards R, Friend SH et al. Large T antigens of many polyomaviruses are able to form complexes with the retinoblastoma protein. J Virol 1990; 64:1353-1356.

54. Harris KF, Christensen JB, Imperiale MJ. BK virus large T antigen: interactions with the retinoblastoma family of tumor suppressor proteins and effects on cellular growth control. J Virol 1996; 70:2378-2386.

55. Shivakumar CV, Das GC. Interaction of human polyomavirus BK with the tumor-suppressor protein p53. Oncogene 1996; 13:323-332.

56. Sheppard HM, Siska IC, Espiritu C et al. New insights into the mechanism of inhibition of p53 by simian virus 40 large T antigen. Mol Cell Biol 1999; 19:2746-2753.

57. Baysal BE, Farr JE, Goss JR et al. Genomic organization and precise physical location of protein phosphatase 2A regulatory subunit A beta isoform gene on chromosome band 11q23. Gene 1998; 217:107-116.

58. Wang SS, Esplin ED, Li JL et al. Alterations of the PPP2R1B gene in human lung and colon cancer. Science 1998; 282: 284-287.

59. Calin GA, di Iasio MG, Caprini E et al. Low frequency of alterations of the alpha (PPP2R1A) and beta (PPP2R1B) isoforms of the subunit A of the serine-threonine phosphatase 2A in human neoplasms. Oncogene 2000; 19:1191-1195.

60. Cadigan KM, Nusse R. Wnt signaling: a common theme in animal development. Genes Dev 1997; 11:3286-3305.

61. Willert K, Nusse R. Beta-catenin: a key mediator of Wnt signaling. Curr Opin Genet Dev 1998; 8:95-102.

62. Ikeda S, Kishida M, Matsuura Y et al. GSK-3b-dependent phosphorylation of adenomatous polyposis coli gene product can be modulated by b-catenin and protein phosphatase 2A complexed with Axin. Oncogene 2000; 19:537-545.

63. Nunbhakdi-Craig V, Craig L, Machleit T et al. Simian virus 40 small tumor antigen induces deregulation of the actin cytoskeleton and tight junctions in kidney epithelial cells. J Virol 2003; 77:2807-2818.

64. Gaillard S, Fahrbach KM, Parkati R et al. Overexpression of simian virus 40 small-t antigen blocks centrosome function and mitotic progression in human fibroblasts. J Virol 2001; 75:9799-9807.

65. Zhao JJ, Gjoerup OV, Subramanian RR et al. Human mammary epithelial cell transformation through the activation of phosphatidylinositol 3-kinase. Cancer Cell 2003; 3:483-495.

66. Beck GR Jr, Zerler BR, Moran E. Introduction to DNA tumor viruses: Adenovirus, simian virus 40, and polyomavirus. In: McCance DJ, ed. Human Tumor Viruses. Washington, DC: ASM Press, 1998:51-86.

67. Loeken MR. Simian virus 40 small t antigen transactivates the adenovirus E2A promoter by using mechanisms distinct from those used by adenovirus E1A. J Virol 1992; 66:2551-2555.

68. Theile M, Grabowski G. Mutagenic activity of BKV and JCV in human and other mammalian cells. Arch Virol 1990; 113:221-233.

69. Theile M, Strauss M, Luebbe L. SV40-induced somatic mutations: possible relevance to viral transformation. Cold Spring Harbor Symp Quant Biol 1980; 44:377-382.

70. Ray FA, Peabody DS, Cooper JL et al. SV40 T antigen alone drives karyotype instability that precedes neoplastic transformation of human diploid fibroblasts. J Cell Biochem 1990; 42:13-31.

71. Stewart N, Bacchetti S. Expression of SV40 large T antigen, but not small t antigen, is required for the induction of chromosomal aberrations in transformed human cells. Virology 1991; 180:49-57.

72. Trabanelli C, Corallini A, Gruppioni R et al. Chromosomal aberrations induced by BK virus T antigen in human fibroblasts. Virology 1998; 243:492-496.

73. Tognon M, Casalone R, Martini F et al. Large T antigen coding sequences of two DNA tumor viruses, BK and SV40 and nonrandom chromosome chances in glioblastoma cell lines. Cancer Genet Cytogenet 1996; 90:17-23.

74. Lazutka JR, Neel JV, Major EO et al. High titers of antibodies to two human polyomaviruses, JCV and BKV, correlate with increased frequency of chromosomal damage in human lymphocytes. Cancer Lett 1996; 109:177-183.

75. Neel JV, Major EO, Awa AA et al. Hypothesis: "Rogue cell"-type chromosomal damage in lymphocytes is associated with infection with the JC human polyoma virus and has implications for oncogenesis. Proc Natl Acad Sci U.S.A. 1996; 93:2690-2695.

76. Ricciardiello L, Baglioni M, Giovannini C et al. Induction of chromosomal instability in colonic cells by the human polyomavirus JC virus. Cancer Res 2003; 63:7256-7262.

77. Simmons DT, Melendy T, Usher D et al. Simian virus 40 large T antigen binds to topoisomerase I. Virology 1996; 222:365-374.

78. Dean FB, Bullock P, Murakami Y et al. Simian virus 40 (SV40) DNA replication: SV40 large T antigene unwinds DNA containing the SV40 origin of replication. Proc Natl Acad Sci USA 1987; 84:16-20.

79. Li D, Zhao R, Lilyestrom W et al. Structure of the replicative helicase of the oncoprotein SV40 large tumour antigen. Nature 2003; 423:512-518.

80. Shein HM, Enders JF. Transformation induced by simian virus 40 in human renal cell cultures. I. Morphology and growth characteristics. Proc Natl Acad Sci U.S.A. 1962; 48:1164-1172.

81. Koprowski H, Ponten JA, Jensen F et al. Transformation of cultures of human tissue infected with simian virus 40. J Cell Comp Physiol 1962; 59:281-292.

82. Jensen F, Koprowski H, Pagano JS et al. Autologous and homologous implantation of human cells transformed in vitro by simian virus 40. J Natl Cancer Inst 1964; 32:917-932.

83. Chen W, Hahn WC. SV40 early region oncoproteins and human cell transformation. Histol Histopathol 2003; 18:541-550.

84. Purchio AF, Fareed GC. Transformation of human embryonic kidney cells by human papovavirus BK. J Virol 1979; 29:763-769.

85. Grossi MP, Caputo A, Meneguzzi G et al. Transformation of human embryonic fibroblasts by BK virus, BK virus DNA and a subgenomic BK virus DNA fragment. J Gen Virol 1982; 63:393-403.

86. Rinaldo CH, Myhre MR, Alstad H et al. Human polyomavirus BK (BKV) transiently transforms and persistently infects cultured osteosarcoma cells. Virus Res 2003; 93:181-187.

87. Vasavada R, Eager KB, Barbanti-Brodano G et al. Adenovirus type 12 early region 1A proteins repress class I HLA expression in transformed human cells. Proc Natl Acad Sci U.S.A. 1986; 83:5257-5261.

88. Corallini A, Pagnani M, Viadana P et al. Induction of malignant subcutaneous sarcomas in hamsters by a recombinant DNA containing BK virus early region and the activated human c-Harvey-ras oncogene. Cancer Res 1987; 47:6671-6677.

89. Corallini A, Pagnani M, Caputo A et al. Cooperation in oncogenesis between BK virus early region gene and the activated human c-Harvey-ras oncogene. J Gen Virol 1988; 69:2671-2679.

90. Pagnani M, Corallini A, Caputo A et al. Co-operation in cell transformation between BK virus and the human c-Harvey-ras oncogene. Int J Cancer 1988; 42:405-413.

91. Pater A, Pater MM. Transformation of primary human embryonic kidney cells to anchorage independence by a combinant of BK virus DNA and the Harvey-ras oncogene. J Virol 1986; 58:680-683.

92. Corallini A, Giannì M, Mantovani C et al. Transformation of human cells by recombinant DNA molecules containing BK virus early region and the human activated c-H-ras or c-myc oncogenes. Cancer Journal 1991; 4:24-34.

93. Takemoto KK, Linke H, Miyamura T et al. Persistent BK papovavirus infection of transformed human fetal brain cells. I. Episomal viral DNA in cloned lines deficient in T-antigen expression. J Virol 1979; 29:1177-1185.

94. Hahn WC, Counter CM, Lundberg AS et al. Creation of human tumour cells with defined genetic elements. Nature 1999; 400:464-468.

95. London WT, Houff SA, Madden DL et al. Brain tumors in owl monkeys inoculated with a human polyomavirus (JC virus). Science 1978; 201:1246-1249.

96. London WT, Houff SA, MacKeever PE et al. Viral induced astrocytomas in squirrel monkeys. In: Sever JL, Madden DL, eds. Polyomaviruses and Human Neurological Disease. New York: Alan R. Liss, 1983:227-237.

97. Chen J, Tobin GJ, Pipas JM et al. T antigen mutant activities in vivo: roles pf p53 and pRB binding in tumorigenesis of the choroid plexus. Oncogene 1992; 7:1167-1175.

98. Van Dyke TA, Finlay C, Miller D et al. Relationship between simian virus 40 large tumor antigen expression and tumor formation in transgenic mice. J Virol 1987; 61:2029-2032.

99. Gee GV, Manley K, Atwood WJ. Derivation of a JC virus-resistant human glial cell line: implications for the identification of host cell factors that determine viral tropism. Virology 2003; 314:101-109.

100. Corallini A, Altavilla G, Carra' L et al. Oncogenicity of BK virus for immunosuppressed hamsters. Arch Virol 1982; 73:243-253.

101. Walker DL, Padgett BL, zu Rhein GM, et al. Human papovavirus (JC): Induction of brain tumors in hamsters. Science 1973; 181:674-676.

102. Del Valle L, Gordon J, Ferrante P et al. JC virus in experimental and clinical brain tumorigenesis. In: Khalili K, Stoner GL, eds. Human polyomaviruses: molecular and clinical perspectives. New York: Wiley-Liss, 2001:409-430.

103. Varakis JN, zu Rhein GM, Padgett BL et al. Experimental (JC virus-induced) neuroblastomas in the Syrian hamster. J Neuropathol Exp Neurol 1976; 35:314.

104. Ohashi T, zu Rhein GM, Varakis J et al. Experimental (JC virus-induced) intraocular and extraorbital tumors in the Syrian hamster. J Neuropathol Exp Neurol 1978; 37:667.

105. Padgett BL, Walker DL, zu Rhein GM et al. Differential neuro-oncogenicity of strains of JC virus, a human polyomavirus, in newborn Syrian hamsters. Cancer Res 1977; 37:718-725.

106. Miller NR, McKeever PE, London WT et al. Brain tumors of owl monkeys inoculated with JC virus contain the JC virus genome. J Virol 1984; 49:848-856.

107. Major EO, Mourrain P, Cummins C. JC virus-induced owl monkey glioblastoma cells in culture: biological properties associated with the viral early gene product. Virology 1984; 136:359-367.

108. Cicala C, Pompetti F, Carbone M. SV40-induced mesotheliomas in hamsters. Am J Pathol 1993; 142:1524-1533.

109. Small JA, Khoury G, Jay G et al. Early regions of JC virus and BK virus induce distinct and tissue specific tumors in transgenic mice. Proc Natl Acad Sci U.S.A. 1986; 83:8288-8292.

110. Dalrymple SA, Beemon KL. BK virus T antigens induce kidney carcinomas and thymoproliferative disorders in transgenic mice: J Virol 1990; 64:1182-1191.

111. Brinster RL, Chen HY, Messing A et al. Transgenic mice harboring SV40 T-antigen genes develop characteristic brain tumors. Cell 1984; 37:367-379.

112. Palmiter R, Chen H, Messing A et al. SV40 enhancer and large-T antigen are instrumental in development of choroid plexus tumours in transgenic mice. Nature 1985; 316:457-460.

113. Feigenbaum L, Hinrichs SH, Jay G. JC virus and simian virus 40 enhancers and transforming proteins: role in determining tissue specificity and pathogenicity in transgenic mice. J Virol 1992; 66:1176-1182.

114. Fiori M, Di Mayorca G. Occurrence of BK virus DNA in DNA obtained from certain human tumors. Proc Natl Acad Sci USA 1976; 73:4662-4666.

115. Pater MM, Pater A, Fiori M et al. BK virus DNA sequences in human tumors and normal tissues and cell lines. In: Essex M, Todaro G, zur Hausen H, eds. Viruses in Naturally Occurring Cancers. Book A. Cold Spring Harbor Conferences on Cell Proliferation. New York: Cold Spring Harbor Laboratory Press, 1980:329-341.

116. Corallini A, Pagnani M, Viadana P et al. Association of BK virus with human brain tumors and tumors of pancreatic islets. Int J Cancer 1987; 39:60-67.

117. Caputo A, Corallini A, Grossi MP et al. Episomal DNA of a BK virus variant in a human insulinoma. J Med Virol 1983; 12:37-49.

118. Pagnani M, Negrini M, Reschinglian P et al. Molecular and biological properties of BK virus-IR, a BK virus variant rescued from a human tumor. J Virol 1986; 59:500-505.
119. Calos MP, Miller JH. Tansposable elements. Cell 1980; 20:579-595.
120. Doerries K, Loeber G, Meixenberger J. Association of polyomavirus JC, SV40 and BK with human brain tumors. Virology 1987; 160:268-270.
121. Flaegstad T, Andresen PA, Johnsen JI et al. A possible contributory role of BK virus infection in neuroblastoma development. Cancer Res 1999; 59:1160-1163.
122. Knoll A, Stoehr R, Jilg W et al. Low frequency of human polyomavirus BKV and JCV DNA in urothelial carcinomas of the renal pelvis and renal cell carcinomas. Oncol Rep 2003; 10:487-491.
123. Monini P, Rotola A, Di Luca D et al. DNA rearrangements impairing BK virus productive infection in urinary tract tumors. Virology 1995; 214:273-279.
124. Geetha D, Tong BC, Racusen L et al. Bladder carcinoma in a transplant recipient: evidence to implicate the BK human polyomavirus as a causal transforming agent. Transplantation 2002; 73:1933-1936.
125. Zambrano A, Kalantari M, Simoneau A et al. Detection of human polyomaviruses and papillomaviruses in prostatic tissue reveals the prostate as a habitat for multiple viral infections. Prostate 2002; 53:263-276.
126. Negrini M, Rimessi P, Mantovani C et al. Characterization of BK virus variants rescued from human tumours and tumour cell lines. J Gen Virol 1990; 71:2731-2736.
127. Monini P, Rotola A, De Lellis L et al. Latent BK virus infection and Kaposi's sarcoma pathogenesis. Int J Cancer 1996; 66:717-722.
128. Peterman TA, Jaffe HW, Beral V. Epidemiologic clues to the etiology of Kaposi's sarcoma. AIDS 1993; 7:605-611.
129. Williams RL, Risau W, Zerwes HG et al. Endothelioma cells expressing the polyoma middle T oncogene induce hemangiomas by host cell recruitment. Cell 1989; 57:1053-1063.
130. O'Connel K, Landman G, Farmer E et al. Endothelial cells transformed by SV40 T antigen cause Kaposi's sarcoma like tumors in nude mice. Am J Pathol 1991; 139:743-749.
131. Corallini A, Possati L, Trabanelli C et al. Tumor-host interaction mediates the regression of BK virus-induced vascular tumors in mice: involvement of transforming growth factor-beta 1. Carcinogenesis 2003; 24:1435-1444.
132. Arthur RR, Grossman SA, Ronnett BM et al. Lack of association of human polyomaviruses with human brain tumors. J Neuro-Oncol 1994; 20:55-58.
133. Volter C, zur Hausen H, Alber D et al. Screening human tumor samples with a broad-spectrum polymerase chain reaction method for the detection of polyomaviruses. Virology 1997; 237: 389-396.
134. MacKenzie J, Perry J, Ford AM et al. JC and BK virus sequences are not detectable in leukaemic samples from children with common acute lymphoblastic leukemia. Brit J Cancer 1999; 81:898-899.
135. Kim JY, Koralnik IJ, LeFave M et al. Medulloblastomas and primitive neuroectodermal tumors rarely contain polyomavirus DNA sequences. Neuro-oncology 2002; 4:165-170.
136. Rencic A, Gordon J, Otte J et al. Detection of JC virus DNA sequence and expression of the viral oncoprotein, tumor antigen, in brain of immunocompetent patient with oligoastrocytoma. Proc Natl Acad Sci USA 1996; 93:7352-7357.
137. Caldarelli-Stefano R, Boldorini R, Monga G et al. JC virus in human glial-derived tumors. Hum Pathol 2000; 31:394-395.
138. Del Valle L, Gordon J, Enam S et al. Expression of human neutropic polyomavirus JCV late gene product agnoprotein in human medulloblastoma. J Natl Cancer Inst 2002; 94:267-273.
139. Boldorini R, Caldarelli-Stefano R, Monga G et al. PCR detection of JC virus DNA in the brain tissue of a 9-year-old child with pleomorphic xanthoastrocytoma. J Neurovirol 1998; 4:242-245.
140. Krynska B, Del Valle L, Croul S et al. Detection of human neurotropic JC virus DNA sequence and expression of the viral oncogenic protein in pediatric medulloblastomas. Proc Natl Acad Sci USA 1999; 96:11519-11524.
141. Krynska B, Otte J, Franks R et al. Human ubiquitous JCV(CY) T-antigen gene induces brain tumors in experimental animals. Oncogene 1999; 18:39-46.
142. Del Valle L, Gordon J, Assimakopoulou M et al. Detection of JC virus DNA sequences and expression of the viral regulatory protein T-antigen in tumors of the central nervous system. Cancer Res 2001; 61:4287-4293.
143. Del Valle L, Delbue S, Gordon J et al. Expression of JC virus T-antigen in a patient with MS and glioblastoma multiforme. Neurology 2002; 58:895-900.
144. Del Valle L, Enam S, Lara C et al. Detection of JC polyomavirus DNA sequences and cellular localization of T-antigen and agnoprotein in oligodendrogliomas. Clin Cancer Res 2002; 8:3332-3340.

145. Boldorini R, Pagani E, Car PG et al. Molecular characterisation of JC virus strains detected in human brain tumours. Pathology 2003; 35:248-253.

146. Safak M, Barrucco R, Darbinyan A et al. Interaction of JC virus agnoprotein with T antigen modulates transcription and replication of the viral genome in glial cells. J Virol 2001; 75:1476-1486.

147. Endo S, Okada Y, Orba Y et al. JC virus agnoprotein colocalizes with tubulin. J Neurovirol 2003; 9 Suppl 1:10-14.

148. Enam S, Del Valle L, Lara C et al. Association of human polyomavirus JCV with colon cancer: evidence for interaction of viral T-antigen and beta-catenin. Cancer Res 2002; 62:7093-7101.

149. Gan DD, Reiss K, Gorrill T et al. Involvement of Wnt signaling pathway in murine medulloblastoma induced by human neurotropic JC virus. Oncogene 2001; 20:4864-4870.

150. Galdenzi G, Lupo A, Anglani F et al. Is the simian virus SV40 associated with idiopathic focal segmental glomerulosclerosis in humans? J Nephrol 2003; 16:350-356.

151. Arrington AS, Butel JS. SV40 and human tumors. In: Khalili K, Stoner GL, eds. Human Polyomaviruses: molecular and clinical perspectives. New York: Wiley-Liss, 2001:461-489.

152. Gazdar AF, Butel JS, Carbone M. SV40 and human tumours: myth, association or causality? Nature Rev Cancer 2002; 2:957-964.

153. Vilchez RA, Butel JS. SV40 in human brain cancers and non-Hodgkin's lymphoma. Oncogene 2003; 22:5164-5172.

154. Mendoza SM, Konishi T, Miller CW. Integration of SV40 in human osteosarcoma DNA. Oncogene 1998; 17:2457-2462.

155. Pacini F, Vivaldi A, Santoro M et al. Simian virus 40-like DNA sequences in human papillary thyroid carcinomas. Oncogene 1998; 16:665-669.

156. Lednicky JA, Garcea RL, Bergsagel DJ et al. Natural simian virus 40 strains are present in human choroid plexus and ependymoma tumors. Virology 1995; 212:710-717.

157. Capello D, Rossi D, Gaudino G et al. Simian virus 40 infection in lymphoproliferative disorders. Lancet 2003; 361:88-89.

158. De Sanjose S, Shah KV, Domingo-Domenench E et al. Lack of serological evidence for an association between simian virus 40 and lymphoma. Int J Cancer 2003; 104:522-524.

159. Engels EA, Sarkar C, Daniel RW et al. Absence of simian virus 40 in human brain tumors from Northern India. Int J Cancer 2002; 101:348-352.

160. Gordon GJ, Chen CJ, Jaklitsch MT et al. Detection and quantification of SV40 large T-antigen DNA in mesothelioma tissues and cell lines. Oncol Rep 2002; 9:631-634.

161. MacKenzie J, Wilson KS, Perry J et al. Association between simian virus 40 DNA and lymphoma in the United Kingdom. J Natl Cancer Inst 2003; 95:1001-1003.

162. Mayall F, Barratt K, Shanks J. The detection of simian virus 40 in mesotheliomas from New Zeland and England using real time FRET probe PCR protocols. J Clin Pathol 2003; 56:728-730.

163. Shah KV. Does SV40 infection contribute to the development of human cancers? Rev Med Virol 2000; 10:31-43.

164. Strickler HD and The International SV40 Working Group. A multicenter evaluation of assays for detection of SV40 DNA and results in masked mesothelioma specimens. Cancer Epidemiol Biomark Prev 2001; 10:523-532.

165. Carbone M, Bocchetta M, Cristaudo A et al. SV40 and human brain tumors. Int J Cancer 2003; 106:140-142.

166. Engels EA, Gravitt PE, Daniel RW et al. Absence of simian virus 40 in human brain tumors from Northern India; response to letter from Carbone et al. Int J Cancer 2003; 106:143-145.

167. Rollison DEM, Helzlsouer KJ, Alberg AJ et al. Serum antibodies to JC virus, BK virus, simian virus 40, and the risk of incident adult astrocytic brain tumors. Cancer Epidemiol Biomark Prev 2003; 12:460-463.

168. Engels EA, Rodman LH, Frisch M et al. Childhood exposure to simian virus 40-contaminated poliovirus vaccine and risk of AIDS-associated non-Hodgkin's lymphoma. Int J Cancer 2003; 106:283-287.

169. zur Hausen H. SV40 in humans cancers: an endless tale? Int J Cancer 2003; 107:687.

170. Testa JR, Carbone M, Hirvonen A et al. A multi-institutional study confirms the presence and expression of simian virus 40 in human malignant mesotheliomas. Cancer Res 1998; 58:4505-4509.

171. Vilchez RA, Butel JS. Simian virus 40 and its association with human lymphomas. Curr Oncol Rep 2003; 5:372-379.

172. Vilchez RA, Kozinetz CA, Arrington AS et al. Simian virus 40 in human cancers. Am J Med 2003; 114:675-684.

173. Brugge JS, Butel, JS. Role of simian virus 40 gene A function in maintenance of transformation. J Virol 1975; 15:619-635.

174. Martin RG, Chou JY.Simian virus 40 functions required for the establishment and maintenance of malignant transformation. J Virol 1975; 15:599-612.
175. Osborn M, Weber K. Simian virus 40 gene A function and maintenance of transformation. J Virol 1975; 15:636-644.
176. Tegtmeyer P. Function of simian virus 40 gene A in transforming infection. J Virol 1975; 15:613-618.
177. Coleman WB, Tsongalis GJ. The role of genomic instability in the development of human cancer. In: Coleman WB, Tsongalis GJ, eds. The Molecular Basis of Human Cancer. Totowa: Humana Press, 2002:115-142.
178. Reinartz JJ. Cancer genes. In: Coleman WB, Tsongalis GJ, eds. The Molecular Basis of Human Cancer. Totowa, NJ: Humana Press, 2002:45-64.
179. Shimamoto T, Ohyashiki K. Chromosomes and chromosomal instability in human cancer. In: Coleman WB, Tsongalis GJ, eds. The Molecular Basis of Human Cancer. Totowa: Humana Press, 2002:143-158.
180. Lengauer C, Kinzler KW, Vogelstein B. Genetic instabilities in human cancers. Nature 1998; 396:643-649.
181. Galloway DA, McDougall JK. The oncogenic potential of herpes simplex viruses: evidence for a 'hit and run' mechanism. Nature 1983; 302:21-24.
182. Schlehofer JR, zur Hausen H. Induction of mutations within the host cell genome by partially inactivated herpes simplex virus type 1. Virology 1982; 122:471-475.
183. Porcu P, Ferber A, Pietrzkowski Z et al. The growth-stimulatory effect of simian virus 40 T antigen requires the interaction of insulin-like growth factor 1 with its receptor. Mol Cell Biol 1992; 12:5069-5077.
184. Cacciotti P, Libener R, Betta P et al. SV40 replication in human mesothelial cells induces HGF/Met receptor activation: a model for viral-related carcinogenesis of human malignant mesothelioma. Proc Natl Acad Sci USA 2001; 98:12032-12037.
185. Cacciotti P, Strizzi L, Vianale G et al. The presence of simian virus 40 sequences in mesothelioma and mesothelial cells is associated with high levels of vascular endothelial growth factor. Am J Respir Cell Mol Biol 2002; 26:189-193.
186. Catalano A, Romano M, Martinotti S et al. Enhanced expression of vascular endothelial growth factor (VEGF) plays a critical role in the tumor progression potential induced by simian virus 40 large T antigen. Oncogene 2002; 21:2896-2900.
187. Carbone M, Pass HI, Miele L et al. New developments about the association of SV40 with human mesothelioma. Oncogene 2003; 22:5173-5180.
188. Carbone M, Rizzo P, Grimley PM et al. Simian virus-40 large T-antigen binds p53 in human mesotheliomas. Nature Med 1997; 3:908-912.
189. De Luca A, Baldi A, Esposito V et al. The retinoblastoma gene family pRb/p105, p107, pRb2/p130 and simian virus-40 large T-antigen in human mesotheliomas. Nature Med 1997; 3:913-916.
190. Bocchetta M, Miele L, Pass HI et al. Notch-1 induction, a novel activity of SV40 required for growth of SV40-transformed human mesothelial cells. Oncogene 2003; 22:81-89.
191. Waheed I, Guo ZS, Chen GA et al. Antisense to SV40 early gene region induces growth arrest and apoptosis in T-antigen-positive human pleural mesothelioma cells. Cancer Res 1999; 59:6068-6073.
192. Bright RK, Kimchl ET, Shearer MH et al. SV40 Tag-specific cytotoxic T lymphocytes generated from the pheripheral blood of malignant pleural mesothelioma patients. Cancer Immunol Immunother 2002; 50:682-690.
193. Procopio A, Strizzi L, Vianale G et al. Simian virus-40 sequences are a negative prognostic cofactor in patients with malignant pleural mesothelioma. Genes Chrom Cancer 2000; 29:173-179.
194. Bocchetta M, Di Resta I, Powers A et al. Human mesothelial cells are unusually susceptible to SV40-mediated transformation and asbestos co-carcinogenicity. Proc Natl Acad Sci U S A 2000; 97:10214-10219.
195. Carbone M, Burck C, Rdzanek M et al. Different susceptibility of human mesothelial cells to polyomavirus infection and malignant transformation. Cancer Res 2003; 63:6125-6129.
196. Dubes GR. Asbestos mediates viral DNA transformation of mouse cells to produce multilayered foci. Proc Am Assoc Cancer Res 1993; 34:185.
197. Cristaudo A, Foddis R, Bigdeli L et al. SV40: a possible co-carcinogen of asbestos in the pathogenesis of mesothelioma? Med Lav 2002; 93:499-506.
198. Dopp E, Poser I, Papp T. Interphase FISH analysis of cell cycle genes in asbestos-treated human mesothelial cells (HMC), SV40-transformed HMC (MET-5A) and mesothelioma cells (COLO). Cell Mol Biol 2002; 48:271-277.
199. Foddis R, De Rienzo A, Broccoli D et al. SV40 infection induces telomerase activity in human mesothelial cells. Oncogene 2002; 21:1434-1442.

200. Stratton K, Almario DA, McCormick MC. SV40 contamination of polio vaccine and cancer. Immunization Safety Review Committee, Board of Health Promotion and Disease Prevention, Institute of Medicine of the National Academies. Washington DC: National Academies Press, 2002 (www.nap.edu)

201. Vilchez RA, Kozinetz A, Butel JS. Conventional epidemiology and the link between SV40 and human cancers. Lancet Oncol 2003; 4:188-191.

202. Imperiale MJ, Pass HI, Sanda MG. Prospects for an SV40 vaccine. Semin Cancer Biol 2001; 11:81-85.

203. Xie YC, Hwang C, Overwijk W et al. Induction of tumor antigen-specific immunity in vivo by a novel vaccinia vector encoding safety-modified simian virus 40 T antigen. J Natl Cancer Inst 1999; 91:169-175.

204. Kennedy RC, Shearer MH, Watts AM et al. CD4+ T lymphocytes play a critical role in antibody production and tumor immunity against simian virus 40 large tumor antigen. Cancer Res 2003; 63:1040-1045.

205. Cho KB, Chong KY. Absence of mutation in the p53 and the retinoblastoma susceptibility genes in primary cervical carcinomas. Virology 1993; 193:1042-1046.

206. Lee YY, Wilcznyski SP, Chumakov A et al. Carcinoma of the vulva: HPV and p53 mutations. Oncogene 1994; 9:1655-1659.

207. Goedert JJ, ed. Infectious causes of cancer. Totowa: Humana Press, 2000.

208. Newton R, Beral V, Weiss RA, eds. Infections and human cancer. Cancer Surveys vol 33. Cold Spring Harbor: Cold Spring Harbor Laboratory Press, 1999.

209. McNally RJQ, Cairns DP, Eden OB et al. An infectious aetiology for childhood brain tumours? Evidence from space—Time clustering and seasonality analyses. British J Cancer 2002; 86:1070-1077.

210. Larsen LS. Brain tumors incidence rising; researchers ask why. J Natl Cancer Inst 1993; 85:1024-1025.

211. Mortimer EA Jr, Lepow ML, Gold E et al. Long-term follow-up of persons inadvertently inoculated with SV40 as neonates. N Engl J Med 1981; 305:1517-1518.

212. Geissler E. SV40 and human tumors. Prog Med Virol 1990; 37:211-222.

213. Carroll-Pankhurst C, Engels EA, Strickler HD et al. Thirty-five year mortality following receipt of SV40-contaminated polio vaccine during the neonatal period. Brit J Cancer 2001; 85:1295-1297.

214. zur Hausen H. Viruses in human cancers. Science 1991; 254:1167-1173.

215. zur Hausen H. Viral oncogenesis. In: Parsonnet J, ed. Microbes and Malignancy. New York: Oxford Press, 1999:107-130.

CHAPTER 24

Epidemiologic Studies of Polyomaviruses and Cancer:
Previous Findings, Methodologic Challenges and Future Directions

Dana E.M. Rollison

Abstract

Polyomavirus infection became the focus of epidemiologic studies of cancer several decades ago, soon after the discovery of simian virus 40 (SV40) in 1960 and its ability to induce tumors in experimentally infected animals in 1961. Between 1963 and 2003, eight case-control and eleven cohort studies investigated the possible associations between polyomavirus infection and multiple types of cancer, including lymphoma, brain tumors, and mesothelioma. Two of these studies included measures of infection with the human polyomaviruses, JC virus and BK virus. Overall, the results from these studies were mostly null, although limitations in study design and exposure assessment complicate their interpretation. This chapter includes a review of results from previous epidemiologic studies of polyomavirus infection and human cancer, discussion of the methodologic challenges in study design, and proposed future directions for epidemiologic research.

Introduction

Polyomavirus infection became the focus of epidemiologic studies of cancer several decades ago, soon after the discovery of simian virus 40 (SV40) in 1960[1] and its ability to induce tumors in experimentally infected animals in 1961.[2] Early polio vaccines were prepared from virus pools grown in monkey kidney tissue which harbored SV40, resulting in the accidental contamination of polio vaccines administered to millions of Americans in the late 1950s to early 1960s.[3] Fraumeni and colleagues were the first to address the concern that widespread exposure to SV40-contaminated polio vaccine may be associated with increased cancer incidence in their cohort study published in 1963.[4] Findings from this initial study were reassuring, since there were no increases in cancer incidence observed within states thought to have the highest levels of SV40 polio vaccine contamination. However, only four years had elapsed since the widespread exposure to SV40 at the time of this study, and the possibility remained that a cancer epidemic was forthcoming.

Subsequent epidemiologic studies of SV40 exposure and cancer published in the late 1960s,[5,6] 1970s[7,8] and early 1980s[9] were mostly negative. Concern was quieted until the advent of polymerase chain reaction (PCR) techniques and the subsequent detection of SV40 genomic sequences in ependymomas and osteosarcomas by Bergsagel et al in 1992.[10] The literature quickly expanded with reports of PCR-detected SV40 sequences in several types of cancer, including brain tumors, mesothelioma, hematologic malignancies, and other types of cancer, as reviewed

Polyomaviruses and Human Diseases, edited by Nasimul Ahsan. ©2006 Eurekah.com and Springer Science+Business Media.

in previous chapters in this book. In response to the renewed concern over the possible association between SV40 exposure and cancer, several cohort studies incorporating longer follow-up time were conducted and published in the 1990s.[11-16] As before, findings from these cohort studies were mostly negative, but all were predicated on the assumption that human exposure to SV40 was limited to those individuals who were vaccinated for polio in 1955-63. Epidemiologic studies conducted up to this point have been previously reviewed (refs. 17,18).

Eight additional epidemiologic studies of polyomaviruses and cancer were published in 2003, seven of which incorporated some measure of exposure to SV40.[19-25] Two studies included measures of infection with the related human polyomaviruses, JC virus (JCV) and BK virus (BKV), as potential risk factors for cancer.[24,26] These viruses are highly prevalent in the human population and have the same transforming capabilities as SV40. This chapter includes a review of results from previous epidemiologic studies of polyomavirus infection and human cancer, discussion of the methodologic challenges in study design, and proposed future directions for epidemiologic research.

Previous Findings

The results from case-control and cohort studies of polyomavirus infection and cancer are presented separately in Tables 1 and 2, respectively, and studies are ordered chronologically within these two tables. When comparing results across studies, it is important to consider several sources of heterogeneity in the study designs, including selection of cases and controls for case-control studies (i.e., hospital-based versus population-based), the type of cancer studied (i.e., cancer site, incidence vs. mortality, adult vs. pediatric), the geographic location of the study (differences in SV40 exposure vary by country), length of follow-up (length of time between exposure and outcome), and adjustment for potential confounders (i.e., approaches to teasing apart age and cohort effects). Variations in methods of exposure assessment are important considerations in the interpretations of these results, thus the case-control and cohort studies discussed below are grouped by method of exposure assessment.

Case-Control Studies (Table 1)

Maternal or Childhood Polio Vaccination and Childhood Cancers

The earliest case-control studies investigated the association between childhood cancer and receipt of polio vaccine potentially contaminated with SV40 by either the mother during pregnancy or the child after birth. Stewart and Hewitt[6] (1965) observed no association between polio vaccination as recorded on the medical records and deaths from childhood leukemia or other cancers in the United Kingdom. Using the same measure of exposure in Australia, Innis (1968) observed no increased risks of childhood cancer in children immunized against polio at ages younger than 1 year, and a significant increase in childhood cancer risk associated with polio immunization at ages greater than 1 year.[5] Farwell et al[16] (1979) conducted a case-control study in Connecticut and observed an overall increase in childhood tumors of the central nervous system (CNS) associated with maternal receipt of injected polio vaccine (IPV) during pregnancy, an increase which was statistically significant for medulloblastomas.[7] This increased risk of medulloblastomas was not replicated in a cohort study of incidence rates in Connecticut conducted years later and reviewed below.

Self-Reported History of Polio Vaccination and Adult Cancers

Self-reported history of polio vaccination was not associated with multiple subtypes of adult non-Hodgkin's lymphoma (NHL) in a population-based case-control study in San Francisco (2003).[23] Results remained unchanged after restriction of analyses to individuals vaccinated prior to 1963 and those vaccinated in childhood.[23] Similarly, a hospital-based case-control study of adult gliomas conducted within three U.S. cities (2003) did not observe a statistically significant association with self-reported history of polio vaccination, regardless of route of administration, year of vaccination, or year of birth.[19]

Table 1. Case-control studies of the association between surrogate measures of polyomavirus infection and cancer

First Author, Year Study Location	Study Design	Study Population	Measure of Exposure to Polyomaviruses	Cancer Site(s) Studied: Results (OR = odds ratio, 95% CI = 95% confidence interval)
Brenner, 2003[19] Boston, Pittsburgh, and Phoenix, USA	Hospital-based case-control	782 cases (adult patients diagnosed with a brain tumor in 1994-98 at 3 hospitals in U.S.) and 799 matched controls (patients admitted to same hospitals with nonmalignant disease)	Self-reported history of polio vaccination (used as a surrogate marker for exposure to SV40)	Adult gliomas (489 cases): OR = 1.08, 95% CI = 0.75-1.56 Adult meningiomas (197 cases): OR = 1.10, 95% CI = 0.68-1.82 Adult acoustic neuromas (96 cases): OR = 1.46, 95% CI = 0.63-3.38 No significantly increased risks were observed when data were stratified by oral vs. injected vaccine or vaccination in 1954-62 vs. 1963+
de Sanjose, 2003[20] Spain	Hospital-based case-control	520 cases (adult patients diagnosed with lymphoma in 4 hospitals in Spain) and 587 matched controls (hospitalized patients without lymphoma)	SV40 capsid antibodies, measured by ELISA	Adult B-cell lymphoma (485 cases): OR = 0.59, 95% CI = 0.37-0.94 Adult T-cell lymphoma (35 cases): OR = 0.76, 95% CI = 0.22-2.57 Adult Hodgkin's lymphoma (57 cases): OR = 2.04, 95% CI = 0.96-4.33
Holly, 2003[23] San Francisco, USA	Population-based case-control	1,157 cases (incident adult cases of NHL diagnosed in 1988-95, identified through SEER) and 2,402 matched controls (selected through random digit dialing)	Self-reported history of polio vaccination (used as a surrogate marker for exposure to SV40)	Small lymphocytic NHL (152 cases): OR = 0.68, 95% CI = 0.46-0.99 REAL follicular NHL (352 cases): OR = 0.97, 95% CI = 0.73-1.3 Diffuse small cleaved-cell NHL (68 cases): OR = 0.71, 95% CI = 0.41-1.2 Diffuse mixed small cleaved & large-cell NL (75 cases): OR = 0.69, 95% CI = 0.39-1.2 REAL diffuselarge-cell NHL (510 cases): OR = 0.82, 95% CI = 0.64-1.0 No differences in risk were observed for those vaccinated before vs. after 193, or at age < 10 vs. > 10 years

continued on next page

Table 1. *Continued*

First Author, Year Study Location	Study Design	Study Population	Measure of Exposure to Polyomaviruses	Cancer Site(s) Studied: Results (OR = odds ratio, 95% CI = 95% confidence interval)
Priftakis, 2003[26] Sweden	Case-control	57 cases (pediatric patients diagnosed with childhood ALL in 4 centers in Sweden in 1980-2001) and 37 controls (children born in similar years who did not develop ALL)	JCV and BKV DNA in dried bloodspots from Guthrie cards, measured by PCR	Childhood acute lymphoblastic leukemia: No JCV or BKV DNA detected in the dried blood spots from Guthrie cards for all cases and controls
Rollison, 2003[24] Washington County, MD, USA	Nested case-control	44 cases (adults diagnosed with a malignant brain tumor in 1975-2000 within an ongoing cohort of approx. 33,000) and 88 matched controls (cancer-free individuals from same underlying cohort)	Capsid antibodies to JCV and BKV; neutralizing antibodies to SV40	Adult brain tumors (44 cases): JCV positive vs. negative: OR = 1.46, 95% CI = 0.61-3.50 BKV positive vs. negative: OR = 0.66, 95% CI = 0.22-1.95 SV40 positive vs. negative: OR = 1.00, 95% CI = 0.30-3.32 Glioblastomas (28 cases - subset of total): JCV positive vs. negative: OR = 2.38, 95% CI = 0.64-8.86 BKV positive vs. negative: OR = 0.53, 95% CI = 0.14-2.04
Farwell, 1979[7] CT, USA	Case-control	52 cases (one third of children born in CT in1956-62 and diagnosed with a CNS tumor before age 20, identified through state cancer registry) and 38 matched controls (cancer-free children selected from birth certificates)	Maternal vaccination with IPV during pregnancy with case or control child, as reported by the treating obstetrician (used as a surrogate marker for exposure to SV40)	Childhood CNS tumors (52 cases): 19 (37%) exposed cases vs. 8 (21%) exposed controls (p = 0.15) Childhood medulloblastomas (15 cases - subset of total): 10 (67%) exposed cases vs. 8 (21%) exposed controls (p < 0.01)

continued on next page

Table 1. Continued

First Author, Year Study Location	Study Design	Study Population	Measure of Exposure to Polyomaviruses	Cancer Site(s) Studied: Results (OR = odds ratio, 95% CI = 95% confidence interval)
Innis, 1968[5] Australia	Hospital-based case-control	816 cases (children diagnosed with cancer in 1958-67 in hospitals in Sydney and Brisbane) and 816 matched controls (children admitted to the same hospitals for conditions other than cancer	Vaccination for polio (IPV) in infancy or early childhood, as recorded on medical records (used as a surrogate marker for exposure to SV40)	Cancer in children under 1 year of age (110 cases): 29 (26%) exposed cases vs. 28 (25%) controls Cancer in children 1 year of age and older (706 cases): 618 (88%) exposed cases vs. 569 (81%) exposed controls (p < 0.0005)
Stewart, 1965[6] England, Wales and Scotland	Case-control	2,107 cases (children who died of leukemia or other cancer at ages 9 and younger in 1956-60) and 2,107 matched controls (cancer-free children, method of selection is not described)	Poliomyelitis immunization (IPV) as recorded on the Oxford survey (used as a surrogate marker for exposure to SV40)	Childhood leukemia (999 deaths): 270 (27%) exposed cases vs. 259 (26%) exposed controls Childhood cancers other than leukemia (1108 deaths): 259 (23%) exposed cases vs. 265 (24%) exposed controls

Abbreviations: ALL, acute lymphocytic leukemia; BKV, BK virus; CI, confidence interval; CNS, central nervous system; ELISA, enzyme-linked immunosorbent assay; IPV, injected polio vaccine; JCV, JC virus; NHL, non-Hodgkin's lymphoma; OR, odds ratio; PCR, polymerase chain reaction; SEER, Surveillance, Epidemiology and End Results; SV40, simian virus 40.

Serologic Markers of Polyomavirus Infection and Adult Cancers

Two recent studies incorporated measures of antibodies to SV40.[20,24] No association was observed between SV40 neutralizing antibodies measured in the blood collected years prior to diagnosis and adult brain tumors in a case-control study nested within a Maryland cohort (2003).[24] The prevalence of SV40 antibodies in this study population was low (11%). Similarly, de Sanjose and colleagues[20] (2003) observed no association between SV40 antibodies measured by ELISA and adult cases of NHL in a hospital-based case-control study conducted in Spain, with a seroprevalence of 8%.

Only two epidemiologic studies incorporated measures of JCV and BKV infection, both of which were case-control studies.[24,26] In the same nested case-control study described above, no statistically significant associations were observed between prediagnostic circulating antibodies to JCV or BKV, as measured by ELISA, and adult brain tumors.[24] Pritakis and colleagues investigated JCV and BKV genomic sequences in dried bloodspots from Guthrie cards in childhood cases of ALL and controls, and found no JCV or BKV sequences in any of the study samples.[26]

Cohort Studies (Table 2)

Detection of SV40 Contamination in Polio Vaccine Lots

As mentioned in the introduction, Fraumeni et al[4] (1963) were the first to publish epidemiologic data on the association between SV40 exposure and cancer. Based on actual measurements of SV40 in stored polio vaccine lots and knowledge of which lots were distributed to individual U.S. states, each state was classified as having had no, low, or high levels of SV40 contamination in polio vaccines distributed in 1955. Mortality rates from leukemia and other cancers were compared for time periods before, during and after the polio vaccination campaign, separately for states with different levels of SV40 contamination. Trends in mortality rates over time did not indicate any increases in childhood cancer associated with mass polio vaccination.[4]

Maternal or Childhood Polio Vaccination and Childhood Cancers

Heinonen et al[8] followed more than 50,000 children born to women in 1959-60 for childhood cancer incidence and mortality through age four, and compared these rates among children born to mothers who reported vaccination for polio during pregnancy to rates among children born to mothers that reported no vaccination.[8] Although small numbers of cases were observed, there was a statistically significant increased risk of childhood cancer overall (14 cases occurred in children of exposed mothers versus 10 in children of unexposed mothers), and neural tumors specifically.[8] In contrast, a 35-year follow-up of more than 1,000 neonates who were experimentally administered IPV or oral polio vaccine (OPV) at 1-3 days of age in 1960-62 observed no increased risks of cancer deaths overall.[9,11,27]

Year of Birth

Eight subsequent cohort studies investigated the association between SV40 exposure and cancer risk by comparing population-based cancer incidence rates among birth cohorts with the highest probability of exposure to SV40-contaminated vaccine to rates among those with the lowest probability of exposure. These studies were conducted in different countries, with emphasis on different cancer sites. Additionally, the complexity of statistical methods used to assess the association between birth year and cancer ranged from a presentation of rates without a measure of association[13] to the use of age-period-cohort models.[25] Despite the heterogeneity in study designs, findings from these studies were reasonably consistent. No statistically significant increases in overall or site-specific cancer incidence were observed among birth cohorts potentially exposed to SV40-contaminated polio vaccine in Germany,[13] Sweden[14] or Denmark,[22] with the exception of ependymomas among children 0-4 years of age in Denmark.[22] Among birth cohorts with the highest probability of exposure to SV40-contaminated

Table 2. Cohort studies of the association between surrogate measures of SV40 infection and cancer

First Author, Year Study Loc.	Description of Cohort	Case Definition and Method of Ascertainment	Measure of SV40 Exposure	Length of Follow-Up	Cancer Site(s) Studied: Results (RR = relative risk, 95% CI = 95% confidence interval)
Engels, 2003[22] Denmark	All children born in 1946-52, 1955-61, or 1964-70	Cancer incidence through 1997, ascertained through Danish Cancer Registry	Birth year of 1946-52 (high probability of IPV years from exposure in infancy) or 1955-61 (high probabilityof IPV exposure in childhood)	Up to 42 1955	All cancers (43,973 cases): RR = 0.82, 95% CI = 0.78-0.88 Mesothelioma (57 cases): RR = 0.82, 95% CI = 0.26-2.61 Ependymoma (104 cases): RR = 1.23, 95% CI = 0.80-1.88 Choroid plexus tumors (14 cases): RR = 0.30, 95% CI = 0.08-1.16 Osteosarcomas (100 cases): RR = 0.93, 95% CI = 0.52-1.65 Non-Hodgkin's lymphoma (1,703 cases): RR = 0.89, 95% CI = 0.75-1.04 Among the subset of cancers diagnosed in children ages 0-4 years, a significant increased risk of ependymoma was observed (RR = 2.59, 95% CI = 1.36-4.92), based on 28 exposed cases and 14 unexposed cases, whereas increased risks were not observed for other cancers diagnosed in this age group
Engels, 2003[21] USA	Adults (15+ years), born in 1958-61 or 1964-67, registered in the AIDS Cancer Match Registry	Non-Hodgkin's lymphoma diagnosed 4-27 months after AIDS onset, in 1980-96, as recorded in the AIDS Cancer Match Registry	Birth year of 1958-61 (high probability of IPV exposure)	Up to 38 years from 1958	Non-Hodgkin's lymphoma (846 cases): RR = 0.97, 95% CI = 0.79-1.20 Risk estimates were similar for different NHL sites and histologies

continued on next page

Table 2. *Continued*

First Author, Year Study Loc.	Description of Cohort	Case Definition and Method of Ascertainment	Measure of SV40 Exposure	Length of Follow-Up	Cancer Site(s) Studied: Results (RR = relative risk, 95% CI = 95% confidence interval)
Strickler, 2003[25] USA	Individuals alive at any time between 1975 and 1997	Cancer incidence through 1997, ascertained through SEER	Individuals 25-54 years of age between 1975 and 1997 (most likely to have received polio vaccine)	Up to 42 years from 1955	Mesothelioma: In an age-period-cohort model, incidence rates remained stable or declined between 1975 and 1997 for individuals ages 25-54 years, those most likely to have been exposed to SV40-contaminated polio vaccines, whereas incidence rates increased among males 75 years and older, those least likely to have been exposed to vaccine
Carroll-Pankhurst, 2001[11] Mortimer, 1981[9] Fraumeni, 1970[27] OH, USA	1,073 neonates who were experimentally administered IPV or OPV at 1-3 days of age in 1960-62	Cancer incidence and death up through 1981 was ascertained through personal correspon-dence in 1981, and cancer deaths through 2003 were ascertained through the National Death Index	Records of vaccine administration (IPV or OPV) from the original experimental study	35 years	Cancer deaths through 2003 (4 total deaths): 4 observed deaths vs. 3.2 expected RR = 1.26, 95% CI = 0.34-3.23 Leukemia deaths (2 -subset of total): 2 observed vs. 0.5 expected RR = 4.19, 95% CI = 0.51-15.73 Testicular cancer deaths (2- subset of total): 2 observed vs. 0.1 expected RR = 36.98, 95% CI = 4.47-133.50
Fisher, 1999[12] USA	All people 20-24 years of age in 1979 (born in 1955-59; n=2,013,344) and all people 20-24 yrs of age in 1987 (born in 1963-67; n=2,111,190)	Cancer incidence through 1993, ascertained through SEER	Birth year of 1955-59 (period of mass IPV vaccination)	Up to 38 years from 1955	All cancers (11,276 cases): % increase in incidence (exp vs. unexp) = -11.0% Ependymomas & choroid plexus tumors (32 cases): % increase in incidence (exp vs. unexp) = 19.6% Other brain tumors (661 cases): % increase in incidence (exp vs. unexp) = -8.4% Osterosarcomas (98 cases): % increase in incidence (exp vs. unexp) = 9.8% Mesotheliomas (8 cases): % increase in incidence (exp vs. unexp) = 178.0%

continued on next page

Table 2. *Continued*

First Author, Year Study Loc.	Description of Cohort	Case Definition and Method of Ascertainment	Measure of SV40 Exposure	Length of Follow-Up	Cancer Site(s) Studied: Results (RR = relative risk, 95% CI = 95% confidence interval)
Strickler, 1999[16] CT, USA	CT only: all children 0-4 yrs old in 1950-69 Entire U.S.: All children born in 1947-52 or 1956-62 and all children born in 1964-69	CT only: medulloblastoma incidence in children 0-4 years old, identified by state cancer registry Entire U.S.: medulloblastoma incidence through 1993, identified using SEER	CT only: birth year of 1950-54 or 1955-64 (before and during wide-spread polio vaccination) Entire U.S.: see below[15]	19 years	Medulloblastoma in children 0-4 years old (CT only): Incidence rate was higher among children who were 0-4 in 1955-59 as compared to those who were 0-4 in 1950-54 (p=0.16) and as compared to those who 0-4 in 1960-69 Medulloblastoma (entire U.S.): Exp. in infancy: RR = 0.74, 95% CI = 0.55-1.00 Exp. in childhood: RR = 0.57, 95% CI = 0.34-0.94
Strickler, 1998[15] USA	All children born in 1947-52 or 1956-62 and all children born in 1964-69	Cancer incidence through 1993, ascertained through SEER	Birth year of 1947-52 (high probability of IPV exposure in infancy) or 1956-62 (high risk of IPV exposure in childhood)	24-26 years	Ependymoma (22 cases): Exp. in infancy: RR = 1.06, 95% CI = 0.69-1.63 Other brain cancers (4,162 cases): Exp. in infancy: RR = 0.90, 95% CI = 0.82-0.99 Osteosarcomas (522 cases): Exp. in infancy: RR = 0.87, 95% CI = 0.71-1.06 Mesotheliomas (71 cases): Exp. in infancy: RR = 3.00, 95% CI = 0.67-13.11 Similar risks were observed for exposure in childhood
Olin, 1998[14] Sweden	All children born in 1946-53 and all children born in 1941-45 and 1954-58	Cancer incidence through 1993, ascertained using the national cancer registry	Birth year of 1946-53 (70% of children born in 1946-49 and 59% of children born 1950-53 received IPV)	30-39 years	Brain cancer incidence per 100,000 females: 8.4 in exposed vs. 9.7 in unexposed, RR = 0.87 Brain cancer incidence per 100,000 males: 8.4 in exposed vs. 7.7 in unexposed, RR = 1.10 Osteosarcoma incidence per 100,000 females: 0 in exposed vs. 0.45 in unexposed Osteosarcoma incidence per 100,000 males: 0.10 in exposed vs. 0 in unexposed Mesothelioma incidence per 100,000 females: 0.20 in exposed vs. 0 in unexposed Mesothelioma incidence per 100,000 males: 0.27 in exposed vs. 0.30 in unexposed, RR = 0.89

continued on next page

Table 2. *Continued*

First Author, Year Study Loc.	Description of Cohort	Case Definition and Method of Ascertainment	Measure of SV40 Exposure	Length of Follow-Up	Cancer Site(s) Studied: Results (RR = relative risk, 95% CI = 95% confidence interval)
Geissler, 1990[13] Germany	All children born in 1959-61 (n = 885,783) and all children born in 1962-64 (n = 891,321)	Cancer incidence through 1988, ascertained using the National Cancer Registry	Birth year of 1959-61 (86% of neonates born in 1959-61 received OPV)	22 years	All cancers: 2,544 in the exposed cohort (28.7 per 10,000) vs. 2,685 in the unexposed cohort (30.1 per 10,000) Incidence rates were slightly higher in the exposed vs. the unexposed cohorts for glioma, medulloblastoma, and oligodendroglioma; rates were lower in exposed vs. unexposed for ependymomas and meningiomas
Heinonen, 1973[8] USA	50,897 children born to women in 1959-65 in 12 hospitals	Incident cases of childhood cancer in the first year of life; deaths from cancer in ages 1-4; incident cases ascertained through clinical follow-up	Self-reported maternal vaccination to polio during pregnancy (IPV), confirmed by attending physicians	4 years	All childhood cancers (24 cases): 14 cases occurred in 18,342 children born to exposed mothers (7.6 per 10,000) vs. 10 cases in 32,555 children born to unexposed mothers (3.1 per 10,000) (p< 0.05) Childhood neural tumors (8 cases -subset of total): 7 cases among children of exposed mothers (3.9 per 10,000) vs. 1 case among children of unexposed mothers (0.3 per 10,000) (p<0.01) Childhood leukemia (8 cases –subset of total): 4 cases among children of exposed mothers vs. 4 cases among children of unexposed mothers (difference was not statistically significant)

continued on next page

Table 2. Continued

First Author, Year Study Loc.	Description of Cohort	Case Definition and Method of Ascertainment	Measure of SV40 Exposure	Length of Follow-Up	Cancer Site(s) Studied: Results (RR = relative risk, 95% CI = 95% confidence interval)
Fraumeni; 1963 [4] USA	Estimates of the number of children, ages 6-8, living in each state in 1955 (a surrogate for the number of children vaccinated for polio at ages 6-8 years in May-June 1955 as part of national campaign); states were grouped by estimated per capita dose of SV40-Salk vaccine administered during the campaign (none, low, high)	Deaths from leukemia and other cancers among children in 1950-59, identified from death certificates on file at the National Vital Statistics Division, U.S. Public Health Service	Residence in a state with low or high per capita dose of SV40-contaminated IPV, as determined by testing of stored vaccine lots	4 years	Childhood leukemia mortality: States with no estimated SV40 polio vaccine contamination had lower mortality rates among children who were 6-8 in 1955 both before and after the introduction of polio vaccination, perhaps reflecting differences in cancer mortality reporting across states; rates did not increase after the introduction of vaccine for states with none, low, or high estimated levels of SV40 contamination of polio vaccines Mortality from all childhood cancers except leukemia: Similar to leukemia mortality rates, states with no estimated vaccine contamination had lower mortality rates for all other childhood cancers; in the states with low or high contamination, mortality rates decreased one year before the introduction of polio vaccine, increased one year after, and decreased thereafter, whereas mortality rates declined over time in states with no estimated SV40 contamination

Abbreviations: CI, confidence interval; IPV, injected polio vaccine; NHL, non-Hodgkin's lymphoma; OPV, oral polio vaccine; RR, relative risk; SEER, Surveillance, Epidemiology and End Results; SV40, simian virus 40.

polio vaccine in the U.S., there were no statistically significant increases in all cancers combined, all brain tumors combined, ependymomas, medulloblastomas, osteosarcomas, or mesotheliomas.[12,15,16,25] Additionally, there was no evidence of an increased risk of non-Hodgkin's lymphoma among HIV-positive individuals born in the period of SV40-contaminated polio vaccination.[21]

Methodologic Challenges

Previous epidemiologic studies of polyomaviruses and cancer were diverse in their design and approach, and consequently had different methodologic strengths and limitations. Understanding the challenges specific to studies of polyomaviruses and cancer will improve the design of future epidemiologic studies.

Study Design

Both case-control and cohort designs have inherent strengths and limitations that are particularly relevant to the question of polyomaviruses and cancer. The cohort design is an obvious approach to investigate the effects of a population-wide polio vaccination campaign that occurred within a specific time period (i.e., the years during which polio vaccine was contaminated with SV40). However, most of the cancers that are hypothesized to be related to polyomaviruses are extremely rare (brain tumors, mesothelioma, childhood cancers), thus the case-control study is more efficient for obtaining adequate sample sizes. In contrast, JCV and BKV infections are highly prevalent in the general population, which limits the ability to detect differences in cancer risk, a limitation that applies to both case-control and cohort studies.

The cohort design establishes that exposure preceded the disease, thus ensuring that the measure of exposure is not influenced by the state of disease. This temporal sequence may be especially important for the investigation of immunologic markers of polyomavirus infection in cancer studies. For example, a case-control study of polyomavirus antibody levels and cancer could include cases whose disease and/or treatment may have altered their current polyomavirus infection status and immune response. The cohort study would include measurements of antibodies conducted prior to cancer diagnosis, uninfluenced by the disease. Additionally, the temporal sequence established in cohort studies allows for the investigation of a "hit-and-run" mechanism, which has been proposed for JCV carcinogenesis.[28] Although the timing of exposure assessment relative to diagnosis may be a strength of the cohort design, it is often not feasbile to obtain detailed measures of exposure from large cohorts at baseline.

A final consideration in study design pertains to the selection of appropriate controls in case-control studies. Although hospital-based case-control studies facilitate the collection of large numbers of rare cancers, hospital-based controls may introduce selection bias. Nonmalignant conditions for which controls may be hospitalized could be related to polyomavirus infection. The magnitude of potential bias is difficult to assess, given that little is known about risk factors for JCV and BKV infection and reactivation. This paucity of information on risk factors for polyomavirus infection also limits the ability to adjust for known confounders (factors associated with both polyomavirus infection and cancer), which is important in all epidemiologic studies.

Exposure Measurement

Exposure measurement is perhaps the greatest methodologic challenge in epidemiologic studies of polyomaviruses and cancer. Different surrogate markers of polyomavirus infection have been used in previous studies, with a considerable range in validity. In the particular case of SV40, exposure to polio vaccine in 1955-63 has been the most frequently used surrogate marker for SV40 exposure, whether measured by medical records, self-report, or simply year of birth. Measurement error may be introduced at several levels, first with the actual assessment of vaccination that may result from use of incomplete medical records or individuals' difficulty in recalling vaccinations that occurred more than 35 years ago. Birth year is not entirely specific, since not everyone who was born in 1955-63 was vaccinated for polio. Even if vaccination with polio is well-documented, levels of SV40 contamination varied from vaccine lot to lot, and not everyone who was exposed to the virus necessarily developed an active infection. Finally, comparing cancer incidence rates among different birth cohorts assumes that there was no human exposure to SV40 after 1963.

An alternative marker of past and/or present polyomavirus infection is the expression of antibodies. Two case-control studies reviewed in this chapter used an ELISA assay to measure antibodies to JCV and BKV[24] or SV40.[20] The feasibility of this approach is appealing for use in large serum banks that can be linked to population-based cancer registries. However, there are several points to consider when measuring antibodies. First, polyomavirus antibodies are cross-reactive, specifically with respect to SV40, thus any samples that test positive for SV40 should be investigated further to rule out cross-reactivity with JCV and/or BKV.[29] For SV40, expression of capsid antibodies may indicate exposure to inactivated virus in the absence of active infection, resulting in misclassification of the exposure. As mentioned earlier, JCV and BKV antibodies are highly prevalent in the general population, with greater than 70% of adults expressing antibodies to both JCV and BKV.[30] An exposure with such high prevalence limits the statistical power to detect differences in cancer risk. Use of more refined exposure measures could increase specificity, in turn increasing statistical power. Examples of more refined measures include antibodies to T-antigen, as opposed to capsid proteins, and different subclasses of antibodies, including IgA as a potential marker of reactivation of infection.

More direct measures of active polyomavirus infection include detection of virus in the blood and viral shedding in the urine. Only one study reviewed here investigated polyomavirus sequences in the blood using PCR, and no sequences were found in any case or control samples.[26] Although all of these samples may have been truly negative, the effect of long-term storage on the ability to detect polyomavirus sequences from blood is unknown. Viral shedding is not possible to measure in most cohort studies, since urine is not routinely banked. Multiple types of blood and urine specimens may be taken from participants in a case-control study, although the effects of cancer and its treatment on reactivation of polyomavirus infection are poorly understood.

Future Directions

Future epidemiologic studies of polyomavirus infection and cancer can be greatly enhanced by parallel developments in other fields, including the identification of risk factors for polyomavirus infection and reactivation that may be used to assess potential selection bias and control for confounding, the development of more sensitive and specific biomarkers of infection, and studies of the effects of cancer treatment on reactivation of infection and immune response. Future case series may identify subpopulations of patients with higher prevalence of tumors that contain SV40 sequences, suggesting that these subgroups have a greater susceptibility to polyomavirus-associated cancers. These individuals could be the focus of epidemiologic studies with increased statistical power. For example, SV40 sequences have been identified from tumors arising in patients with Li-Fraumeni syndrome.[31] Since cancers such as brain tumors are much more common in Li-Fraumeni patients than in the general population,[32] an epidemiologic cohort study of polyomavirus-associated brain tumors would have more statistical power if conducted among Li-Fraumeni patients than among the general population.

As the natural history of polyomavirus infections are elucidated, including the reactivation of latent infection or "hit-and-run" mechanisms, these concepts can be incorporated into large cohort studies of serum banks with long follow-up time. Future hospital-based case-control studies should be designed with multiple control groups to address the possibility that some nonmalignant conditions may be associated with polyomavirus infection. The resources of all case-control studies should be pooled to obtain large numbers of extremely rare cancers, such as mesothelioma. Finally, more studies need to address infections with JCV and BKV in relation to cancer.

Conclusion

Results from previous epidemiologic studies of SV40 and cancer have been mostly null. Methodologic challenges in study design and exposure assessment limit the interpretation of these results, especially in light of laboratory evidence that these viruses are oncogenic in experimental animals and have been reported to be present in human tumors. However limited, the consistency of null findings across several studies argues against a large effect of SV40 exposure on cancer risk. Future studies should incorporate more sophisticated measures of SV40 infection as they are developed in the laboratory. Epidemiologic data on JCV and BKV infection in relation to cancer are sparse and warrant further study. The accidental contamination of polio vaccines with SV40 in the late 1950s may not have resulted in a cancer epidemic, but infection with polyomaviruses, including JCV and BKV, cannot be excluded as risk factors for cancer.

References

1. Sweet BH, Hillemann MR. The vacuolating virus, SV40. Proc Soc Exp Biol Med 1960; 105:420-427.
2. Eddy BE, Borman GS, Berkeley WH et al. Tumors induced in hamsters by injection of rhesus monkey kidney cell extracts. Proc Soc Exp Biol Med 1961; 107:191-197.
3. Shah K, Nathanson N. Human exposure to SV40: Review and comment. Am J Epidemiol 1976; 103(1):1-12.
4. Fraumeni Jr JF, Ederer FE, Miller RW. An evaluation of the carcinogenicity of simian virus 40 in man. JAMA 1963; 185(9):713-718.
5. Innis MD. Oncogenesis and poliomyelitis vaccine. Nature 1968; 219(157):972-973.
6. Stewart AM, Hewitt D. Aetiology of childhood leukaemia. Lancet 1965; 2(7416):789-790.
7. Farwell JR, Dohrmann GJ, Marrett LD et al. Effect of SV40 virus-contaminated polio vaccine on the incidence and type of CNS neoplasms in children: A population-based study. Trans Am Neurol Assoc 1979; 104:261-264.
8. Heinonen OP, Shapiro S, Monson RR et al. Immunization during pregnancy against poliomyelitis and influenza in relation to childhood malignancy. Int J Epidemiol 1973; 2(3):229-235.
9. Mortimer Jr EA, Lepow ML, Gold E et al. Long-term follow-up of persons inadvertently inoculated with SV40 as neonates. N Engl J Med 1981; 305(25):1517-1518.
10. Bergsagel DJ, Finegold MJ, Butel JS et al. DNA sequences similar to those of simian virus 40 in ependymomas and choroid plexus tumors of childhood. N Engl J Med 1992; 326(15):988-993.
11. Carroll-Pankhurst C, Engels EA, Strickler HD et al. Thirty-five year mortality following receipt of Br J Cancer 2001; 85(9):1295-1297.
12. Fisher SG, Weber L, Carbone M. Cancer risk associated with simian virus 40 contaminated polio vaccine. Anticancer Res 1999; 19(3B):2173-2180.
13. Geissler E. SV40 and human brain tumors. Prog Med Virol 1990; 37:211-222.
14. Olin P, Giesecke J. Potential exposure to SV40 in polio vaccines used in Sweden during 1957: No impact on cancer incidence rates 1960 to 1993. Dev Biol Stand 1998; 94:227-233.
15. Strickler HD, Rosenberg PS, Devesa SS et al. Contamination of poliovirus vaccines with simian virus 40 (1955-1963) and subsequent cancer rates. JAMA 1998; 279(4):292-295.
16. Strickler HD, Rosenberg PS, Devesa SS et al. Contamination of poliovirus vaccine with SV40 and the incidence of medulloblastoma. Med Pediatr Oncol 1999; 32(1):77-78.
17. Rollison DEM, Shah KV. The epidemiology of SV40 infection due to contaminated polio vaccines: Relation of the virus to human cancer. In: Khalili K, Stoner GL, eds. Human polyomaviruses: Molecular and clinical perspectives. Wiley-Liss Inc., 2002:561-584.
18. Strickler HD, Goedert JJ. Exposure to SV40-contaminated poliovirus vaccine and the risk of cancer- -a review of the epidemiological evidence. Dev Biol Stand 1998; 94:235-244.
19. Brenner AV, Linet MS, Selker RG et al. Polio vaccination and risk of brain tumors in adults: No apparent association. Cancer Epidemiol Biomarkers Prev 2003; 12(2):177-178.
20. de Sanjose S, Shah KV, Domingo-Domenech E et al. Lack of serological evidence for an association between simian virus 40 and lymphoma. Int J Cancer 2003; 104(4):522-524.
21. Engels EA, Rodman LH, Frisch M et al. Childhood exposure to simian virus 40-contaminated poliovirus vaccine and risk of AIDS-associated non-Hodgkin's lymphoma. Int J Cancer 2003; 106(2):283-287.
22. Engels EA, Katki HA, Nielsen NM et al. Cancer incidence in Denmark following exposure to poliovirus vaccine contaminated with simian virus 40. J Natl Cancer Inst 2003; 95(7):532-539.

23. Holly EA, Bracci PM. Population-based study of non-Hodgkin lymphoma, histology, and medical history among human immunodeficiency virus-negative participants in San Francisco. Am J Epidemiol 2003; 158(4):316-327.
24. Rollison DE, Helzlsouer KJ, Alberg AJ et al. Serum Antibodies to JC Virus, BK Virus, Simian Virus 40, and the Risk of Incident Adult Astrocytic Brain Tumors. Cancer Epidemiol Biomarkers Prev 2003; 12(5):460-463.
25. Strickler HD, Goedert JJ, Devesa SS et al. Trends in U.S. pleural mesothelioma incidence rates following simian virus 40 contamination of early poliovirus vaccines. J Natl Cancer Inst 2003; 95(1):38-45.
26. Priftakis P, Dalianis T, Carstensen J et al. Human polyomavirus DNA is not detected in Guthrie cards (dried blood spots) from children who developed acute lymphoblastic leukemia. Med Pediatr Oncol 2003; 40(4):219-223.
27. Fraumeni Jr JF, Stark CR, Gold E et al. Simian virus 40 in polio vaccine: Follow-up of newborn recipients. Science 1970; 167(914):59-60.
28. Khalili K, Del Valle L, Otte J et al. Human neurotropic polyomavirus, JCV, and its role in carcinogenesis. Oncogene 2003; 22(33):5181-5191.
29. Viscidi RP, Rollison DE, Viscidi E et al. Serological cross-reactivities between antibodies to simian virus 40, BK virus, and JC virus assessed by virus-like-particle-based enzyme immunoassays. Clin Diagn Lab Immunol 2003; 10(2):278-285.
30. Shah KV. Polyomaviruses. In: Fields BN, Knipe DM, Howley PM, eds. Fields Virology. Philadelphia: Lippincott-Raven, 1996:2027-2043.
31. Malkin D, Chilton-MacNeill S, Meister LA et al. Tissue-specific expression of SV40 in tumors associated with the Li-Fraumeni syndrome. Oncogene 2001; 20(33):4441-4449.
32. Birch JM, Alston RD, McNally RJ et al. Relative frequency and morphology of cancers in carriers of germline TP53 mutations. Oncogene 2001; 20(34):4621-4628.

Index